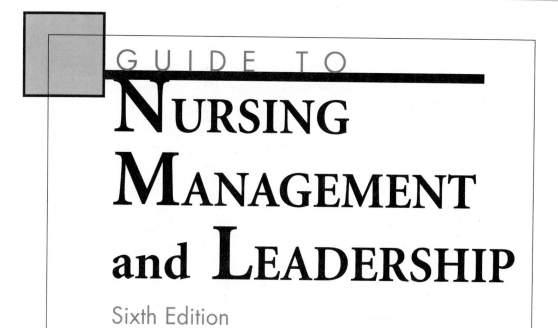

GUIDE TO

NURSING MANAGEMENT and LEADERSHIP

Sixth Edition

GUIDE TO

NURSING MANAGEMENT and LEADERSHIP

Sixth Edition

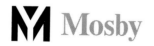 *Ann Marriner Tomey,* RN, PhD, FAAN
Professor
Indiana State University School of Nursing
Leadership and Management Consultant
Terre Haute, Indiana

M Mosby

A Harcourt Health Sciences Company

St. Louis   London   Philadelphia   Sydney   Toronto

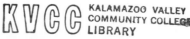

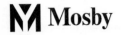 Mosby

Senior Editor: *Susan R. Epstein*
Editorial Assistant: *Graquel Clay*
Project Manager: *John Rogers*
Production Editor: *Mary Turner*
Designer: *Kathi Gosche*
Cover Art: *Kathi Gosche*

SIXTH EDITION
Copyright © 2000 by Mosby, Inc.

Previous editions copyrighted 1980, 1984, 1988, 1992, 1996

Mosby, Inc.
A Harcourt Health Sciences Company
11830 Westline Industrial Drive
St. Louis, Missouri 63146

Printed in the United States of America

International Standard Book Number

0-323-01066-0

00 01 02 03 04 CL/FF 9 8 7 6 5 4 3 2 1

DEDICATION

To H. Keith Tomey

REVIEWERS

ERNESTINE BADY DAVIS, RN, EdD
Professor
RN/BSN Co-Coordinator
Assistant to President of Minority Affairs
University of North Alabama College of Nursing
Florence, Alabama

MARY S. TILBURY, EdD, RN, CNAA
Assistant Professor
Department of Education, Administration, Health
 Policy, and Informatics
University of Maryland School of Nursing
Baltimore, Maryland

PREFACE

Guide to Nursing Management and Leadership is designed to teach nursing students about the management process and leadership and to supply the practicing nurse with practical information about nursing administration. The first edition of this book was written during the 1970s, when nursing education emphasized clinical skills at the expense of managerial expertise and nurses who were interested in leadership and management had to turn to other disciplines. Now there are many books and journals about nursing leadership and management. The first edition was *Guide to Nursing Management*. It was organized around the management process—plan, organize, staff, direct, and control as the conceptual framework. The rapid changes during the 1980s, with the increase in better educated personnel and increased technology to handle management functions, brought about a focus on leadership, which was reflected in *Guide to Nursing Management and Leadership*. Continuous quality improvement, cost containment, free market competition, managed care, technology, increasing diversity, more focus on ethical issues, and the need for teams and transformational leadership were dominant during the 1990s, requiring a major transformation of this book for 2000. The book is now divided into two major sections: leadership and management. The content has been refocused.

I want to express appreciation to the following research assistants for helping update the review of articles, literature, and current practices: Lindsay Acree, Chasity Archer, Kim Arvin, Wendy Brown, Cynthia Cottrell, Bob Davis, Dawn Dunagan, Shelly Eslinger, Jill Fromme, Cindy Gowdy, Cindy Hamilton, Tonya Harper, Tara Hester, Jodie Holtman, Shannon Kirby, Claudia Sue Lofton, Carole Lonneman, Angie Madden, Terri McCollom, Nicole Moore, Dana Morlan, Rita Paitson, Jenny Palmer, Angie Remmel, Amy Robinson, Lynette Smith, Amy Spitler, Alice Staley, Robin Turner, Justin Thomas Vaughn, Dana Wohlwend, and Heidi Woodard.

Thanks to Cindy Gowdy for checking the most recent publication dates of books; Jill L. McCrory, RN, JD, for legal council regarding labor relations; Marsha Ciolli, Nicke Waters, and Sally Zuel for consultation about JCAHO; and Amy Tomey for consultation about OSHA.

I have used literally hundreds of articles and books for the transformation of this edition. The assistance provided by numerous individuals in the University Library has been most helpful. Faculty at the Information Desk readily answered my questions and guided me to appropriate resources. Staff in the Interlibrary Loan unit did an outstanding job of retrieving numerous requested materials within my timelines. Also supportive and attentive to my needs was the staff at the Check-Out, Reserves, and Periodicals Desks. I cannot forget the behind-the-scenes staff who classify materials and maintain the collections, making it possible for all patrons to find the sources they need. I would like to express my appreciation to the following library staff: Information Desk: Melody Allison, Ann Cockerham, Scott Davis, Ralph Gabbard, Steve Hardin, Allen Keathley, Penny Kyker, Valentine Muyumba, Judy Tribble, and Wilma Turetzky; Periodicals Desk: John Lunceford, Jennifer Morrison, and Jim Shoptaw; Check-Out, Reserves, and Interlibrary Loan Desks: Donna Curtis, Teresa Herrington, Jini Jackson, Alison Montgomery, Shirley Risley, Tina Tapy, and Nancy Watkins; and Cataloging: Sally Baker, Cheryl Bealmear, Tieh-peng Chin, Debbie Considine, Mary Griffy, Esther Hedges, Betsy Hine, Larry Lynch, Debra Taylor, and Carol Vanatti. I thank Ellen Watson for her leadership in information and library services and others such as student assistants who are too numerous to mention.

Last but not least, I thank my loving husband, H. Keith Tomey, for enriching my private life while supporting my professional activities and for helping me maintain balance.

Ann Marriner Tomey

CONTENTS

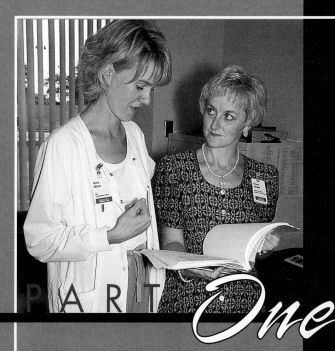

PART *One*

LEADERSHIP

CHAPTER 1

COMMUNICATIONS

Chapter Overview

Chapter 1 describes the communication process, communication systems, barriers to communications, ways to improve communications, communicating with difficult people, assertiveness, transactional analysis, and life positions.

MAJOR CONCEPTS AND DEFINITIONS	
Communication	giving and receiving information via talk, gestures, writing, and so forth
Ideation	decision to share an idea
Encoding	putting meaning into symbols
Transmission	sending the message
Receiving	seeing and hearing transmitted message
Decoding	defining words and interpreting gestures
Feedback	an evaluative response
Grapevine	informal communication system
Informal communications	casual, not according to prescribed ways
Formal communications	according to prescribed rules
Verbal	spoken
Nonverbal	not spoken; body language, tone of voice, facial expressions, posture, gestures, pauses
Assertiveness	the quality of being confident in stating one's opinions or needs
Transactional analysis	a technique for analyzing discussions
Life positions	an individual's assumptions about self in relation to others
Passive	inactive, acted on
Aggressive	active, bold, pushy
Broken record	a technique involving repeating what one wants
Fogging	agreeing with the truth
Negative assertion	accepting negative aspects about oneself
Negative inquiry	asking for more information about oneself

COMMUNICATION PROCESS

All of the manager's functions involve communication. The communication process involves six steps.

Ideation → Encoding → Transmission → Receiving → Decoding → Response ┐
Response ← Decoding ← Receiving ← Transmission ← Encoding ←————————┘

The first step, ideation, begins when the sender decides to share the content of a message with someone, senses a need to communicate, develops an idea, or selects information to share. The purpose of communication may be to inform, persuade, command, inquire, or entertain. Whatever the reason, the sender needs to have a goal and think clearly or the message may be garbled and meaningless.

Encoding, the second step, involves putting meaning into symbolic forms: speaking, writing, or nonverbal behavior. One's personal, cultural, and professional biases affect the goals and encoding process. Use of clearly understood symbols and communication of all the information that the receiver needs to know are important.

The third step, transmission of the message, must overcome interference such as garbled speech, unintelligible use of words, long, complex sentences, distortion from recording devices, noise, and illegible handwriting.

Receiving is next. The receiver's senses of seeing and hearing are activated as the transmitted message is received. People tend to have selective attention (hear the messages of interest to them but not others) and selective perception (hear the parts of the message that conform with what they want to hear), which cause incomplete and distorted interpretation of the communication. Sometimes people tune out the message because they anticipate the content and think they know what is going to be said or are so busy formulating their response that they do not hear the message. The receiver may be preoccupied with other activities and consequently not be ready to listen. Poor listening is one of the biggest barriers in the communication process.

Decoding of the message by the receiver is the critical fifth step. The receiver defines words and interprets gestures during the transmission of speech. Written messages allow more time for decoding while receivers assess the explicit meaning and implications of the message based on what the symbols mean to them. The symbols are subject to interpretation based on one's personal, cultural, and professional biases and may not have the same meaning to the receiver as to the sender. The communication process is dependent on the receiver's understanding of the information.

Response, or feedback, is the final step. It is important for the manager or sender to know that the message has been received and accurately interpreted.

BASIC COMMUNICATION SKILLS

One can *ensure understanding* by *assuming value, clarifying,* and *confirming* and can then *enhance the value* by *identifying the merits, building* on the expressed ideas, and *balancing* the merits and concerns. One should *support* by expressing appreciation and being specific (*Advanced Executive Leadership Skills,* 1981).

Ensuring understanding is facilitated by *assuming value, clarifying,* and *confirming. Assuming value* is an attitude that the person is worth listening to that opens lines of communication so one can understand what the other person thinks and feels. It helps one understand what the other person is saying and why and increases the chances that the other person will listen in return. *Clarification* is used when one is not sure of what the other person is saying by asking a specific question like "What do you mean when you say . . .," by making a statement like "I don't understand what you mean," or by expressing open-ended interest by comments like "and then?" *Confirmation* is used when one thinks there is understanding about what was said and why by checking for understanding and confirmation from the other person that one's understanding is accurate. Repeating what was said indicates one heard what was said but does not necessarily mean one understands. Saying "I understand what you said" indicates one thinks she understands what the other person said, but her understanding may not be the same as the speaker's. Stating one's understanding of what the speaker said and why is a more accurate way of confirming.

Enhancing value differs from criticism by *identifying the merits, building,* and *balancing* instead of rejecting the other's ideas and actions. We often criticize by telling others what we do not like about their ideas, what is wrong, and what will not work. That leads to demoralization, defensiveness, and oppressed innovation. We may be more effective if we do not criticize.

To *enhance value, identify the merits* mentally and ask yourself if you can improve on the idea or action without mentioning concerns. If yes, *build* by specifying the merits verbally and adding value. A merit is anything you like about what the other person said or did or what you want the person to keep doing despite the need for change. A merit may be a part of an idea, a good intention, an important issue that was addressed, or part of an action. If you have difficulty identifying merit, you can ensure understanding by asking the person the value to their idea or act. Most people have good intentions. You can often enhance value by specifying the merits and suggesting slight refinement or changes by suggesting another way to reach the goal without mentioning your concerns. If a merit you have identified can be used as an example of what you want, the change you suggest is an alternative to reaching the goal, or if the person is not strongly committed to the previous idea or act, you can build by suggesting a minor change or refinement. Specify the merits verbally, add value by suggesting a refinement, and check back to confirm that the other person thinks that action is acceptable.

However, if the person asks you for an evaluation or needs to know what is wrong to be able to make necessary changes or if the situation requires a major change, you need to *balance.* You specify the merits and concerns, ask for suggestions or reaction, and check back. Invite suggestions after you identify the merits and your concerns to get the person involved in finding a solution, to get commitment to one's own ideas, and to get the other person's ideas instead of a confirmation of your ideas. Do not invite suggestions unless you do consider them or if you think the person needs to know your ideas for the discussion. After you have invited and received suggestions, give your reaction, confirm or clarify, give another itemized response, and ask for the other person's response.

Supporting promotes cooperation by giving timely and specific feedback about the positive aspects of another's ideas or efforts and by acknowledging the value of the other's contributions to you and others. Most people need recognition for their efforts and accomplishments. There is a direct relationship between support given and cooperation. Less time is wasted if others know what is important to you. However, there are several reasons people are reluctant to support others. Some fear being perceived as weak or insecure, do not see a connection between giving and receiving, or fear generalization for a specific accomplishment to other situations. It is appropriate when someone shows the first signs of improvement or meets minimum requirements not usually met, meets the basic requirements, or exceeds minimum requirements. Give support by expressing appreciation. Be specific to provide recognition, prevent others from misunderstanding your intent, prevent others from thinking you like everything, make your support believable, and let others know you pay attention to what they are doing. By mentioning personal qualities, you reinforce those qualities and earn goodwill and support. By mentioning how others' accomplishments are important to you, you help them know that their efforts make a difference and are valued, make them feel more important, and increase their desire to continue contributing.

COMMUNICATION PRINCIPLES

De Ann Gillies (1994, p. 187) identifies some communication principles. The effectiveness of various media differs with educational level, with the less educated relying more on aural and pictorial media and the more educated relying more on print. People with low self-esteem are more easily influenced by persuasive communications than are people with high self-esteem. People are more likely to hear messages that are compatible with their expectations and are more likely to listen to messages on topics about which they have read. The more trustworthy the speaker, the less manipulative she is perceived to be. Majority opinion is more effective in changing attitudes than expert opinion.

METHODS OF COMMUNICATION

David Whetten and Kim Cameron (1998) present a five *s*'s approach to effective oral and written presentations: *strategy, structure, support, style,* and *supplement.* The strategy develops the purpose for the specific audience and occasion. The structure translates the strategy into specific content. Examples and illustrations are used to support or reinforce ideas. Style, or the way ideas are presented, is as important as the ideas expressed. Supplement means to give informed responses to challenges and questions related to the presentation.

Strategy involves identifying the general and specific purposes, understanding the needs and attitudes of the audience, and designing the message for the audience. The speech should be audience centered. More formal situations call for more formal presentations, while informal situations allow for slang. Both sides of issues should be presented if the audience is uncommitted or hostile.

Structure begins with a forecast of the main ideas to capture the audience's attention and give them a reason to listen or read. It gives the audience an outline of the message, making it easier for them to follow the presentation. Simple to complex, familiar to unfamiliar, and old to new are some ways to structure a presentation. Only a few main points should be made, transitions should be made between main points, and the presentation should end on a high note, calling for action or creating a good feeling.

Support from evidence and visual aids helps establish credibility. It is advisable to use a variety of supports and to keep visual aids simple and effective to aid comprehension and retention.

Style for oral communications involves preparing notes, practicing the presentation with the visual aids, and planning to engage the audience through use of eye contact, physical space, and body movement. Style for written communications involves mechanical and factual precision. Tone is related to word choice and should be adjusted to the formality of the situation. The proper format for the business letter, memo, proposal, or paper should be used.

Supplement the presentation by responding to challenges and questions by being prepared to answer questions in a specific format. First restate the objection. Then state your position. Offer support for your position and speak to the impact of adopting your position.

USE OF COMPUTERS FOR COMMUNICATION

Word processing is commonly used and allows electronic writing, revising, storing, and printing of documents. *Spreadsheet software* allows manipulation of information in columns and rows as in accounting and allows writing, editing, graphing, storing, and printing of the data. *Database software* collects and catalogs information so that lots of well-organized data can be located and displayed. *Graphic software* allows use of clip art, icons, silhouettes, and line drawings to enhance written communications, while *presentation software* creates visual aids such as overheads and slides for oral presentations. *Electronic mail (e-mail)* allows users to send messages instantaneously using one-on-one interchanges, or e-mail can connect staff throughout an organization at one or many sites. It can get information, including graphics and sound, to listservs and newsgroups. *Voice mail* answers the telephone automatically, plays a message, and accepts and stores voice messages. *Calendar and scheduling software* in conjunction with e-mail allows networked users to access each other's schedules. The software can identify common free time and immediately book a meeting. *Chat rooms* can be used for exchange of written messages in real time without having to find a physical location for a meeting. Much committee work can be done asynchronously through e-mail. The *World Wide Web* links computers around the world and is a major source of information (Kreider and Haselton, 1997).

COMMUNICATION SYSTEMS

Study of small-group process has revealed various communication networks (Figure 1-1). The chain system is fast and accurate for simple problems. The middle person in the chain emerges as the leader, and the leadership position is stable. Unfortunately,

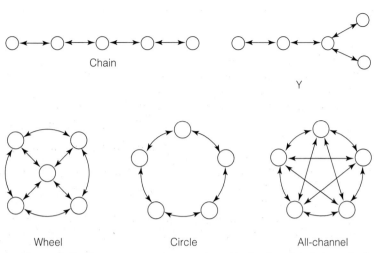

Figure 1-1   Communication systems: chain, Y, wheel, circle, all-channel.

morale is low and so is the flexibility for problem solving.

The leader emerges at the location of highest centrality, which is the fork of the Y and the hub of the wheel. Both provide fast, accurate problem solving. The coordinator, who is centrally located, is generally satisfied, but the peripheral members are less satisfied than members in less efficient systems. The wheel is an efficient, effective communication structure for simple problems.

The circular structure is slow and inaccurate. The structure does not influence the emergence of a leader. Because no one can communicate with everyone, there is no coordinator. However, morale is high, and there is considerable flexibility for problem solving.

When free to do so, groups tend to evolve to the all-channel network as problems become complex and shift back to a wheel structure as problems become simple. Greater amounts of information must be processed as task uncertainty and complexity increase. Consequently, an adaptive structure such as the all-channel system is best for completing complicated and unpredictable tasks. Essentially the right network is the structure that facilitates the communication necessary to accomplish the task.

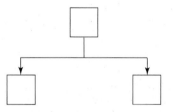

Figure 1-2   Downward communication.

Downward Communication

The traditional line of communication is from the manager down through the levels of management (Figure 1-2). This downward communication is primarily directive and helps coordinate the activities of different levels of the hierarchy by telling staff associates what to do and by providing the information needed by staff associates to relate their efforts to the organization's goals. It includes oral and written indoctrination, education, and other information to influence the attitudes and behaviors of staff associates. Common forms of downward communications are employee handbooks, operating manuals, job description sheets, performance appraisal interviews, employee counseling, a loudspeaker system, letters, memos, messages circulated with paychecks, posters, bulletin boards, in-

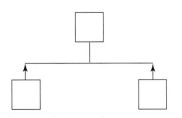

Figure 1-3 Upward communication.

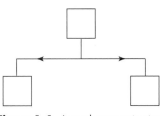

Figure 1-4 Lateral communication.

formation racks, company newspapers, annual reports, the chain of command, the grapevine, and unions. Downward communication contributes to greater staff associate dissatisfaction than upward communication, regardless of the quality of the message.

Upward Communication

Newer management techniques encourage delegation of authority and more personal involvement in decision making, thus creating a need for accurate upward communication (Figure 1-3). Upward communication provides a means for motivating and satisfying personnel by allowing employee input. The manager summarizes information and passes it upward to the next level for use in decision making. That level then summarizes its action and transmits information to the next level. Because each level tends to bias the report by embellishing it with information that puts that level in the best light, there is a natural filtering process as information moves upward. By the time it reaches top management, it is highly refined.

In spite of this bias, staff associates are often in a position to assess the situation more accurately than are their managers. An employee may have a better solution to a problem than the first-line manager, who may know more about a situation than a middle manager, and so on. Consequently, accurate upward communication is important for effective problem solving. Staff associates must feel free to communicate both solicited and unsolicited information upwardly and must have opportunity to do so, or management will lack needed information and both managers and staff associates will be-

come frustrated. Common means for upward communication include face-to-face discussions; open-door policies; staff meetings; task forces; written reports; performance appraisals; grievance procedures; exit interviews; attitude surveys; suggestion boxes; counseling; the chain of command; ombudsmen; informers; the grapevine; unions; and participative, consultative, and democratic management in general.

Lateral Communication

Lateral, or horizontal, communication is between departments or personnel on the same level of the hierarchy and is most frequently used to coordinate activities (Figure 1-4). The need for lateral communication increases as interdependence increases. For instance, it becomes more important when one worker starts a job and someone else finishes it. It is also used by staff to transmit technical information to line authorities, and it may contain subjective and emotional aspects. Committees, conferences, and meetings are often used to facilitate horizontal communication.

Diagonal Communication

Diagonal communication occurs between individuals or departments that are not on the same level of the hierarchy (Figure 1-5). Informal in nature and frequently used between staff groups and line functions and in project types of organizations, it is another facet of multidirectional communication, which is common when communications often flow in all directions at the same time.

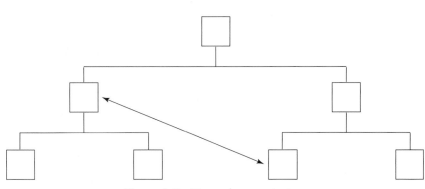

Figure 1-5   Diagonal communication.

The Grapevine

Informal methods of communication coexist with formal channels and are referred to as the grapevine. Informal communication is often rapid and subject to considerable distortion. The grapevine transmits information much faster than the formal channels because it uses cluster chain pathways involving three or four individuals at a time instead of going from one person to another as in manager–staff associate relationships. Communication passes at an increasing rate as individuals from clusters inform other small groups of people who work near each other or have contact with each other. Information spreads most quickly through the grapevine when it is recent, affects personnel's work (for example, pay increases or changes in policies), and involves people they know. People who work near each other or come in contact with each other are likely to be on the same grapevine.

Information becomes distorted for a number of reasons. Grapevine information is often fragmentary and incomplete. Consequently, there is a tendency to supply the missing pieces. Some people seize this opportunity to express feelings of self-importance, thus compensating for feelings of insecurity but also distorting the message. Because the grapevine is informal, with no formal lines of accountability, individuals do not have to answer to their manager for misinforming others.

Managers can learn much by listening to the grapevine and can remedy distortions by using the informal channels to pass on correct information.

BARRIERS TO COMMUNICATION

Thomas Gilovich (1991) indicates that misperception and misinterpretation of random data, misinterpretation of incomplete and unrepresentative data, biased evaluation of ambiguous and inconsistent data, seeing what we want to see, believing what we are told, and imagined agreement of others are *How We Know What Isn't So.*

Faulty reasoning and poorly expressed messages are major barriers to communication. Lack of clarity and precision resulting from inadequate vocabulary, poorly chosen words, platitudes, jargon, awkward sentence structures, poor organization of ideas, and lack of coherence are common. Talking too fast or too slow, slurring words, and not emphasizing important points lead to the faulty transmission of ideas. Memos that are poorly organized, ramble, and lack summaries also complicate the communication process. Words mean different things to different people. Communication is complicated when the sender uses words with which the receiver is not familiar, does not communicate on the receiver's level, or makes the message long and complicated.

If senders lack information or omit facts they do know, they will pass on a distorted or filtered message. Filtering, whether intentional or unintentional, involves a biased choice of what is communicated. For instance, distortion is more likely when subordinates desire promotion, for they may pass on information about their merits and suppress less successful aspects of their work. Fear of the consequences of full disclosure contributes to such omissions. At other times individuals may not communicate some information because they do not believe it is important enough to do so. The receiver becomes confused when nonverbal cues such as facial expressions and posture conflict with the verbal communication or when the sender does not admit to the intent of, or to the emotions underlying, the message.

People use selective perception to hear what they want to hear in terms of their biases. Values, attitudes, and assumptions affect one's perception of the message. Making a value judgment about the worth of a message based on one's opinion of the sender or the expected meaning of the message allows the receiver to hear what she wants to hear. An attitude is a feeling toward someone or something that is based on experience or the lack thereof, and it is a common barrier to communication because of its screening effect.

Uncommunicated assumptions are common and can make a considerable difference between the message sent and the one received. For instance, when program evaluation is mandated, personnel may fear that the results will be used to terminate workers, whereas management's actual intention is to use the results for recruiting purposes. Trust or distrust of the sender also influences how the message is received.

The sender is judged along with the message because the receiver has difficulty separating what she hears from how she feels about the sender. In fact, nonexistent motives can be attributed to the sender. Messages from higher echelons are often considered authoritative, even when they are not intended to be. The higher in the hierarchy a message originates, the greater are its chances of being accepted because of the status of the sender. If the sender has status with the listener, the message is usually considered credible. If the sender does not, the message may be discounted.

Staff associates tend to pay attention to communications from managers, thus facilitating downward communication. Unfortunately, managers may give verbal and nonverbal cues about how busy and unapproachable they are. They probably value communications from higher-level managers more than those from staff associates and may not reward associates for communications. In fact, staff associates are sometimes punished for communicating. Staff associates will be reluctant to report problems or potential problems when they believe these will be viewed as a weakness in their performance appraisal. Similarly, middle managers may not report problems that would reflect unfavorably on their managerial skills.

Status symbols magnify role and status barriers by increasing the psychological distance and the perceived organizational distance. Time pressures also become barriers that prevent communication. Managers do not have time to see all of their staff associates as much as desired, and staff associates may not take the time to report to the manager. Time pressures are also used as an excuse for not listening. Premature evaluation of what is going to be said, preoccupation with oneself, lack of readiness to hear, lack of receptivity to new ideas, and resistance to change interfere with listening. Physical distance, organizational complexity, temperature, noise, physical facilities (such as offices, meeting rooms, and an informal coffee shop), and technical facilities (such as telephones, loudspeakers, and duplicating equipment) also affect communications.

Gender Differences

Deborah Tannen (1990) indicates that women talk about their problems at length, whereas men want to find a solution or laugh them off. Women do rapport-talk, whereas men do report-talk. Women tend to be more talkative than men, initiate turn taking, make more frequent interruptions of others' comments, ask most of the questions, keep the conversations going, and use a larger vocabulary (Douglas, 1996). In *Men Are From Mars, Women Are From Venus,* John Gray (1992) indicates that men want to reason, whereas women want to be heard and validated. When stressed, men become focused and withdrawn, whereas women become emotionally involved and overwhelmed. Women have difficulty supporting a man who is not talking, whereas men have difficulty listening to women without giving advice.

Cultural Differences

Culture is a learned pattern of beliefs, customs, language, norms, and values that is shared by a group of people. How that learned pattern of behavior is expressed distinguishes cultures from each other. Cross-cultural communication involves having respect for, tolerance of, and nonjudgmental attitudes toward people with different attitudes, behaviors, and values; obtaining knowledge of other cultures; and being sensitive to cultural differences. One should assume differences until similarity is indicated; emphasize description rather than evaluation and interpretations; and treat interpretations as working hypotheses to be tested.

Cross-cultural communication occurs when someone from one culture correctly understands a message sent by someone from another culture. Cross-cultural miscommunication occurs when someone from the second culture misinterprets the sender's message. No two people have exactly the same cultural background, so every communication is somewhat intercultural. The greater the cultural differences, the greater the communication challenges and probability that the message sent will not be the message received. As attitudes, behaviors, and values are shared, people change and the cultural process continues (Douglas, 1996; Hein, 1998).

IMPROVING COMMUNICATION

Ideas should be clear before one speaks. What is the purpose of the message? Is it to seek information, inform, persuade, or initiate action? To formulate a message, one must gather the information needed and seek consultation from others as appropriate. Considering the goals and attitudes of the receivers helps the sender convey something of help or value to the receivers. One must also determine the mode of communication—by written or oral messages or through gestures. Face-to-face contact involves nonverbal behavior that further clarifies intent and allows for feedback to validate understanding of the message. Feedback through mutual exchange decreases the chance for misunderstanding. A climate that allows people to say what they think facilitates feedback.

One must also consider the setting in which one communicates and time one's messages for maximal impact. Should the communication be made in public or private? What is the social climate, and what effect will that have on the tone of the communication? What are the customs and practices of the audience, and how does one's message conform to its expectations? It is helpful for the message to refer to something the person has experienced and for it to be timed for immediate use by the receiver. For example, a building evacuation plan will be better received during fire prevention week, when personnel are expecting a fire drill, than at most other times.

Communications should be well organized and expressed in simple words, a clear style, and the shortest sentences possible. Redundancy—the repetition of the message verbatim or its presentation in several different ways—ensures that the message is understood. The amount of redundancy depends on the content of the message and the experience and background of the receiver. Repetition is especially important when the information is important and the directions are complicated. However, redundancy can become a barrier to communication if the message is simple and personnel are familiar with it. Employees are likely to stop listening because they know what is going to be said.

Because actions speak louder than words, the message is more forceful if the sender acts congruously. Communications should be followed up to make sure they were understood, and one should seek to understand as well as to be understood.

Listening, an active process that requires conscious attention, is critical to good communication. Trust is a prerequisite, because nurses will not share feelings with people they do not trust. The speaker must be convinced that disclosures will be kept confidential, that feelings will be respected and not judged, and that the information will be used appropriately and not used against the speaker.

Once trust is established, empathetic listening is needed. We think faster than we talk. Consequently, when listening to another talk, we have time left over for thinking, time that is frequently misused. There is less time for irrelevant thoughts when one concentrates on what is being said. One can think ahead of the speaker, try to guess the points that will be made next, consider what the conclusion will be, listen between the lines, try to understand the speaker's point of reference, review, and summarize the points made.

Active listening involves refraining from talking while trying to understand the speaker's attitude and feelings. One should listen to the whole story, talking as little as possible and avoiding leading questions, arguing, or giving advice. Silent pauses encourage the speaker to continue. Attentiveness is indicated by comments such as "yes," "uh huh," "go on," restatement (repeating what was said), paraphrasing (saying what was said in different words), clarifying (asking the speaker what was meant), reflecting (responding to the feelings communicated), and summarizing (reviewing the major points made). By saying little, receivers can concentrate on listening instead of on what they are going to say in return.

Written communications usually have the advantage of being more carefully formulated than oral communications. They also may save time and money and can be retained as legal records and reference sources. Written communications are sent downward, upward, or horizontally. Policies, procedures, handbooks, annual reports, bulletin boards, and house newspapers are usually directed downward. Attitude and morale surveys, suggestion systems, and written grievances are directed upward. Letters, memos, and reports may be upward, downward, or horizontal communication. Between department heads they are horizontal.

Before writing, one must first consider the purpose of the communication. For a planned and organized message, the writer develops thoughts logically, gives evidence to back up statements, and carefully selects words. Writers must ask themselves whether the communication answers who, what, when, where, and why questions and should appraise the tone of the document. Because writing is not easy, one should expect to edit original drafts.

Dictation is a valuable communication skill. Dictating probably requires more effort at first, but it can soon become easier than writing in longhand. In dictation one must again consider the purpose of the communication and plan and organize one's remarks. One starts dictation by indicating who is dictating what (letter or memo), the subject, type of paper needed (letterhead stationery, memo pad), and the number of copies needed. One should state the format (headings, double space, tabular outline, new paragraph), punctuation (capitalization, hyphen, period, commas, question marks, italics), and spell out unusual or unfamiliar words. Conversational instructions are given as one dictates. For example, "Mary, list the following statements and precede each with a dash." One should not smoke, eat, or chew gum while dictating. Background noises should be reduced as much as possible. Closing the office door during dictation can eliminate interference. Dictation should be given at a normal talking speed, with the words pronounced clearly and correctly. The sender can conclude dictation by saying "end of memo." If one cannot complete the dictation, instructions for the incomplete correspondence should be dictated. The dictator may want to keep a list of what is dictated and mark the items off as they are processed.

Telephone etiquette takes into account the needs of the sender and the receiver. One should answer the telephone promptly and speak clearly and distinctly to identify the agency, unit, and self. One should establish the purpose of the telephone call, determine the appropriate respondent, and ask questions to verify the message. One should answer questions with discretion, describe options appropriately, and identify actions for follow-up. Then the message is documented if indicated. To send a telephone message, one should gather the information needed and anticipate questions, call the number, identify the sender and receiver of the message, state the purpose of the call, exchange information, identify the follow-up, and document the call if indicated (Wywialowski, 1997).

Communications are critical for the functioning of an organization. Nurses need to be familiar with the communication process, communication systems, and directions communications can take. There are numerous barriers to communication. Managers need to know them and ways to overcome them.

Jahari Window

The process of giving and receiving feedback is illustrated by the Jahari Window (Figure 1-6). There are two columns representing the self and two rows representing the group. The left column represents things one knows about oneself. The right column represents things one does not know about oneself. As one solicits more feedback from the group, the pane moves to the right, enlarging the arena area, where what one knows about oneself and others also know is represented. The pane varies as the level of mutual trust and feedback in the group changes. The arena is characterized by free and open exchange of information between self and others.

The second pane, the blind spot, contains information one does not know about oneself but members of the group may know. One communicates to group members in verbal and nonverbal ways of which one may not be aware. The person with the large blind spot interacts primarily by giving feedback but solicits very little. The person may be a poor listener or may be insensitive to the feedback, or she may respond to feedback with undesirable responses like anger, crying, or leaving, which

makes others reluctant to give feedback. Soliciting feedback can decrease this pane.

The third pane, the façade, is where one knows something that the group does not know. The person with the large façade asks questions of the group but does not give information or feedback. The information may be hidden from the group because of fear of rejection, attack, or other hurtful behavior. When one perceives supportive elements in the group and does self-disclosure, the pane can decrease. One needs to disclose some information to test one's assumptions about the supportiveness of the group. Keeping information to oneself may be used to control and manipulate others.

The fourth pane, unknown, is where neither the person nor the group knows. The person neither solicits nor gives feedback. As the arena gets larger through feedback and self-disclosure, the other panes get smaller. However, there will probably always be some unknown information such as intrapersonal dynamics, early childhood memories, and latent potentialities that are unconscious. A receptive attitude to feedback and self-disclosure increase the arena and reduce the blind spot, the façade, and the unknown. The goal is to solicit self-disclosure and feedback to move information from the façade and the blind spot into the arena, making the information available to everyone.

COMMUNICATING WITH DIFFICULT PEOPLE

One requires special communication skills to deal with some personalities, including hostile-aggressive, complaining, negative, unresponsive, and overly nice. Some hostile-aggressive types seem to attack in an abrupt, abusive, intimidating manner that pushes others to acquiesce against their better judgment. These people tend to know what others should do, need to prove themselves right, and lack trust and caring. One must stand up to a hostile-aggressive person or feel overrun and frustrated. It is important to do this without fighting, or the conflict will escalate. It can be advantageous to give the hostile-aggressive person time to run down for a while and then interrupt to stand up for one-

Self		
→ Solicits feedback		
	Things I know	Things I do not know
	Arena	Blind spot
	Façade	Unknown

Group Self-disclosure ↓ or ↓ Gives feedback

Figure 1-6 Jahari Window.
From Jones JE, Pfeiffer JW, editors: *The 1973 annual handbook for group facilitators,* La Jolla, Calif, 1973, University Associates.

self. There may be no opportunity to speak between sentences, thus making it necessary to interrupt before the other person has finished speaking. It is also likely that the other person may interrupt. Then one must state firmly, "You interrupted me," and start again, preferably with a smile. One needs to get the other person's attention to do problem solving. Calling the person by name may help get the person's attention. Deliberately dropping a book is a more dramatic way to get attention. By standing up, one may also get attention. In addition, the other person may be less aggressive when sitting down. Then one needs to state ideas forcefully in a friendly manner that does not belittle the other person. It is important to avoid fighting with the hostile-aggressive person because such a battle will likely be lost. Even if the battle is won, the hostile-aggressive person's righteous anger will likely increase, and the war may be lost. When one stands up to a bully, one may become a friend. When dealing with hostile-aggressive people, it is important to stand up for oneself without fighting.

Exploders are another type of hostile-aggressive personality. Adult tantrums are the grown-up version of childhood tantrums that are a defense mechanism to cope with fear, helplessness, and frustration. Adult tantrums are sudden, almost automatic, responses to feeling threatened. The exploder typically feels angry first and then blaming or suspicious. People act on their perceptions, but people are likely to perceive the same situation differently. Consequently, the other person may be unaware that the exploder has been threatened and be surprised by the outburst. The exploder should be given time to finish the tantrum and regain self-control. If the exploder does not finish, a neutral statement such as "Stop" may interrupt the tantrum. Then one can show that the person is taken seriously by a comment such as "I can see this is important to you. I want to discuss this with you but not like this." Possibly one should change the pace by getting a cup of coffee and seeking a private place for a problem-solving session.

Sniping is an aggressive response to an unresolved problem. It causes distress rather than positive actions. Unfortunately, the unsolved problems

become worse, and the resulting stress causes more difficult behavior such as innuendoes, not-too-subtle remarks, and nonplayful teasing.

First of all, it is important to expose the attack by such comments as "That sounded like a put-down; did you mean it that way?" Usually snipers will deny any attack. Sniping is not possible without a camouflage that works. Standing up to the attack without escalating it will help one proceed with problem solving. It gives the sniper an alternative to a direct contest. It is appropriate to get other points of view that confirm or deny the sniper's criticism, then try to solve any problems that have surfaced. Sniping can be prevented by establishing regular problem-solving meetings.

Complainers may dump on you directly or may complain about other "awful" people. Complaining helps people appear blameless and innocent, at least to themselves. One should listen attentively to the complaints, paraphrase as acknowledgment of what was heard, and confirm one's perception of how the complainer feels. One should not agree with or apologize for the allegations and should avoid the accusation-defense-reaccusation pattern. It is preferable to simply state and acknowledge the facts without comment, then proceed with problem solving.

Negatively thinking people believe that any task that is out of their hands will fail and that others do not care and are self-serving. One should beware of being dragged down by their despair. One can make optimistic but realistic comments about past successes in similar situations but should not try to argue negativists out of their pessimism. It is better not to offer solution-alternatives until the problem has been thoroughly discussed or to ask people to act before they feel ready. During the problem-solving session, the negative events that could occur if the option is implemented should be explored. One should be ready to take independent action if the group refuses to do so and announce these plans without equivocation.

Unresponsive people cannot or will not speak when input is needed from them. It is difficult to know what their silence means. The most important strategy is to get the silent person to speak by asking open-ended questions, waiting calmly for a response, and not talking to fill the silence. If an open-ended question gets no response, one should comment on what is happening, for example, "I'm not getting any feedback from you," and end the observation with another open-ended question such as "What are you thinking?" Attention should be given when the person does speak. If the person never speaks, one should terminate the meeting by stating what will be done because no discussion occurred.

Superagreeable people are equally difficult people because they lead one to believe that they are in agreement but let one down when it comes to taking action. They have strong needs to be liked and accepted and help others feel approved to get approval themselves. They run into trouble when their need for approval conflicts with negative aspects of reality. They commit themselves to actions that they do not complete. Once again, problem solving is important. One must try to learn what prevents people from taking action and let them know that they are valued by telling them so and by asking questions about their interests, hobbies, and family to get to know them better. One should ask them what is not as good as they would like it to be and what could interfere with good relationships. Listening to their humor for hidden messages in teasing remarks and being prepared to do problem solving are also important (Bramson, 1997).

ASSERTIVENESS
Barriers to Assertiveness

Communication styles are passive, aggressive, or assertive. Assertiveness is the best style for nurse managers and the one they should foster in their personnel. However, there are barriers that nurses must overcome to become assertive. The most pervasive barrier is female sex role socialization. Whereas men are characterized as aggressive, competitive, independent, objective, analytical, task oriented, confident, self-disciplined, and emotionally controlled, women are expected to be passive, dependent, subjective, intuitive, empathetic, sensitive, interperson-

ally oriented, weak, inconsistent, and emotionally unstable.

The nursing socialization process and the nature of nursing are additional barriers. Both nursing schools and health care agencies have organizational hierarchies with authority and power concentrated at the top. This arrangement usually promotes compliance and conformity. Nurses are taught to value sacrifice, humility, and service to others. They have been taught not to state their thoughts or feelings. Although they give intimate physical nurturing, they are not to become emotionally involved with clients. Nurses have been socialized into a subservient role. They are expected to follow physicians' orders and to be professional but not to anticipate equal financial reimbursement for their education and responsibilities. They are expected to be a part of the health care team but not to make decisions or policies. They tend to keep so busy that they ignore their own rights.

In addition to these male-female role competition problems, nurses face female-female relationship problems. Men are more competitive with women than with other men, and women are more competitive with women than with men. Consequently, attempts to develop support systems for nurses are not usually successful. Instead, the queen bee and the trashing syndrome emerge.

The queen bee identifies with men, enjoys being told that she is different from most women, and feels superior to other women. The queen bee usually has to work very hard to become a success in a male-dominated society. She is likely to need to be cooperative and nonthreatening to achieve and maintain her successful position. She probably feels little animosity toward the system and the men who allowed her to become successful. Consequently, she is likely to identify with her male colleagues instead of with other women. However, protective of her own position and aware of the high price she paid for it, she makes it no easier for other women to succeed.

Trashing is a form of character assassination that divides women against one another. It is self-destructive and leads to impotent rage. Rather than exposing disagreements to resolve differences, trashing is done to destroy. It can be done to one's face or behind one's back, in public or in private. It questions one's motives, stresses one's worthlessness, and breaches one's integrity. The victim may be ignored, or anything she says or does may be interpreted in the most negative manner. Others' unrealistic expectations about her ensure failure. The trasher may give misinformation to others about what the victim does and thinks or tell her lies about what others think of her. Whatever method is used, it is manipulative, dishonest, and destructive. Women in general and nurses specifically need to become aware of what they are doing to each other, commit themselves to supportive instead of destructive behavior, learn to analyze interpersonal communication, and learn assertive behavior.

TRANSACTIONAL ANALYSIS

Transactional analysis is a technique that can be used by nurses for analyzing and understanding behavior. It was developed by Eric Berne (1996) and popularized by Thomas Harris, Muriel James, and Dorothy Jongeward. Transactional analysis is an outgrowth of the Freudian concepts of id, ego, and superego—elements of the psyche that stimulate, monitor, and control behavior. Berne calls these ego states parent, child, and adult.

Ego States

The *parent* ego state controls and is the source of values, opinions, rules, regulations, and social conscience. The two major types of parent ego states are nurturing parent and critical parent. The nurturing parent guides, teaches, advises, and supplies "how to" information. The critical parent prohibits and supplies "should" and "should not" information. The parent ego state is a result of cultural traditions, social programming, and responsibilities. Parental judgments are drawn heavily from natural parents, older siblings, teachers, and other parent figures.

The *child* ego state is dominated by emotions and is the feeling state. It is the id ego state where strong feelings are triggered by immediate experiences. People are in the child state when they are experiencing childlike natural impulses such as joy, delight, and gaiety or anger, hostility, and rage. The child ego state may be happy or destructive. The natural child is spontaneous, trusting, joyful, living, creative, and adventurous. The adapted child is suppressed and may express anger, rebellion, fear, or conformity.

The *adult* is the ego state that monitors one's behavior. It is the unemotional, thinking, problem-solving state. The adult ego state collects information, sets goals, compares alternatives, makes decisions and plans, and tests reality. The adult ego state is an unemotional state in which rational decision making takes place.

Every individual exhibits behavior from the three ego states at different times. A healthy individual maintains a balance between them. Unfortunately, some people are dominated by one or two of the ego states and are likely to create problems for managers. Parent-dominated individuals may not participate in problem solving because they think they already have the answer and know what is right and wrong. Child-dominated individuals do not engage in rational problem solving either. Screaming and being emotional have helped them get what

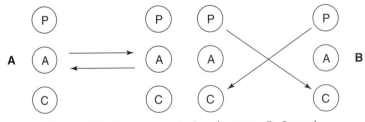

Figure 1-7 Transactions. **A,** Complementary. **B,** Crossed.

they wanted before. It is likely to be difficult to reason with someone dominated by the child ego state. Working with adult-dominated individuals may be boring because they work so hard. A balance between the three ego states produces the healthiest worker.

Transactions

When people interact, they participate as parent, child, or adult. A transaction or an observation unit is an exchange between people that consists of at least one stimulus and one response. Transactional analysis is done to identify the participant's ego state and consists of complementary or crossed types (Figure 1-7). The basic principle of the complementary type is that the response to the stimulus is predictable and expected.

Adult-to-adult transactions are the manner in which much business is conducted (Figure 1-8). For instance, a supervisor says, "Would you please give Mr. Jones his prn medication before you give Mrs. Smith her 8 AM medications?" A staff nurse replies, "Yes, I understand that Mr. Jones is complaining of surgical pain."

Parent-to-parent interaction is often a short-term sharing of opinions (Figure 1-9). One staff nurse says to another, "Those new graduate nurses certainly don't know how to function." The other nurse replies, "That's for sure."

Child-to-child interactions usually involve an emotional exchange (Figure 1-10). As long as both parties are in a child ego state, they are unable to think rationally and solve problems. The first staff nurse says, "I just gave Mrs. Smith her 8 AM medications, and when I went to chart them, you had signed for giving them. Why don't you sign right after you give medications so they won't be repeated!" The second nurse answers, "Why don't you give me a chance to sign before you go and give them again!"

In *parent-to-child* interactions one person takes a psychologically superior position over the other (Figure 1-11). Manager says, "I want to see you in my office." Staff nurse answers, "Yes, ma'am."

Crossed transactions result in closing communications at least temporarily (Figure 1-12). The response may be inappropriate or unexpected and may confuse or threaten the sender of the stimulus. Supervisor says, "Miss Jones, could I see you about this in my office right away?" Miss Jones replies, "No! Can't you see I'm busy? You'll have to wait."

Transactions usually proceed in a programmed series with rituals and procedures being the sim-

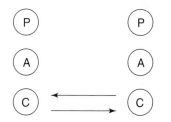

Figure 1-8 Adult-to-adult complementary.

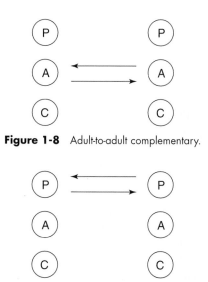

Figure 1-9 Parent-to-parent complementary.

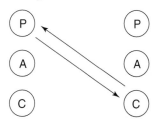

Figure 1-10 Child-to-child complementary.

Figure 1-11 Parent-to-child complementary.

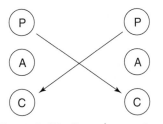

Figure 1-12 Crossed transaction.

plest kinds. Rituals are a series of simple comple-mentary transactions that provide mutual stroking with no real commitment. Most rituals have been used so often that the form has become more im-portant than the content, but they provide structure for greeting people and expressing religious beliefs. Greeting rituals such as "Hi," "How are you?" "I am fine" are not intended to supply information. The person who goes from office to office participating in rituals may get promoted because she is "a good guy." Rituals work for the person who can still get the job done. People who work hard to develop themselves may become apathetic when they realize socializing is more effective for obtaining promo-tions than hard work. Rituals may have started as a series of complementary adult transactions in-tended to manipulate reality, but they have lost their procedural validity over time.

Pastimes are pleasant ways to pass time with others to learn if you have enough in common to warrant further interaction. Common small talk in-cludes topics such as cooking, fashions, costs, sports, recreation, and mutual acquaintances. There is no goal or emotional closeness involved. People who spend too much time participating in pastimes may sense that their lives are happy but empty, whereas the person who spends too little time mak-ing small talk may not have much fun and may feel harassed. Pastimes become a problem for the orga-nization when they are an alternative to work.

Game Playing

In *Games People Play* Eric Berne writes: "A game is an ongoing series of complementary ulterior trans-actions progressing to a well-defined, predictable outcome." Games have a high stroke or recognition potential, but the payoff is usually negative. Games have hidden agendas that prevent both people and organizations from becoming winners. While play-ing games, people dwell on their own sorrows and inadequacies, make mistakes, catch others making mistakes, pass the buck, and fail to meet their obli-gations. People receive negative strokes and get hurt while real problems go unsolved. Productivity is limited because people use their energies to play games instead of to get the job done. Attention is given to past events rather than to the present. While realities of the current situation go unper-ceived, problems go unsolved.

People need strokes, and negative strokes are better than no strokes. Consequently, in work envi-ronments that do not provide positive strokes, people have a need to play games. People who are bored with their jobs are also likely to play games. Games discourage openness, honesty, and intimacy. They take many forms. Games that blame others include "If it weren't for you" and "See what you made me do." Games that attack others include "Blemish," "Now I've got you, you SOB," "Bear Trapper," "Corner," "Rapo," "Uproar," and "Let's you and him fight." Self-pity is reinforced by games such as "Poor me," "Kick me," "Stupid," "Wooden leg," "Harried," and "Lunch bag."

"If it weren't for you" is a blaming game in which people who feel inadequate blame others for their inability to achieve. People who blame their inability to be innovative on rigid policies may fear their own creative abilities. "If it weren't for . . ." is a clue that the game is being played. When managers hear an employee say this, they should suspect that the complainer would not function better under different circumstances but would likely become frustrated and request a transfer or quit. Changes may be made on a trial basis to test suspicions.

"See what you made me do" and "You got me into this" are closely related blaming games. The player avoids responsibility by being vindictive. It is common for workers to blame managers for prob-lems and for democratic managers to blame work-ers for mistakes or poor decisions. The manager de-cides whether or not to use the input from the workers and needs to accept that responsibility.

Many games attack others. The *"Blemish"* player looks for inconsequential, unimportant flaws. Instead of looking at purposes, the player concentrates on minutiae and zeroes in on trivial mistakes. Any positive stroke is discounted with a blemish. Blemish players also play "I was only trying to help you." The victims become resentful and may become the persecutor by playing *"Now I've got you, you SOB."* In this game the persecutor waits for the victim to make a mistake or sets the victim up for failure. The manager may be indulging in this game by setting standards too high to achieve, assigning people to work for which they are not qualified, creating impossible working conditions, or giving incomplete or unclear instructions. The worker may use grievance procedures or lawsuits against managers playing this game.

The *"Bear trapper"* often baits someone with false promises and then lets the trap fall. Organizations play this game in hiring practices when glamorous job descriptions are presented. This tends to result in high turnover. Workers learn the shortcomings of the job and become disillusioned. Presenting both the advantages and disadvantages of jobs is a more realistic approach.

The *"Corner"* player's victim is in a lose-lose situation. No matter what the victim does, it is wrong. A woman manager is damned if she is aggressive because that is not considered feminine and damned if she is not because aggressiveness is a desired managerial quality. A manager can corner someone into not completing work on time by not accepting the work that is done.

"Corner" can lead to *"Uproar."* Uproar often starts with a critical remark and results in an attack-defense dialogue that is often loud.

"Rapo" is a sexual game. A woman may wear revealing clothing and move in provocative ways. When a man responds, she rejects him. This game is problematic when men and women work together. Organizations require concentrating on equality and using human resources regardless of sex.

In *"Let's you and him fight,"* one person gets a second and third person into a fight. When one person tells a second person the "bad" things a third person said about the second, the first person is fostering a fight.

There are several versions of self-pity games. *"Kick me"* players provoke put-downs and make comments such as "I could kick myself for that." *"Stupid"* players collect put-downs about their intelligence. Managers need to give immediate feedback and take corrective actions to prevent the Stupid game. The *"Wooden leg"* player uses a physical or social handicap to avoid work. A deprived background may be used as an excuse to underachieve. The manager needs to set and maintain standards to minimize this game.

Managers play *"Poor me"* games also. *"Harried"* executives work hard to maintain the sense of being OK. They are likely to work nights and weekends to appear competent and confident. "I'm not OK" feelings are hidden by appearing super OK.

The Harried executive may also participate in the *"Lunch bag game."* Managers carry leftovers in a used paper bag and eat at their desk instead of going out to lunch with peers. This technique can be used to make other people feel guilty.

Games always involve putting someone down. To decrease games in organizations, one must stop putting oneself and others down. One should not play the complementary role but should give and receive positive strokes and invest time in activities and intimacy. Managers should integrate the goals of the workers and the organization and decrease boredom through job enrichment and personnel development. With good organization and management, positive strokes can become an intrinsic part of the job. Managers should foster an "I'm OK, you're OK" atmosphere.

Activities such as working and learning are goal directed and have a high stroke potential. They are a highly rewarding way to spend time. Workers must be careful not to take on so many activities that they neglect rituals and pastimes, and managers should not overload themselves with activities and leave the workers with idle time.

Intimacy is an open sharing of experience with others usually by people with close relationships but sometimes by strangers. It is the most rewarding way to spend time. It is also the most risky. Although intimacy is without ulterior motives or exploitation, one needs high self-esteem to risk the openness of intimacy. It requires and fosters the "I'm OK, you're OK" atmosphere.

Life Positions

Life positions are more permanent than ego states. As individuals mature, they make assumptions about themselves and others. They consider themselves as OK or not OK and see others as OK or not OK. Four positions result: *"I'm OK, you're OK,"* *"I'm OK, you're not OK," "I'm not OK, you're OK,"* and *"I'm not OK, you're not OK."* OK feelings are associated with a sense of power, personal worth, well-being, capability, and lovableness. Not-OK feelings result from a sense of inability, weakness, helplessness, worthlessness, anxiety, and a feeling of being insignificant and unlovable. Most people develop a basic life position early in childhood that tends to be reinforced by the person's selective perceptions and reactions to experiences.

In the I'm OK, you're OK position, individuals feel interdependent with others and the environment. They are happy, active people with a positive outlook on life who like reinforcement for being OK but are not dependent on it. They use the happy child and nurturing parent ego states. Because they feel OK about themselves, they have little difficulty feeling others are OK.

People in the I'm OK, you're not OK position do not believe they can rely on anyone but themselves. They think people are worthless and are likely to be enemies and consequently tend to blame others. The critical parent ego state is dominant. A manager in this position possesses a Theory X philosophy, implements a Likert type I system, and supervises people closely because they cannot be trusted.

People in the I'm not OK, you're OK position are burdened with self-defeating attitudes and a lack of confidence. They take a psychologically inferior stand to others and assume that they are less competent and less influential than others.

Individuals in the I'm not OK, you're not OK position are maladjusted. They think they are worthless and so are others. Lacking confidence in themselves and trust in others, they are suspicious and anxious, disconnected from others, alienated from the environment, and miserable, and they tend to give up.

During infancy individuals have a mixture of OK and not-OK feelings, with the not-OK feelings predominating. The infant feels OK when physical needs are met and positive strokes are received. Most of an infant's experiences provide negative strokes and not-OK feelings. Because adults can satisfy the infant's needs, they are viewed as OK. Consequently, for most people the I'm not OK, you're OK position is established early and continues into adulthood. Socialization of women and nurses particularly reinforces the position that they are not OK. Therefore they need a lot of positive reinforcement to move to an I'm OK, you're OK position. Assertiveness can help one achieve and maintain that position. Once it is learned, there will be less passive-aggressive behavior.

Assertive Techniques

Communication styles are commonly passive, aggressive, or assertive. Passive persons are often self-denying and inhibited and allow others to choose for them. Consequently, their goals are not achieved and they feel hurt, anxious, and frustrated. Aggressive persons are self-enhancing at others' expense. They are expressive, choose for others, deprecate others, and achieve their goals by using others. Aggressive behavior generates hatred and sometimes revenge. Assertive persons are self-enhancing. They are expressive, choose for themselves, and can achieve their goals. Consequently, they are likely to feel good about themselves.

Passive persons tend to be at a loss for words, do not say what they really mean, use many apologetic words, and hope people will understand what they want without telling them. They tend to have a weak, hesitant voice, downcast eyes, and fidgety hands, and they nod frequently.

The aggressive person is loud, uses loaded, subjective words, makes accusations, and sends "you" messages that blame others. A flippant, sarcastic style with an air of superiority and rudeness is common. The person is likely to stand with hands on hips, feet apart, narrowed eyes, pointing a finger and talking in a superior, demanding, authoritarian manner.

Assertive persons say what they want in direct statements that say what they mean. They use objective words, send "I" messages, and make honest statements about their feelings. They are attentive listeners who give the impression of caring. They use eye contact and spontaneous verbal expressions with appropriate gestures and facial expressions while speaking in a well-modulated voice.

The style used governs how situations will be handled. Suppose, for instance, that a manager has noticed that a staff nurse has been arriving at work late for the past 3 days. The passive manager may not mention the problem at all. The aggressive manager might say, "How about getting here on time or looking for a new job? What do you think we pay you for anyway?" The assertive manager would be likely to speak to the staff nurse in private and might say, "I've noticed you have been late the past 3 days. Why haven't you been getting to work on time?" The last approach gives an impression of caring and facilitates problem solving.

Assertiveness is the most desirable style for a nurse manager. To achieve assertiveness, one must substitute verbal persistence for silent passivity or verbal abuse. Broken record is a technique managers can use to reach a compromise by indicating what they want and by keeping other people from talking them into what the others want to do. With the broken-record technique managers keep repeating what they want.

Manager: I expect you to get to work on time.

Staff nurse: But I'm a night person. I stay up late, and it's difficult to get up so early to come to work. I'm so tired that I shut off my alarm and go back to sleep. Then when I do get up, I stumble around in the dark to find my clothes so I won't wake my husband.

Manager: You are scheduled to work the day shift this rotation, and I expect you to be at work on time. If you are a night person, would you like to be assigned to the night shift permanently?

Staff nurse: No. I wouldn't be able to see my husband then. He works 9 AM to 9 PM and gets home about 9:30 PM. I would have to come to

work at 10:30 and I could see him for only about an hour. I would get home just in time for him to go to work.

Manager: You are scheduled to work the day shift this rotation, and I expect you to get to work on time. However, we could assign you to the evening shift permanently. Would you want that?

Staff nurse: Working the evening shift would allow me to see my husband after work and to sleep in. Yes, I would prefer the evening shift.

Manager: I will see how quickly we can get your schedule changed to permanent evenings. I do expect you to be here by 7 AM until we get your schedule changed.

Fogging, negative assertion, and negative inquiry are techniques for dealing with criticism, whether it is self-directed or from another source, real or imagined. They help minimize the negative emotional response of anxiety to criticism that manipulates one into defending what one wants to do instead of doing it. Consequently, one feels less at conflict with oneself and more comfortable with both the negative and positive aspects of one's personality.

Fogging is agreeing with the truth, agreeing in principle, or agreeing with the odds rather than denying the criticism, getting defensive, or counterattacking with criticism. It helps desensitize one to criticism and leads to a reduction in the frequency of criticism from others. It sets up psychological distance, is a passive skill, and does not encourage the other person to be assertive. It also encourages a person to listen to what the critic says, to respond only to what the critic says rather than to what is implied, and to consider probabilities. For example:

Staff nurse: You scheduled me to double back from evenings to days twice in a 2-week time schedule.

Manager: I see that I scheduled you to double back the first Wednesday and the second Friday (agreeing with the truth).

Staff nurse: When I double back, I have less than 7 hours of sleep. I get tired, have trouble functioning, and fear making mistakes.

Manager: I understand that you get tired when you double back and fear making mistakes. It seems logical that one would make more mistakes when tired than when alert (agreeing with the odds).

Staff nurse: We need a policy to prevent having just one shift off between shifts.

Manager: I agree. We do need staffing policies that would provide for adequate rest periods between shifts (agreeing in principle).

With negative assertion people assertively accept negative aspects about themselves. This reduces the need to seek forgiveness for one's mistakes or the need to counterattack with criticism.

Staff nurse: Your new uniform really reveals how fat you are.

Manager: I'm overweight because I eat too much. I eat just about everything in sight except the kitchen sink. I've even seen the cat get worried (negative assertion).

Staff nurse: Well, that new uniform sure makes you look like a blimp.

Manager: These new styles don't complement my figure (negative assertion).

Negative assertion is not appropriate for physical or legal conflicts or for relating to people on a close interpersonal basis. The persistence of the critic will determine if one needs to use other assertive techniques.

Negative inquiry fosters assertiveness in the critic. In an unemotional manner, the criticized person asks for more information that may be negative. This provides a basis for problem solving and consequently reduces repetitive criticism.

Staff nurse: You don't look good today.

Manager: Is it me or what I'm wearing?

Staff nurse: It's your face. You look so tired.

Manager: I don't feel tired. What about my face makes me look tired?

Staff nurse: Your eyes look so tired. They're so dark. There are bags under them.

Manager: What can I do to make them look less tired?

Staff nurse: If the problem isn't fatigue, I guess you could use a creme cosmetic over the bags and use light instead of dark-colored eye shadow.

Assertive behavior is more than demanding your rights from others and keeping others from manipulating. In a social sense assertiveness is the ability to communicate with others about who you are, how you live, what you do, and what you want and the ability to make them feel comfortable talking about themselves. Free information—information offered without being asked for—gives you something to talk about and reduces awkward silences. Self-disclosure reveals how you think, feel, and react to others' free information. This social conversation allows you to discover mutually rewarding relationships or to identify people with whom you have few common interests.

CHAPTER SUMMARY

Chapter 1 covered the following:
Communication Process
Basic Communication Skills
Communication Principles
Methods of Communication
Use of Computers for Communication
Communication Systems
    Downward Communication
    Upward Communication
    Lateral Communication
    Diagonal Communication
    The Grapevine
Barriers to Communication
    Gender Differences
    Cultural Differences
Improving Communication
    Jahari Window
Communicating With Difficult People
Assertiveness
    Barriers to Assertiveness
Transactional Analysis
    Ego States
    Transactions
    Game Playing

Life Positions
Assertive Techniques

REFERENCES

Advanced executive leadership skills, Stamford, Conn, 1981, Xerox Learning Systems.

Barr L, Barr N: *The leadership equation,* Austin, Tex, 1989, Eakin Press.

Berne E: *Games people play,* New York, 1996, Ballantine.

Bramson RM: *Coping with difficult people,* New York, 1997, Doubleday.

Douglas LM: *The effective nurse,* St. Louis, 1996, Mosby.

Gillies DA: *Nursing management: a systems approach,* Philadelphia, 1994, WB Saunders.

Gilovich T: *How we know what isn't so,* New York, 1991, Free Press.

Gray J: *Men are from Mars, women are from Venus,* New York, 1992, HarperCollins.

Harris TA: *I'm OK—you're OK: a practical guide to transactional analysis,* New York, 1969, Harper & Row.

Hein EC: *Contemporary leadership behavior: selected readings,* Philadelphia, 1998, Lippincott.

James M, Jongeward D: *Born to win,* 1996, Perseus Press.

Jones JE, Pfeiffer JW, editors: *The 1973 annual handbook for group facilitators,* La Jolla, Calif, 1973, University Associates.

Kreider NA, Haselton BJ: *The systems challenge,* Chicago, 1997, American Hospital.

Pfeiffer JW, Jones JE, editors: *A handbook of structured experiences for human relations training,* Vol II, La Jolla, Calif, 1974, University Associates.

Tannen D: *You just don't understand: women and men in conversation,* New York, 1990, Ballantine Books.

Whetten DA, Cameron KS: *Developing management skills,* Reading, Mass, 1998, Addison-Wesley.

Wywialowski EF: *Managing client care,* ed 2, St. Louis, 1997, Mosby.

BIBLIOGRAPHY

Brown SJ: Communication strategies used by an expert nurse, *Clin Nurs Res* 3:43-56, Feb 1994.

Davidhizar R, Dowd S: The dynamics of rumours in the clinical setting, *Nurs Standard* 11:40-43, Dec 18, 1996.

Davis LL, Cos RP: Looking through the constructivist lens: the art of creating nursing work groups, *J Prof Nurs* 10:38-46, Jan-Feb 1994.

Dowd SB, Davidhizar R, Dowd LP: Rumors and gossip: a guide for the health care supervisor, *Health Care Supervisor* 16:65-70, Sept 1997.

Fiesta J: Communication—are you listening? *Nurs Manage* 25:15-16, Sept 1994.

Hanna B: Improving communication . . . "over the sink," *Nurs Manage* 25:88F-88H, July 1994.

Heineken J: Patient silence is not necessarily client satisfaction: communication problems in home care nursing, *Home Healthcare Nurse,* 16:115-121, Feb 16, 1998.

Jones-Schenk J, Hartley P: Organizing for communication and integration, *JONA* 23:30-33, Oct 1993.

Kolber R: Team building: a strategy to enhance cohesiveness, *Recruitment Retention Report* 7:1-6, Jan 1994.

McClellan MA, Henson RH, Schmele J: Introducing new technology: confusion or order? *Nurs Manage* 25:38-39, July 1994.

McMahon B: The functions of space, *J Adv Nurs* 19:362-366, Feb 1994.

Mertens R, Jans B, Kurz X: A computerized nationwide network for nosocomial infection surveillance in Belgium, *Infect Control Hosp Epidemiol* 15:171-179, March 1994.

Minnick A, Pischke-Winn K, Sterk MB: Introducing a two-way wireless communication system, *Nurs Manage* 35:42-47, July 1994.

Newman J: Managing cultural diversity: the art of communication, *Radiologic-Technology* 69:231-46, 249, Jan-Feb 1998.

Peterson LW et al.: Communicating with staff nurses, *Nurs Manage* 26:36-38, June 1995.

Piscopo B: Organizational climate, communication, and role strain in clinical nursing faculty, *J Prof Nurs* 10:113-119, March-April 1994.

Ribeiro VE, Blakeley JA: The proactive management of rumor and gossip, *JONA* 25:43-50, June 25, 1995.

Roberts GW: Nurse/patient communication within a bilingual health care setting, *Br J Nurs* 3:60-64, 66-67, Jan 27-Feb 9, 1994.

Simpson RL: Technology: nursing the system: ensuring patient data, privacy, confidentiality and security, *Nurs Manage* 25:18-20, July 1994.

Soet JE, Basch CE: The telephone as a communication medium for health education, *Health Educ Behav* 24:759-772, Dec 1997.

Williams D, Brown DL: Automation at the point of care, *Nurs Manage* 25:32-35, July 1994.

CASE STUDY

The institution where you work is rightsizing and carefully evaluating productivity. The workers know that something is going on but are not informed. Consequently, they are imagining scenarios and rumors are rampant. One day a normally quiet, shy person explodes in your presence. She screams about the unfairness of cutting wages and laying off people. What might be the causes of her behavior? How should you deal with her behavior as it is occurring? What will you do regarding rumors?

CASE STUDY

A staff nurse who is frequently late to work works with you. How will you assertively problem solve the situation with the nurse?

Critical Thinking Activities for this chapter begin on page 469.

CHAPTER 2

STRESS MANAGE-MENT

Chapter Overview

Chapter 2 presents sources of stress, stress response, symptoms of stress, stress control, relaxation, time management, delegation, procrastination, and ways to maximize organization time.

MAJOR CONCEPTS AND DEFINITIONS	
Stress	the body's nonspecific response to any demand
Eustress	a positive form of stress that adds excitement and challenge
Distress	a negative form of stress that threatens effectiveness
Delegation	to entrust a task to another person who serves as one's representative
Responsibility	obligation; what must be done to complete the task
Authority	power to make final decisions and give commands
Accountability	liability for satisfactory completion of work
Planning	preparing a scheme for doing
Time management	controlling use of time for maximum productivity

STRESS MANAGEMENT
Sources of Stress

Adjustment to change is stressful. Many events in life produce individual stress reactions. Death of a spouse or close family member, divorce, marital separation, marriage or remarriage, and personal injury or illness are highly stressful events. Change in the health of a family member, pregnancy, gain of a new family member, marital reconciliation, increased arguing with spouse, sexual difficulties, changes in financial state, mortgages, trouble with in-laws, a son or daughter leaving home, and the death of a close friend are stressful. Changes in living conditions and personal habits, such as changes in work, residence, school, recreation, church activities, social activities, sleeping habits, and eating habits, cause stress. Even personal achievements, vacations, and holidays are stressful. These personal stressors can affect one's job performance.

In addition to the personal stressors, there are many sources of stress at work. Dismissal and retirement are highly stressful. Business readjustments such as changing jobs or responsibilities, changes in working hours or conditions, and problems with the boss are stressful. Even outstanding achievement is stressful. Poor physical working conditions; physical danger; work overload; time pressures; responsibility for people; role ambiguity and conflict; conflicts with superiors, peers, and subordinates; restrictions; little participation in decision making; overpromotion or underpromotion; and lack of job security are stressors common to jobs.

Nurses face stress with life-and-death situations; heavy workloads involving physical and mental strain; knowledge of how to use numerous pieces of equipment and the consequences of equipment failure; reporting to numerous bosses; communication problems between staff members, physicians, families, and other departments; and awareness of the serious consequences of mistakes. A hospital is one of the most stressful work environments.

People often needlessly increase their own stress. The difference between demands people place on themselves or perceive from others and the resources they perceive as available to meet the demands is a threat or stress. Individuals are typed by the demands they place on themselves. Type A people set high standards, are competitive, and put themselves under constant time pressure. They are very demanding of themselves even in leisure and recreation activities. Type B people are more easy-going and relaxed. They are less competitive and more likely to accept situations than fight them.

Stress Response

Stress is impossible to avoid. It is a nonspecific response of the body to any demand. There are two types of stress: (1) eustress, a positive force that adds excitement and challenge to life and provides a sense of well-being, and (2) distress, a negative force caused by unrelieved tension that threatens effectiveness. Whether one will experience eustress or distress largely depends on the person's perceptions, physical activity or inactivity, mental activity or inactivity, sound nutrition, and meaningful relationships.

A stressor is anything an individual perceives as a threat. Stressors produce a state of stress by disrupting homeostasis. There are three stages in the stress response (Box 2-1). First, the alarm reaction is the mobilization of resources to confront the threat. Second, in the resistance stage, there is a large increase in energy consumption. Once the reserve energy has been used, the body needs time to recover and to replenish the supply. When stress continues for long periods of time, the energy is used but not replaced and the third stage, exhaustion, results.

Consequently, unrelieved stress interferes with one's physical and mental well-being. After the stress event the body returns to a state of equilibrium. Stable periods for bodies to restore adaptive energy allow one to meet new stressful situations.

Box 2-1   THREE STAGES IN STRESS RESPONSE

Alarm reaction—mobilization of resources to confront threat
Resistance stage—increase in energy consumption
Exhaustion—depletion of the body's energy reserves

Symptoms of Stress

Numerous symptoms indicate that stress is becoming distress. These include but are not limited to those shown in Box 2-2.

High stress levels accumulated over several months are likely to result in physical and psychological reactions. The amount of stress necessary before one manifests symptoms varies, depending on factors such as heredity, habits, personality, past illnesses, and previous crises and coping mechanisms. Well-educated, intelligent, creative people in management are at high risk for burnout. They may become workaholics but get little accomplished, experience chronic fatigue, feel they do not want to go to work, take increasing amounts of sick time, become negative, blame and criticize others, engage in backbiting, and talk behind others' backs.

Stress Control

Nurse managers can prevent and control burnout by setting personal and professional goals, establishing priorities, practicing good health habits and relaxation techniques, improving their self-esteem by obtaining the skills they need, and using support systems.

Values clarification.   Values clarification is a useful activity. Values should be chosen freely from alternatives with thoughtful consideration to the consequences of each alternative. They should be cherished and shared with others. The value should be integrated into one's lifestyle, and actions should be consistent with the values. To help clarify one's values, one may assign priorities to a list of values such as the following:

Affection	Pleasure
Duty	Power
Expertise	Prestige
Health	Security
Independence	Self-realization
Leadership	Service
Parenthood	Wealth

Box 2-2　**SYMPTOMS OF STRESS**

Fatigue	Nightmares
Depression	Early morning waking
Tearfulness	Feeling of not being able to get anything done
Restlessness	Feeling that everything is too much
Nervousness	Forgetfulness
Withdrawal or sudden gregariousness	Lack of concentration
Irritability	Tendency to be demanding
Anger	Loss of appetite or overeating
Feeling of being unloved	Indigestion
Insecurity	Constipation or diarrhea
Feeling of vague anxiety	Nausea
Pessimism	Coughing
Self-criticism	Headaches
Frequent frustration	High blood pressure
Loss of interest in going out	Rapid pulse
Loss of interest in people and things	Heart palpitation
Decrease in self-care	Perspiration
Disorganization	Aching neck and shoulder muscles
Inability to relax or rest	Low back pain
Accidents	Allergy problems
Arthritis	Dermatitis
Asthma	Influenza
Colds	Hives
Colitis attacks	Menstrual distress
	Ulcers

One can also list in order of priority characteristics such as the following:

Ambitiousness	Honesty
Broadmindedness	Imagination
Cheerfulness	Independence
Cleanliness	Logic
Courage	Lovingness
Forgiveness	Responsibility
Helpfulness	

Goal setting. Goals should be consistent with one's values, and one should consider goal alternatives. To do this, one considers why a goal is desired. One may want a promotion for recognition or for economic reasons. If the promotion is not forthcoming, one may receive recognition through community service. Money might be generated through wise investments or fees for community services. The achievement of desired outcomes through different approaches increases flexibility and decreases stress caused by unmet goals.

Stress avoidance and regulation. When reappraising situations, one should avoid troublesome transactions. The frequency of stress-inducing situations should be minimized. Every change takes energy. Therefore during periods of high stress, routines and habits should be maintained as much as possible. One should be cautious about moving and starting a new job at the same time one is getting a divorce. That also would be a particularly poor time to try to stop smoking or lose weight. Unnecessary changes should be prevented during periods of high stress. Deliberately postponing some changes helps one deal with unavoidable change constructively and reduces the need for multiple adjustments at one time. However, increasing positive sources of tension that foster growth, such as learning a sport, can help offset the deleterious effect of negative tension.

Time blocking. Time blocking is the setting aside of specific time for adaptation to a stressor. To reduce the stress from having been promoted to a management position, you can set aside time for reading about management or for observing a manager. This helps ensure that concerns are addressed and tasks accomplished. It decreases anxiety, time urgency, and feelings of frustration. Define off-limit times and set aside time when you will not be interrupted by phone calls or individuals except for emergencies. Schedule free time, exercise time, and put social events on the calendar like you would a business appointment.

Time management. Time management helps control stress. Much time can be conserved when one knows one's value system and acts consistently with it, sets goals, and plans strategies for accomplishment of those goals. One can also use organizers such as to-do lists and calendars to plan good use of one's time.

Assertiveness. When one asserts oneself, one increases self-esteem and reduces anxiety, thus reducing stress. As with time management, assertiveness involves thinking through goals and acting consistently with one's values through the use of effective work habits and by setting limits on others' attempts to block one's goals. It involves stating what one wants and how one feels, making requests, taking compliments, handling put-downs, and setting limits. An assertive person makes eye contact with others, stands straight, sits in an open, listen-ing posture, and speaks in a clear voice. Assertive people choose for themselves and achieve desired goals through self-enhancing behavior that reduces stress.

Feeling pauses. Feeling pauses are useful. One should take time to identify a feeling, label it, distinguish between thinking and feeling, and accept the feeling for what it is rather than talking oneself into what it should be. One should be aware if one is feeling the following:

Amusement	Hope
Calmness	Joy
Care	Love
Compassion	Passion
Elation	Relaxation
Excitement	Satisfaction
Forgiveness	Thrill
Happiness	

One should also acknowledge negative feelings such as the following:

Anger	Fear
Anxiousness	Frustration
Confusion	Hurt
Depression	Jealousy
Embarrassment	Restlessness
Envy	Terror

Then one should determine whether the feeling is appropriate for the situation and decide how to express the feeling in a safe and appropriate way. Feelings can be expressed in "I feel" messages rather than "You" messages that blame or attack others. Feelings can be talked about with an uninvolved person. One can fantasize about how one would like to handle the situation better the next time. Negative feelings may be acted out symbolically by punching a pillow, drawing a picture, or writing a poem. One may set aside negative feelings by getting involved in something pleasant, such as exercise, hobbies, music, television, or talking to a friend. Feelings can also be experienced vicariously by getting involved in another's experience through reading a book, watching a movie, or listening to someone.

Inner shouting. Inner shouting is the process of shouting "I feel . . ." inside one's head; the person blurts the feeling out spontaneously rather than saying it quietly. Anger should be viewed as a symptom. Pains should be focused on to help one take responsibility for feelings of hurt and humiliation.

Anchoring. Anchors are associated feelings that are initiated either by an event or by the memory of that event. Anchors may be sounds, sights, smells, tastes, or touches that stimulate positive or negative feelings. Birds chirping may remind one of happy, lazy mornings with the family. One may recall an awful accident at the sight of blood. One might remember fall walks through the woods with a lover at the smell of dry leaves. A taste may revive memories of grandma's home cooking. A light touch to the face may remind one of earlier loving moments and cause one to experience a sense of well-being. Our lives are filled with anchors that cause associations. We can use anchoring in a useful way to experience desired feelings. Because touch can be inconspicuous and easy to replicate, one can associate a positive feeling with a familiar touch to the body. This may be so simple as clasping one's hands and being reminded of soft music, beautiful colored glass, and the peaceful sanctuary of church. Exact pressure at a very specific spot makes the anchor work most accurately and should be done when one desires to bring back a pleasurable feeling.

Sorting. Sorting is choosing the interpretation of an event. One can have an optimistic or pessimistic interpretation of events. Is the glass half full or half empty? We become what we think and therefore can make ourselves happy or miserable. To be more happy and fun loving, one should focus on the positive aspects of situations.

Thought stopping. Thought stopping helps get rid of negative thinking. Excessive rehearsals in our minds of negative past events are unhelpful thoughts that waste time, reduce our self-esteem, and encourage maladaptive behavior patterns. To prepare for thought stopping, one should think of beautiful, pleasant experiences: a sunrise, a water-fall, a flower, a pet, favorite music, baking bread, holding hands. One should also identify not-so-helpful thoughts: I'm stupid; I'm fat; Nobody likes me. One should identify the negative thoughts that are most bothersome. In private one can think about a negative thought momentarily and suddenly yell, "Stop!" while clasping one's hands or hitting one's head or leg. One startles oneself, and the thought escapes. Immediately one should insert a pleasant thought. If the negative thought returns, the procedure can be repeated. It is reinforced when the negative thoughts are stopped. Thoughts lead to feelings that can lead to behaviors, so by changing the way one thinks, one can change the way one behaves. Thought stopping should not be used, however, when physical or emotional safety and grieving are involved.

Compartmentalization. Compartmentalization of thought is the deliberate decision to think negative thoughts at specified times of the day. During the allotted time one thinks about worry, guilt, or jealousy. One does not allow oneself to think these thoughts at other times of the day.

Environmental changes. Environmental changes can be designed to reduce stress. This may be as extreme as changing jobs or residence or as minor as painting a room a favorite color or adding a picture, candle, or basket. The short time inconvenience of remodeling may be worth the long-term stress reduction. Temporary changes in jobs can add variety and stimulation.

Humor. Humor related to an attitude toward life is most likely to reduce stress. There is a cluster of qualities that characterize this frame of mind, including flexibility, spontaneity, unconventionality, shrewdness, playfulness, humility, and irony. These are qualities that can be developed. Flexibility is the ability to examine all sides of the issues. One should try to look at a situation from several different viewpoints: the boss's, the subordinate's, the client's. Spontaneity is the ability to swing from one mood to another quickly. One might practice the body language of several emotions, including fear, anger, sadness, and love. One can free oneself from current values, places, and occupations through unconventionality and imagine living a day as a favorite animal, a famous historical person, an Eskimo, a Native American, or an astronaut. Shrewdness is refusal to believe that people or things are what they appear to be. One can think of a list of people and things and give an example of how each is not what it seems to be. Playfulness is the ability to see life as an amusing game. One can visualize life as a game and give the game a name. One should identify times of various emotions—fun, enjoyment, fear, anger, sadness—and chart wins and losses. Humility is a willingness to question the importance of one's values, ideas, achievements, and existence. One must consider the meaning of one's life and consider how difficult situations have brought happiness and how happy relationships have included suffering. Irony is the ability to see that situations are not black or white.

Centering. Centering helps reduce stress by bringing the mind and body back into balance. With left-sided dominance, intuitive, aesthetic, and creative functions are reduced under stress. To center oneself, one is to put one's tongue on the centering button, which is about a quarter of an inch behind the upper front teeth. This spot apparently stimulates the thymus gland, weakens the effect of stress, and balances the cerebral hemispheres. Other activities that seem to balance the two hemispheres of the brain include reading a poem in a rhythmic fashion; listening to a person with a soothing voice; listening to classical music; listening to natural sounds such as cats purring, birds chirping, or brooks or waterfalls babbling; looking at pictures of pleasant landscapes or smiling people making caring gestures; swinging one's arms during a vigorous walk; and taking a shower. Good posture is also beneficial.

Nutrition. Good nutrition helps maintain the body for full functioning. Eating a balanced diet, taking vitamin supplements, and drinking plenty of water are important. In general, people in the United States need to reduce fat and cholesterol, sugar, salt,

and food additive consumption. Their diets contain high levels of fat and cholesterol, which are abundant in red meats, eggs, cheese, and prepared foods. Excessive consumption of fat is associated with cardiovascular diseases. They are obtaining an increasing proportion of their calories from sugar, which is associated with obesity, tooth decay, diabetes, and heart disease. There is a growing concern that additives and pollutants are related to cancer. These food additives include preservatives, coloring, flavoring, and stabilizers that extend shelf life and make processed food taste better. In addition, pesticides and other chemical pollutants are health hazards.

The increasing consumption of saturated fats and sugar, coupled with a decrease in activity levels, contributes to a widespread occurrence of obesity. In general, people in the United States need to increase exercise while decreasing caloric intake, particularly from fats and sugars. At the same time, the percentage of calories from foods containing fiber, such as fresh fruits, vegetables, and whole grains, should be increased. Canned, frozen, and prepared foods are usually devoid of their original fiber content and often have sugar and salt added. The grains we eat have often been refined to white flour and rice, thereby losing much of the roughage. Although improving eating habits may not prevent stress, it is one way to maintain the level of fitness needed to fight stress.

Exercise. Regular, vigorous exercise can also help one withstand chronic stress. Aerobic exercise elevates the heart rate during and for a period after the exercise. The range of elevation necessary to produce an aerobic effect is from 60% to 80% of the maximal heart rate the person can achieve, which is calculated at 220 minus the person's age in years. Jogging, cycling, and swimming are particularly good aerobic exercises. Dance allows one to stretch and strengthen muscles and to reduce tension.

Regular exercise develops greater capacities in several areas of function. It increases the strength of cardiac contractions, the size of the coronary arteries, the blood supply to the heart, the size of the heart muscle, and the blood volume per heartbeat.

It decreases the heart rate at rest and with exertion and reduces vulnerability to cardiac dysrhythmias. It increases the blood oxygen content, blood volume, and efficiency of peripheral blood distribution and return. Exercise increases the blood supply to the lungs and the functional capacity during exercise. It increases lean muscle mass and functional capacity during exercise. Exercise also reduces strain and nervous tension resulting from psychological stress and reduces the tendency for depression.

Sleep.   Sleep is also important for dealing with stress. Sleep needs decrease with age, and people may awaken several times during the night as they grow older. This should not be confused with insomnia, which is a prolonged inability to sleep. There are three types of insomnia: (1) initial, when it takes more than 15 minutes to fall asleep; (2) intermittent, with awakening during the night and difficulty returning to sleep; and (3) terminal, with early morning awakening and inability to go back to sleep.

Physical, emotional, and nutritional factors may contribute to insomnia. A lack of physical exercise, digestive problems, heart trouble, and high blood pressure interfere with sleep. Disturbing emotional states such as anger, fear, guilt, depression, and anxiety create tension that interferes with sleep. An unbalanced diet, alcohol, caffeine consumption, and a large meal shortly before bedtime can interfere with sleep.

To foster a good night's sleep, the day's activities should be tapered off before getting ready for bed. Regular exercise promotes deep sleep but should not be done for a couple of hours before bedtime. Likewise, biofeedback and meditation have stress-reducing properties that foster sleep but should not be done before bedtime because they can boost energy and alertness. Chocolate, cola, coffee, tea, and other foods and beverages containing caffeine should be restricted, particularly in the evening. Overeating, particularly heavy foods, should also be avoided at night. The bed should be associated with sleep, and the room should be dark and quiet.

Relaxation

Abdominal breathing.   There are numerous techniques that can be used to foster relaxation. Abdominal breathing is a quick method. When stressed, people tend to breathe in short, shallow breaths. Consequently, the lungs do not fill up completely. The remaining air is stale, and oxidation of tissues is incomplete. Muscle tension results. Without being conspicuous, one can take a few abdominal breaths almost anywhere at any time. It is best to do abdominal breathing for 5 to 10 minutes once or twice a day while sitting upright. It may be done during normally low times or to reverse the stress response when it has been triggered. To do abdominal breathing, one should inhale slowly through the nose while keeping the back straight. First the abdomen expands, then the chest, and finally the shoulders. Then one should exhale slowly and hold the breath for a second or two before starting another inhalation.

Massage.   Massage can relieve tension, provide a passive form of exercise, and foster tactile communication. It stimulates relaxation and flexibility. Self-massage can be done from a chair. It can be done as a full-body massage or to a part of the body that is particularly tense. To do a full-body massage, one may start by placing both hands on the top of the head and moving them in slow circular motions down the back of the head, neck, and shoulder area. The neck and shoulder are common sites for tension. They may be most easily massaged by crossing hands over so that the right hand massages the left shoulder and the left hand massages the right shoulder. Then the hands are returned to the top of the head and moved forward in circular motions over the forehead, face, neck, and chest. To relax the right arm, one grasps the fingertips of the right hand with the left hand and moves up the hand and arm to the shoulder in circular motions with the fingers on top and the thumb on the underside. Then one massages down the right side of the chest. The procedure is repeated up the left arm and down the left side. Then hands are placed on the lower abdomen with fingertips touching. Circular motions are used up to the chest.

The low back is another area that is commonly tense, particularly from sedentary work. One places the hands on the lower back with fingertips touching at the coccyx. The fingertips then massage up as high as one can reach. A foot should be massaged with the massage continuing up the foot, over the ankle, and up the calf and thigh. Then the massage should be repeated on the other foot and leg. This full-body massage can be done after a warm bath at bedtime to foster sleep.

Progressive relaxation. Progressive relaxation may also be used to foster sleep. It is the conscious contraction and relaxation of muscles. By deliberately tensing muscles, one can learn to identify what muscles are tight and learn to relax them. It can be used before, during, or after an anxious situation. If done routinely once or twice a day, it can help keep one's level of anxiety down.

Progressive relaxation can be done in a standing, sitting, or lying position. There is greater likelihood of falling asleep in a lying position. In a sitting position, one should keep the head squarely on the shoulders, back against the chair, feet on the floor, legs uncrossed, and hands on the lap in a relaxed position. During progressive relaxation one tenses specific muscles to a maximal degree and notices how the tight muscles feel for about 5 seconds. Then the muscle is relaxed, and the pleasant feeling of relaxation is enjoyed for about 10 seconds. For a head-to-toe progression, one starts by wrinkling up the forehead and noticing where it feels particularly tense. Then one relaxes that part slowly, identifies the muscles that are relaxing, notices the difference between tension and relaxation, and enjoys the relaxed feeling. Box 2-3 contains abbreviated instructions for other body parts.

With experience in progressive relaxation, one can also learn to relax without tension. One first concentrates on relaxing each body part and then on generalized relaxation with deep breathing. One takes a deep breath, holds it, and then exhales slowly while relaxing the entire body from head to toe, saying "relax" so that the "x" is said as the focus reaches the toes.

Biofeedback. Biofeedback uses mechanical devices to gain self-regulation to control autonomic

Box 2-3   PROGRESSIVE MUSCLE RELAXATION

Close eyes tightly.
Wrinkle nose.
Place teeth together and press lips against teeth into a forced smile.
Press tongue hard against the roof of the mouth.
Clench teeth.
Pucker lips.
Pull chin toward chest.
Put head back as far as it will go.
Press head to right shoulder.
Press head to left shoulder.
Hold arm out straight, make a fist, and tighten the whole arm or pull elbow tightly into side.
Repeat with the other arm.
Push shoulder blades toward each other.
Pull chest in.
Pull stomach in.
Tighten muscles in lower abdomen, buttocks, and thighs and raise self in the chair.
Push foot against the floor, then point toes toward the head and repeat with the other leg and foot.

responses. The galvanic skin response uses electrodes attached to the fingertips to measure skin resistance, which is moisture of the skin that indicates nervousness. Arteries contract under stress and dilate with relaxation. A thermistor on the finger detects changes in peripheral skin temperature that are associated with activity of the smooth muscles in peripheral arteries. This skin temperature is particularly useful for control of migraine headaches. The electroencephalograph uses electrodes attached to the scalp to detect electrical activity on the brain's cortex. Different brain wave patterns are associated with different states of mind. The electromyograph uses electrodes attached to the forehead or forearm to measure muscle tension from electrical impulses generated by muscles. People with migraine and tension headaches, hypertension, and gastrointestinal problems have responded well to biofeedback. Because the instruments convert skin resistance, skin temperature, brain waves, and muscle tension into readily observable signs, people can tell if they are controlling their body responses or not. They can also learn to read and interpret body signals without the use of instruments to modify their responses.

Autogenic training: self-hypnosis. Autogenic training produces deep relaxation through self-hypnosis. These regular but brief sessions of passive concentration on physiologically adapted stimuli reduce other extraneous stimuli and have helped people with asthma, arthritis, constipation, hypertension, migraine headaches, and sleep disturbances.

To do self-hypnosis, one should lie down with eyes closed in a quiet room and take a few deep breaths. Each autogenic training session should last 2 to 20 minutes, preferably 20 minutes 2 or 3 times a day. There are six phrases. When learning autogenic training, only one phrase should be added at a time once a week.

The first phrase focuses on heaviness, the next on warmth, then on heartbeat, breath, the solar plexus, and the forehead. Supporting phrases such as "I am relaxing" or "I am at peace" are interspersed between induction phrases. For the heaviness induction, one systematically concentrates on

thinking that each part of the body feels heavy: "My face is heavy. I am relaxing. My neck is heavy. I am at peace. My shoulders are heavy. I am resting. My chest is heavy. I am quiet." For the warmth induction phrase, one substitutes "warm" for "heavy" in the previous phrases. The heart induction phrase is, "My heartbeat is calm and regular." Then one concentrates on, "My breathing is relaxed and comfortable." Next one puts one's hands on one's abdomen to create warmth and repeats, "My solar plexus is warm." Finally, one thinks, "My forehead is cool." To return to an alert state, one takes a few deep breaths and thinks, "I will arise refreshed and alert," then moves one's arms and legs, opens one's eyes, and slowly gets up.

Meditation. Meditation focuses attention on an experience, helps one become aware of one's response, and facilitates the integration of the physical, mental, emotional, and spiritual aspects of one's life. There are many methods for meditating. One may focus on an object such as a candle, chant, listen to music, or meditate on one's own breath. To meditate on one's breath, one can count while breathing: one on inhalation, two on exhalation, three on inhalation, and four on exhalation. That process can be repeated until the allotted time for meditation is over. Usually people experience an inner calm and sense of well-being from meditation.

Visualization and mental imagery. Visualization and mental imagery can be used to relax. One starts in a relaxed position and visualizes pleasant thoughts. One can meditate on a visualized colored object such as a blue sky, white cloud, green tree, red apple, or pink flower. One can imagine being in a favorite place such as on a sandy beach, in the mountains, or in front of a fireplace in a favorite room listening to music. One can concentrate on the sights, sounds, smells, tastes, and feelings of the pleasant thoughts.

Poetry. Poetry reading or writing is useful for reducing tension, particularly if one is depressed and movement and verbalizing have not worked sufficiently. Poems are chosen for their rhythm, their mood, and the feelings expressed. Poems can be read in a one-to-one or group meeting. Discussions about the meaning can help verbalize feelings.

Music. Soft classical music can help release feelings and emotions and bring about relaxation.

Baths. Water is a relaxant. One should fill the bathtub with water that is body temperature and immerse oneself up to one's neck for about 15 minutes.

Enhancing Self-Esteem

Positive affirmations can be used to enhance one's self-esteem. One can become more comfortable with positive thoughts about oneself and decrease the amount of self-devaluation. Several methods can be used. One might imagine positive scenes and see oneself as one wants to be. One can repeat positive affirmations such as "I am happy," "I am healthy," or "I am beautiful." One can also write positive affirmations on cards, put them in conspicuous places, and read them often. People may take turns making positive comments about each other.

Support Groups

Support systems are synergistic. One can accomplish more through support groups than alone. Support groups provide a feeling of being accepted, valued, loved, and esteemed and a sense of belonging. In addition to providing emotional support, support systems help provide a social identity and are a source of information, services, and material aid.

There are several types of support systems. Usually the family is the natural support system that constitutes the primary support group. Peer support groups are also important. They are composed of people who have had similar experiences, have adjusted, and want to share their insight. A head nurse may receive support from other head nurses or a jogger from other joggers. Religious organizations provide a congregation that sets guidelines for living, shares values, and provides traditions. Voluntary service groups and self-help groups provide support for specific purposes such as to

lose weight, to stop drinking alcohol, to quit smoking, or to adjust to a mastectomy or a stoma. Family, friends, and peers are usually sought out before professional support systems, but the helping professions are available when support from others is inadequate.

It is extremely important that managers take excellent care of their own well-being. They can function at their best if they are healthy. They need considerable energy to be supportive of others and will not have strength to share if they are hurting. Likewise, staff nurses need a sense of health and well-being to provide the best nursing care. Managers are responsible for providing care to the caregivers.

The manager should help protect personnel from undue stress. Personnel may be taught identification of stress symptoms and stress management. Annual physical examinations could be required. Vacations are provided and encouraged. Counseling and referral services can be provided as support systems. Nutrition, educational, and health promotional programs are presented, and nutritious food is served in the cafeteria. Exercise programs can be provided and encouraged. Managers should monitor stress levels and intervene when necessary.

TIME MANAGEMENT

If productivity were a function of time only, one would expect all to produce equally. And yet, although everyone has the same number of hours in a day and the same number of days per week, some people accomplish more than others. Granted, some people work longer and harder than others to accomplish more, but some just make better use of their time. Because nurses work long hours, they should work smarter—not harder—to get more done in less time.

PERSONAL TIME MANAGEMENT

Stephen Covey (1989) speaks to *The 7 Habits of Highly Effective People: Powerful Lessons in Personal Change.* He says one needs to start by being proactive and accepting responsibility for one's actions and attitudes. The more one exercises freedom to choose responses, the more proactive one becomes.

Then opportunities are fed and problems are starved.

Second, one should begin with the end in mind. One should begin with a clear understanding of the desired direction and destination. Things are created mentally before they are created physically. Quality is designed and built in. Ineffective people use old habits and environmental conditions. They may climb the ladder to success only to find once they get to the top that the ladder is against the wrong wall.

Third, put first things first. Personal management is organizing and managing according to personal priorities to get where you want to go. It is important to give less time to things that are urgent but not important like pressing matters and nonproductive meetings and to spend more time on things that are important but not urgent like relationships, prevention, planning, preparation, taking opportunities, and recreation.

Fourth, think win-win. Effectiveness is often accomplished by cooperative efforts of two or more people. A win-win attitude explores options until a mutually satisfactory solution is reached. Desired results, guidelines, accountability, resources, and consequences are made explicit. It is an abundance mentality that builds on synergy rather than a scarcity mentality that leads to win-lose strategies.

Fifth, seek first to understand, then to be understood. Communications are important to building win-win relationships. Our perceptions come from our experiences. Credibility problems usually involve differences. Empathetic listening is therapeutic. Once people feel they are understood, they lower their defenses. Once one understands the other person's point of view, it is easier to problem solve a win-win solution.

Sixth, synergize. Synergy comes from teamwork or creative cooperation. Diversity can produce a synergy, where the whole is greater than the sum of its parts. Synergy results from bringing different perspectives together in a spirit of mutual respect to seek the best solution.

Seventh, sharpen the saw. The longer one saws, the duller the saw gets and the harder one works to get less and less accomplished. People need physical, spiritual, mental, and social and emotional self-renewal. One needs to give a priority to a balanced program for self-renewal.

Habits involve knowledge, attitudes, and skills. Effective habits can be learned, and ineffective habits can be unlearned. As one practices the seven habits of highly effective people, one is changed from the inside out.

In *First Things First* Covey (1994) teaches the six steps to empowerment by putting first things first. Start by connecting to the mission. Write a personal mission statement. Identify up to seven roles. Second, review your roles. Third, identify your goals related to each role. Concentrate on relationships, prevention, preparation, planning, seizing opportunities, and recreation. Fourth, organize your week by prioritizing activities to reach your goals for each role. Schedule your priorities on your calendar. Fifth, exercise integrity toward the first things in your life. Start each day by previewing the day, prioritizing, and being sensitive to important commitments. Watch for opportunities to live your mission. Sixth, evaluate, learn, and live.

In *Fast Cycle Time* Christopher Meyer (1993) discusses how to align purpose, strategy, and structure for speed instead of working faster. He indicates that analyzing strategy and core processes enables management to detect and correct problems earlier and leverage knowledge toward improved innovations and increased value.

MAXIMIZE MANAGERIAL TIME
Inventory Activities

Nurse managers may start a plan for maximizing use of their time by conducting an inventory of their activities. After recording what they did every 15 minutes for a typical week, they assess how they spent their time. How much time was spent in which activities? Was the way the time was spent determined by conscious decisions, habit, work demands, default, or spontaneity? What do they like to do? What activities do they want to increase? What do they want to decrease? How can they reduce the time wasters (Box 2-4)?

Box 2-4	TIME WASTERS

Poor planning	Unorganized office visits
Failure to establish goals	Poorly planned meetings
Failure to set objectives	Lack of delegation
Failure to plan strategies to accomplish goals	Lack of information
Unwillingness to say no	Poor communication
Ineffective use of transition times	Lack of feedback
Cumbersome paperwork	Procrastination
Poor filing system	Indecisiveness
Poor reading skills	Haste
Poor listening and memory techniques	Management by crisis
Telephone interruptions	

Set Goals

Next, nurses determine their short-, medium-, and long-range goals. What do they want to accomplish? What do they want to do soon? Which goals must be completed before others? Which will take the longest to achieve? Setting priorities helps resolve goal conflicts and directs how they will spend their time.

Plan Strategies

Once they have determined and ranked their goals, they plan strategies for how to accomplish them. What activities must they do? What are low-priority activities that can be eliminated? Next the nurse manager schedules activities. A tickler box with divider cards for months and weeks can be used by filing task cards behind the appropriate month and week card. As they look at their major responsibilities for a whole year, they may have some flexibility in determining when certain jobs are done and can use those to help balance the workload around tasks that have to be done at certain times, such as preparing the budget. Various calendar systems can also be used: one may do major project planning on a year-at-a-glance calendar; desk ink blotters that depict a month at a time can help regulate that month's work; a week-at-a-glance or a day-at-a-glance calendar is convenient for carrying in one's

purse. Daily work sheets depicting what work should be done during which hour may also be useful. Computer scheduling is increasingly popular.

Plan Schedule

Nurse managers need to assess their peak and low times to plan a detailed schedule more effectively. Are they most alert and creative in the early morning or late at night? Are they slow starters in the morning? Do they reach a low energy point in the middle of the afternoon? The nurse's prime internal time—the most creative time for working alone—is a good time to schedule work that should not be interrupted. When is their prime external time, their best time to work with others? If they reach a low point in the afternoon, that may be a good time to schedule office visits. They may offer their guests a cup of coffee or tea, which tends to facilitate communication, sip on their own drinks, and listen.

Time should be set aside for certain activities each day. Scheduled activities are recorded. Scheduled and unscheduled times are noted, and contact and thinking times are identified. The secretary may be given available hours for scheduling office visits.

A few minutes at the beginning of each day should be allowed for planning. A running list of what the nurse manager needs to do in order of importance can be made each morning to plan what will be done that day. Desk-organizing files—which are merely folders with such labels as urgent, return calls, dictate, read, file, and low priority—can help determine what to do each day. Scheduled free time can be used to deal with these activities. A few minutes at the end of the day are used to evaluate what happened.

Say No

Learning how to say no graciously especially regarding low-priority work saves time. It is advisable for nurse managers to acknowledge the request, state and explain their position, check back for understanding with the other person, and avoid defensiveness. For example, when asked to speak at a meeting, they might respond, "I would love to discuss our institutional goals with your committee. However, I have another commitment at that time. Barbara Jones and Sue Smith are both very familiar with the institutional goals. Perhaps you could ask one of them to speak. Does that sound agreeable to you?"

Use Transition Times

Managers can accomplish much during transition times. Incoming mail may be read while one is on hold when returning phone calls. Reports can be read while commuting to and from work, or audiotapes can be listened to while driving. Isometric exercises can be done at almost any time. Lunch and coffee breaks may be used for personal business. Because many people are watching their weight, lunch breaks may be better used for exercise such as walking and jogging or for meditation than for eating a large lunch.

Accelerate Learning

Leaders and managers need to be familiar with relevant information. An accelerated learning program includes *clear, realistic learning goals* that can be achieved in days. It is often better to quickly learn and act on the available information in a few days or weeks rather than to wait to retrieve all of the information and wait for months or years to act. *Collect the information in one place.* Discard irrelevant and redundant materials and rapidly skim the rest. Organize the materials into a logical sequence and use speed-reading techniques to reread it. *Group the material into small study units.* Abstract the study unit information into a short paragraph. *Format the material* into a style you will study repeatedly. *Review the material* preferably at least twice a day to quickly comprehend and memorize it. Accelerated learning can help leaders learn a large volume of information without anxiety and overload (Bennis, Mason, and Mitroff, 1993).

Improve Reading

Learning speed-reading techniques such as tapping, L pattern, S swirl, area reading, and reading for meaning can help overcome common reading problems of single-word fixation, involuntary regression by rereading, subvocalization of words as one reads, and inability to concentrate.

Improve Memory

Listening and memory techniques also save time. When listening for understanding, one should assume value in what the speaker is saying by being attentive, delaying judgment, maintaining eye contact, and using attentive body language. One then needs to assess the content of the information by focusing on central ideas, looking for relationships between ideas, and selecting an organizing structure such as main and supporting ideas, advantages and disadvantages, or putting information into chronological order. One should analyze the information by listening to what is being said, identifying how it is being said by inferring emotions from body language and tone of voice, and considering the speaker's motivation for saying it. Distractions may have to be reduced so the listener can concentrate.

Verbal, physical, and mental techniques can be used to stimulate memory (Box 2-5). Repeating, clarifying, and summarizing are effective verbal techniques. Physical techniques for stimulating memory are note taking, filing, and follow-up

Box 2-5   MEMORY TECHNIQUES

Verbal Techniques	Physical Techniques	Mental Techniques
Repeating	Note taking	Focusing
Clarifying	Filing	Imaging
Summarizing	Follow-up memos	Linking
		Locating
		Chunking

memos. Focusing, imaging, linking, locating, and chunking are mental techniques.

Focusing by putting attention on one thing at a time helps block out distractions.

Imaging creates a vivid mental image that helps one remember something. When introduced to Leona Dean, the nurse might picture her leaning on a dean of a specific school to help remember her name.

Linking makes associations between things that make them easier to remember later. Associations may be cause and effect, parts of a whole, or things that are near each other, logically go together, contrast with each other, or happen concurrently. Creating an association that leads from point one to point two to point three and creating an image of those associations will help one remember a speech.

Locating is a memory technique that uses a known structure, often one's home, to arrange and remember information by putting it in specific locations. One might progress through an orientation program by visualizing the hallway in the office and thinking of who is in each office as one walks through the hall and what service that person provides new staff.

Chunking helps one remember by dividing large amounts of information into smaller, more manageable pieces. One could chunk information needed into separate sections of a report, or the nurse could locate what items are needed in specific, separate offices.

Critical Thinking

Critical thinking is needed to excel in the information age. It is a reflective problem solving style of thinking. One should *focus on the right questions*, define terms, and list critical issues. *Analyze arguments* by identifying and examining assumptions, positions, reasons, and conclusions. *Question, challenge,* and *clarify* by asking who, what, when, where, and why questions. Distinguish between facts and inferences. Request more information as needed. *Judge the credibility of the sources.* Consider the reputation, expertise, and possible conflicts of interest of the source. *Use logic,* including inductive and deductive reasoning. Evaluate the related research. *Use high-level thinking strategies* like analyzing, clarifying, comparing, inferring, and problem solving.

Avoid faulty thinking such as overgeneralization, use of selected cases instead of a wide-based foundation of facts, and use of inadequate sources. Emotion-laden words that elicit strong emotions can camouflage weaknesses. Highly ambiguous language and poorly defined terms can lead to multiple interpretations. Unrelated and irrelevant points can cause distractions from the key points of an argument. Repetition in a variety of places by a number of people becomes more believable regardless of its truthfulness. Acceptable statements make unacceptable conclusions more believable. Expert opinion is not necessarily the truth. Denigration of opponents is sometimes used to discredit another's arguments, so conclusions should be separated from the person presenting the issues.

Streamline Paperwork

Much time can be saved by streamlining paperwork. Scheduling a block of time to answer mail prevents interruptions. If the situation warrants, a standard reply can be used. Some responses can be made on the query memo if no file copy is needed, and typing carbon responses to letters onto the back of the query letter saves filing time and space. Keeping as little as possible and only what is needed saves time. Color coding is useful, and recording of destruction dates on files reduces the need to review the materials later. Dictation usually takes less time than writing by hand, and calls can be used when a record is not necessary. Computerization and e-mail also save time. Invisible information (spoken word) can be recorded on a steno pad kept by the phone with each page dated sequentially. Unfortunately that information is difficult to move to priority areas. A spiral-bound message pad with no carbon required can be used to tear off the top sheet and send wherever needed while still keeping a chronological record. The disadvantage is that there is little space for writing on the form. Recycled paper by each phone can be used when a permanent record is not needed. Some calendar systems have forms for recording conversations and can be treated like phone message sheets. Selective reading by scanning tables of contents and reading summaries at the end of long responses and reports saves time. Managers should not concentrate on details unless necessary, because they are quickly forgotten. Scanning for major points is often adequate.

Use Computers for Time Management

Computers can replace a hodgepodge of record-keeping procedures with a uniform system. With the use of a computer, printer, and accounting and payable software, information can be entered one time into a database and sent electronically anywhere that the technology is available. A graphical interface program can merge a computerized mailing list of names and addresses into letters, address envelopes and mailing labels, do mathematical calculations on the screen while the letter is being composed, spell check the entire document, identify more interesting words using the on-screen thesaurus, print out multiple copies, make global changes in all documents if the letter is revised, and preview the letter on the screen before printing it. It can also check a calendar for a date or schedule an appointment; set an alarm for the appointment; dial a phone number; send and receive faxes; calculate figures; address envelopes; create a macro of often-used addresses or phrases; create, save, and delete files; and locate a file and insert it into another

document. Computer software can be used to organize projects and keep and track the progress relative to performance objectives. Files should be saved frequently and backed up on hard disk and floppy disk or tape. Computer files can duplicate the paper files. Clutter should be removed from both computer and paper files. Portable printers and fax machines or a phone jack and a fax-modem board inside a portable computer allow receiving and sending data anywhere the technology is available (Allen, 1995; Lively, 1996).

Use Telephone Calls

Telephone calls instead of office visits or correspondence save time. Secretaries can screen calls so that other activities are not interrupted and, in fact, may be able to handle much of the business. A call-back system can be used to complete the business the secretary cannot handle. If late morning and late afternoon are chosen for returning calls, calls are likely to be kept short, because people are eager to eat lunch or to go home.

Paging and beeping systems, call forwarding, call back, call waiting, speed dialing, three-way calling, voice mail, and conference calls make telephoning more efficient. A long cord or portable phone allows one to move around and work while using the telephone. Car phones can be used during transition times.

Forms for telephone messages are less likely to get lost than scraps of paper. It is helpful for phone messages to be collected in one place. A secured pen or pencil by the phone is convenient. One should keep a list of commonly called phone numbers handy. If major topics for conversation are outlined before making a call, it is less likely that one will forget something and need to call back. One can set the tone of the call. A businesslike call started by "What can I do for you?" will accomplish more in less time than a friendly call started with "How are you?" Conference calls also save time by focusing more on business than socializing. The purpose for the conversation helps determine whether a meeting or a conference call is necessary.

Schedule Office Visits

Secretaries may also screen office visits. Again, they may be able to handle much of the business themselves. When managers schedule reception hours, secretaries can schedule appointments for the appropriate length of time and inform managers of the purpose of the meeting so that they can be adequately prepared. One may need to close the office door to complete a task without interruptions. Sitting with one's back to the door may decrease interruptions because people will notice that the manager is busy.

Control Visit Time

The length of a meeting can be better controlled if it is not in the manager's office. Managers may go to the staff associates' work area or meet visitors in a reception area, where they are free to leave whenever they desire. By standing up when someone drops into the office, managers prevent the visitor from sitting down, thus controlling the situation. They can assess the priority, make an appointment for another time, keep the visit short, or invite the visitor to sit down for a longer discussion. Many drop-in visits can be prevented by scheduling lunch with staff associates on a regular basis. This allows the manager opportunity to keep informed, discuss matters of common interest, and eat lunch at the same time. Staff can be informed through memos and routing slips.

Use Meetings Effectively

Managers spend considerable time in meetings, much of which is wasted. Meetings are used for participative problem solving, decision making, coordination, information sharing, and morale building. Managers first consider the purpose of the meeting; if it is not necessary, they do not conduct it. Key participants are identified, and if they cannot attend, the meeting is not held. People who do not need to attend are not invited. Managers should consider alternatives to a meeting, such as a memo, telephone call, or conference. Staff associates can represent the manager at some meetings both to save managerial time and to develop the staff associates. Managers may limit their time in meetings by attending only that segment when they are to make a contribution. Scheduling meetings before lunch and quitting time facilitates ending meetings on time. A centrally located meeting place saves travel time. The purpose of the meeting should be clearly defined, and an agenda should be circulated before the meeting.

Meetings should start on time, because time is expensive. Starting a meeting 15 minutes late for 20 people who earn $10 an hour costs $50 in downtime. Stating the purpose of the meeting and following the agenda are the manager's responsibilities. The manager should start with high-priority items so that only low-priority items will be left over. The manager should control interruptions, restate conclusions, make assignments and deadlines clear, and end the meeting on time. If the business is completed early, the manager dismisses the meeting. Minutes are circulated preferably within a day after the meeting; this allows people to be informed without having to attend the meeting unless their input is specifically needed. Minutes also remind participants of their assigned tasks.

Delegation

The manager decides what task should be done, when, where, and by whom. Responsibility and authority should be assigned. The manager needs to evaluate the risk involved in delegating by assessing the criticality of the expected results and the confidence in resources. The planning strategy ascertains specifications, including the expected results, rationale, requirements, and constraints. The delegated authority should be specified, and support needed should be anticipated. When communicating the delegated assignment, the manager should ensure understanding, give and receive feedback, and address concerns. To monitor the delegated assignment, the manager should set up a milestone-tracking system, review scheduled status reports, and give feedback on the interim reports.

Support is provided by responding to the delegatee's needs, acknowledging the status reports, and being available for guidance and problem solving. The manager should intervene only when the action seems warranted and, even then, by avoiding interference and explaining one's actions. Reverse delegation can be avoided by clarifying specifications, transferring authority, and expressing confidence in the delegatee. The results should be evaluated by examining the specifications, evaluating the monitoring results, and giving feedback on the final results. Establishing routines improves learning curves, success, and productivity. Routines can reduce tension, errors, and wasted time. The manager decides what to delegate, selects the appropriate person, communicates the responsibilities to that person, grants authority with the responsibility, provides support, monitors the situation, and evaluates the results.

Reasons for delegating. Delegation saves time and can help develop others. Delegation maximizes the use of the talents of staff associates. It uses latent abilities in personnel that contribute to their growth and development. Staff members learn by doing. Their involvement tends to increase their motivation and commitment to accomplish goals while freeing the manager to manage. This also reduces managerial costs.

The four rights of delegation. The four rights of delegation are (1) task, (2) person, (3) communication, and (4) feedback. The right task should be within the scope of the person's practice and consistent with the job description. The right person should have the appropriate license or certificate, an appropriate job description, and demonstrated skill and is checked off on the skill checklist to delegate in the first place and to accept the delegated responsibility in the second place. The right communication should be clear, concise, complete, and correct. The right feedback should ask for input, get the person's recommended solution to the problem, and recognize the person's efforts (Hansten, 1998).

Delegation decision-making process. A National Council of State Boards of Nursing position paper (http://www.ncsbn.org/files/delegati.html) describes the assessment, planning, implementation, and evaluation of delegation. First, the nurse practice act should permit the delegation, authorize task(s) to be delegated, and authorize the nurse to decide delegation. The delegator needs the appropriate education, skills, and experience; the appropriate scope of authority; and demonstrated and documented evidence of current competency. The delegatee needs appropriate education, skills, and experience and demonstrated and documented evidence of current competency. The delegator needs to assess the needs of the patient, the circumstances, and availability of adequate resources. Then the delegator needs to plan for the task(s) to be delegated by specifying the knowledge and skills required to do the nature of each task, by requiring documented or demonstrated current competency to do each delegated task, and by determining the implications for the patient and others. To ensure appropriate accountability, the delegator accepts accountability for the performance of delegated task(s) and verifies that the delegatee accepts the delegation and accountability for the delegated task(s). Then the delegator supervises performance of the task by providing directions and clear expectations about how the task(s) is to be performed; monitoring the performance to ensure compliance to established standards of practice, policies, and procedures; intervening as necessary; and ensuring documentation of the task(s). Finally, the delegator evaluates the delegation process, evaluates the patient and the performance of the task(s), and receives and gives feedback. The delegator adjusts the plan as necessary.

Conditions that facilitate delegation. Several conditions facilitate delegation. First, managers need to understand the concept of delegation and have a generally positive attitude toward people. They need to overcome feelings of loss of prestige through delegation and develop a positive atmosphere for their staff. They should help achieve results through effective communication instead of by doing the job themselves. Thus they concentrate on the accomplishment of overall goals and objectives rather than the day-to-day details.

Top management clarifies policies, goals, and objectives, and these are further developed by each succeeding lower level. For example, top management sets the overall budget, but each department then works with its own budget. Specifying goals and objectives directs personnel and determines priorities and the use of resources. Management by objectives promotes this.

Job descriptions provide a definition of the responsibility and authority involved with each position. Everything that must be done for the organization to meet its goals is part of someone's job. Consequently, job descriptions are based on the functional needs of the agency and clarify the responsibility of the individual's position and the objectives of the work.

Before writing job descriptions, management decides which assignments to delegate. To do so, managers should be aware of the capabilities and characteristics of their staff associates. Testing of employees to learn what they can and cannot do and providing the necessary training help overcome many personnel failures. Staff members are often asked to perform skills for which they are not qualified or in which they are not interested. People tend to put off tasks they find unpleasant and then do them poorly. It is not necessary to delegate equally. By knowing individual capabilities, the manager can delegate according to the associate's interests and abilities.

Job descriptions are not always advantageous in small or rapidly changing organizations because those staffs often assume different roles at different times. Generalization is more common than the specialization required in larger, more stable organizations. Some employees outperform the requirements of their job descriptions, whereas others are not able to do some of the duties described. Job descriptions can be redefined according to the person's capability and organizational needs. If employees are unable to handle the required duties, they may be transferred to another area, given further training, supplied with an assistant to supplement their weak areas, or fired.

Controls based on goals, rather than means, are important. The manager checks on how well the delegated responsibilities are being performed, and the staff know whether or not they are meeting their responsibilities. Performance standards clarify how the manager measures achievement. These standards cover the quantity and quality of work expected and the time allowed for its accomplishment. The standards should be broad enough to allow individuality. If the standards are perceived as reasonable and fair by both manager and staff associate, they will both be happier with their jobs. Staff associates like their work to be noticed and appreciated. The manager meets their need for recognition and appreciation by having a general knowledge of what is happening, using an open door policy, expressing willingness to give assistance and support, and taking a personal interest in their problems. A "snoopervisor," however, is not appreciated.

It is the manager's responsibility to assess the results of delegation. One of the most satisfactory ways of being aware of what is happening is by being among the staff associates. Formal and informal meetings, systems of reporting, quality control, and statistical sampling are other means. Although inspection is perceived as unpleasant, most staff associates accept it as necessary. However, they do object to unnecessary inspections that disturb routines.

Even though people may receive satisfaction by knowing that they are doing a good job, having those efforts recognized by others is appreciated. Managers err if they do not give praise for work well done. People should also be rewarded for their continued contributions to the agency through raises and promotions. If staff associates err, they should be corrected—the sooner the better. But when staff associates participate in goal setting, when the emphasis is on the goal rather than individual personalities, and when training is a continuous process, corrections that otherwise would have been made by the manager may be unnecessary. The system encourages self-correction.

Learning to live with differences may be difficult for managers, especially if they once performed their staff associates' tasks and now find that they are being done differently. It is even more threatening when the staff associate does a better job than the manager once did. It has to be recognized that there will be differences in quantity and quality of work accomplished and methods used between the manager and staff associate or between staff associates.

Responsibility, authority, and accountability. Assignment of responsibility, delegation of authority, and creation of accountability are the three concepts most often mentioned in relation to the delegation process (Box 2-6). Responsibility denotes obligation. It refers to what must be done to complete a task and the obligation created by the assignment. The manager and the staff associate must understand the activities for which the staff associate is responsible, what results are expected, and how performance is to be evaluated. Managers need a clear idea of what they want done before they can communicate that to others. To clarify them for themselves, the managers may put their ideas in writing. By so doing, they are then less likely to give incomplete directions. The assignment of responsibility is not complete, however, until the staff associate decides to accept the obligation.

Authority is the power to make final decisions and give commands. People to whom responsibility has been assigned need the authority to direct the performance of delegated duties. They need authority of sufficient scope to include all related activities without frequent consultation with their manager. The granting of too little authority is a common problem, because organizational policies and procedures are often limiting, and sometimes the person may have little control over the actions of others.

People with delegated authority perform for the manager. Although authority is delegated so that the staff associates can fulfill their responsibilities, the manager maintains control over the delegated authority and may recall it. Delegation of authority involves the staff associate's knowledge, abilities, skills, and potential contribution and the manager's guidance. During the initial phase of delegating authority, staff associates present their ideas and plans. The manager raises questions, explores alternatives, and helps identify potential problems and ways to prevent them. Then mutual agreement is reached. The manager offers continuing support by providing staff, resources, and information needed by the staff associate for the completion of the delegated responsibility. Good communications, sharing of information, and feedback are important.

Accountability refers to liability. Staff associates incur an obligation to complete work satisfactorily and to use authority appropriately when they accept delegated responsibility. They are accountable to their manager. Managers are accountable for the performance of the task, the selection of the person to complete it, and both the staff associate's and their own performance. Head nurses are responsible for delegation to team leaders, who are accountable for delegation to team members. Each remains accountable for the work delegated.

Reasons for underdelegating. There are numerous reasons for underdelegating. Managers may think they can do the job more quickly themselves, resent interruptions to answer questions, or not want to take the time to check what has been done. They may get cooperation from other departments more easily than from staff associates or be unwilling to take risks for fear of being blamed for others' mistakes.

Some managers do not have confidence in their staff associates and are afraid that their staff associates will not keep them adequately informed. Or

---

Box 2-6   ASPECTS OF DELEGATION

Responsibility
Authority
Accountability

they may not trust their staff associates and complain that they lack training and sufficient experience. They may argue that their staff associates have little understanding of the organizational objectives and are specialists without the general knowledge needed for problem solving. In some cases, they may even be afraid that their staff associates will outperform them.

Therefore managers may like to do the work themselves and think that they can do it better. They receive personal recognition for and satisfaction from the work and prefer to do the real things instead of just plan with others. Such people often expect perfection, consider themselves indispensable, and desire to dominate. They are afraid of losing power and prestige and are aware that their poor operating procedures and practices may be exposed.

Reasons for not accepting delegation. Staff associates have their reasons for not accepting delegation. Some are dependent on their manager and find it easier to ask the boss. Others lack self-confidence and fear failure and criticism. This fear is often related to how mistakes have been handled. Emphasis on the mistake itself is more threatening than using the situation as a learning experience.

Lack of guidelines, standards, and control are additional problems. Duties are not always clearly defined, authority not specified, or necessary information and resources not readily available. Some staff associates are already overworked. The incentives are inadequate, and they do not want to perform work if their manager receives the credit.

PROCRASTINATION
Reasons for Procrastination

Reasons for procrastination may be divided into two basic categories: emotional reasons and nonemotional reasons. Box 2-7 lists some of the most common reasons in each category.

Emotional reasons. There are several emotional causes of procrastination. People may fill present moments with trivia to escape an overwhelming task or choose a pleasant task to escape an unpleasant one. Procrastination can be used as an excuse for poor work with comments such as "I just couldn't get to it until the last minute." Some play victims of circumstances to gain sympathy. Although it is preferable to delegate than to play "poor me," there are those who try to get someone else to do the job through procrastination.

Nonemotional reasons. Lack of goals, goals without deadlines, and unrealistic time estimates are some reasons for procrastination. Some people have insufficient information to do a job, do inadequate

---

Box 2-7   REASONS FOR PROCRASTINATION

Emotional Reasons	Nonemotional Reasons
To escape an overwhelming task	Lack of goals
To escape an unpleasant task	Goals without deadlines
To excuse poor work	Unrealistic time estimates
To gain sympathy	Insufficient information
To get someone else to do the job	Inadequate follow-up
	Interruptions
	Overcommitment

follow-up, or have so many interruptions they cannot get a job done. Others are just so overcommitted that they do not have time to do everything they have agreed to do.

Techniques to Stop Procrastination

Dividing and conquering, or breaking a large job down into smaller, more manageable tasks, is a good way to overcome procrastination. Doing a start-up task to get in the mood and taking advantage of moods help. Starting with what one does not like to do and the highest priorities and giving oneself incentives are helpful. Considering the consequences of not doing the job can motivate some people into action.

Consider using the money you earn by doing things you like to do to hire someone to do what you do not like to do. Consider switching jobs with someone or divide up the job so you do what you like to do, such as the review of the literature, while someone else does what she likes to do, such as the statistical analysis of the data. Make a commitment to someone to help overcome procrastination.

It is appropriate to ask yourself, "What's the best use of my time now?" Then set goals, plan realistic time schedules, and gather the necessary information to do the job. Avoid overcommitment and give yourself rewards for jobs well done. Box 2-8 summarizes techniques to help stop procrastination.

MAXIMIZE ORGANIZATION TIME
Plan

Much time can be saved through appropriate organizational planning. The purpose for the existence of the agency should be determined, and the goals and objectives should be defined and ranked in order of importance. Nurse managers determine who is responsible for coordinating activities, who makes what decisions, and who needs to be informed about certain decisions. They also determine what decisions need to be made before others, what action needs to be taken first, and what deadlines must be set. The determining and ranking of goals focus activities and prevent people from spending time doing inappropriate or unimportant tasks. People who are adequately informed of what is expected of them do not waste time wondering what they are supposed to do. Making time estimates and setting time limits help regulate work flow. Through appropriate planning, problems can be prevented. The decreased amount of time spent in crisis management increases the time available for creative work.

Organize

The manager structures the agency to accomplish the tasks necessary to meet the agency's goals. Organizational charts help clarify who is responsible to whom and for what. Job descriptions further clarify these matters. Multiple bosses, confusion over who is responsible and who has authority for

---

Box 2-8   TECHNIQUES TO STOP PROCRASTINATION

Break a large job into smaller tasks.	Ask yourself, "What's the best use of my time now?"
Do a start-up task.	Set goals.
Take advantage of your moods.	Set realistic time schedules.
Consider the consequences of not doing the task.	Gather necessary information.
Consider hiring someone to do the task.	Avoid overcommitment.
Consider switching jobs with someone.	Give yourself rewards.
Make a commitment to someone or a wager with someone.	

what, and duplication of tasks can be prevented with planning. Autonomy and independence reduce the amount of time otherwise spent in conflict management. Policies and procedures help clarify expectations.

Staff

Selection of well-qualified staff is critical for time saving because they require less supervisory time for development and corrective action. Staff development further reduces time lost by better preparing staff to do their jobs. Appropriate use of personnel through assessment of work to be done, careful planning of the number and mix of personnel, and matching staff members' interests and abilities to the job further reduce waste. When nurses' interests are matched to the organizational goals and they feel appreciated, they are likely to have increased job satisfaction. Consequently there is little absenteeism and less turnover. Nurse managers should watch for chronic absenteeism, try to determine the reason, and correct it. They also expect punctuality, because tardiness is a loss of time. If nurse managers find that employees' personal problems are affecting their work, they should refer personnel for appropriate assistance so that they will have more energy to do their jobs.

Direct

It is nurse managers' responsibility to delegate what a less qualified, lower-paid person can handle. They identify the task to be delegated, determine the best person to do the job, and communicate the assignment clearly. They allow the staff associate to help determine how the task will be accomplished and keep authority commensurate with responsibility. They set controls, monitor results, and provide support as needed. It is essential that managers teach others how to do the work instead of doing it themselves. They can save considerable time by streamlining communication systems and by not holding any more meetings than necessary. Nurse managers should also facilitate open communications and as-

sertive behavior and handle conflict immediately before it drains time and energy.

Control

Nurse managers set standards, monitor results, and give feedback. They adjust closeness of supervision to the needs of the employee, take disciplinary action as soon as it is justified, and fire personnel who are not meeting minimum standards. Good management conserves time and energy. Lack of it leads to management by crisis.

CHAPTER SUMMARY

Chapter 2 covered the following:
Stress Management
    Sources of Stress
    Stress Response
    Symptoms of Stress
    Stress Control
        Values clarification
        Goal setting
        Stress avoidance and regulation
        Time blocking
        Time management
        Assertiveness
        Feeling pauses
        Inner shouting
        Anchoring
        Sorting
        Thought stopping
        Compartmentalization
        Environmental changes
        Humor
        Centering
        Nutrition
        Exercise
        Sleep
    Relaxation
        Abdominal breathing
        Massage
        Progressive relaxation
        Biofeedback
        Autogenic training: self-hypnosis
        Meditation

Visualization and mental imagery
Poetry
Music
Baths
Enhancing Self-Esteem
Support Groups
Time Management
Personal Time Management
Maximize Managerial Time
Inventory Activities
Set Goals
Plan Strategies
Plan Schedule
Say No
Use Transition Times
Accelerate Learning
Improve Reading
Improve Memory
Critical Thinking
Streamline Paperwork
Use Computers for Time Management
Use Telephone Calls
Schedule Office Visits
Control Visit Time
Use Meetings Effectively
Delegation
Reasons for delegating
The four rights of delegation
Delegation decision-making process
Conditions that facilitate delegation
Responsibility, authority, and accountability
Reasons for underdelegating
Reasons for not accepting delegation
Procrastination
Reasons for Procrastination
Emotional reasons
Nonemotional reasons
Techniques to Stop Procrastination
Maximize Organization Time
Plan
Organize
Staff
Direct
Control

REFERENCES

Allen KR: *Time and information management that really works,* Los Angeles, 1995, Affinity.
Bennis W, Mason RO, Mitroff II: *High-speed management,* San Francisco, 1993, Jossey-Bass.
Covey SR: *The 7 habits of highly effective people: powerful lessons in personal change,* New York, 1989, Simon & Schuster.
Covey SR: *First things first,* New York, 1994, Simon & Schuster.
Hansten RI: *Clinical delegation skills: a handbook for professional practice,* ed 2, Gaithersburg, Md, 1998, Aspen.
Lively L: *Managing information overload,* New York, 1996, AMACOM.
Meyer C: *Fast cycle time,* New York, 1993, Free Press.

BIBLIOGRAPHY

Adams JL: *Conceptual blockbusting: a guide to better ideas,* ed 3, Redwood City, Calif, 1990, Addison-Wesley.
Badger JM: 14 tips for managing stress on the job, *Am J Nurs* 95:31-33, Sept 1995.
Barter M, Furmidge ML: Unlicensed assistive personnel: issues relating to delegation and supervision, *JONA* 24:36-40, April 1994.
Barter M, McLaughlin FE, Thomas SA: Registered nurse role changes and satisfaction with unlicensed assistive personnel, *JONA* 27:29-38, Jan 1997.
Benson H: *The relaxation response,* New York, 1992, Random House.
Brooks E, Wilkinson JM, Popkess-Vawter S: Promoting situational support for nurses in practice, *Image J Nurs Sch* 26:305-307, Winter 1994.
Burka JB, Yuen LM: *Procrastination: why you do it, what to do about it,* Reading, Mass, 1990, Addison-Wesley.
Cautela JR, Goden J: *Relaxation,* Champaign, Ill, 1978, Research Press.
Chillot R: 25 tips to recharge your memory, *Prevention* 51:114-119, Feb 1999.
Christensen W, Stearns EI: *Microcomputers in management,* ed 2, Rockville, Md, 1990, Aspen.
Collins MA: The relation of work stress, hardiness, and burnout among full-time hospital staff nurses, *J Nurs Staff Development* 12:81-85, March-April 1996.
DesCamp KD, Thomas CC: Buffering nursing stress through play at work, *West J Nurs Res* 15:619-627, Oct 1993.

Dick M, Anderson SE: Job burnout in RN-to-BSN students: relationships to life stress, time commitments, and support for returning to school, *J Cont Educ Nurs* 24:105-109, May-June 1993.

Duquette A et al.: Factors related to nursing burnout: a review of empirical knowledge, *Issues Ment Health Nurs* 15:337-358, July 1994.

Erbin-Roesemann MA, Simms LM: Work locus of control: the intrinsic factor behind empowerment and work excitement, *Nurs Econ* 15:183-190, July-Aug 1997.

Eskreis TR: Seven common legal pitfalls in nursing, *Am J Nurs* 98:34-40, April 1998.

Gandee RN, Knierim H, McLittle-Marino D: Stress and older adults: a mind-body relationship, *J Phys Educ, Recreation & Dance* 69:19-22, Nov-Dec 1998.

Girdano D, Everly G: *Controlling stress and tension,* ed 5, Needham Heights, Mass, 1997, Allyn & Bacon.

Hacker BA: Psychologically speaking: procrastination and its effect on job and career change, *Revolution: J Nurse Empowerment* 3:88-89, 92, Spring 1993.

Hasten R, Washburn M: Delegation: how to deliver care through others, *Am J Nurs* 92:87-89, March 1992.

Hasten R, Washburn M: How to plan what to delegate, *Am J Nurs* 92:71, April 1992.

Hasten R, Washburn M: What do you say when you delegate work to others? *Am J Nurs* 92:48, July 1992.

Hasten RI: Delegation: learning when and how to let go, *Nurs 91* 21:126, April 1991.

Hinds PS et al.: A comparison of the stress-response sequence in new and experienced pediatric oncology nurses, *Cancer Nurs* 17:61-71, Feb 1994.

Jackson I: Coping with stress, *Nurs Times* 93:31-32, July 1997.

Klein R: *Manage your time/market your business,* New York, 1995, AMACOM.

Krejci JW: Changing roles in nursing: perceptions of nurse administrators, *JONA* 29:21-29, March 1999.

Lachman VD: Care of the self for the nurse entrepreneur, *Nurs Adm Q* 22:48-59, Winter 1998.

Ladouceur ME: Four dimensions, *Executive Excellence* 11:11, Jan 1994.

LaFleur C: Easing stress during a move, *Nurs Manage,* pp 32c-32k, Aug 1998.

Lee V, Henderson MC: Occupational stress and organizational commitment in nurse administrators, *JONA* 26:21-28, May 1996.

MacKenzie RA: *The time trap: how to get more done in less time,* New York, 1975, McGraw-Hill.

McConnell EA: *Burnout in the nursing profession,* St. Louis, 1982, Mosby.

Meade J: On-screen sidekick can help to organize your work, *HR Magazine* 39:36-42, Jan 1994.

Milton D, Benjamin S: Providing alternatives in your health system, *Healthcare Forum J* 41:32-34, Nov-Dec 1998.

Narasi B: A tool for living through stress, *Nurs Manage* 25:73-75, Sept 1994.

National Council of State Boards of Nursing position paper (http://www.ncsbn.org/files/delegati.html), accessed June 5, 1999.

Overell S: Stress arousal 'good for employees and business,' *People Management* 4:17, Feb 1998.

Parsons LC: Delegation decision making: evaluation of a teaching strategy, *JONA* 27:47-51, Feb 1997.

Parsons LC: Delegation skills and nurse job satisfaction, *Nurs Econ* 16:18-26, Jan-Feb 1998.

Petermann BA, Springer P, Farnsworth J: Analyzing job demands and coping techniques, *Nurs Manage* 26:51-53, Feb 1995.

Roberts KT, Whall A: Serenity as a goal for nursing practice, *Image J Nurs Sch* 28:359-364, Winter 1996.

Rogers AC: Vulnerability, health and health care, *J Adv Nurs* 26:65-74, July 1997.

Rondeau KV: Procrastination means lost productivity . . . ten suggestions for eliminating employee workplace procrastination, *Can J Med Technol* 55(2):74-76, 1993.

Schwab L: Individual hardiness and staff satisfaction, *Nurs Econ* 14:171-173, May-June 1996.

Selye H: *The stress of life,* ed 2, New York, 1978, McGraw-Hill.

Selye H: *Stress without distress,* New York, 1978, McGraw-Hill.

Thomas SP, Droppleman P: Channeling nurses' anger into positive interventions, *Nurs Forum* 32:13-21, April-June 1997.

CASE STUDY

A number of nurses on your staff are married, raising small children, taking classes toward a degree, and feeling stressed. They are starting to develop some negativism. How will you approach this problem?

CASE STUDY

You are the charge nurse on the 3-to-11 shift. When you return from your dinner break, the ward clerk reports the following:

1. Mrs. Jones's intravenous (IV) fluid has infiltrated.
2. The operating room staff are on their way to take Mr. Anderson to surgery. He has not received his preoperative medication yet.
3. A parent has asked if her daughter, who is a new surgical patient, should have bright red blood on her dressing.
4. Two patients have not received their meal trays yet.
5. Someone spilled a bouquet of flowers in a patient's room.

   The other registered nurse (RN) is busy with his own patients. You have yourself, a ward clerk, and an IV-certified licensed practical nurse (LPN) to whom you can delegate. Decide who should do what and in what priority. Using Worksheet 2-1 on page 475, justify your decision.

Critical Thinking Activities for this chapter begin on page 474.

CHAPTER 3

DECISION-MAKING PROCESS AND TOOLS

CHAPTER OBJECTIVES

- List the five steps in the decision-making process.
- Identify at least six techniques to increase creativity.
- Describe at least two ethical positions that can be used to consider moral dilemmas.
- List at least five decision-making tools.
- Identify at least three models that can be used to describe phenomena.
- Describe how to use a Gantt chart.
- Describe how computers can be applied in nursing.
- Compare advantages and disadvantages of group participation in decision making.

Chapter Overview

Chapter 3 outlines the decision-making process, critical thinking, creative decision making, consultation, ethics, moral reasoning, ethics committees, decision-making tools, computers, group factors in decision making, and committee aspects of decision making.

MAJOR CONCEPTS AND DEFINITIONS	
Decision-making process	the process of selecting one course of action from alternatives
Critical thinking	the ability to question philosophically and exercise careful judgment when evaluating a situation
Creativity	intellectual inventiveness
Consultation	an interactive, helping relationship between two parties
Ethics	a moral philosophy that examines how means are related to ends and how to control means to serve human ends
Tool	an instrument used to accomplish an end
Model	an abstraction or representation of something more complex
Probability	the likelihood of an event's occurrence
Simulation	an imitation of an event or process
Game theory	a simulation of system operations
Gantt chart	a tool used to visualize multiple tasks that need to be done
Decision tree	graphic tool to visualize alternatives available, chance events, and probable consequences
PERT	program evaluation and review technique
CPM	critical path method to calculate time estimate for activities
Queuing theory	a mathematical technique used to determine efficiency of intermittent services
Linear programming	matrix algebra or linear mathematical equations used to determine the best way to use limited resources for maximal results
Computer	an electronic machine that performs rapid calculations or compiles, correlates, and selects data by means of stored instructions and information
Vroom and Yetton model	a tool used to identify autocratic, consultative, and group decision processes

DECISION-MAKING PROCESS

Decision making, the process of selecting one course of action from alternatives, is a continuing responsibility of nurse managers. They are confronted by a variety of situations. Hospital or agency policies provide guidelines for dealing with routine situations. Exceptional instances, however, can make decisions more difficult and may require

Box
3-1
DECISION-MAKING PROCESS

1. Identify the problem and analyze the situation.
2. Explore the alternatives.
3. Choose the most desirable alternative.
4. Implement the decision.
5. Evaluate the results.

a mature sense of judgment. Problem solving is a skill that can be learned, and because staff nurses can learn by observing their leaders, good decision making by the leader may do more than solve immediate problems; more important for the long term, it can foster good decision making by staff nurses.

Decision making relies on the scientific problem-solving process: identifying the problem, analyzing the situation, exploring alternatives and considering their consequences, choosing the most desirable alternative, implementing the decision, and evaluating the results (Box 3-1).

Identify the Problem and Analyze the Situation

The first step in the decision-making process is defining the problem. What is wrong? Where is improvement needed? Sometimes the problem seems obvious and can be dealt with routinely. If the employee repeatedly reports late to work or abuses the privilege of sick leave, the manager can respond in accordance with agency policies. However, when managers are concerned only with the infraction, they may be dealing with the effect rather than the cause of the problem. Consequently, similar situations may continue. It is important to define the factors that are causing the problem. For instance, two staff nurses may each complain about the intrusion of the other into her work. Initially the problem may appear to be a personality clash or a political power struggle. However, the cause may be the manager's failure to define the job responsibilities of each nurse. As long as the manager concen-

trates on the symptom instead of the problem, the difficulties will arise. It is only when the real problem has been identified that effective decision making can be initiated.

Nurse managers can identify the problem by analyzing the situation. All too frequently decisions are made and implemented before all the facts have been gathered. To prevent this the manager should have a questioning attitude. What is the desirable situation? What are the presenting symptoms? What are the discrepancies? Who is involved? When? Where? How? With answers to these questions managers can develop tentative hypotheses and test them against what they know. Progressive elimination of hypotheses that fail to conform to the facts reduces the number of causes to be considered. Feasible hypotheses should be further tested for causal validity. When managers believe they have identified the cause or causes of the problem by analyzing available information, they should begin exploring possible solutions.

Explore the Alternatives

There are usually a number of ways to solve a problem. Some may be quick and economical but less effective than their alternatives. Others may be more effective but less economical. If various alternatives are not explored, the course of action is limited.

When solving a problem, managers should determine first whether the situation is covered by policy. If it is not, they must draw on their education and experience for facts and concepts that will help them determine alternatives. Using one's experience is probably the most common approach to solving problems, but it may be inadequate. The more experience the manager has had, the more alternatives may be suggested to solve a variety of problems. However, health care changes rapidly, and solutions to yesterday's problems may not work today. Consequently, managers should look beyond their own experiences and learn how others are solving similar problems. This can be done through continuing education, professional meetings, review of the literature, correspondence, and brainstorming with staff. Inductive and deductive reasoning are both appropriate.

Choose the Most Desirable Alternative

The number and quality of alternatives depend largely on the creativity and productivity of managers and their staff. Leadership that prevents immediate acceptance of an apparently obvious solution and facilitates group exploration of decision-making opportunities (such as problems to solve) usually increases the number of alternatives and the quality of problem solving.

Eagerness to reach a decision may lead to premature solutions; on the other hand, considering only a few alternatives in haste blocks good decisions. Avoidance of the real problem, lack of clear problem definition, insufficient data, early statement of attitude by a status figure, mixing of idea generation and idea evaluation, lack of staff commitment because the superior who makes the decision does not implement it, and decisions made by large groups also interfere with reaching effective solutions.

One alternative is not always clearly superior to all others. The manager must try to balance such factors as patient safety, staff acceptance, morale, public acceptance, cost, and risk of failure. Criteria for calculating the value of decisions are useful. The following questions may be asked: Will this decision accomplish the stated objectives? If it does not, it should not be enforced and another option should be used. Does it maximize effectiveness and efficiency? One should use available resources before seeking outside assistance. Finally, can the decision be implemented? If not, it obviously will not solve the problem.

Implement the Decision

After a decision has been made, it must be implemented. A decision that is not put into action is useless. The manager will need to communicate the decision to appropriate staff associates in a manner that does not arouse antagonism. The decision and procedures for its implementation can be explained in an effort to win the cooperation of those responsible for its implementation. The manager will need to select the staff associate to implement the decision and provide the direction to initiate action. Managers may need to control the environment so staff associates can function as planned. Once the decision has been implemented, it should be evaluated.

Evaluate the Results

The final step of decision making is evaluation of the results of the implementation of the chosen alternative. Evaluative criteria may have to be developed. Audits, checklists, ratings, and rankings can be used to review and analyze the results. Because solutions to old problems sometimes create new problems, making and evaluating additional decisions may be required.

The decision-making and problem-solving models and the nursing process are very similar (Box 3-2). They are all scientific problem solving.

CRITICAL THINKING

Elements of reasoning are essential dimensions that provide general logic to reason. They include purpose or goal; central problem or question at issue; point of view or frame of reference; empirical dimension; conceptual dimension; assumptions, implications, and consequences; and inference and conclusion (Box 3-3).

Purpose or Goal

All reasoning has purpose and requires clarity, significance, achievability, and consistency of purpose.

Central Problem or Question at Issue

All reasoning is an attempt to solve a problem, figure something out, or answer a question. To answer a question or solve a problem one must understand what it requires. Clarity, significance, relevance, and answerability of the question are needed.

| Box 3-2 | DECISION-MAKING AND PROBLEM-SOLVING MODELS AND NURSING PROCESS | |

Decision Making	Problem Solving	Nursing Process
1. Identify the problem and analyze the situation.	1. Assess—define the problem.	1. Assess.
2. Explore the alternatives.	2. Plan—generate a list of alternatives and evaluate for cost, feasibility, and risk.	2. Select nursing diagnosis.
3. Choose the most desirable alternative.	3. Choose the best solution.	3. Plan care.
4. Implement the decision.	4. Implement the apparent best solution.	4. Implement the care plan.
5. Evaluate the results.	5. Evaluate the effectiveness of the action.	5. Evaluate outcomes.

Box 3-3 ELEMENTS OF CRITICAL THINKING AND REASONING

Purpose or goal
Central problem or question at issue
Point of view or frame of reference
Empirical dimension
Conceptual dimension
Assumptions
Implications and consequences
Inference and conclusions

Data from Paul R: *Critical thinking*, Santa Rosa, Calif, 1993, Foundation of Critical Thinking.

Point of View or Frame of Reference

All reasoning is done from a point of view. Reasoning is improved when multiple relevant points of view are sought and when those points of view are articulated clearly, empathized with logically and fairly, and applied consistently and dispassionately.

Empirical Dimension

Reasoning is only as sound as the evidence on which it is based. The evidence should be clear, relevant, accurate, adequate, fairly gathered and reported, and consistently applied.

Conceptual Dimension

Reasoning is only as relevant, clear, and deep as the concepts that form it. Concepts should be clear, deep, neutral, and relevant.

Assumptions

All reasoning is based on assumptions. Reasoning can only be as sound as the assumptions on which it is based. Assumptions should be clear, consistent, and justifiable.

Implications and Consequences

All reasoning has implications, consequences, and direction. Understanding the implications and consequences is important to reason through a decision or issue. One must consider the clarity, completeness, precision, reality, and significance of articulated implications.

Inference and Conclusions

All reasoning has inferences by which one draws conclusions and gives meaning to the data. Reasoning is only as sound as the inferences it makes and the conclusions to which it comes. Inferences should be clear and justifiable. Conclusions should be consistent, profound, and reasonable.

CREATIVE DECISION MAKING
The Creative Process

The creative process has steps similar to those of the problem-solving process, but the emphasis is different (Box 3-4). Decision making stresses choice of a solution, whereas the creative process emphasizes the uniqueness of the solution. Creativity is a latent quality, activated when a person becomes motivated by the need for self-expression or by the stimulation of a problem. Thus the first phase of the creative process is a *felt need*. Similarly, when decision makers are confronted with a problem, they start seeking a solution.

The second phase of creative problem solving is a work stage known as *preparation,* from which creative ideas emerge. Innovation is partially dependent on the number of options considered. By exploring relationships between potential solutions, one may identify additional solutions. Many decisions are made after slight preparation and therefore result in commonplace solutions. Superficial analysis of obvious information does not facilitate creative answers. Extensive use of libraries for data collection is useful; the creative person may take notes on readings, develop them into files with other clippings and ideas, review these materials, and combine the most appropriate aspects of old solutions into new answers.

Incubation, the third phase, is a period for pondering the situation. Repetition of the same thoughts with no new ideas or interpretations is a sign of fatigue and indicates that it is a good time to start the incubation period. Switching one's attention provides a necessary respite, and yet the un-conscious mind continues to deal with the problem. A time should be set to reexamine the situation and review the data collected during the preparation phase.

Illumination is the discovery of a solution. It may come to mind in the middle of the night or during the performance of another task. It is recommended that the idea be written down so the details can be preserved. Having paper and pencil readily available at all times (including in the bedside stand) is helpful.

It is rare for an illumination to be ready for adoption. *Verification,* the fifth and final phase of creative decision making, is the period of experimentation when the idea is improved through modification and refinement. The advantages and disadvantages of each alternative must be weighed; resources and constraints such as personnel, finances, facilities, and equipment have to be evaluated, and potential technical and human problems should be considered. Some decisions have failed at implementation because potential problems were not anticipated and dealt with. It would be unfortunate for an otherwise useful alternative to be rejected for a disadvantage that could be easily overcome. By comparing the advantages and disadvantages of the options, the manager can choose the most desirable alternative.

Encouraging Creativity

The thinking mechanism of the human brain has been conceptualized as having two sides. The right side is intuitive and conceptual and is used for uninhibited creative thinking. The left side is analytical and sequential. If we use the analogy of driving a car, the right side of the brain is a green light that keeps us going until we have generated a multiplicity of ideas. The left side is a red light that says, stop and question whether this is worthwhile. The judicial left side of the brain analyzes and evaluates the creative ideas generated by the right side of the brain. We need to use both sides. We are usually socialized to use the left side more than the right side, but the right side can be stimulated. Box 3-5 lists some creative thinking techniques.

Box 3-4   **CREATIVE DECISION-MAKING PROCESS**

Felt need
Preparation
Incubation
Illumination
Verification

Convergent thinking. The problem is divided into smaller and smaller pieces to find a more manageable perspective.

Divergent thinking. One's view of the problem is expanded. The problem is considered in different ways.

Forced association. The situation requiring improvement is identified. Participants use free association to generate a list of words associated with the situation. Then a list of associated words is generated. The participants look for relationships between the original list and the associated list. The lists are critically analyzed to choose words useful for addressing the situation requiring improvement.

Think tanks. Five to eight people are gathered together in an exotic or different place to stimulate innovation. A relaxed atmosphere is encouraged to stimulate divergent and unusual ideas. The problem or goal is clearly stated. This is particularly useful for future projections.

Brainstorming. Under favorable circumstances a group working together can identify more ideas

Box 3-5　CREATIVE THINKING TECHNIQUES

Brainstorming
Brainwriting
Collective notebook technique
Convergent thinking
Delphi technique
Divergent thinking
Drawing
Forecasting alternative future scenarios
Lists
Meditation
Modeling
Reverse brainstorming
Stepladder technique
Synetics
Visualization

than an individual or that group of individuals working separately. Brainstorming is a technique leaders can use to create a free flow of ideas. They should encourage the members to contribute a large number of freewheeling ideas without fear of criticism or ridicule. This can improve the quality of ideas offered and result in new combinations through rearrangement, reversal, substitution, and other modifications.

Brainstorming seems to work best for simple and specific problems. Complex problems can be divided into parts that are handled separately. If the problem is too complex, the discussion may lack focus and be very time-consuming. Brainstorming may be most useful when group members understand at least part of the problem. Although the session may not produce a viable solution, its stimulation may continue beyond the meeting and cause employees to take another look at their routinized activities.

Creativity is probably fostered best in a permissive atmosphere in which mutual respect prevails and people are encouraged to express their views and ideas even if they are at variance with current policies and practices. A free interchange of ideas with considerable borrowing and adaptation fosters the production of creative ideas. This is a divergent way of thinking that apparently generates the largest number of creative ideas when people look for what can be used from "wild" ideas rather than criticizing them because they will not work.

Reverse brainstorming. This encourages convergent thinking to break down ideas into smaller parts and analyze and focus on a particular problem or part of a problem. It is done verbally and works best for auditory or verbally oriented people.

Brainwriting. Brainwriting encourages free association and recording of ideas without verbal interaction. A problem is identified. Participants are given a blank piece of paper and told to write at least four ideas, suggestions, solutions, and so forth. The paper is then passed to someone else. Reading others' ideas is intended to stimulate more ideas, which are then written on the page. The process continues until no one can think of anything else to write.

Collective notebook technique. A problem is identified, and participants are instructed to record thoughts and ideas about the problem for a specified period. Each participant gives her notebook to another person, who reads it, looks for patterns, and synthesizes the content. The participants then meet, analyze the results, and make recommendations to solve the problem.

Stepladder technique. This technique structures the entry of group members into the group to ensure that each member contributes to the decision-making process. Initially two group members try to solve a problem. Then a third member joins the core group and presents a preliminary solution to the problem. The entering person's presentation is discussed by all three persons. The process is repeated as group members are added.

Each member is given the group's task and time to think about it before presenting to the group. The entering person presents preliminary solutions before the group comes to a final decision. There is a discussion after each entering person presents. The final decision is delayed until all members of the group have presented and are available to participate in the final decision.

The Delphi technique. The Delphi technique allows members who are dispersed over a geographical area to participate in decision making without meeting face to face. A problem is identified, and members are asked to suggest potential solutions through the use of a questionnaire. Members anonymously return the first questionnaire, and the results are centrally compiled. Each member is sent a copy of the results; after viewing them, members are asked for their suggestions again. Review of the results of the first questionnaire typically triggers new solutions or stimulates changes in original positions. This process continues until consensus is reached. Little change usually occurs after the second round.

The Delphi technique insulates group members from one another's influence and does not require physical presence, so it is particularly appropriate for scattered groups. Unfortunately, it is time-consuming and may not develop as many alternatives as the other techniques.

Lists. The checklist method is used to assemble criteria on a checklist, sort it, prioritize it, eliminate items, and add others. An attribute list records characteristics. They are then rearranged in possible combinations of ideas. The SCAMPER technique lists verbs that are idea generating. Scamper is an acronym for substitute, combine, adapt, modify, put to other uses, eliminate, and reverse.

Drawing. Drawings can be used to evoke and record creative insight because intuitive consciousness communicates more readily in symbols and impressions than in words.

Synetics. Synetics is the joining together of apparently irrelevant elements. A problem is identified, and a brief analysis given. The problem is then simplified to clarify it and reinterpreted in analogy or metaphor. The group then plays with the analogy. The analogy or metaphor chosen to represent the problem is considered in depth. The problem is thus redefined in a new light.

Visualization. Free association can be used to create a big dream approach. First, desired outcomes are visualized and then visually run backward to identify a new approach. Imagine what you would like: a phone that tells you who is calling before you answer it, that shows who is talking to you, that you do not have to touch to answer, that rings wherever you are (office, home, car, beach). Once you have imagined what you want, you can begin dreaming about how to make your dream a reality. This technique allows you to pretend that you already have what you want and facilitates concentration on the outcomes.

Forecasting alternative future scenarios. The future is often more a matter of choice than of chance. The choice is enhanced by forecasting potential scenarios—status quo, least preferred, most preferred, and not likely—and selecting the most desired. The process includes assessing the present situation, identifying its strengths and weaknesses, recognizing the driving forces in the environment, constructing possible alternative future scenarios, identifying the preferred future, developing a plan of action, implementing the plan, and evaluating the implementation.

Self-interrogation checklist. Questions are used to stimulate new perspectives about a situation. Questions help define and refine situations. They help obtain information, assess options, generate new ideas, and make decisions. Questions could include, Is it practical? Is it cost-effective? Is it efficient? Is it effective? Can we do more? Can we streamline? Can we improve the situation?

Modeling. Look at how others are doing what you wish to do. However, be cautious: what works for someone else, somewhere else, may not work for you here and now. Similarly, what worked for you somewhere else or at some other time may not work now. Seek out what can be used or adapted, given the current situation and the preferred future.

Meditation. The optimal state for peak performance of athletes is relaxed concentration, or "playing loose." Meditation can generate a more focused state of relaxed attention.

Developing Creative Thinking Attitudes

People need to be open-minded about new ideas and the ideas of others. Inquiring minds are never satisfied. Creative people are not unduly concerned about the opinions of others, because many great ideas are first ridiculed and later accepted. People need to put aside critical, analytical, and judicial thinking while working creatively and move beyond their personal habits and attitudes. After numerous ideas have been generated, they can be judged, and the best selected. Trust, acceptance, and good humor help create an environment conducive to creative problem solving. Creative people have an inner motivation, mental ability, objectivity, tolerance for complexity, enjoyment of risk taking, and ability to find problems.

Blocks to Creativity

Negative attitudes, self-censorship, lack of confidence, lack of effort, habits, conformity, and reliance on authority all block creativity.

CONSULTATION

Consultation is a helping relationship. It is a process of interaction between the consultant, who has the specialized knowledge and skills, and the consultee, who asks for assistance with problem solving. It has a beginning and an end and is a temporary, voluntary, educational relationship. The consultee identifies a problem and seeks help from an expert. Because the consultant is usually not a part of the hierarchical structure of the organization, the consultant is an outsider who advises. Implementation of the recommendations depends on the consultee, thus giving the process a take-it-or-leave-it quality. The consultative process usually involves problem solving, but the consultant may play several roles: helping identify problems, educating staff about related issues, identifying obstacles to problem solving, offering advice about how to solve problems, acting as a change agent, developing interpersonal relationships, mediating conflicts, or performing tasks that organizational members do not have the skill to perform. The consultant typically collects and analyzes data, recommends or intervenes, and then terminates the relationship.

Consultants become known by doing something and telling others about it, volunteering to present workshops and speeches, publishing books and articles, being active in professional organizations, circulating flyers and announcements, and being included in lists of consultants.

An internal consultant knows the system, history, political realities, norms, and language better than an outside consultant and will probably devote more time to the problem. Internal consultants are viewed as less costly because they are usually not compensated extra for consultative services. Unfortunately, there are disadvantages to hiring internal consultants. They may be part of the problem; lack perspective to see the whole; have no independence of movement; have no adequate power base; encounter resistance because of their relationship with the hierarchy, vested interest, or organizational politics; or have a limited background.

An external consultant has a more diverse background, brings new ideas and a different perspective to the situation, is independent of the power structure, and is consequently high powered. Unfortunately, the external consultant does not know the history and politics of the institution and may not care about them.

Once it has been determined that there is a need for consultation, what the purpose is, and who the consultant should be, a contractual agreement is necessary. The agreement may be verbal or written, but it should determine the fee, hours of the consultant's time, expected outcome, and criteria for termination. The fee may be negotiated as a flat fee, a fee based on hours spent at the agency that includes travel and preparation time, or an hourly rate for all the time the consultant spends on the project, including research and report writing. The hours are largely controlled by the compensation structure. The consultant may have a regular schedule or be "on call." In most cases the outcome is accepted whether it is judged acceptable or not. A common outcome is a written analysis with recommendations, decisions reached, systems devised or revised, and projects completed. Usually the termination occurs at a natural closure point such as the resolution of the problem or completion of the project. However, contingency plans should be made in case there are personality conflicts or the project takes too long and exceeds the budget.

ETHICAL ASPECTS OF DECISION MAKING

Ethics is a moral philosophy, a science of judging the relationship of means to ends, and the art of controlling means so they will serve human ends.

It involves conflict, choice, and conscience. When there is a conflict, there is a choice between conflicting alternatives. The choice is influenced by values. Values are learned first from important adults and are modified by association with people of different values. Value modification and reinforcement are lifelong processes. A value is consciously prized and cherished, freely chosen from alternatives, and acted on in a variety of ways. Ethical choices must also consider wants, needs, and rights: people may want what they do not need. Someone may want a dessert but not need it; in fact, it may be harmful. People often need what others also need. One who needs food to prevent starvation may have a right to receive food from people who have plenty but not from someone who would starve without it. That would infringe on the other person's rights, and duty and rights are correlated: it is one's duty to protect rights. A legal obligation is legislated, but it may not be ethical. A moral dilemma occurs when a decision has equally unsatisfactory alternatives.

Ethical Theories

Deontological (from the Greek deon or duty) theories focus of the intent of the action and are duty and rights based. Emphasis is on the dignity of human beings. The intention of the action rather than the end of the action is considered.

Teleological (from the Greek telos or end) theories derive the rules and norms for conduct from utilitarian consequences of actions. They favor the common good. Right has good consequences and bad has bad consequences. The greatest amount of good and the largest amount of happiness are good.

Principlism is an emerging theory that includes ethical principles. The ethical principles control ethical decision making more than the ethical theories. The principles are moral norms, including autonomy, beneficence, fidelity, justice, nonmaleficence, paternalism, respect for others, utility, and veracity. Each principle can be used individually, but they are often used in concert.

Ethical Principles

Autonomy involves personal freedom, freedom of choice, and responsibility for one's choices. Informed consent and progressive discipline recognize autonomy.

Beneficence indicates that the actions one takes should be in an effort to promote good. This principle can support providing extensive, painful treatments to increase quantity and quality of life or allowing a person to die without life support. It can be used to promote employees' positive attributes instead of their shortcomings.

Fidelity is keeping one's commitments and promises. One should not make a promise to a patient or worker that cannot be kept.

Justice means treating people equally and fairly. Equals should be treated equally, and unequals should be treated according to their differences. It is useful to apply when making decisions about competition for scarce resources or benefits. Pay raises should reflect performance as well as time of service. Holidays, vacation time, and attendance at conferences should reflect performance as well as who is next on the list.

Nonmaleficence means if you cannot do good at least do no harm. Nurses may need to remember that even pain and suffering can bring about good for the patient when they are performing painful procedures for the patient's benefit. Performance appraisals should emphasize the employee's good qualities and give positive direction for improved performance instead of destroying self-esteem.

Paternalism allows one to make decisions for another, limits freedom of choice, and is seen as an undesirable principle. Most see it as justified only to keep another person from harm. It is not appropriate for a paternalistic manager to set the personal goals for employees.

Respect for others is considered the highest principle that incorporates all of the principles. Respect for others acknowledges the rights of people to make their own decisions and to live by their decisions. It transcends cultural, gender, and racial issues.

Utility indicates that what is best for the common good outweighs what is best for the individual.

It could justify paternalism. One using utility needs to be careful not to become less humanistic.

Veracity indicates that people should tell the truth. It applies to telling patients and staff the truth so they can make well-informed decisions (Grohar-Murray and DiCroce, 1997; Marquis and Huston, 1996; Swansburg and Swansburg, 1999; Yoder-Wise, 1999).

Ethical Positions

There are several ethical positions that do not solve dilemmas. However, they do provide ways to structure and clarify them.

Utilitarianism is a community-oriented position that focuses on the consequences and prefers the greatest amount of good and happiness for the most people, or the least amount of harm.

In contrast, *egoism* seeks solutions that are best for oneself without regard for others. One's own pleasure is the concern.

Formalism considers the nature of the act and the related principles without thought to personal position or consequences of the actions: be honest; remember the golden rule.

Rule ethics expects obedience to laws, rules, professional codes, and authority.

Fairness considers distribution of benefits and liabilities from the viewpoint of the least advantaged. Benefit to the least advantaged is the norm in this type of decision making.

Ethical Relationships

There are also models for ethical relationships. In the *priestly model* the manager is paternalistic and makes decisions without considering others' values or seeking others' input. Although nurses may have expertise that qualifies them to make some decisions, they have no right to make moral decisions affecting other people. Autocratic leadership may use the priestly model. The *engineering model* suggests that one person presents facts to another and sets aside her own code of ethics to do what the other wants; staff working for line authority may provide an example of this model. The *contractual* *model* provides a contract that identifies general obligations and benefits for two or more people. It deals with the morals of both parties and is appropriate for superior-subordinate relationships. In the *collegial model* individuals share mutual goals and reach decisions through discussion and consensus. When there are shared values, this model helps build teams and minimize conflict (Veatch, 1980).*

To make an ethical decision, one must first consider what is intended to be a means and an end and then determine what good or evil is found in the means and the end. If a major evil is intended either as a means or an end, it is an unethical decision.

If the ramifications of the decision are probable but not willed as a means or an end, there are several factors to consider. The good or evil of each alternative should be evaluated: a necessary good outweighs a useful good; paying workers' wages outweighs paying for profit sharing. Urgency increases the necessity; therefore physical needs must be met before self-actualizing needs. An agency should provide adequate wages for food and shelter before providing continuing education. The probability of an outcome should be considered: a possible negative outcome is outweighed by a probable good; one will work to earn a living even though there is a slight risk of back strain. The intensity of one's influence is considered because one's impact on someone else may have undesirable consequences; for instance, if an employee is fired for incompetence, it may cause a hardship for the employee's family. If the manager did not tell the employee what was expected or how to do the job, the manager would have been a considerable factor in that employee's poor job performance. Firing the employee would seem evil. If, however, the staff associate is frequently tardy or absent through no fault of the manager, the consequences of firing the worker seem justified. If there is no proportionate reason for permitting an evil, the act is unethical. If there is an alternative that provides more good and

less risk of evil, it should be chosen; if there is not, there is proportionate reason for risking an evil (Aroskar, 1980).

MORAL REASONING

Levels of moral development have been identified as (1) premoral or preconventional when behavior is motivated by social or biological impulses with no sense of obligation to rules; (2) conventional when the person accepts standards of the group with little critical reflection, uses literal obedience to the rules, and feels obligation; and (3) autonomous when the person thinks and judges for himself, considers the purpose and consequences of the rules, and does not accept the group standards without reflection.

Moral choice involves selecting one of two or more values that conflict. Ten universal moral values are distributive justice, law, liberty, life, property, punishment, roles and concerns of affection, roles and concerns of authority, sex, and truth.

The level of moral development determines what a person finds valuable, how she defines the value, and why she finds it valuable. First, a person considers the power of the person involved. Second, she looks at satisfying her own needs. Third, the individual considers relationships with others and then sees life as inherently worthwhile aside from other considerations. Moral judgment is necessary but not sufficient for mature moral action. People may do wrong even when they know better.

ETHICS COMMITTEES

Complex ethical issues regarding patient care and policy making must be addressed. Institutional ethics committees deal with ethical questions that often require painful choices for patients, particularly for infants and those elderly adults who are unable to make their own decisions.

The following issues must be addressed within the institution's philosophy, both when forming an institutional ethics committee and through ongoing study and evaluation of the existing committee: responsibility, accountability, economic costs, efficacy,

---

*Robert Veatch's models for ethical medicine are discussed in Aroskar MA: Ethics of nurse-patient relationships, *Nurse Educ* 5:18, 1980.

role of the committee in patient care decisions, privacy for the patients and families, and committee composition, structure, meetings, and access. Nursing should be represented on the committee. Ethics committees are likely to deal with such ethical issues in nursing practice as do-not-resuscitate orders, patients' rights, professional practice issues, death and dying, and allocation of resources.

DECISION-MAKING TOOLS

Most decisions involve varying degrees of uncertainty. Leaders and managers use research of various kinds to minimize the uncertainty of their decisions.

Probability Theory

Probability theory can be applied when risk or uncertainty is present in a decision. It operates on the assumption that factors occur in accordance with a predictable pattern. For example, if a person tosses a coin 200 times, we can predict that it will show heads 100 times and tails 100 times. Deviations can be set within a predictable margin. Inferences based on statistical analysis of existing data can be used to predict results.

Sometimes a sample of the population may be analyzed. Measures of probable error become increasingly important when one is dealing with a sample because the smaller the probable error, the greater the amount of confidence that can be put in the findings. One must consider the reliability of sampling and the additional time and expense involved in collecting more information. Probability can become a substitute for otherwise unknown information: when probabilities can be substituted for unknowns, the margin of error for the solution may be limited but not completely removed.

There are three criteria that assume that previous experience is necessary to work with probability. In the "maximax" criterion managers maximize the maximum possible gain. Managers are optimistic about the factors influencing their decision and select the option from which they can achieve the best results. This is a dangerous criterion in that it

does not consider possible complications. When applying the "maximin" criterion, managers are pessimistic and expect the worst possible results. They select the option that allows them to maximize the least favorable results. They consider what complications can occur for each option, assume that everything that can go wrong will go wrong, and select the alternative that offers the best results when everything possible goes wrong. The "minimax" criterion can be applied when managers have made a decision they regret. Something unexpected prevented them from achieving the most favorable results; managers then subtract the complication from the most favorable results and try to minimize their regrets.

Uncertainty arises when the manager has to make a decision for which there is no historical data on which to calculate probabilities. Under uncertain conditions there is no best criterion to apply. The manager considers objective and subjective options according to her own optimistic or pessimistic philosophy and guesses which alternative will render the most desirable results.

Simulation, Models, and Games

Simulation is a way of using models and games to simplify problems by identifying the basic components and using trial and error to determine a solution. Through simulation the manager may compare alternatives and their consequences. The computer may be used to help solve simulations. These methods may be used to study organizational changes, scheduling, assembly line management, and time sequences.

A model represents something else, most commonly objects, events, processes, or systems. It is a technique of abstraction and simplification for studying something under varying conditions. Manipulation is used to test the impact of proposed changes on the system without disturbing the subject of the model. Almost all quantitative methods used to guide decision making are models. They are particularly useful because of their convenience and low cost compared with manipulating real occurrences. Although models vary considerably in the accuracy with which they represent real situations, they increase predictive capabilities over such methods as guesswork and intuition.

Models are developed to describe, explain, and predict phenomena. The critical element of model building is conceptualization. Consequently, models can provide abstractions that facilitate communication. Models vary in the degree of abstraction used: a life-size mannequin is a realistic model that nursing students use to learn to make occupied beds; a model of a building or a piece of equipment built to scale is quite concrete, whereas blueprints or photographs, organizational charts, and mathematical models are abstract.

The more variables added to the model, the more realistic but cumbersome it becomes. The objective of modeling is to provide a simplified, abstract version of reality. Managers must strive for the appropriate level of abstractness. They may base their decision on an oversimplified model if they do not attempt to expand their knowledge of the situation. Simplified models may be useful for quantitative analysis and prediction, but one must be cautious, because a person with the least knowledge of a situation may be the most certain about how to solve the problem. If description and understanding are important, more comprehensive models should be developed. Continuing to research a problem may contribute to a more realistic model, but it may also delay the decision too long. The cost of gathering additional information may be prohibitive; therefore balancing the cost of model refinement against the benefits obtained is required.

Game theory is a simulation of system operations. The player tries to develop a strategy that will maximize gains and minimize losses, regardless of what the competitor does. War games are commonly used to train personnel and to test plans and equipment under field conditions. Management games are used primarily to train personnel rather than to solve competitive problems. They are particularly useful for training in decision making by simulating real-life operations in a laboratory setting.

Gantt Chart

Gantt charts, named for their developer, Henry Gantt, are highly developed schedules that allow one to visualize multiple tasks that have to be done. A Gantt chart is a grid with columns for tasks, assigned responsibility, and time frame, which may be minutes, hours, days, weeks, months, years, or decades, depending on the longevity of the project. A line is drawn through the time frame while a task is in process. An X is put at the point where that task is completed. One typically works backward from due dates.

A person is told on Monday that a report is due Friday at 4 PM. The person needs to collect information, type the report on the computer, revise the report, and submit it. The person will use 3 days to collect the information and 1 day to type or word process it, incubate the ideas overnight, do any revision needed Friday morning, and submit the report Friday afternoon (Figure 3-1).

Task	Responsible	Mon	Tue	Wed	Th	Fr
Collect information	ME	---------	---	---		
Type report	ME				X	
Revise report	ME					X
Submit report	ME					X

Figure 3-1 Gantt chart.

Decision Trees

A decision tree is a graphic method that can help managers visualize the alternatives available, outcomes, risks, and information needs for a specific problem over a period of time. It helps them to see the possible directions that actions may take from each decision point and to evaluate the consequences of a series of decisions. The process begins with a primary decision having at least two alternatives. Then the predicted outcome for each decision is considered, and the need for further decisions is contemplated. The matrix resembles a tree as the decision points are diagrammed (Figure 3-2).

The results diagrammed on the tree are founded on the manager's experience and judgment but may be supported by computational data. For complex problems probability statistics may be used to explore further factors that favor or oppose expected events. Although the decision tree does not depict an obviously correct decision, it allows managers to base their decision on a consideration of various alternatives and probable consequences. It helps them realize that subsequent decisions may depend on future events. Decision trees are useful for short- and medium-range planning, as well as for decision making. Unfortunately, decision trees for longer than 2 or 3 years become cumbersome and speculative.

In Figure 3-3 the nursing staff decides to have a ward picnic for the psychiatric patients. The alternatives are to hold the picnic indoors or outdoors, and the chance events are rain or no rain. If the picnic is scheduled indoors and it rains, the patients may be crowded but dry; there will be no bugs; and the staff will be proud of their decision. If the picnic is scheduled indoors and it does not rain, the patients may feel crowded; the room may seem stuffy; the party will lack a picnic atmosphere; and the staff may regret not scheduling it outside. On the other hand, if the picnic is scheduled outdoors and it rains, the participants will get wet; the food will be ruined; and spirits will be dampened. If the picnic is scheduled outdoors and it does not rain, it will be a pleasant experience.

Program Evaluation and Review Technique

Program evaluation and review technique (PERT) is a network system model for planning and control under uncertain conditions. It involves identifying the key activities in a project, sequencing the activities in a flow diagram, and assigning the duration of each phase of the work. It is particularly appropriate for one-of-a-kind projects that involve extensive research and development.

PERT recognizes that certain tasks must be completed before the total project can be completed and, furthermore, that subtasks must be completed before others can be started. The key events are identified, numbered, labeled, or numbered and labeled on the flow chart. The activities that cause the progress from one event to another are indicated by arrows, with the direction of the arrow showing the direction of the work flow.

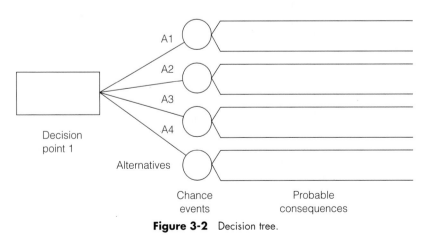

Figure 3-2 Decision tree.

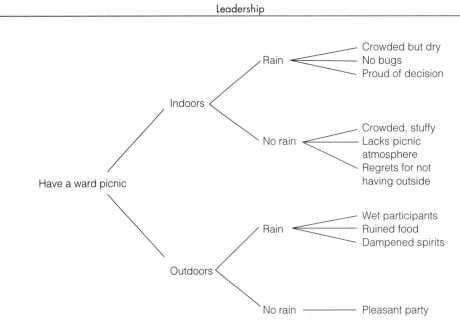

Figure 3-3 Decision tree for psychiatric ward picnic.

PERT also deals with the problem of uncertainty with respect to time by estimating the time variances associated with the expected time of completion of the subtasks. Three projected times are determined: (1) the optimistic time (t_0), which estimates the completion time without complications; (2) the most likely time(t_m), which estimates the completion time with normal problems; and (3) the pessimistic time(t_p), which estimates the completion time given numerous problems. Thus the shortest, average, and longest times needed to complete an activity are calculated. The expected time (t_e) is calculated from these figures by the following formula:

$$t_e = \frac{t_0 + 4(t_m) + t_p}{6}$$

If the optimistic time is 2 weeks, the most likely time 4 weeks, and the pessimistic time 6 weeks, the expected time is

$$t_e = \frac{2 \text{ weeks} + 4(4 \text{ weeks}) + 6 \text{ weeks}}{6} =$$

$$\frac{24 \text{ weeks}}{6} = 4 \text{ weeks}$$

The PERT model helps the manager determine priorities (Figure 3-4). Use of resources can be considered when setting priorities. Assignments may be changed temporarily, overtime may be allowed, or temporary help hired to facilitate the activity flow and to manipulate the time required to move from one event to another.

Critical Path Method

Critical path method (CPM), closely related to PERT, calculates a single time estimate for each activity, the longest possible time. A cost estimate is figured for both normal and crash operating conditions. Normal means the least-cost method, and crash refers to conditions in less-than-normal time. Simple sequences can be worked out manually, and more complex ones by computer. CPM is particularly useful where cost is a significant factor and experience provides a basis for estimating time and cost. Managers can observe the critical path and compare the progress with the projected dates.

Network analysis techniques facilitate planning and result in objective plans by making it possible to identify the critical path and show interrelationships between parts, thus facilitating improvements

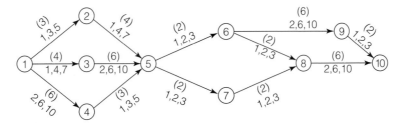

Figure 3-4   PERT model. This PERT model indicates that subtask 1 must be completed before 2, 3, and 4 can be done; 2, 3, and 4 before 5; 5 before 6 and 7; 6 before 9; 6 and 7 before 8; and 8 and 9 before 10. A coding system can be used to determine what the numbers mean. For example, 1 = program planned, 2 = staff informed. Arrows show direction of work flow. Optimistic, most likely, pessimistic, and expected times are recorded for each activity. The expected time is in parentheses.

in structure and communications. They are particularly useful for task force or project forms of organization and for projects.

Queuing Theory

Queuing theory deals with waiting lines or intermittent servicing problems. It is a mathematical technique for determining the most efficient balance of factors related to intermittent service. It is particularly applicable when units to receive service arrive in a random fashion but the time required for service is predictable. It balances the cost of waiting versus the prevention of waiting by increasing service; it acknowledges that although delays are costly, eliminating them may be even more costly. Decreasing or eliminating the waiting line to reduce waiting line costs causes an increase in cost of labor and physical facilities. The time of arrival is an important factor in determining the optimal size of facilities and staffing. Sometimes actual observations may be made, and tallies kept, of how many units or clients require service each hour of the workday or during certain seasons. For example, through observation one may determine that many junior and senior high school students attend sexually transmitted disease (STD) or family planning clinics during after-school hours. The STD or family planning clinics in a small college community may have fewer demands for service during holiday seasons and summer vacation because many students have returned to their hometown communities. The manager may adjust staffing accordingly. In the hospital setting the manager may choose to use part-time

people or split shifts to help compensate for an increased workload during the morning, when most patients are bathed and once-a-day treatments are given, and again during late afternoon or early evening, when most patients are admitted.

When observations cannot be made for an extended period to determine a stable pattern of workload, the Monte Carlo technique may be applied. It provides a large sample of random numbers that may be generated by a computer to determine rather precise predictions of servicing load per hour.

Linear Programming

Linear programming uses matrix algebra or linear mathematical equations to determine the best way to use limited resources to achieve maximal results. The technique is based on the assumption that a linear relationship exists between the variables and that the limits of the variations can be calculated. Three conditions are necessary for linear programming. First, either a maximal or minimal value is sought to optimize the objective. The value may be expressed as cost, time, or quantity. The manager may wish to minimize time and expense while maximizing quantity and quality of production. She may wish to reduce the time lost through inefficient allocation of resources or minimize the number of people required to do a job. Second, the variables affecting the goal must have a linear relationship; the ratio of change in one variable to the change in another variable must be constant. If it takes 3 minutes to do a task, it should take 15 minutes to do the task 5 times. Third, constraints or obstacles to the relationships of the variables exist. Linear programming would not be needed if there were no restrictions.

Simple allocations can often be made by observation and experience, but in large operations the problems may be complex and involve thousands of possible choices. Linear programming is a sophisticated shortcut technique in which a computer can be used to determine solutions. It may be used to determine a minimal-cost diet for meeting certain nutritional standards or for assigning community health nurses to territories. A school of nursing might use this technique to determine class sizes, class hours, and instructors by feeding information into a computer equation containing such variables as a student's desire or requirement to enroll in particular classes, number of students, number of professors qualified to teach the course, and the hours available to conduct the course. Because linear programming depends on linear relationships and many decisions do not involve them, the manager may need to apply nonlinear programming.

Advantages and Limitations of Quantitative Tools for Decision Making

Quantitative tools lend themselves to a rational, systematic approach to problem solving for decisions that can be expressed mathematically. They encourage disciplined thinking. They are not limited to the six or seven variables the human mind can consider at one time, and they may evaluate thousands of interrelationships simultaneously. Decisions made with the use of quantitative tools are likely to be superior to those that rely heavily on judgment. Unfortunately, many managerial problems involve intangible, nonmeasurable factors that reduce the effectiveness of the tools. The mathematical expressions are based on assumptions; if those assumptions are not true for a given situation, the tool becomes useless.

COMPUTERS

Computers provide several advantages over paper-based record systems. Information can be stored in smaller areas, search and analytical tasks can be performed, and information can be obtained fast and efficiently. Unfortunately, if used improperly, computers can magnify weaknesses in an organization.

Computers can be applied in nursing in three major categories: (1) clinical systems, (2) management information systems, and (3) educational systems. In clinical systems computers help with patient histories, medical records, and patient monitoring. Computerized record systems can improve the usability of patient information because data from the chart can be rearranged to be useful to various health care professionals. Physicians can enter their diagnoses, protocols, and notes directly into the computer, saving nurses transcribing time. The instructions can be printed out at the appropriate auxiliary department. Nurses can also record their notes directly into the computer and spend less time and energy accumulating and summarizing data to develop care plans. Standard screens with standard choices increase efficiency for recording observations and doing care plans. Nurses are made aware of changes that require their intervention quickly because information from ancillary departments can be sent automatically to the nursing station terminal. The computer can sort and analyze data and facilitate communication about the patients among health care providers.

An integrated clinical system allows patient data to be quickly available to health care providers. The system should be easy to use, have standardized data elements, have data repositories and archival systems for information that should be retained long term, and should have stand-alone or departmental system accessibility to patient information. *Emergency department* systems can triage patients based on assessment criteria. The system can calculate the level of severity based on the assessment and historical data entered by the triage person. The data can be readily available to all clinical personnel like those in the laboratory, pharmacy, and radiology departments. The marketing and planning departments can use the statistics to evaluate the market share information. The *laboratory system* allows ordering, collecting, analyzing, and storing of laboratory information, as well as reporting of results. *Pharmacy systems* can be used to order, check allergies, check dosage based on the patient's height and weight, check drug-to-drug interactions, check drug-to-food interactions, label medications, do inventory control, do drug utilization monitoring, and dispense medications. It allows medication cart fill, update, and check functions, printing of written orders, electronic recording of administration of medications, and an alert system for when medications are overdue. *Radiology systems* allow for ordering, scheduling, recording results, and tracking radiology exams. They can generate notices to send to patients and schedule repeat exams. Transcription can be done electronically with electronically attached signature. Some transcription systems allow for fill in the blanks to eliminate excessive typing. It can also track the location of various exam results and has the capability to store images directly on the radiology system, making digitized images readily available. *Cardiology systems* are similar to radiology systems and can be used for the collection, analysis, and reporting of cardiology exams. Transcription capabilities, ability to display and store digitized images, and telemedicine to transmit the report to physicians are desirable.

Dietary systems can assess nutritional status and facilitate ordering and preparing diets. They can create, maintain, and print menus, enter modifiers about restrictions or limitations to basic diets, place a diet on hold for a period of time, print a worksheet for the tray preparation area, and print out diet information for patient and family education.

Respiratory therapy systems can be used to order equipment and treatments, schedule procedures, document responses to treatments, and record interventions. The system can track routine cleaning and maintenance of equipment and disposable and reusable equipment and supplies.

Computer systems can also be used in *operating rooms, ambulatory clinics, physician offices,* and *case management systems.* They are good for scheduling and materials management. Transcription and patient billing are useful functions. Systems can handle scheduling of appointments with several different services with one phone call, which can also obtain basic information like insurance information, which can be verified later. They can track missed appointments.

Patient care documentation systems are the largest application of computer systems in health care. Point of care or bedside systems document patient assessments, treatments, medication administration, response to treatments and medications, and other progress notes. They can be used in home care, as well as critical care. They allow for integration of care by several care providers.

Patient monitoring systems record patient responses and can alert nurses to changes. Computers can record the patient's progress on paper or on the monitor, sound an alarm, and often transmit information from the patient's bedside to monitors at the nursing station. In addition to monitoring patients continuously and detecting changes, computers can analyze and interpret the data. Through computer monitoring, nurses can respond quickly to changes in patients' conditions.

Computers have many applications in management information systems. They can be used for tracking patient acuity and calculating patient care requirements and for patient classification systems, inventory control, supplies and material management, staff scheduling, policy and procedure changes and announcements, patient charges, budget information and management, personnel records, statistical reports, administrative reports, memos, and record location and tracking.

In educational systems computer-assisted instruction allows students to proceed at their own speed, provides immediate feedback, and allows dissemination of information to remote areas.

When using computers as decision-making tools, nurses should take advantage of good commercial software that is available and should investigate the possibility of using existing systems. Securing the confidentiality of patient and personnel records by carefully locking up diskettes or by constructing a password system is very important (Kreider and Haselton, 1997).

The Vroom and Jago model (1988) is a computer-friendly revision of the Vroom and Yetton model (1973) (Box 3-6). It provides an additional number of problem attributes, deletes the decision rules, changes dichotomous variables to continuous variables, and provides mathematical formulas to determine decisions.

Box 3-6   VROOM AND YETTON NORMATIVE MODEL

Vroom and Yetton address decision making as a social process and emphasize how managers do rather than should behave in their normative model. They identify the following alternative decision processes: A = autocratic, C = consultative, G = group, I = first variant, and II = second variant.

Types of Management Decision Styles*

AI	You solve the problem or make the decision yourself, using information available to you at that time.
AII	You obtain the necessary information from your subordinate(s), then decide on the solution to the problem yourself. You may or may not tell your subordinates what the problem is in getting the information from them. The role played by your subordinates in making the decision is clearly one of providing the necessary information to you, rather than generating or evaluating alternative solutions.
CI	You share the problem with relevant subordinates individually, getting their ideas and suggestions without bringing them together as a group. Then you make the decision that may or may not reflect your subordinates' influence.
CII	You share the problem with your subordinates as a group, collectively obtaining their ideas and suggestions. Then you make the decision that may or may not reflect your subordinates' influence.
GII	You share a problem with your subordinates as a group. Together you generate and evaluate alternatives and attempt to reach agreement (consensus) on a solution. Your role is much like that of chairman. You do not try to influence the group to adopt "your" solution, and you are willing to accept and implement any solution that has the support of the entire group.

(GI is omitted because it applies only to more comprehensive models outside the scope of the article.)

Decision Rules

Vroom identifies seven rules that do most of the work of the model. Three rules protect decision quality, and four protect acceptance.*

1. The information rule
If the quality of the decision is important and if the leader does not possess enough information or expertise to solve the problem by herself, AI is eliminated from the feasible set. (Its use risks a low-quality decision.)

2. The goal congruence rule
If the quality of the decision is important and if the subordinates do not share the organizational goals to be obtained in solving the problem, GII is eliminated from the feasible set. (Alternatives that eliminate the leader's final control over the decision reached may jeopardize the quality of the decision.)

3. The unstructured problem rule
In decisions in which the quality of the decision is important, if the leader lacks the necessary information or expertise to solve the problem by herself, and if the problem is unstructured, i.e., she does not know exactly

what information is needed and where it is located, the method used must provide not only for her to collect the information but also to do so in an efficient and effective manner. Methods that involve interaction among all subordinates with full knowledge of the problem are likely to be both more efficient and more likely to generate a high-quality solution to the problem. Under these conditions AI, AII, and CI are eliminated from the feasible set. (AI does not provide for her to collect the necessary information, and AII and CI represent more cumbersome, less effective, and less efficient means of bringing the necessary information to bear on the solution of the problem than methods that do permit those with the necessary information to interact.)

4. *The acceptance rule*
If the acceptance of the decision by subordinates is critical to effective implementation, and if it is not certain that an autocratic decision made by the leader would receive that acceptance, AI and AII are eliminated from the feasible set. (Neither provides an opportunity for subordinates to participate in the decision, and both risk the necessary acceptance.)

5. *The conflict rule*
If the acceptance of the decision is critical, and an autocratic decision is not certain to be accepted, and subordinates are likely to be in conflict or disagreement over the appropriate solution, AI, AII, and CI are eliminated from the feasible set. (The method used in solving the problem should enable those in disagreement to resolve their differences with full knowledge of the problem. Accordingly, under these conditions, AI, AII, and CI, which involve no interaction or only "one-on-one" relationships and therefore provide no opportunity for those in control to resolve their differences, are eliminated from the feasible set. Their use runs the risk of leaving some of the subordinates with less than the necessary commitment to the final decision.)

6. *The fairness rule*
If the quality of decision is unimportant and if acceptance is critical and not certain to result from an autocratic decision, AI, AII, CI, and CII are eliminated from the feasible set. (The method used should maximize the probability of acceptance because this is the only relevant consideration in determining the effectiveness of the decision. Under these circumstances, AI, AII, CI, and CII, which create less acceptance or commitment than GII, are eliminated from the feasible set. To use them is to run the risk of getting less than the needed acceptance of the decision.)

7. *The acceptance priority rule*
If acceptance is critical and not ensured by an autocratic decision, and if subordinates can be trusted, AI, AII, CI, and CII are eliminated from the feasible set. (Methods that provide equal partnership in the decision-making process can provide greater acceptance without risking decision quality. Use of any method other than GII results in an unnecessary risk that the decision will not be fully accepted or receive the necessary commitment on the part of subordinates.)

As one asks the diagnostic questions and applies the rules to specific situations, one may eliminate all but one decision style from the feasibility set. However, it is more likely that several decision styles could be used and still protect both the decision quality and acceptance requirements. Then the time factor is used to determine which of the feasible options will require the least time.

Vroom and Yetton focus on three classes of outcomes that influence the ultimate effectiveness of decisions: (1) the quality of the decision, (2) acceptance of the decision by the subordinates, and (3) available time needed to make the decision. The authors found that managers can diagnose a situation quickly and accurately by answering seven questions.*

Continued

Problem Attributes	Diagnostic Questions
A. The importance of the quality of the decision	Is there a quality requirement such that one solution is likely to be more rational than another?
B. The extent to which the leader possesses sufficient information/expertise to make a high-quality decision by herself	Do you have sufficient information to make a high-quality decision?
C. The extent to which the problem is structured	Is the problem structured?
D. The extent to which acceptance or commitment on the part of subordinates is critical to the effective implementation of the decision	Is acceptance of decision by subordinates critical to effective implementation?
E. The prior probability that the leader's autocratic decision will receive acceptance by subordinates	If you were to make the decision by yourself, is it reasonably certain that it would be accepted by your subordinates?
F. The extent to which subordinates are motivated to attain the organizational goals as represented in the objectives explicit in the statement of the problem	Do subordinates share the organizational goals to be obtained in solving this problem?
G. The extent to which subordinates are likely to be in conflict over preferred solutions	Is conflict between subordinates likely in preferred solutions?

CHAPTER SUMMARY

Chapter 3 covered the following:
Decision-Making Process
    Identify the Problem and Analyze the Situation
    Explore the Alternatives
    Choose the Most Desirable Alternative
    Implement the Decision
    Evaluate the Results
Critical Thinking
    Purpose or Goal
    Central Problem or Question at Issue
    Point of View or Frame of Reference
    Empirical Dimension
    Conceptual Dimension
    Assumptions
    Implications and Consequences
    Inference and Conclusions
Creative Decision Making
    The Creative Process

Encouraging Creativity
    Convergent thinking
    Divergent thinking
    Forced association
    Think tanks
    Brainstorming
    Reverse brainstorming
    Brainwriting
    Collective notebook technique
    Stepladder technique
    The Delphi technique
    Lists
    Drawing
    Synetics
    Visualization
    Forecasting alternative future scenarios
    Self-interrogation checklist
    Modeling
    Meditation

REFERENCES

Aroskar MA: Ethics of nurse-patient relationships, *Nurse Educ* 5:18, 1980.

Grohar-Murray ME, DiCroce HR: *Leadership and management in nursing,* Stamford, Conn, 1997, Appleton & Lange.

Kreider NA, Haselton BJ: *The systems challenge,* Chicago, 1997, American Hospital.

Marquis BL, Huston CJ: *Leadership roles and management functions in nursing: theory and application,* Philadelphia, 1996, Lippincott.

Paul R: *Critical thinking,* Santa Rosa, Calif, 1993, Foundation of Critical Thinking.

Swansburg RC, Swansburg RJ: *Introductory management and leadership for nurses,* Boston, 1999, Jones & Bartlett.

Vroom V: A new look at managerial decision making, *Organizational Dynamics* 1(4):69, 1973.

Vroom VH, Jago AG: *The new leadership: managing participation in organizations,* Englewood Cliffs, NJ, 1988, Prentice Hall.

Vroom VH, Yetton PW: *Leadership and decision-making,* Pittsburgh, 1973, University of Pittsburgh Press.

Yoder-Wise PS: *Leading and managing in nursing,* St. Louis, 1999, Mosby.

BIBLIOGRAPHY

Anderson CA: Ethics committees and quality improvement: a necessary link, *J Nurs Care Qual* 11(1):22-28, 1976.

Begley AM: Acts, omissions, intentions and motives: a philosophical examination of the moral distinction between killing and letting die, *J Adv Nurs* 28(4):865-973, 1998.

Blanchard KH, Peale NV: *The power of ethical management,* New York, 1989, Fawcett.

Booth D, Carruth AK: Violation of the nurse practice act: implications for nurse managers, *Nurs Manage,* pp 35-39, Oct 1998.

Bosnan J, Roper JM: The reality of political ethical conflicts: nurse manager dilemmas, *JONA* 27:42-46, Sept 1997.

Chally PS, Loriz L: Decision making in practice, *Am J Nurs* 98:17-20, June 1998.

Coleman D, Khanna R, editors: *Groupware: technology and applications,* Upper Saddle River, NJ, 1995, Prentice Hall PTR.

Curtin LL: Ethics, health professionals and health reform, *Nurs Manage* 25:28-30, July 1994.

Curtin LL: Ethics for, in, and about nursing administration, *Nurs Manage* 25:25-28, Dec 1994.

Curtin LL: A case of entrapment, *Nurs Manage* 26:56-58, March 1995.

Curtin LL: Why good people do bad things, *Nurs Manage* 27:63-65, July 1996.

Curtin L, Flaherty MJ: *Nursing ethics: theories and pragmatics,* Bowie, Md, 1999, Robert J Brady.

Davis AJ, Aroskar MA: *Ethical dilemmas and nursing practice,* ed 4, New York, 1997, Appleton & Lange.

Dowd SB, Dowd LP: Maintaining confidentiality: health care's ongoing dilemma, *Health Care Superv* 15(1):24-31, 1996.

Jones A, Ridener AJ, Smith KG: Preparing for change: emergency department queuing theory and computer simulation, *Top Emerg Med,* pp 40-46, June 1997.

Millette BE: Using Gilligan's framework to analyze nurses' stories of moral choices, *West J Nurs Res* 16(6):660-674, 1994.

Parsons LC: Delegation skills and nurse job satisfaction, *Nurs Econ* 16:18-26, Jan-Feb 1998.

Quinn CA, Smith MD: *The professional commitment: issues and ethics in nursing,* Philadelphia, 1987, WB Saunders.

Sullivan PA: Common-sense ethics in administrative decision making, *JONA* 21:21-23, Oct 1991.

Trott MC: Legal issues for nurse managers, *Nurs Manage* 29:38-42, Jan 1998.

Warzlawick P, Winkland J, Fisch R: *Change: principles of problem formation and problem resolution,* New York, 1984, WW Norton.

Zielstorff RD: *Computers in nursing,* Rockville, Md, 1982, Aspen.

CASE STUDY

Your organization has limited funds for personnel raises. You represent your unit on the agency budget committee. Should you give everyone the same dollar amount raise, thus giving a lower percentage raise to personnel with larger salaries? Should you give the same percentage raise across the board, thus giving people with higher salaries more money? Should the raises be stratified, giving different categories of people different dollar or percentage raises? What are other options?

CASE STUDY

You are the nurse manager of a home health care agency. Because of your computer management programs you know how many supplies have been used in specific time frames and can anticipate how much of what will be needed in the future. Using the Vroom and Yetton normative model in Box 3-6, analyze the problem attributes and determine if you should use an autocratic, consultative, or group decision process to make a fast, economical, quality, and acceptable decision regarding ordering supplies for the unit.

Critical Thinking Activities for this chapter begin on page 478.

CHAPTER 4

MOTIVATION AND MORALE

CHAPTER OBJECTIVES

- Put Maslow's five needs into Alderfer's three categories of growth, relatedness, and existence needs.
- Identify at least five hygiene and five motivation factors in Herzberg's theory.
- Describe Vroom's expectancy theory.
- Explain how Skinner's positive reinforcement theory works.
- Describe ways people deal with perceived inequities.
- List at least three beliefs each for McGregor's Theory X and Theory Y.

Chapter Overview

Chapter 4 explains theories of motivation, including Taylor's monistic theory, Maslow's hierarchy-of-needs theory, Alderfer's modified need hierarchy, McClelland's basic needs theory, Herzberg's motivation-hygiene theory, or two-factor theory, Argyris's psychological energy theory, Vroom's expectancy theory, Skinner's positive reinforcement theory, equity theory, intrinsic motivation, McGregor's Theory X and Theory Y, Likert's participative management theory, and Theory Z. Historical development of motivation theory, morale, burnout, and job satisfaction are discussed.

MAJOR CONCEPTS AND DEFINITIONS	
Burnout	a state of emotional exhaustion
Climate	prevailing conditions affecting life
Dissatisfaction	discontent
Motivation	given impetus to incite or impel or to spur on
Intrinsic	essential, inherent, not dependent on external circumstances
Extrinsic	not inherent, not essential, external, extraneous
Job satisfaction	contentment with one's work

MOTIVATION

Why do people work? Why do some employees achieve high productivity while others are content with mediocrity or less? What can a manager do to stimulate intrinsic and extrinsic motivation? These questions are important to the manager. They elicit complex and uncertain answers. Unfortunately, there are no simple rules that a manager can follow to stimulate the staff.

Taylor's Monistic Theory

Monistic theory is derived from the principles of scientific management. Frederick Taylor, a pioneer in this field, believed that if energetic people with high productivity learn that they earn no more than a lazy worker who does as little as possible, they will lose interest in giving optimal performance. Taylor argued that an incentive is needed to prevent this loss. It should be possible to earn more by producing more, so that pay would depend on productivity. Incentives such as merit increases, bonus systems, profit sharing, savings sharing, and piece rates

are examples of monistic methods. With implementation of payment by piece rate, the employer must be certain that wage costs do not increase more rapidly than production. This system can place considerable pressure on the worker and create tensions that lead to undesirable behavior. Payment by piece rate almost certainly guarantees that some workers will be paid more than others. A larger paycheck may increase one's self-esteem and even serve as a status symbol, but the amount of motivation provided by money is questionable.

Maslow's Hierarchy of Needs

In contrast to Taylor's belief that money is a primary motivator, Abraham Maslow maintained that people are motivated by a desire to satisfy a hierarchy of needs. Maslow hypothesized that satisfaction of the basic physiological needs triggers the emergence of more abstract needs and that a satisfied need is no longer a motivator. The five basic needs he identified are physiological, safety/security, social/belonging, esteem, and self-actualization (Figure 4-1).

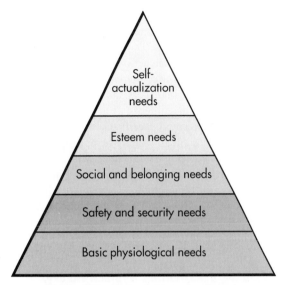

Figure 4-1 Maslow's hierarchy of needs.
Modified from Maslow, Abraham II, *Motivation and personality,* © 1954, © 1987, © 1970 by Abraham H. Maslow. Adapted by permission of Prentice-Hall, Inc, Upper Saddle River, NJ.

Existence needs
Relatedness needs
Growth needs

Physiological needs.   The body needs water, food, oxygen, elimination, rest, exercise, sex, shelter, and protection from the elements. People have a strong drive for self-preservation, and whenever their basic physiological needs are threatened, the needs become prepotent. These needs are relatively independent and must be met repeatedly to remain fulfilled. In an affluent society the physiological needs are probably not the most common motivators. The nurse manager should determine whether physiological needs are being met. Personnel should not be overworked. Meal breaks and rest breaks should be provided. Pay should be adequate for food, shelter, health care, and recreation.

Safety/security needs.   People need physical, emotional, and financial safety. They need a stable environment in which they are protected against the threats of danger and deprivation. People do not want to worry about inadequate income because of loss of job, accident, or old age. Arbitrary management actions, favoritism toward or discrimination against employees, and unpredictable administra-

tion of policy are dangerous to safety needs and should be avoided.

Social/belonging needs.   Social needs include a feeling of belonging, acceptance by one's peers, recognition as an accepted member of a group, being an integral part of the operation, giving and receiving friendship, and affectionate relations with others. A cohesive work group is likely to be more effective than an equal number of people working separately. Yet management, fearing hostility toward its objectives, may control situations to prevent *esprit de corps.* Thwarting of the social needs, however, may stimulate resistance and antagonism that further defeat management's objectives.

Esteem needs.   Achievement, competence, knowledge, independence, status, recognition, prestige, appreciation, reputation, and respect contribute to one's self-confidence and self-esteem. Management can help meet these needs by giving praise when it is deserved and through the use of constructive evaluations, pay raises, and titles. Unlike the lower physiological and safety needs, the esteem needs are not so easily satisfied.

Self-actualization needs.   It is doubtful that one ever achieves all that of which one is capable. Feelings of accomplishment, responsibility, importance, challenge, advancement, and new experiences and opportunities for growth contribute to self-fulfillment.

Alderfer's Modified Need Hierarchy

Clayton Alderfer proposes a modified need hierarchy theory that collapses Maslow's five hierarchical levels into three (Box 4-1). His existence-relatedness-growth (ERG) theory suggests that in addition to a satisfaction-progression process, in which people are constantly frustrated in their attempts to satisfy one level of needs, they can redirect their energy toward a lower-level need. Alderfer's model is less rigid than Maslow's and suggests that more than one need may be operative (Box 4-2).

McClelland's Basic Needs Theory

David McClelland has identified three basic needs that all people have in varying degrees: the need for achievement, power, and affiliation (Box 4-3). The need for achievement involves a desire to make a contribution, to excel, and to succeed. People with high achievement needs are eager for responsibility, take calculated risks, and desire feedback about their performance. People who have a high need for power want to be in control and desire influence over others. They are more interested in personal prestige and power than effective performance. For contrast, people with high affiliation needs desire working in human environments and seek out meaningful friendships. They want to be respected and avoid decisions or actions that oppose group norms. They are more interested in high morale than productivity. Managers should match personnel needs with assignments. If a project has well-defined objectives and specific tasks, a person with a high achievement need may be appropriate. If a project involves unpleasant tasks with personnel (such as retrenchment), a person with high power needs may do the job best. A person with high affiliation needs would not want to make decisions that would alienate peers but would be good for fostering morale.

Herzberg's Motivation-Hygiene Theory, or Two-Factor Theory

Frederick Herzberg found that work motivators include achievement, growth, responsibility, advancement, recognition, and the job itself. According to Herzberg, if people are satisfied with their job, they are receiving positive feedback, developing skills, and improving their performance. Herzberg maintains that employees can be motivated by giving them challenging work in which they can assume responsibility (Figure 4-2 and Box 4-4).

Dissatisfaction results when people perceive that they are being treated unfairly in pay, benefits, status, job security, supervision, and interpersonal relationships. Herzberg classifies all of the above as hygiene factors and argues that they are not motivators because they do not cause any improvement in attitudes or performance. They can only prevent

Box 4-2   COMPARISON OF MASLOW'S HIERARCHY OF NEEDS AND ALDERFER'S EXISTENCE, RELATEDNESS, AND GROWTH

Maslow	Alderfer
Self-actualization needs Esteem needs	Growth needs
Social/belonging needs	Relatedness needs
Safety/security needs Physiological needs	Existence needs

Box 4-3   MCCLELLAND'S BASIC NEEDS THEORY

Need for
Achievement
Affiliation
Power

Box 4-4   HERZBERG'S MOTIVATION-HYGIENE THEORY

Maintenance factors	Motivational factors
Dissatisfiers	Satisfiers
Hygiene factors	Motivators
Job contest	Job content
Extrinsic factors	Intrinsic factors

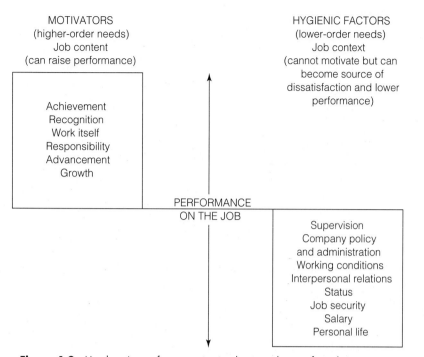

MOTIVATORS
(higher-order needs)
Job content
(can raise performance)

HYGIENIC FACTORS
(lower-order needs)
Job context
(cannot motivate but can
become source of
dissatisfaction and lower
performance)

Achievement
Recognition
Work itself
Responsibility
Advancement
Growth

PERFORMANCE
ON THE JOB

Supervision
Company policy
and administration
Working conditions
Interpersonal relations
Status
Job security
Salary
Personal life

Figure 4-2 Herzberg's two factor motivation hygiene theory of needs motivation.
From Claus KE, Bailey JT: *Power and influence in health care,* St. Louis, 1977, CV Mosby.

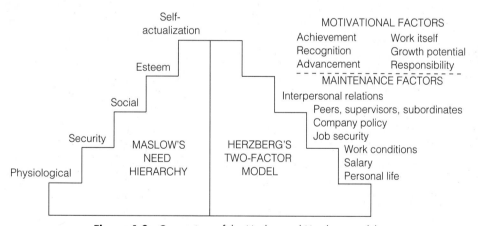

Self-
actualization

Esteem

Social

Security

Physiological

MASLOW'S
NEED
HIERARCHY

HERZBERG'S
TWO-FACTOR
MODEL

MOTIVATIONAL FACTORS

Achievement   Work itself
Recognition   Growth potential
Advancement   Responsibility

MAINTENANCE FACTORS

Interpersonal relations
Peers, supervisors, subordinates
Company policy
Job security
Work conditions
Salary
Personal life

Figure 4-3 Comparison of the Maslow and Herzberg models.
From Donnelly JH Jr, Gibson JL, Ivancevich JM: *Fundamentals of management: functions, behavior, models,*
ed 4, Dallas, 1990, Business Publications. © by Business Publications, Inc.

dissatisfaction and poor morale. Hygiene factors do not make a job more interesting. If people are highly motivated and find their job interesting and challenging, they can tolerate dissatisfaction with hygiene factors (Figures 4-3 and 4-4).

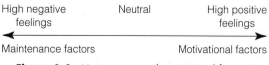

High negative   Neutral   High positive
feelings   feelings

Maintenance factors   Motivational factors

Figure 4-4 Maintenance and motivational factors.

Argyris's Psychological Energy Theory

Chris Argyris believes that people will exert more energy to meet their own needs than those of the organization. The greater the disparity between the individual's and the organization's goals, the more likely it is that the employee will feel dissatisfaction, tension, conflict, apathy, or subversion. Argyris suggests that management match personnel and jobs by taking advantage of people's talents and interests, make jobs interesting and challenging, help personnel satisfy their needs for self-actualization, improve interpersonal relationships, and use a management style consistent with Theory Y (which will be discussed later).

Vroom's Expectancy Theory

Victor Vroom popularized the expectancy theory during the 1960s. It is based on Kurt Lewin's field theory and has been expanded by Lyman Porter and others. Expectancy theory states that motivation is dependent on how much people want something and their estimate of the probability of getting it (Figure 4-5).

Valence is the strength of a person's preference for something. It may be negative or positive from −1 to +1. If the person does not want something, there is a negative valence. If the person is indifferent, the valence is 0. A positive valence indicates a desire for something (Figure 4-6, *A*).

Expectancy is the probability of getting something through specific actions. If a person believes that an action will result in an outcome, expectancy has a value of 1. If no probability is perceived, the expectancy is 0. Expectancy varies from one situation to another (Figure 4-6, *B*).

If someone has a high valence and a high expectancy, the motivation will be high. If there is a low valence and a low expectancy, the motivation will be low. If one is high and the other low, moderate motivation will result.

The expectancy theory has been further developed to include the value of the outcome factor. To be highly motivated, a person needs to find an outcome attractive, believe that certain actions will lead to the desired outcome, and assess that the result is worth the effort. Consequently, to motivate personnel, managers should clarify connections between work and outcome and should reward desirable behavior.

Skinner's Positive Reinforcement Theory

Operant conditioning and behavior modification are other names for B.F. Skinner's positive reinforcement theory. Behavior may be strengthened or weakened depending on what follows it. Positive reinforcement strengthens behavior. Withholding positive reinforcers weakens behavior, whereas intermittent reinforcement increases resistance to ex-

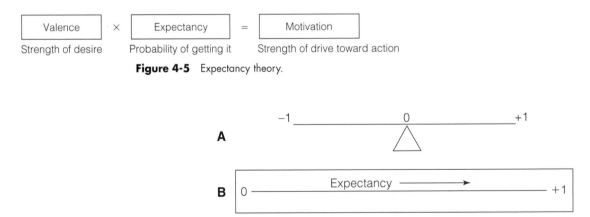

Valence	$\times$	Expectancy	$=$	Motivation
Strength of desire		Probability of getting it		Strength of drive toward action

Figure 4-5   Expectancy theory.

Figure 4-6   Ranges of valence and expectancy. **A,** Valence. **B,** Expectancy.

tinction. Punishment will help reduce behavior, but it cannot teach new behaviors, and it may condition avoidance.

Accentuating the positive with plenty of praise and positive feedback may increase the frequency of desired behavior. If, however, a subordinate admits to less than desirable behavior, the manager may respond, "I appreciate your honesty," while reminding the worker of the goal.

When desired results are not obtained, managers should analyze the situation. First, they should assess the working environment for interference. Do the employees have adequate time to complete the task? Does the system allow nurses to maximize their efficiency, or must they spend most of their time running to central supply to gather materials that should have been readily available? If managers do not locate the cause of the problem in the environment, they must ask themselves if the employees have been properly utilized. Do they have the knowledge and skills necessary to do the job? If not, can they be taught? If they cannot be taught, can they be replaced and assigned other duties?

Equity Theory

During the 1960s Jo Stacy Adams and others studied perceptions of equity and inequity. They found that employees assess fairness by considering their input and the psychological, social, and financial rewards in comparison with those of others. Perceived inequity causes tension. The amount of the tension was found to be proportional to the magnitude of the perceived inequity. Tension motivates people to reduce its cause. Consequently, the strength of the motivation to reduce the perceived inequity is proportional to the cognitive dissonance. To reduce the inequity, people may alter input or output, cognitively distort input or output, change the basis for comparison, or leave. If people feel overworked and underpaid, they are likely to decrease their productivity. Less often, employees feel overrewarded and strive to improve their performance. People resist changing their bases of comparison or distorting their perceptions. People

do not usually leave an organization unless there is extreme inequity. If the comparison is equal, people feel that they are treated fairly. If not, they are motivated to take corrective action. Managers should be attentive to the perceived equity of the reward system (Box 4-5).

Intrinsic Motivation

Edward Deci has studied intrinsic motivation. He found that some activities are ends in themselves, not just means to ends. There is no apparent reward except the activity itself. Intrinsically motivated behavior seems to be stimulated by people's needs for feeling competent and self-determining. When there is no stimulation, people will seek it. When they are overstimulated, they back away, regroup, and reaffirm competence. People engage in a process of seeking and conquering to feel competent and self-determined. When people's feelings of competence and self-determination are enhanced, their intrinsic motivation will increase. If their perceptions of competence and self-determination are diminished, their intrinsic motivation will decrease. Extrinsic rewards have a controlling aspect that may

---

Box 4-5 EQUITY THEROY

A person compares her input/output with and perceives relation to a reference person.

$$IP = IRP$$
$$OP = ORP$$
Equity

$$IP < IRP$$
$$OP < ORP$$
Inequity

$$IP > IRP$$
$$OP > ORP$$
Inequity

IP = Inputs of the person
OP = Outputs of the person
IRP = Inputs of reference person
ORP = Outputs of reference person

decrease intrinsic rewards. Insufficient extrinsic rewards tend to increase intrinsic motivation because people try to reduce cognitive dissonance. Consequently, managers should foster stimulation through means such as continuing education and special projects.

McGregor's Theory X and Theory Y

Douglas McGregor has classified traditional management theories as Theory X. They are based on the assumption that people will avoid work if possible because they dislike it; consequently, most people must be directed, controlled, coerced, and threatened. Theory X assumes that people want direction, have little ambition, avoid responsibility, but want security. A manager with a Theory X philosophy would probably use fear and threats to motivate personnel, supervise closely, delegate little responsibility, and not consider personnel participation in planning.

McGregor maintains that if people behave as described in Theory X it is because of what the system has done to them—not because of their inherent nature. He believes that as long as managerial strategies are based on Theory X, managers will fail to discover, let alone use, the potentials of their personnel.

McGregor classifies the newer developments in management as Theory Y. In this theory McGregor makes the assumption that people like and enjoy work, are self-directed, and seek responsibility. It maintains that most people have imagination, ingenuity, creativity, and other intellectual capacities that are only partially utilized. A manager with a Theory Y philosophy will use positive incentives such as praise and recognition, give general supervision, provide opportunities for individual growth, delegate responsibilities, and encourage participation in problem solving. Job enlargement and decentralization are additional motivational techniques that may stimulate personnel's performance to the extent that it exceeds the requirements stated in the job description (Box 4-6).

Likert's Participative Management Theory

Rensis Likert believes that effective managers are highly sensitive to their staff associates, use communication to keep the group working as a unit, and foster supportive relationships between all group members. Participative management is a human relations theory that may use management by objectives and job-enrichment approaches.

Theory Z

The Japanese form of participative management is known as Theory Z. The major firms of Japan are organized into *Zaibatsu*, small groups of 20 to 30 firms representing each important industrial sector.

Box 4-6 **MCGREGOR'S THEORY X AND Y**

X	Y
People dislike work.	Work is natural.
People must be directed to do work.	People will exercise self-control.
People want to avoid responsibility.	People enjoy responsibility.
People believe that achievement is irrelevant.	People value achievement.
People are dull and uncreative.	People have potential, imagination, and creativity.
Money is the reason for working.	Money is only one reason for working.
People lack desire to improve quality.	People want to improve quality.

Each firm hosts satellite companies that provide a service or manufacture a subassembly for the host firm. Employees are hired to work for the host firm until retirement. After slow evaluation and promotion in nonspecialized careers, employees are retired at age 55. They then work on a part-time basis for a satellite company. Women work temporarily and serve as a buffer to the job security of the male work force. Their schedules are flexible so they can care for their families, and they are laid off in slack periods.

Concern for the worker is apparent. Japanese companies form inclusive personal and professional relationships and provide social support. Because personnel anticipate lifetime relationships, they are cautious about interpersonal conflicts. Cooperation is stressed. Collective decision making is practiced. Through the ritual *ofringi,* ideas pass from manager to manager for approval. This helps establish trust and cooperation. Objectives and the procedures to achieve them are implicitly described. Quality circles are formed when 2 to 10 employees meet to identify problems, explore options, and make decisions. Quality circles have increased worker productivity, enhanced job satisfaction, and reduced turnover in addition to solving identified problems. Decisions are made by consensus. Because it takes so much time to reach a consensus, only policy and behavior changes are dealt with. Responsibility is also collective. An emphasis is placed on developing all aspects of the employees, and they are rewarded with regular pay bonuses based on the company's performance.

The Japanese Theory Z managers focus on the four soft S's of management: staff, skills, style, and superordinate goals. Staff is the workers. Skills are the capabilities of the organization or key personnel. Style refers to the cultural style of the organization or how managers achieve goals. The superordinate goals are the guideposts as determined by the personnel.

Less attention is given to the hard S's: system, structure, and strategy. The system is the mechanism whereby information circulates through the organization. Structure is the organization, and strategy is the plan of action.

Historical Development of Motivation Theory

Traditional management theory is based on McGregor's Theory X. Traditional theory addresses itself to Maslow's primary physiological and safety needs and employs the monistic theory for reinforcement. The latter, according to Herzberg, helps meet some of the hygiene needs but does not provide motivation.

Newer developments in management are based on McGregor's Theory Y. Maslow's secondary needs of belonging, esteem, and self-actualization are more prepotent than the primary needs for most personnel. Because a satisfied need is no longer a motivator, hygiene factors such as money and working conditions do not serve as motivators. People are more interested in autonomy, responsibility, achievement, recognition, variety in work, and efforts for self-actualization. Argyris has suggested that personnel may become more self-actualized if their personal goals are consistent with the goals of the organization. Talents and interests should be considered when assigning jobs. And then, according to Skinner, positive reinforcement will further increase desired behaviors.

Participation is a major factor in newer management techniques. Personnel are encouraged to contribute to decisions, goals, and plans. Decentralization is supported to the point of management by objectives, allowing personnel to define their own objectives and to determine how they plan to achieve them. The supervisor approves the goals, makes sure they are consistent with the organization's goals, and evaluates personnel using their own objectives as the standard. Modern managers delegate duties and assist others to work more effectively. They help each person develop her own talents and try to maintain a close relationship between the interests and skills of the individual and the requirements of the job. Job enrichment and job rotation may be used to help develop personnel fully. When personnel are actively striving toward esteem and self-actualization and when their goals are consistent with those of the organization, there is likely to be a noticeable effect on the accomplishment of the organization's goals and productivity.

Morale

Morale is a state of mind related to cheerfulness, confidence, and discipline. A person who works confidently, courageously, and with discipline demonstrates high morale. A person who is cowardly, disorderly, devious, fearful, and rebellious demonstrates low morale. Morale is related to productivity, quality, job satisfaction, and motivation. Morale is related to leadership style and the interpersonal and communication skills of the leader. Recognition and praise contribute to high morale.

Replacing competition with an effort to outdo one's own previous accomplishments is helpful. That leads to continuous improvement. One sees others as benchmarks while trying to improve one's own performance and appreciates one's own importance. This replaces the old competitive paradigm of the game where the goal is winning; the others are enemies; and I am separate and better than they. The transformational leader helps others gain enthusiasm from shared accomplishments and permission to take risks. This encourages initiating, asserting, engaging, collaborating, appreciating, and supporting toward a high-focused energy.

Organizational morale is the attitudes of the workers toward the quality of their work lives. Each work environment is unique, and each worker's view of the quality of life is uniquely related to how it satisfies one's needs. Managers should survey workers' perceptions of the importance of job factors and their satisfaction with those factors. Common factors affecting morale, in alphabetical order, are as follows (Morrison, 1993, p. 301):

Absence of apathy

Absence of undue stress associated with the job

Advancement based on merit

Career goal progress

Confidence in the management

Development and utilization of skills, talents, and abilities

Economic well-being (salary, benefits)

Employee commitment, involvement, and influence

Employee state of mind

Impact of job on personal life

Physical working environment

Relations with supervisor and work group

Respect for the individual

Union-management relations

Because both the individual worker and the work environment are changing, managers need to constantly monitor the work environment regarding morale and job satisfaction. Increased interpersonal conflict; criticism of policies, procedures, and rules and disregard of rules; decreased productivity; decreased quality of work; and increased lateness, absenteeism, and job turnover are signs of low morale. Managers can observe, listen, and ask related questions to assess morale.

There are age-related differences related to morale. Younger people make commitments to the job more slowly than older adults do. They are concerned about career decisions rather than just working. Because they often have been raised under more permissive conditions than older people have, they respond well to participative leadership styles rather than an autocratic environment. Challenge, opportunity to learn, and involvement are more important to the younger worker, while security becomes increasingly important as the worker grows older. Money is important but is not always the most important factor. Automation has eliminated most of the need for physical labor and endurance that were important in the past. Young people tend to be loyal to their profession but not necessarily to the job or boss. They tend to want to prove themselves, push for opportunities, and be recognized.

It is natural for older workers to refer to how it was done in the past. They need consistent and frequent feedback to help them through change. They have been through a variety of leadership styles, may be suspicious of new leadership, and need open and direct communication. It is preferable to ask them for what the manager wants and needs specifically. They seem to respect high standards. They respond favorably to having their knowledge and experience used. They like to know that seniority counts. Habits, routines, and work schedules may be ingrained and difficult to change.

Manager morale is important too. The first 3 months on a new job are very important for setting an impression. Projecting confidence and enthusiasm and building relationships are important. Each worker should be respected and treated fairly and equally to develop credibility. Managers should act as a buffer for outside stressors, should save time for planning, and should not make changes too quickly. Managers should involve people in decisions and slowly introduce innovations to help maintain good morale. They should get to know the business and the people, communicate the goals and expectations clearly, clarify values and priorities, and motivate, delegate to, and reward people. It is very important for managers to replenish their energy by eating a balanced diet, exercising, resting, and relaxing to help maintain their morale.

Burnout

Burnout is a syndrome of physical and emotional exhaustion that leads to negative attitudes and behaviors. The major cause is stress. It leads to the signs of low morale and job dissatisfaction. Prevention is the best strategy. Managers should try to prevent overwhelming situations. One should appraise the situation, set priorities, and focus on what work needs to be done. Meeting goals can reduce stress. When one is busy doing what one can, achieving goals, feeling comfortable with what one is doing, and getting recognition for work well done, one will probably use less energy for being stressed. Open communications, identifying negative feelings and talking them through, good nutrition, physical exercise, rest and relaxation, and stress management should help prevent burnout. The manager can help create a pleasant work environment, set realistic goals, make realistic demands on self and others,

acknowledge people's good work, prioritize, identify and talk about negative feelings, rotate undesirable, popular, and unpopular tasks, and facilitate good nutrition, exercise, rest and recreation, and various relaxation and stress management techniques (Morrison, 1993).

Personal hardiness through commitment, control, and challenge helps prevent burnout. Commitment is a tendency to involve oneself in whatever one does to find purpose and meaning in events, things, and people. Control is influence over the surroundings, events, and people. One believes one can influence life events rather than feel helpless. Challenge is anticipation of change as an opportunity instead of a threat. Stress management techniques help prevent burnout. Exercise, good nutrition, rest, and relaxation are helpful. Setting limits on commitment to work and giving attention to meaningful relationships and satisfying activities are important.

Burnout is a state of emotional exhaustion. It is characterized by depletion of energies, disillusionment, doubts, depersonalization, and frustration, leading to loss of purpose, ideas, and energy. A person with burnout may feel alienated, apathetic, and exhausted. The person is at high risk of developing symptoms of stress, including backaches, headaches, indigestion, and lowered resistance. Family difficulties and social problems may develop. Burnout leads to excessive absenteeism and turnover.

Factors contributing to burnout include but are not limited to long hours, dissatisfaction with quality of work, lots of paperwork, lack of appreciation, lack of support, low pay, sense of powerlessness, and few advancement opportunities.

Improving job design, personnel policies, and staff relationships are appropriate. A stress management workshop including delegation, time management, meditation, relaxation techniques, and yoga could help. A multifaceted worker-support program including exercise programs; nutrition instruction; stress management; health promotion education such as hypertension screening, stop-smoking activities, and weight loss plans; and individual counseling helps.

Job Satisfaction

Job dissatisfaction contributes to higher turnover rates and decreased productivity. Considerable time and money are required to recruit and select a replacement for someone who leaves a position. It takes time to socialize the new employee to the organization's norms. This orientation period is expensive because of educational expenses and decreased productivity. Other employees must carry more than their share of the load until the new individual can work to capacity, and group redevelopment is necessary after each change in membership. For all these reasons job satisfaction is a concern for nursing administrators.

Job dissatisfaction has been shown to be correlated with absenteeism and turnover. Herzberg maintains that satisfiers and dissatisfiers are mutually exclusive; he classifies the sense of achievement, recognition for achievement, the work itself, responsibility, advancement potential, and possibility of growth as motivators or satisfiers and matters such as working conditions, policies, supervision, interpersonal relations, salary, status, and job security as hygiene factors or dissatisfiers. He concludes that hygiene factors cannot motivate employees but can only prevent dissatisfaction. Herzberg's work remains controversial.

Maslow's theory shows insight into Herzberg's findings. It suggests that hygiene factors can be motivators and that only when hygiene factors are satisfied do satisfiers such as responsibility become motivators. Several research studies have indicated that people at lower educational, socioeconomic, and occupational levels and minority members tend to place more emphasis on hygiene or extrinsic job factors, whereas people at higher educational, socioeconomic, and occupational levels and whites are more concerned with motivators or intrinsic factors. In accordance with Maslow's theory, physiological and safety needs are apparently prepotent for lower socioeconomic groups, whereas these needs have probably been satisfied for people at higher educational and occupational levels, such as nurses, for whom esteem and self-actualization needs have become prepotent.

Researchers disagree about the effects of supervision on job satisfaction. Employees' attitudes toward supervision are influenced by their perception of the supervisor's role, their self-perception, and their level of development. These individual differences necessitate that supervision be an adaptive leadership process.

The desire for influence in decision making is also affected by individual differences. Even though people presumably desire some control over their environment, this desire is not equally strong for all people. Vroom found that authoritarians are relatively unaffected by participating in decision making but that participation in decision making generally has a favorable effect on job satisfaction. Role ambiguity, the result of a failure to inform an individual of what is needed to do the job, is relatively common. Even if the role is clear, an employee in that role may resign if role conflict is present and persists. Role conflicts may result from a number of factors and are affected by individual differences. Likewise, job satisfaction is multidimensional and subject to individual differences.

Women seem to show more variation than men in their job attitudes. Women emphasize working conditions, hours and ease of work, supervision, and social aspects of the job, whereas men emphasize wages, opportunity for advancement, company management and policies, and task interest. College-educated women rank the importance of motivators such as achievement, recognition, and responsibility significantly higher than female clerical workers without college degrees. People tend to have more job satisfaction before the age of 20 years and after the age of 35 years than during the period between. Younger people tend to be more interested in income, whereas older people are interested in security.

Nurses surveyed about their sources of satisfaction identify a sense of achievement, recognition, challenging work, responsibility, advancement potential, autonomy, authority, pleasant work environment, agreeable working hours, and adequate staffing all as satisfiers. Nurses stress the importance of respected hospital administrators, supportive nursing administrators, trustful managers, fair evaluations, and adequate feedback. Poor planning, poor communication, inadequate explanations of decisions affecting jobs, unclear rules and regulations, unreasonable pressure, excessive work, workload negatively affecting work quality, understaffing, uncooperative physicians, nonnursing duties, and unqualified managers are all sources of dissatisfaction. Reduced productivity, increased absenteeism, and rapid turnover are expensive consequences of job dissatisfaction but can be reduced if the nursing administrator fosters job satisfaction through organization and management (Marriner, 1982).

CHAPTER SUMMARY

Chapter 4 covered the following:
Motivation
    Taylor's Monistic Theory
    Maslow's Hierarchy of Needs
        Physiological needs
        Safety/security needs
        Social/belonging needs
        Esteem needs
        Self-actualization needs
    Alderfer's Modified Need Hierarchy
    McClelland's Basic Needs Theory
    Herzberg's Motivation-Hygiene Theory, or Two-Factor Theory
    Argyris's Psychological Energy Theory
    Vroom's Expectancy Theory
    Skinner's Positive Reinforcement Theory
    Equity Theory
    Intrinsic Motivation
    McGregor's Theory X and Theory Y
    Likert's Participative Management Theory
    Theory Z
    Historical Development of Motivation Theory
Morale
Burnout
Job Satisfaction

REFERENCES

Claus KE, Bailey JT: *Power and influence in health care,* St. Louis, 1977, CV Mosby.

Donnelly JH Jr, Gibson JL, Ivancevich JM: *Fundamentals of management: functions, behavior, models,* ed 4, Dallas, 1990, Business Publications.

Marriner A: *Contemporary nursing management,* St. Louis, 1982, CV Mosby.

Maslow AH II: *Motivation and personality,* ed 3, Upper Saddle River, NJ, 1987, Prentice-Hall.

Morrison M: *Professional skills for leadership: foundations of a successful career,* St. Louis, 1993, Mosby.

BIBLIOGRAPHY

Albrecht M, Goeppinger J, Anderson MK et al.: The Albrecht nursing model for home healthcare, *JONA* 23:51-54, Jan 1993.

Baard PP, Neville SM: The intrinsically motivated nurse: help and hindrance from evaluation feedback sessions, *JONA* 26:19-25, July-Aug 1996.

Beaulieu R et al.: Empowerment and commitment of nurses in long-term care, *Nurs Econ* 15:32-41, Jan-Feb 1997.

Breisch LR: Motivate! *Nurs Manage,* pp 27-29, March 1999.

Deci E, Ryan RM: The support of autonomy and the control of behavior, *J Pers Soc Psychol* 53:1024-1037, Dec 1987.

Douglass LM: *The effective nurse leader and manager,* St. Louis, 1996, Mosby.

Festinger L: *A theory of cognitive dissonance,* Evanston, Ill, 1957, Row, Peterson.

Gillies DA: *Nursing management: a systems approach,* Philadelphia, 1994, WB Saunders.

Goodell TT, Coeling HVE: Outcomes of nurses' job satisfaction, *JONA* 24:36-41, Nov 1994.

Grohar-Murray ME, DiCroce HR: Leadership and management in nursing, Stamford, Conn, 1997, Appleton & Lange.

Harris W: Withering on the vine: ten ways to ensure your employees become stagnant, *Supervision* 60:12+, Jan 1999.

Hausfeld J, Gibbons K, Hotlmeier A et al.: Self-staffing: improving care and staff satisfaction, *Nurs Manage* 25:74-80, Oct 1994.

Herzberg F: One more time: how do you motivate employees? *Harv Bus Rev* 46:53-62, Jan-Feb 1968.

Huber D: *Leadership and nursing care management,* Philadelphia, 1996, WB Saunders.

Hurst KL, Croker PA, Bell SK: How about a lollipop? A peer recognition program, *Nurs Manage* 25:68-72, Sept 1994.

Irvine DM, Evans MG: Job satisfaction and turnover among nurses: integrating research findings across studies, *Nurs Res* 44:246-251, July-Aug 1996.

Kielson DC: The new paradigm for competition, *Futurist* 28:64, Nov-Dec 1994.

Kovner CT et al.: Nursing care delivery models and nurse satisfaction, *Nurs Adm Q* 19:74-85, Fall 1994.

Laabs J: Killing the spirit—one worker goes from committed, to wanting to be committed, *Workforce* 77:47, Nov 1998.

Maslow AH: *Motivation and personality,* New York, 1987, Prentice Hall.

Mason JE: Superb customer service comes from within, *Nurs Manage,* p 31, Sept 1998.

McGregor DM: *The human side of enterprise,* New York, 1960, Harper and Row.

McClelland DC: Managing motivation to expand human freedom, *Am Psychology* 33:201-210, March 1978.

McConnell CR: The evolving role of the health care supervisor: shifting paradigms, changing perceptions, and other traps, *Health Care Superv* 15(1):1-11, 1996.

McNeese-Smith DK: Job satisfaction, productivity, and organizational commitment, *JONA* 25:17-25, Sept 1995.

McNeese-Smith DK: The influence of manager behavior on nurses' job satisfaction, productivity, and commitment, *JONA* 27:47-54, Sept 1997.

Morrison RS, Jones LD, Fuller B: The relation between leadership style and empowerment on job satisfaction of nurses, *JONA* 27:27-34, May 1997.

Ouchi WG: *Theory Z: how American business can meet the Japanese challenge,* Reading, Mass, 1981, Addison-Wesley.

Pierce LL, Hazel CM, Mion LC: Effect of a professional practice model on autonomy, job satisfaction and turnover, *Nurs Manage* 27:48M-48T, Feb 1996.

Seyle H: *The stress of life,* New York, 1956, McGraw-Hill.

Swansburg RC: *Management and leadership for nurse managers,* Boston, 1996, Jones & Bartlett.

Swansburg RC, Swansburg RJ: *Introductory management and leadership for nurses,* Boston, 1999, Jones & Bartlett.

Tappen RM: *Nursing leadership and management: concepts and practice,* Philadelphia, 1995, FA Davis.

Vance A, Davidhizar R: Motivating the paraprofessional in long-term care, *Health Care Superv* 15(4):57-65, 1997.

Vroom V: *Work and motivation,* New York, 1964, Wiley.

CASE STUDY

You have identified that Ann has a high need for achievement, Betty for power, and Carl for affiliation. What assignments will you give them to meet those needs and motivate them?

Critical Thinking Activities for this chapter begin on page 481.

CHAPTER 5

POWER, POLITICS, NEGOTIA- TIONS, AND LABOR RELATIONS

CHAPTER OBJECTIVES

- Identify at least five sources of power.
- Describe ways to communicate with legislators.
- Describe the process by which a bill becomes a law.
- Describe principled negotiations.
- Compare hard and soft negotiation tactics.
- Describe the four phases of unionization.
- Explain the decertification process.
- Identify advantages and disadvantages of collective bargaining.

Chapter Overview

Chapter 5 describes power, authority, politics, sources of power, power relations, kinds of power, negotiations, labor relations, labor laws, unionization, nurse managers' role in collective bargaining, and advantages and disadvantages of collective bargaining.

MAJOR CONCEPTS AND DEFINITIONS

Power	one's capacity to influence others
Formal power	power related to position
Informal power	power related to personal power
Reward	something given in recompense for a good deed
Coercive	restraining, constraining, or curbing in nature
Legitimate	logically correct
Referent	a type of power based on identification with a leader and what that leader symbolizes
Expert	skillful, having knowledge and training
Information	knowledge, access to information
Connection	coalition
Authority	legitimate power determined by structure
Politics	authoritative allocation of scarce resources
Negotiation	bargaining process
Labor relations	relations between the workers and management
Unionization	organization of workers
Collective bargaining	organization of workers to bargain for working conditions
Synergy	the sum is greater than the individual parts

POWER, AUTHORITY, AND POLITICS

Power and authority are closely related and often confused. Power is one's capacity to influence others, whereas authority is the right to direct others. One's power may be greater or less than the authority of the position. Authority is obtained through position power, but several other sources of power exist (Box 5-1). Politics uses legitimate power.

Sources of Power

Reward. Much of a manager's power comes from the ability to reward others for complying. When the staff associate perceives that managers have the ability to provide something valued, the manager has reward power. Sources of reward power include money, desired assignments, provision of personal space, or the acknowledgment of accomplishments. Rewards contribute to an independent system.

**Box
5-1   SOURCES OF POWER**

Reward	Referent
Coercive	Expert
Legitimate	Information and connection

Coercive power. Coercive power is the opposite of reward power and is based on fear of punishment if one fails to conform. Undesired assignments, embarrassment in front of others, withheld pay increases, and termination are sources of coercive power that contribute to a dependent system.

Legitimate power. Their official positions in the organizational hierarchy give managers legitimate power. Legitimate power gives the manager the right to influence and the staff associate an obligation to accept that influence. The director of nursing has more legitimate power than the manager, who in turn has more legitimate power than the head nurse. Cultural values that give a person the right to prescribe appropriate behavior for another (such as parents for children), social structures involving a hierarchy of authority, and election processes to legitimize a person's right to an office are bases for legitimate power.

Referent power. Referent power is based on identification with a leader and what that leader symbolizes. The leader is admired and exerts influence because the followers desire to be like the leader.

Expert power. People gain expert power through knowledge, skills, and information. Their expertise gains them respect and compliance. Knowledge of the organization and its rules, regulations, and work flow helps one to acquire power over others who need the knowledge to meet their responsibilities (Loveridge and Cummings, 1996).

Information. Information power comes from knowledge and access to information.

Connection. Connection power comes from coalitions and interpersonal relations.

Sources of Personal Power

Expand your personal resources. Start by taking good care of yourself. Eat a well balanced diet. Rest. Relax. Exercise. Develop relationships. Develop hobbies and interests. Have fun. Develop and focus on your goals. Recognize opportunities. Be assertive. Learn how to collect and review accurate information. Be a proactive decision maker. Expand your personal resources by broadening your skill base and continuing your education. Show up to do networking and develop political alliances and coalitions. Ninety percent of success may be showing up and volunteering.

Sources of Interpersonal Power

Connection power. This is a power based on connections with a powerful person or others as a way to get accurate and reliable information. One can expand the network of communication contacts to increase connection power by joining listservs and professional organizations and volunteering for committee work.

Information power. Information is power if used strategically. Increase information power through connections and try to get on routing lists.

Group decision-making power. Synergy can be created when people come together to make decisions and go forth as a united front. Increase decision-making power by volunteering for problem-solving task forces.

Sources of Position Power

Centrality. Access to information in a communication network increases position power. Increase centrality power by getting centrally located and by having information routed through you.

Criticality.   Criticality increases position power. It is determined by (1) how dependent others are on the work performed by the position, (2) the number of others performing the same tasks, and (3) the level of knowledge and skills required by the position. General-purpose positions have less power than highly technical and specialized positions, which fewer people can do. One can increase criticality by increasing technical sophistication of one's job, making part of one's job responsibilities unique, and by taking on tasks that are critical to the work processing.

Flexibility.   Flexibility or discretion allows one to exercise judgment. It is associated with the life cycle of a position. It is more difficult to routinize new tasks than old tasks. The number of rules governing a position increases with the number of people occupying the position over time. Flexibility is associated with novelty and variety. The more routine the work and the fewer tasks assigned to a person the easier it is to routinize, and the less powerful the position is. One can increase flexibility power by getting involved in new projects, participating in decision-making processes, initiating new ideas, reducing the percentage of routine activities in one's job, expanding task novelty and variety, and seeking unusual jobs rather than maintenance-oriented, repetitive jobs.

Relevance.   Positions related to central objectives and issues of the organization have more position power. The trainer or mentor, evaluator, and advocate or representative are relevantly powerful positions. Trainers reduce uncertainty for new employees and tend to be appreciated by those who have benefited from the training. Evaluators are powerful by virtue of the dependence on good evaluations for organizational rewards. Advocacy identifies a person with important causes. One can increase relevance power by becoming involved in activities central to the priorities of the organization and by expanding one's work domain.

Visibility.   A key to success is excellent performance multiplied by visibility. Direct contact with face-to-face communication is a way to have visibility. A good presentation of a report will get more visibility than writing the report. Participating in problem-solving task forces gives one visibility. Name recognition gives visibility and can be addressed by introducing oneself to others, using business cards, sending out information with a signed cover note, sending a note of congratulations or appreciation to colleagues as appropriate, and sharing good ideas with appropriate parties in person with a follow-up memo.

Informal Sources of Power

Informal sources of power are related to one's personal power rather than position power. Some people have situational power because they happen to be in the right place at the right time. Others have personal power because of their unique characteristics.

Education, experience, drive, and decisiveness are viewed positively and help establish credibility. The person with these qualities may be viewed as reliable, and therefore others are willing to cooperate. Attractiveness gains an individual access to people who will help promote the cause, because people enjoy being around others who have a happy temperament, generate a sense of well-being, and foster goodwill in others. Personal appearance, good manners, body language, posture, gestures, eye contact, and speech with a firm, confident voice contribute to personal power. Location also influences others, because individuals communicate more with people who are located near them in the organization, and communication increases their opportunities to influence. For instance, full voting membership on powerful committees places one in close proximity for persuading other members and provides the opportunity to confront, negotiate, and solve problems. In general, people are most comfortable with others who have similar values, beliefs, and customs. Social pressure from people who share social norms encourages others to conform to those norms. Coalitions strengthen one's power base. Consequently, friendships and associations with people can be a source of power.

Interpersonal relationships also provide access to the informal communication network. Doing favors for others so that they owe you favors creates an obligation-based power. One may gain power by default when there is no one else available or by autonomy when the decision is one's own to make. Control of resources such as information, procedures, equipment, and personnel also strengthens one's power base. Religion, politics, race, and national origin are bases for establishing power in some situations but interfere with power bases in others. For example, a nurse of a certain faith may be given priority for a job on the staff of an institute run by that faith, but religion may be held against the person seeking position at a hospital affiliated with another religion or denomination.

Organizational informal power is enhanced by expertise, career goal setting, and communication skills plus understanding the organization, a sense of unity with the organizational goals, mentoring, networking, coalition building, negotiating, collaborating, fostering collegiality, and using an empowering attitude.

Power Relations

Power is interpersonal. It is a dependence relationship. Person x has power over person y to the extent that y depends on x for goal attainment. The power varies inversely to the availability of goals outside the particular interpersonal relationship. If nurses want to work for a hospital but do not care whether they work for one head nurse or another, they reduce the head nurses' power. Motivational investment in the goals being mediated is a variable. The nurse who wants to work in intensive coronary care is far more dependent on one head nurse than the nurse who is willing to work on several units. Cost of goal achievement is also a factor. Nurses may not be willing to work straight nights to work on the unit of their choice. A staff nurse may not be willing to hassle with a grievance procedure to get what is deserved. Sources of dependence are numerous: knowledge, skills, interpersonal relations, and organizational authority.

Predictable behaviors occur when there is a conflict of interest between people with power. Coalition is a technique to strengthen one's power. It involves uniting to gain a sense of strength. Whether coalition occurs or not, there will probably be bargaining in an attempt to negotiate the conflict. One may leave the situation if bargaining is ineffective or adjust to lessened power if alternative positions are not readily available.

It is useful to assess one's power in a relationship before engaging in conflict. Although there is no magic formula to assess one's power, there are considerations that help identify one's power in relation to that of others. Who is the most powerful? The person who appears the most powerful may not be. Communication patterns help assess who actually has the power. The person who structures the options has more power, whereas the person who does more accommodating probably has less power. The person with the least interest in maintaining the relationship has more power. Those who gain the most from ritualized patterns have the most power, because institutionalized norms reinforce the existing power structure, and people who try to maintain the status quo are probably protecting their own power. People who are aware of their sources of power can use that knowledge, but people are often unaware of their sources of power and consequently are unable to use those sources effectively.

Kinds of Power

In *Power and Innocence* Rollo May has identified five kinds of power. Exploitative power is the most destructive type. It subjects people to whatever use the power holder chooses. Slavery is an example. Manipulative power is influence over another person that may have been invited because of the person's desperation and anxiety. Operant conditioning is an example of manipulative power. Competitive power is energy used against another. One person wins and another loses, although neither the gain nor the loss is necessarily related to merit. An example is the competition of several people for one position. One person wins, and the others lose—even if they were well qualified for the job. Nutrient power, such as parents' caring for their children, teachers' caring for students, and politicians' caring for their constituents, is influence used for others. Integrative power is cooperative power with others. A person can possess the five types of power at different times (Box 5-2).

Authority

Authority is legitimate power. It is determined by structure, which involves rules, roles, and relations. Rules legitimize authority and tend to suspend the subordinate's critical faculties. Subordinates tend to do unquestioningly what the superior with legitimate authority tells them to do. Role is position or office. Authority is inherent in the position, not in the person. Relations are related to credibility, which is obtained through knowledge and expertise.

Authority is traditionally structured as line or staff. Line authority refers to levels of authority and superior-subordinate relationships, and it therefore provides the framework for the organization. Staff authority has no command privileges. It has only the right to advise or assist managers in the performance of their duties. Staff members provide assistance when requested, must sell their ideas to the manager over whom they have no authority, and must sell their ideas up the line to managers who have the line authority to implement the ideas. More recently, functional authority, or authority of the specialist, has emerged. Functional authority is normally limited to the performance of defined duties for a limited period of time.

It is preferable for a manager's power to be equitable to the authority of the position. Knowledge,

Box 5-2	KINDS OF POWER

Exploitative
Manipulative
Competitive
Nutrient
Integrative

experience, drive, and decisiveness help achieve power. Being attractive, visible, and available are sources of informal power. More formal sources of power available to nurse managers are control of resources, reward and coercive power, association with other powerful people, and legitimate power derived from the managerial position. The nurse manager's knowledge of sources of power can help her assess and use them.

Power and Gender

Gender differences are noted in relation to power. There has been a tendency to socialize women into family and societal roles to facilitate others' success. Men have generally been socialized to relate to others' rank and status. Power is likely to be perceived within the nursing profession differently from outside the profession. Nurses are commonly stereotyped as "superwomen," "iron maidens," or "mothers." Superwomen often are isolated and overcommitted, demanding perfection and refusing to delegate. Iron maidens tend to be distant, competitive, and controlling. They may critically sabotage collaboration. Mothers tend to be passive, sacrificing peacemakers who foster dependence. These roles may be perceived as dysfunctional in a male-dominated organization (Cummings, 1995).

Gendering of occupations is apparent in health care, with most physicians being men and most nurses being women. Men had limited opportunities in nursing until after World War II. Then nursing education for men was facilitated through financial support from GI bills. Men in nursing have often experienced role strain. Female nurses have often expected male nurses to function like orderlies by assisting with lifting and transferring patients and by doing male procedures. As society begins to challenge gender-specific occupations, we may begin to see more men in nursing (Hein, 1998).

Empowerment

Empowerment is the process of gaining control. One can use physical, psychological, and material resources to empower oneself. Maintaining one's physical health provides a basis for personal power. A balanced diet, exercise, rest, and relaxation help one maintain good health, making it easier to become more powerful.

Personal psychological resources are also important for gaining control. One should schedule activities to maintain one's mental health and emotional balance. One needs a strong self-concept and a clear understanding of one's strengths and weaknesses. Effective decision making and creative problem solving demonstrate power. One needs to be able to admit mistakes and look for solutions instead of someone to blame. Maintaining a positive outlook is important to one's power.

Material resources may include money, clothing, supplies, or personnel. Much power is derived from control of material resources. An awareness of what material resources are needed and how to get them is important to empowerment.

One can help empower oneself by developing expertise through formal education, continuing education, in-service classes, and reading. Joining a professional organization, attending meetings, and reading professional journals help develop both information and connection power. One can seek legitimate power by seeking a position or promotion to a position with greater authority and to where one can use reward or perhaps coercive power.

Empowerment means providing freedom that allows people to successfully do what they want to do rather than getting them to do what the managers want them to do. Removing controls and constraints empowers people. Managers design work situations to energize and stimulate intrinsic encouragement. People then perform because of intrinsic motivation instead of external rewards. Empowered employees tend to be more satisfied, productive, and innovative. They are likely to produce higher quality products and services than nonempowered employees. Nurse managers can empower employees by letting those closest to the situation do the decision making, encouraging personal growth and achievement of organizational goals, recognizing excellence and expertise, and emphasizing the importance of contributions of individuals. This may help develop self-confidence and higher self-esteem. Patients can be given cognitive

and decisional control too. Clients can be informed of what is happening and what is expected in the future. They can be allowed to make decisions based on information and their goals.

Managers and nurses may have difficulty empowering others because of negative attitudes about others, personal insecurities, or a desire for power. Some managers may think that subordinates avoid work, are not competent, are not interested, and will not accept responsibility. The manager may fear subordinates' making mistakes, getting the recognition, or even doing better than the manager could do. Some people have a high need to control and direct and may fear confusion if they do not closely snoopervise. And then empowerment is not completely controlled by the manager; some people refuse to feel empowered no matter how much a manager does to empower others.

David Whetten and Kim Cameron (1998) have identified five dimensions of empowerment based on research by Gretchen Spreitzer (1992) and Aneil Mishra (1992): a sense of (1) self-efficacy, (2) self-determination, (3) personal consequences, (4) meaning, and (5) trust. When people have self-efficacy, they feel competent and confident. People need to believe that they have the ability and the necessary effort and support to do the task. Having a choice is necessary for self-determination. A sense of self-control is a desired personal consequence. People need to make a sense of meaning out of a task to get committed to it. Then people get a sense of trust and feel they will be treated fairly.

Whetten and Cameron (1998, p. 387) have identified nine prescriptions for fostering empowerment as "(1) articulating a clear vision and goals, (2) fostering personal mastery experiences, (3) modeling, (4) providing support, (5) creating emotional arousal, (6) providing necessary information, (7) providing necessary resources, (8) connecting to outcomes, and (9) creating confidence." The best ways to articulate a vision are through metaphors, real-life examples, stories, and word pictures. SMART goals are specific, measurable, aligned, reachable, and time bound. Vision and goals should be associated with personal values. Success breeds success. Managers need to help employees develop an awareness and belief that they can succeed. Finding opportunities for small successes or a small-wins strategy can help build self-confidence and lead to bigger successes. Managers can divide large problems into smaller ones and assign simpler tasks before more complex ones. Managers can role model by demonstrating correct and desirable behavior and can give recognition to others' successes. Feedback about good performance, praise, thank-you notes, and recognition ceremonies provide support. It is also important to provide social and emotional support. Counseling and training can help empower people through changes. They can also help replace negative emotions like anxiety, fear, and complaints with positive emotions like anticipation, excitement, and passion. Information is a power tool that helps empower people with self-determination, personal control, and trust to work more productively in harmony with the manager's goals. If people are given relevant information instead of too much, overload is less likely to occur. People need task-related information and the resources necessary to do their jobs. Connecting an individual's work with organizational outcomes helps develop a sense of self-efficacy and personal consequence. According to Whetten and Cameron (1998, p. 394), (1) reliability, (2) fairness, (3) caring, (4) openness, and (5) competence contribute to a sense of confidence and trustworthiness. Authentic, honorable, and trustworthy behavior contributes to confidence in employees and managers.

Empowered Delegation

Research results show a positive correlation between participation and acceptance of change, commitment, desire for more work, productivity, and satisfaction. Quality of decisions can be improved through empowered delegation by using more information closer to the problem than the manager alone has. Whetten and Cameron (1998, p. 397) have identified "five dimensions of empowerment: a sense of competence, choice, impact, value, and security." Unfortunately, when poorly done, delegation can have negative consequences that inhibit empowerment, subvert the ability to get the tasks accomplished, take more time, increase frustration

and stress, and create chaos. Managers need to consider when to delegate to whom and how.

Based on Victor Vroom and Philip Yetton (1973) and Vroom and Arthur Jago (1974), Whetten and Cameron (1998, p. 398) have identified five questions managers should ask when making delegation decisions:

> Do subordinates have the necessary (or superior) information or expertise? Is the commitment of subordinates critical to successful implementation? Will subordinates' capabilities be expanded by the assignment? Do subordinates share with management and each other common values and perspectives? Is there sufficient time to do an effective job of delegating?

Also ask, who can ensure the necessary quality?

A manager may make an autocratic decision (tell and sell) when she knows the relevant information, especially if others do not; when the workers do not share the same values and goals and their commitment is not necessary; when time is limited; and when the manager can address the necessary quality. Managers may consult with others but make the decision with or without incorporating ideas expressed (tell and listen) when interaction helps clarify the situation; the interaction will increase commitment; dysfunctional conflicts are unlikely; and time is not critical. The manager may participate in group decisions when the manager has important information to share; no one else could provide the necessary leadership; the manager's presence does not interfere with the expression of ideas; and the time is well spent developing others. The manager may delegate when the group collectively has the necessary information; its commitment is important; it has the same goals as management; it can ensure the necessary quality; and time is not critical.

Whetten and Cameron (1998, pp. 400-403) also have identified the following 10 principles regarding how to delegate:

1. "Begin with the end in mind." (p. 400) It is important for the manager to specify the

results desired from the delegation. It is motivating to specify the importance of the task.

2. "Delegate completely." (p. 400) The manager should be clear about to whom accountability is being assigned; for what task; when the work is to be completed; and how and to whom the results are to be reported. The level of initiative should be clarified when the assignment is made. Does the worker need to wait to be told what to do? This is not very empowering. Can the worker formulate ideas and ask permission to implement the ideas? Empowerment is constrained. Can the worker collect information, determine courses of action, and present options to the manager to decide or make recommendations for approval? This is progressively more empowering. Can workers act and then report what was done? Can mature workers initiate action and then report routinely? This is the most empowering and most likely to produce high motivation and satisfaction with quality results if the workers are mature problem solvers.

3. "Allow participation in the delegation of assignments." (p. 401) When workers understand the assignment and its importance to the organizational goals; have the knowledge and skills necessary to do the job; find the assignment consistent with their values and interests; and have input into what is delegated to them when, they are more likely to willingly accept delegated tasks.

4. "Establish parity between authority and responsibility." (p. 401) Balance responsibility with authority to do the job.

5. "Work within the organizational structure." (p. 401) Delegate down through the hierarchy. Do not skip people in line authority to get to the people closest to the situation.

6. "Provide adequate support for delegated tasks." (p. 402) Give people what they need to do the job or explain why desired resources are not available.

7. "Focus accountability on results." (p. 402) Close monitoring of the process "destroys the five dimensions of empowerment: self-efficacy, self-determination, personal control, meaningfulness, and trust."

8. "Delegate consistently." (p. 402) Use delegation to empower and develop others, not to get rid of unpleasant tasks.

9. "Avoid upward delegation." (p. 403) Ask workers to make recommendations rather than to ask for advice or assistance. If asked for advice, respond with questions like "What do you think we should do?"

10. "Clarify consequences." (p. 403) Identify the impact the task has had on the organization and consumers. Give rewards for success even if they are so simple as a thank you for a job well done.

Not all employees want to be empowered. Some resist delegation. One might ask oneself if the request is delegation or dumping. Has the employee been taught how to do what was delegated? Has there been recent practice? Is there a reward for not doing the task? Is there punishment for doing the delegated task? Once those issues have been satisfied and the employee is performing at or above the minimum standard, there is little the manager can do except give attention to other employees. The resistant employee is likely not to receive additional delegations or new assignments, thus forfeiting learning opportunities, and will become self-limited for promotional opportunities (Hein, 1998).

Politics

Politics is the authoritative allocation of scarce resources. It requires legitimate power to distribute goods, services, and other resources that are less abundant than desired. A political system is a social system that gets people to do what they would not ordinarily want to do. There are several theories that help explain the dynamics of political systems. According to *game theory,* politics is a fascinating game with rules, referees, and players on opposing sides. *Elite theory* purports that political power is concentrated with people who hold top positions in large, centralized institutions. These people tend to have a unified purpose because of similar social backgrounds and interests and consequently have stable power. *Pluralist theory* explains that political life is based on competition between interest groups. The influence of political groups is determined by their political organization, strategies, and leadership. These competitive relationships are unstable because interest groups and related alliances are short-lived and new coalitions and interest groups develop as old ones decline. The power of interest groups is limited by dependence on other groups and the need for compromises. *Exchange theory* states that political behavior is based on the exchange of resources. People decide what they want, what it will cost, and whether they have the resources to exchange for it.

Stages of political development.   The following are stages of political development and activism for individual nurses and the profession of nursing (Cohen, Mason, Kovner et al., 1996; Yoder-Wise, 1999):

- Apathy—The nurse has little to no interest in politics and does not belong to a professional organization.

- Buy-in—The nurse recognizes the importance of activism within professional organizations and may join a professional organization but is not active.

- Self-interest—The nurse uses professional organizations for networking to further her own career and the interests of the profession.

- Political sophistication—The nurse moves beyond self-interest to activism on behalf of the public through holding offices in professional organizations at local and state levels.

- Leading the way—The nurse provides leadership on broad issues often by serving in elected and appointed positions in professional organizations.

Levels of political participation.   There are levels of political participation ranging from apathetic in-

activists who engage in no political activity to complete activists who engage in numerous activities. As nurses become involved in politics, they can expand their influence beyond a single vote. Spectator political activities include gathering political information, displaying bumper stickers or wearing buttons, initiating political discussions, trying to persuade others, and voting. As one becomes increasingly involved, one can make financial contributions, attend political meetings, and contact political leaders. Activists become active members in political parties, attend caucus meetings, contribute time to political campaigns, solicit funds, and run for offices.

Nurse managers can encourage others to become more politically active by educating them in issues, posting and circulating information, and encouraging staff discussion of political topics. They can educate and encourage others to work with legislators by providing formal classes on the legislative process, a list of key contacts, and information about voting records. The nurse manager can encourage participation in professional organizations, consumer groups, boards, legislative committee meetings and hearings, and political functions. Staff members can be sent to testify at hearings and be assigned to attend political activities. The manager can generally support political activities, exemplify political involvement, encourage others to vote, and grant release time for political participation.

Communicating with legislators.   Nurse administrators have found that communicating with legislators, building coalitions, being knowledgeable about current issues, providing testimony, solving problems, educating and involving other nurses, and knowing the legislator before needing help are the most successful political strategies. Less effective political strategies include mass mailings, petitions, demonstrations, and reliance on others to protect nurses' interests. Factors that have contributed to unsuccessful political outcomes include emotionalism, lack of preparation, lack of unity among nurses, failure to build an adequate power base, failure to attend political meetings, failure to contact policy makers until too late, lack of publicity, and lack of feedback from politicians, other nurses, and community members.

Legislators spend so much time in sessions and at committee meetings that it can be difficult to reach them by telephone. A letter is a written record that requires a written reply and is more likely to reach the legislator. Letters should be kept brief, preferably one and not more than two pages. A personal letter is more effective than a form letter or a petition. The title and number of the bill one is addressing and a brief interpretation of it should be included. One's position should be stated succinctly. The name and address of the writer should be legible, and when possible writers should identify themselves as nurses and voters in the legislator's district. One must use discretion in selecting a time to discuss an interest with a legislator. It is preferable not to talk to legislators who are engrossed in activities related to another bill; one should wait until they can give their full attention to one's concerns. Appointments are set up ahead of time. The nurse should prepare a short, well-written statement of what legislative action is preferred and why, specifying the direct impact it will have on the legislator's constituents. The points should be concise and accompanied with news clippings, research reports, and other supportive documentation. It is preferable to deal with one issue at a time.

One should know the party of which the legislator is a member and address him as a representative or senator, as appropriate, to show respect. One should be specific and reasonable about what is wanted and should ask legislators to do only what is within their power. A dialogue can be continued by writing to express gratitude for the meeting and by sending new information as it becomes available.

Organizing political meetings. Nurse managers can take the initiative to organize political meetings. It is best to start with a small group with political and organizing experience. The group should include all organizations and important people willing to be involved. One should compile lists of members of organizations, agency directories, officers, names from newspaper articles, and so on. Personal time and money will be needed to type, copy, and mail invitations, as well as for refreshments, room rental, supplies such as name tags and agendas, and follow-up correspondence.

The meeting should be held at a neutral meeting site. A map should be included with the invitation. A self-addressed, stamped response postcard and request for correction of address and telephone number should also be enclosed. Brief handouts and name tags should be prepared in advance of the meeting. A minimum of food should be served. The atmosphere of the political meeting should be kept comfortable and professional.*

The legislative process. Because the legislative process is complex and technical, nurses need to know the process to determine when to intervene. The state legislative process is similar to the national process that follows. First, legislation is introduced. These legislative proposals originate in a number of ways, but most originate in the executive branch. However, either individuals such as members of Congress or groups such as interest groups may introduce legislation.

Next, there is committee referral. A bill is considered read for the first time when it is referred to a committee. Only a member of Congress can introduce legislation in the committee. There is no limit to the number of bills a member may introduce. In the House of Representatives and the Senate, a bill is numbered according to its place in the order of introduction, referred to committee, labeled with the sponsor's name, and printed by the Government Printing Office. Bills are prefixed with HR when introduced in the House of Representatives and S when introduced in the Senate. After referral to a standing committee, most legislation is referred to a subcommittee. Most bills go no further. Each bill introduced must pass the House of Representatives and the Senate in identical form within 2 years to become a law.

After referral to a standing committee and a subcommittee, hearings are held by the subcommittee. Often only a few members of the subcommittee who have a special interest in the subject will par-

---

*From Davis CK, Oakley D, Sochalski JA: Leadership for expanding nursing influence on health policy, *JONA* 12:15-21, Jan 1982.

ticipate in the hearings. The chairperson uses the agenda, funds, and staff to expedite, delay, or modify legislation. The subcommittee usually schedules public hearings and invites testimony from private and public witnesses. Interested individuals submit written requests to testify. Once they are informed of when to testify, rescheduling is not allowed. If one cannot be present at the designated time, one may file a written statement for the record of the hearing. Witnesses who share common positions are urged to consolidate testimony and designate a single spokesperson. Groups with similar concerns that are unwilling to have a single spokesperson may form panels. Panelists are allowed a 6-minute presentation of the key points in their written documents and are urged to avoid repeating other presentations. All witnesses are required to file a written statement with the committee at least a day before the scheduled appearance or the preceding Friday if the testimony is to be on Monday or Tuesday. The statement should be typed on letter-size paper and include a summary of the principal points. Witnesses should not read their written statements but should summarize the key points in no more than 6 minutes. Once the testimony has been given, each subcommittee member may ask questions.

If, after the hearing, the subcommittee members decide the legislation should go further, they consider the language line by line and section by section to determine the language of the final bill, which is then recommended to the full committee.

When presenting the bill to the floor of the House or Senate, the full committee justifies its actions in a written report that accompanies the bill. Bills that are unanimously voted out of committee have a good chance on the floor. However, dispute is likely to occur on the floor if there has been a divided committee.

After a bill has passed one house, it is sent to the other, where the same process takes place. If the second house approves the bill as it was passed by the first, it is sent to the president for his signature. However, if the bill was revised or amendments added, the bill must be returned to the originating chamber for approval of the changes. If that body refuses to approve the revised bill, both versions are sent to a conference committee. The bill is sent to the president for signature or veto after the differences are reconciled and there is a final vote of acceptance by the conference committee. In the case of a presidential veto, both houses can override the veto to make the bill law.*

NEGOTIATION

Two major ways of negotiating have been identified: hard and soft. The hard negotiator wants to win and believes that the side that takes an extreme position and holds out longer benefits more. Unfortunately, hard negotiators often exhaust themselves and their resources and harm relationships. On the other hand, the soft negotiator prevents conflict and makes concessions quickly to reach an agreement. The soft negotiator ultimately feels exploited and bitter.

Positional bargaining is typical; each side takes a position and argues for it. Negotiations then involve taking and giving up positions successively. The more one defends a position, the more committed one becomes to it and the more difficult it becomes to revise the position. Egos become involved, and "saving face" is an issue. Besides producing unwise agreements, positional bargaining is inefficient. The more extreme the opening position and the smaller the concessions, the longer it takes to reach an agreement. Positional bargaining also damages ongoing relationships.

Principled negotiation is another option for negotiation that is neither hard nor soft. This method decides issues on their merits, looks for mutual gains, and insists on fair standards. It is hard on merits and soft on people. There are four basic points to principled negotiations: (1) separate the people from the problem, (2) focus on interests instead of positions, (3) generate a variety of options before deciding what to do, and (4) insist that the result be based on an objective standard (Box 5-3). Roger Fisher and William Ury (1981) discuss these strategies in detail in *Getting to Yes.*

---

*The legislative process is discussed in more detail in Kalisch BJ, Kalisch PA: *Politics of nursing,* Philadelphia, 1982, JB Lippincott.

Box 5-3 PRINCIPLED NEGOTIATIONS

1. Separate the people from the problem.

2. Focus on interests, not positions.

3. Generate a variety of options before deciding what to do.

4. Insist on objective data.

During the analysis phase one tries to gather and organize data and to diagnose the situation. One notes the people problems, hostile emotions, unclear communications, interests, and options and standards already identified. During the planning phase each of the four principles is again considered and additional options and criteria are generated. During discussions differences in perceptions, feelings such as frustration and anger, and difficulties in communication can be identified and addressed. There can be mutual exploration of how to meet each party's concerns by using objective standards. Negotiations that focus on interests, mutually satisfying options, and fair standards are likely to reach sound agreements.

When separating the people from the problem, understanding others' thinking is critical because that thinking is the problem. Activities include discussing each other's perceptions, trying to put yourself in their shoes, avoiding blaming them for your problem, getting them involved and committed through participation, and making your proposal consistent with their values. It is also important to understand both your and their emotions; make the emotions explicit and acknowledge them as legitimate; let them ventilate; do not react to their emotional outbursts; and use symbolical gestures of friendship such as shaking hands, embracing, eating together, apologizing, and sending a note of congratulations or sympathy.

Communications are critical to negotiations. Listen actively and acknowledge what is being said. Speak calmly to be understood. Speak about yourself instead of about them. Speak with a purpose.

Build working relationships and face the problem, not the people.

Focus on interests instead of positions, because the conflicts between needs, desires, concerns, and fears are the problem. Look for shared and compatible interests, as well as conflicting ones. Realize that each side has multiple interests and that the most powerful interests are the basic human needs for security, belonging, recognition, and control.

Next, invent options for mutual gain. Separate inventing options from judging them. During brainstorming, generate as many ideas as possible without judging them. After brainstorming, note the most promising ideas and invent improvements on them. Later, evaluate the ideas and the ramifications of implementing them. Then decide on the best options. Each side may want different things from the same item, so look for ways to dovetail differing interests. Try to make the desired option so appealing that the decision is easy.

Finally, insist on objective criteria for reaching wise agreements amicably and efficiently. Look for fair standards and fair procedures such as parliamentary procedure.

Some players will not play fairly. Some assert their position, attack your ideas, and even attack you. First, do not attack the idea; look behind it to see what the person's interest is. Second, do not defend your idea; invite criticism and advice instead. Third, reframe the attack on you as an attack on the problem. When attacked, do not counterattack. Break the vicious cycle by refusing to attack. Avoid pitting your strength against theirs directly. Instead of resisting their force, channel their energy into exploring interests, generating options that are mutually acceptable, and finding independent standards. Some negotiators use dirty tricks such as deliberate deception by misrepresenting the facts, using ambiguous authority, and seeking dubious intentions. They employ psychological warfare by using stressful situations, personal attacks, and threats.

Positional pressure tactics such as refusal to negotiate, extreme demands, escalating demands, and calculated delay are also common devices. Other dirty tricks include ridicule to undermine the psychological space of others. To counter ridicule, try to keep a relaxed body posture, pleasant smile, and steady gaze. "Smoke screen" uses ambiguous or inappropriate questioning. Simply state that the question is irrelevant to the issue. "Over the barrel" is when one uses the weaknesses of the other to force concessions. Attempt to hide weak spots and desensitize areas of vulnerability. Seduction implies future promises that something good will happen. Flattery is a form of seduction that causes a loss of power. However, exchanging pleasant opening statements before negotiating is acceptable. Gender can be used as a weapon. Illness and helplessness bring out an impulse to help. Guilt causes discomfort. A definitive statement like "I know you are an intelligent person" limits the freedom of another person. Self-definition like "I am an abused person" is an excuse for not taking responsibility for one's own behavior. Paternalism is an attempt to convince the other party that the action will be for that person's good. Favors, flattery, and gifts are forms of ingratiation. Aggressive takeover is when someone assumes authority and rapidly makes a decision. Saying, "I need time to think about this" helps stop an aggressive takeover. Pacifists win because they refuse to fight (Marquis and Huston, 1996). There are three steps in negotiating the rules when the other side uses dirty tricks (Box 5-4): (1) recognize the tactic, (2) raise the issue explicitly, and (3) question the tactic's legitimacy and desirability by using principled negotiations. Again, separate the people from the problem. Focus on interests instead of positions. Invent options for mutual gain, and insist on objective criteria (Fisher and Ury, 1981).

Peter Block (1987) describes negotiating with allies and adversaries in *The Empowered Manager*. He presents a grid with agreement increasing up the vertical axis and trust increasing to the right along the horizontal axis (Figure 5-1). Adversaries are represented by low agreement and low trust in the lower left quadrant; opponents are represented by low agreement and high trust in the lower right quadrant. Allies are indicated by high agreement and high trust in the upper right quadrant, and bedfellows are indicated by high agreement and low trust in the upper left quadrant. Fence sitters are represented by low trust and medium agreement

| **Box 5-4** | **THREE STEPS IN NEGOTIATING** |

1. Recognize the tactic.
2. Raise the issue explicitly.
3. Question the tactic's legitimacy and desirability.

between adversaries and bedfellows on the left side of the grid.

Adversaries, with whom we have low agreement and low trust, use much of our time and psychic energy. They become adversaries only after our attempts to negotiate agreement and trust have failed. Steps in dealing with adversaries include the following: (1) State your vision of the project. (2) State in a neutral way your best understanding of the adversary's position. (3) Identify your own contribution to the problem, such as having lobbied against them, discounted their position, gone around them, or talked to a higher authority. (4) End the meeting with your plans and no demand.

Opponents are people whom we trust but who disagree with our goals and purposes. Opponents can bring out the best in us by challenging us and making us clarify our beliefs and strategies. The steps for dealing with opponents are as follows: (1) reaffirm the quality of your relationship and mutual trust, (2) state your position, (3) state in a neutral way what you think your opponent's position is, and (4) do problem solving.

One has high agreement and high trust with *allies.* They should be treated as friends; one can discuss doubts and vulnerabilities with them. The basic strategy when dealing with allies is to bring them into the organization and treat them as members. Steps include the following: (1) affirming agreement, (2) reaffirming the quality of the trusting relationship, (3) acknowledging doubts and vulnerabilities related to the project, and (4) asking for advice and support.

One has high agreement and low trust with *bedfellows.* There is a tendency to become manipulative toward people we do not trust. One is careful

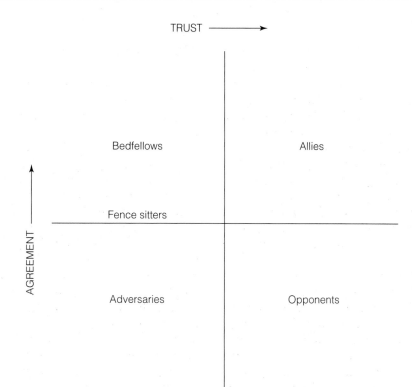

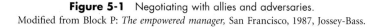

Figure 5-1 Negotiating with allies and adversaries.
Modified from Block P: *The empowered manager,* San Francisco, 1987, Jossey-Bass.

about how much information to share. The issue is trust, not agreement. To work with bedfellows, (1) reaffirm the agreement, (2) acknowledge caution, (3) be clear about what one wants from the bedfellow, such as keeping one informed, (4) ask what the bedfellow wants and expects, and (5) try to agree about how to work together.

Fence sitters do not take a stand for or against us; they exhibit doubt, risk, and uncertainty. To deal with fence sitters, (1) state your position, (2) ask for the fence sitter's position, (3) apply gentle pressure to get a decision and express frustration with neutrality, and (4) ask what it would take to get the fence sitter's support (Block, 1987).

Using our power in organizations and politics through principled negotiations with people with whom we have more or less agreement and trust can advance nursing.

Negotiation Process

Negotiations may result around emotional issues such as anxiety, fear of rejection, need for recognition or status, and personal need deprivation. Substantive issues concern policies, rules, and regulations. To do negotiations, parties must recognize that a conflict of interest or incompatibility exists. The relationship should be voluntary, and both parties should desire an agreement that satisfies both parties.

One starts negotiations by creating a dialogue. Exchanging ideas and information helps make the negotiating process a collaborative problem-solving process allowing parties to communicate openly, seek to understand each other, and identify mutually agreeable solutions. Even though it may be impossible to reach total agreement, dialogue increases the chances of producing productive and viable options. To create the dialogue, one needs to probe, offer ideas, build on ideas, and constructively criticize. Probing asks questions to get information from the other party, determine the other party's ideas and needs, ensure understanding, and respond to the concerns. By discovering and understanding the needs of the other party, it becomes possible to work toward mutually acceptable solutions instead of becoming locked into a fixed position. Probing helps avoid miscommunications and is useful when one needs to verify or uncover information or to make a decision based on what was said. A probe is a statement or question used to get more information. Open probes encourage people to speak freely. They are often who, what, when, where, why, how questions or "explain to me" or "tell me" statements. Closed probes elicit a yes or no response and often include words like could, would, are, is, or will. Open probes are better for identifying others' needs and ideas and clarifying when one is not sure what the other person is meaning. Closed probes can be used to ensure understanding by stating your understanding and then using a closed probe to ask for confirmation.

There are two steps to offer ideas so they will more likely be heard. First, indicate your intent, and then present your reasons before your conclusions. Your intent may be that you want to introduce or present an idea or support an idea. Indicating intent gives you time to prepare what you want to say before you say it and prepares the other person to hear what you are about to say. You might say something like "I have a question" or "I would like to make a suggestion." However, do not state your intent if you plan to offer a criticism or opposing idea, because that would greatly reduce the chances of the other person listening. Because most people stop listening when they hear the bottom line, you should give your reasons before your conclusions. That way the other person is more likely to hear your rationale for your opinions.

There are two steps to build on another person's idea when you want to increase its usefulness. First, acknowledge the connection, and then add value. You might say something like, "Your comment made me think about . . . ." Then you can

add value by suggesting a modification or a different approach to the other person's idea. You retain a significant part of the content or intent of the other person's idea rather than dismissing it for your own idea.

When you disagree with the other person's idea or opinion, you may want to constructively criticize. First, you state the merits, and then you state your concerns. Then ask for ways to retain the merits and eliminate the concerns. For example, if you were negotiating the redecorating of a wing of a building or a room in your home and you liked the decorator's ideas but thought the cost was too high, you might say, "I love the color scheme and the furnishing. However, the price estimates are about 20% over the budget. Can you think of ways to cut back on the costs?"

It is not uncommon to encounter obstacles, impasses, and even counterproductive tactics. You should break an impasse by stating your desire to continue and by initiating a change of pace; for example, you can say, "Let's take a 5-minute break and then continue trying to resolve this problem," or "Let's meet again after lunch." Maintain a positive and collaborative tone.

Counterproductive tactics should be confronted. Counterproductive tactics or dirty tricks are underhanded and adversarial to negotiation. They are attempts to strengthen one's position while weakening the other person's position. They undermine the relationship between the parties and the agreement. They are numerous and have been previously discussed. When confronting counterproductive tactics, first confirm the behavior, and then express the impact on you or the negotiation. Make sure you are confirming the person's behavior, not your judgment of that behavior. Express how the behavior makes you feel. Speak to how it affects the negotiation process. Express the impact in ways that allow the other person to change without losing face.

To plan your strategy, analyze the situation. Identify the who, what, when, and where. Determine the facts about the issue and consider the relationship. Next, organize the information by anticipating the needs and identifying the common ground and options. Then synthesize the approach by examining consequences of options and plan the discussion.

When negotiating, state the purpose and review the situation. Then explore the ideas and needs. Examine ideas from both points of view. Combine ideas. Rework solutions. Reverse perspectives. Uncover dissatisfactions. Restate the desire to satisfy needs. Determine the best alternative. Set terms and conditions. Summarize the agreement, and confirm the next steps (*Negotiating self-taught,* 1984). Then write a follow-up letter specifying your understanding of the agreement.

LABOR RELATIONS
Why Employees Join Unions

Employees join a union essentially to increase their power to get certain responses from management. Management's actions or inactions have probably caused the employees to reach their limit of tolerance. Poor working conditions and job inequities in wage increments, promotion, and benefits cause distress. Poor quality of immediate supervision, arbitrary treatment from management, and poor communications between employer and employee are major reasons for unionization. Instead of quitting their jobs and giving up their seniority, security, and friends to move to another job, employees form a union.

Labor Law

In 1935 the National Labor Relations Act (NLRA), or the Wagner Act, was passed in an effort to end the depression. It prevented some employers from cutting wages in the hopes that higher worker incomes and increased spending would lessen the severity of the economic depression. Unfortunately, some employers went bankrupt because they could not reduce wages. Employers could not legally fire employees who sought unionization. The NLRA created the National Labor Relations Board (NLRB) to investigate and initiate administrative proceedings against employers who violated a law that listed employer violations only.

In 1887 the Nurses' Associated Alumnae of the United States and Canada was formed, and in 1911 it became the American Nurses Association (ANA). In 1946 the ANA started the Economic Security Program to help state associations bargain collectively. The "no strike" pledge adopted at the start of the program hampered nurses' bargaining position. The "strike" policy was rescinded in 1968 (Decker and Sullivan, 1992).

Because the NLRA was biased toward unions, it was amended in 1947 by the Taft-Hartley Act, or Labor Management Relations Act. It listed union restrictions to restore equality between employers and employees. Nonprofit health care institutions, however, were exempted from the law. The unions developed public relations problems when some of them went on strike during the war and when unions were blamed for the postwar inflation (Dienemann, 1990).

In 1959 the laws were further modified by the Landrum-Griffin Act, or Labor-Management Reporting and Disclosure Act, to safeguard against corrupt financial and election procedures used by some unions. The Union Members' Bill of Rights resulted.

The Equal Pay Act of 1963 indicated that men and women performing equal work should receive equal compensation.

The Civil Rights Act of 1964 prohibits discrimination and promotes employment based on ability and merit. It specifically mentions race, color, religion, sex, and national origin. Equal employment opportunity legislation is to prevent discrimination. Affirmative action plans are to actively seek to correct past injustices.

The Age Discrimination and Employment Act (ADEA) of 1967 promotes employment of older people based on their ability rather than age, and the 1978 amendment increased the protected age to 70. Although statistics show a trend toward earlier retirement, Congress voted to remove the age restriction except in certain categories in 1987.

The Rehabilitation Act of 1973 provides affirmative action to recruit, hire, and advance qualified handicapped people. Congress passed the Americans With Disabilities Act (ADA) in 1990 to eliminate discrimination against people with physical or mental impairments, including physical disabilities, cancer, diabetes, and human immunodeficiency virus, and recovering alcoholics and drug users.

The Vietnam Veterans Act of 1973/1974 addressed employment rights and privileges for veterans. It allowed some nurses to get reemployed after serving in the Persian Gulf war even though there was a nursing surplus at the time.

In 1974, Public Law 93-360, the Nonprofit Health Care Amendments to the Taft-Hartley Act, extended federal collective bargaining rights to private sector employees. It created notification procedures that must precede a strike and ensured employees of the right to join, or refrain from joining, a union. The 1974 amendments to the NLRA resulted in the following changes:

- Required unions to give a 10-day prestrike notice

- Did not permit a strike or lockout during the notice period

- Required unions to give advance written notice of contract termination or modification to the employer and to a federal mediator and Conciliation Service

- Required mediation by a federal mediator and Conciliation Service

- Allowed a board of inquiry to be established to settle disputes

- Allowed employees to be held exempt from a requirement to join or financially support a union for bona fide religious grounds

This extended the legal protection of nurses for collective bargaining. Because of declining union membership in manufacturing industries, unions welcomed the expanded market (Gillies, 1994; Vestal, 1995).

Taft-Hartley Amendments give the NLRB the responsibility to determine the composition and size of bargaining units. However, all NLRB decisions are subject to review by 12 federal Circuit Courts of Appeal, which did reject separate bargaining units for registered nurses. In 1984 the NLRB made a landmark decision to recognize two broad units of professional and nonprofessional employees (St. Francis Hospital II NLRB 948, 1984), which the Federal Court of Appeals overturned in 1987. In 1987 the NLRB designated eight bargaining units: registered nurses, employed physicians, all other professionals, technical employees, skilled maintenance employees, business office and clerical staff, security guards, and all other nonprofessional employees. Nursing homes, psychiatric hospitals, and rehabilitation facilities were exempt. The NLRB had never used its rule-making power to establish bargaining units before. In May 1989 the American Hospital got injunctive relief against the rules, and the Chicago Federal District Court issued a permanent injunction against the rule in July 1989. However, in April 1990 the U.S. Court of Appeals for the Seventh Circuit reversed the lower court's decision. In 1991 the U.S. Supreme Court upheld the NLRB ruling that unions can organize eight separate groups of hospital employees. This opened the market of the minimally unionized health care industry to unions (Grohar-Murray and DiCroce, 1997; Management Science Associates, 1997; Marquis and Huston, 1996, 1998; National Labor Relations Act, 1935; Tappen, 1995; Vestal, 1995).

The Family and Medical Leave Act (FMLA) of 1993 was intended to cover pregnancy and maternity leave but became very broad. The act requires employers with 50 or more employees to provide up to 12 weeks per year of unpaid, job-protected leave. Eligible workers must have been employed for at least 12 months and completed 1250 hours of service during the 12 months immediately preceding the leave. A worker is entitled to a leave for the following circumstances: (1) for the birth of the worker's child, (2) for adoption or foster placement of a child with the worker, (3) to provide care for a child, spouse, or parent with a serious health condition, and (4) when the worker is unable to perform functions of the job position because of a serious health condition. The worker then has the right to return to work in the same or an equivalent position with equivalent benefits, compensation, and conditions of employment and to take leave on a reduced time or intermittent basis if medically necessary for a serious health condition of the worker, child, spouse, or parent. The employer can require the worker to use accrued paid vacation and sick leave time in lieu of part of the 12 weeks of unpaid leave. The employer must continue to pay health benefits for the duration of the leave. Records are to be maintained with the medical information, kept confidential and separate from the personnel file (Grohar-Murray and DiCroce, 1997).

In 1994 the U.S. Supreme Court decision National Labor Relations Board (NLRB) v. Health Care and Retirement Corporation of America was that licensed practical nurses employed by Heartland Nursing Home in Urbana, Ohio, were considered "supervisors" who acted in the interest of their employer when performing patient care duties and were consequently not eligible for protection under the amended NLRA. In 1996 the NLRB did a reinterpretation of the NLRA and issued a decision containing a detailed analysis of nursing duties defining true supervisory work according to labor law. In the NLRB decision (not the Supreme Court decision), nonsupervisory employees continue to have the right to organize for collective bargaining purposes (Grohar-Murray and DiCroce, 1997; Hein, 1998; Marquis and Huston, 1998).

NLRA Section 7 about employee rights states the following:

> Employees shall have the right to self-organization, to form, join, or assist labor organizations, to bargain collectively through activities for the purpose of collective bargaining or other mutual aid or protection, and shall also have the right to refrain from any or all such activities except to the extent that such right may be affected by an agreement requiring membership in a labor organization as a condition of employment as authorized in section 8(a)(3).

NLRA Section 2(11) defines supervisor as follows:

> The term "Supervisor" means any individual having authority, in the interest of the employer, to hire, transfer, suspend, lay off, recall, promote, discharge, assign, reward or discipline other employees, or responsibility to direct them, or to adjust their grievances, or effectively to recommend such action, if in connection with the foregoing the exercise of such authority is not of a merely routine clerical nature, but requires the use of independent judgment.

This has implications for nursing, particularly as registered nurses are supervising more and more unlicensed personnel. This eliminates many nurses from bargaining units.

Title VII prohibits an employer from engaging in conduct that creates a hostile or offensive working environment on the basis of race, religion, gender, or national origin. To state a claim of harassment or discrimination, a plaintiff must establish that the behavior endured by her at her place of work was severe and pervasive enough to alter the conditions of her employment and to create an abusive working environment. The behavior complained to be harassment or discrimination usually takes the form of an action or inaction by a supervisor. The U.S. Supreme Court placed vicarious liability upon employers for the actions or inactions of their supervisors in the context of sexual harassment. If an employee is being harassed by anyone who is a supervisor, the employer is vicariously liable for the harassment. This is true whether the harassment is in the form of sexual favors or jokes or tangible job detriment such as a cut in pay, termination, or demotion. The only defense the employer will have is claiming an effective antiharassment policy was in place and that the employees failed to use the policy or to avoid harm otherwise. These rulings have not been extended beyond the areas of sexual discrimination as of 1999. Supervisors are not individually liable for Title VII, ADA, or ADEA violations because they are not "employers" as that term is defined in Title VII, ADA, or ADEA (McCrory, 1999).

The 1999 ANA House of Delegates supported affiliation with the American Federation of Labor Congress of Industrial Organizations (AFL-CIO), a federation of trade and professional unions. The AFL-CIO's constitution requires that federation members do not raid other federation unions. That would provide the state nurses associations (SNAs) some protection and allow more time and resources for educating, organizing, and representing registered nurses instead of fending off other unions. The 1999 ANA House of Delegates also recommended establishment and funding of a Task Force on Workplace Advocacy to develop and evaluate models by which the ANA and SNAs could ensure that nurses not represented by a collective bargaining unit will have access to workplace advocacy (1999 ANA House of Delegates materials).

Unfair labor practices by management. The NLRA's section 8(a) prohibitions on management are known as the unfair labor practices. They include interference, 8(a)(1); domination, 8(a)(2); discrimination, 8(a)(3); discrimination, 8(a)(4); and refusal to bargain, 8(a)(5). Restraining, coercing, or otherwise interfering with employees during the exercise of their right to organize is an unfair labor practice. Management may not contribute financial or other support or otherwise dominate or interfere during the development or administration of a labor organization. The employer may not discriminate in hiring or tenure or other terms of employment to encourage or discourage membership in a labor organization. Nor can the employer discriminate against an employee for filing charges or giving testimony. The employer is also forbidden to refuse to bargain with representatives of the employees.

Unfair labor practices by unions. Before 1935 management's power had few limitations. From 1935 to 1947 managers had to contend with unfair labor practice limitations, but no such unfair labor practices were defined for labor organizations. In 1947 the Labor Management Relations Act amended the NLRA and added restrictions for labor organizations. These include interference, 8(b)(1); induced discrimination, 8(b)(2); refusal to bargain, 8(b)(3); strikes and boycotts, 8(b)(4); initiation fee, 8(b)(5); featherbedding, 8(b)(6); and recognition picketing, 8(b)(7). Labor organizations may not restrain or coerce an employer in the selection of a representative for collective bargaining. The union may not cause an employer to discrimi-

nate against an employee who is not a member of the union. Nor can a union representative of the employees refuse to bargain with the employer. With adherence to required notification procedures, an employee organization may strike against the employer when negotiations have failed. A primary boycott is a strike action taken by union members against their employer. The illegal or protected status of strikes or boycotts depends on the union objectives and the tactics used. Labor unions may not force an employer to join any organization or cease using specific products or doing business with someone, thus making "hot cargo" clauses illegal. Hot cargo agreements are stipulations on the employer's use of products that give the union power over other organizations. A secondary boycott that is directed at a customer or supplier of the employer is also illegal. An employee group may not force an employer to bargain with them if the employees are represented by another bargaining agent. Labor organizations may not force "any employer to assign particular work to employees in a particular labor organization . . . rather than to employees in another labor organization," and they may not honor strike lines against other employers by refusing to cross the picket lines. Informational picketing is not barred because it does not disrupt the employer's operation. Recognition picketing to get an employer to recognize an employee group is lawful except when the employer has recognized another labor organization, when it is within 12 months preceding a valid election, and when picketing has been conducted without a petition. The union may not charge discriminatory or excessive initiation fees or cause an employer to pay for services not performed, a practice called featherbedding.

UNIONIZATION
Organizing Phase

To form a union, an organizer must establish internal contacts. In a hospital or other health care agency the organizer needs at least one nurse on each shift to assist with unionization. The organizer should be known by a majority of the nurses, be knowledgeable about related laws, and be able to use free time for organizing. The organizers ascertain the level of interest informally by listening, asking questions, and supplying information. After an assessment period, the organizers meet, discuss the prevailing climate, identify the frustration level, enumerate the kinds and extent of employment problems, and assess the nurses' interest in unionization. If interest is minimal, further organizing efforts should be postponed. If nurses show interest in organizing, the campaign is planned.

There must be commitment from the nurses before a formal organization can be established. To achieve this, the organizers hold informational meetings. Coordination of efforts, development of unity, identification of problems and concerns, education about collective bargaining, and active participation of nurses are the tasks to be accomplished in the organizing meetings. The organizers should work in nonwork areas on their own time. The organizers contact the labor organization that they want to represent them for information and authorization cards. The labor organization can send a letter to the employer informing management that the nurses within that agency are organizing and that the activity is protected by law. Box 5-5 contains a list of questions that the manager can ask to help determine whether staff members are in the organizing phase.

Recognition Phase

The organizers must get at least 30% of the nurses to be represented to sign individual authorization cards before the labor organization can act on behalf of the group. Handing out authorization cards is solicitation but cannot be prohibited by management anywhere in the agency during nonworking time. Recognition of the labor organization by the employer is necessary before collective bargaining can begin. Some employers will recognize the labor organization on a voluntary basis when given proof of the majority representative status. However, employers often refuse to recognize the labor organization voluntarily on the basis of a good faith doubt of majority representation. Thus it becomes necessary to obtain certification from the NLRB.

The NLRB does not start an election until requested to do so by an employee organization. A *petition* for an election must be accompanied by designation cards signed by 30% of the employees

| Box 5-5 | QUESTIONS TO HELP DETERMINE WHETHER STAFF ARE IN THE ORGANIZING PHASE |

A "Yes" answer to the following questions may indicate that personnel are in the organizing phase:
- Have you seen union authorization cards anywhere on the agency premises?
- Have you heard of any union-sponsored meetings outside the organization?
- Have you heard of any employee meetings being held at an employee's home?
- Has there been an increase in the number of peer work social activities?
- Have you noticed a repeated presence of strangers or ex-employees mingling with employees outside the agency as employees are coming to and going from work?
- Have you seen employees talking together in small groups and either breaking up their conversation and walking away or becoming silent as you or other members of management approach?
- Has there been any significant increase in the number of employee complaints about wages or conditions of employment?
- Has there been an increase in employee complaints regarding schedules, staffing levels, content or frequency of in-service education programs, or unclear and overlapping job classifications?
- Has there been a change in the rate of turnover?
- Are you aware of any other factors that appear to be out of the ordinary and seem to be separating administration from employees?

in the bargaining group to indicate a substantial show of interest. Labor organizations usually obtain signatures from at least 50% of the potential members before they file a petition.

A *preliminary hearing* is held before an election is scheduled. This provides participants an opportunity to express their opinions. The regional director of the NLRB assesses that the employer is under the board's jurisdiction; determines that other criteria are met; determines the bargaining unit and voter eligibility; and sets the date, hours, and place for the *election.* The election usually takes place during working hours on the employer's premises about a month after the hearing. All employees in the bargaining unit who were on the employer's payroll during a given payroll period in the recent past are allowed to vote. This rule prevents hiring people to vote in the election.

The number of bargaining units within an agency is held to a minimum. Appropriate bargaining units include the following: (1) technical employees, such as x-ray technicians, surgical technicians, and licensed practical nurses; (2) service and maintenance employees, such as employees doing kitchen work, laundry, and housekeeping; (3) business office clerical employees, such as receptionists, clerks, and switchboard operators; and (4) professional employees, such as nurses.

Spouses and children of the employers, temporary employees, and managerial employees are not eligible to vote. People who have the authority to hire, fire, and direct others are considered managers. This may include nurse managers, head nurses, and charge nurses. As a member of management, the director of nursing is ineligible to vote.

During the preelection period, the employer is required to post NLRB election notices stating the time, date, and place of the election. On election day the field examiner from the regional board sets up the election machinery and does not allow electioneering around the polling place. Eligible employees cast secret ballots. Ballots are counted in the regional office. The tabulation of votes is forwarded to the office of the General Counsel in Washington, D.C., and the General Counsel decides the election. If employees no longer want to be represented by the labor organization, they can initiate a decertification election with a requisite 30% show of interest. If a bargaining unit is denied because of the vote tabulation, the labor organization is not permitted to seek certification among the same people until after a 12-month moratorium, and the management group should rectify the problems identified during the organization. If a union wins the election, both parties prepare to negotiate.

Contract Negotiation Phase

The piecemeal, total, and combination approaches are used for contract negotiations. The piecemeal is a step-by-step approach that tries to settle the issues one by one. The total approach considers nothing settled until everything is settled. This allows for calculation of the effects of the interdependent variables on each other. The combination method uses both approaches. The step-by-step method is used to progress from the easy to the hard issues. The decisions are not irrevocable, trading takes place, and decisions are reworked until negotiations are acceptable to both parties. The union representatives present the solutions to the members for a ratification vote to accept or reject the offer. If the solutions are accepted, the employee and management representatives sign the agreement, and it becomes binding. If they are rejected, the representatives reassemble to continue negotiating the contract.

During contract negotiations the union is on the offensive and management is on the defensive. The union makes most of the demands, whereas management defends itself against them and prepares for a strike. The threat of a strike strengthens the union negotiator's position.

Strikes in the health care field require more special and elaborate notification procedures than those in other industries. This allows for the delay of new admissions or referral to other facilities. Alternative health care plans are made for ambulatory patients. Some hospitalized patients may be transferred to other agencies, and supervisory personnel are scheduled to care for the remaining patients.

The NLRB categorizes collective bargaining into three groups: illegal, voluntary, and mandatory.

Illegal topics violate the NLRA and other laws. Voluntary subjects need not be negotiated unless both sides consent to do so. Voluntary issues include size of the bargaining team, union dues, management salaries, and patient charges. Mandatory subjects are related to conditions of employment, work hours, and remuneration.

Contracts often start with a preamble that states both parties' objectives and a pledge of cooperation. Near the beginning there is a statement of the employer's recognition of the union as the bargaining representative for specific employees with specification of employees who are excluded.

A union security clause requires new workers to join the union. Union security is protected by establishing a closed shop, union shop, agency shop, or maintenance-of-membership arrangement in the contract. The closed shop requires the employer to hire and retain only union members in good standing. However, this is prohibited by the Labor Management Relations Act of 1947 for employers and employees in industries affecting interstate commerce. A union shop requires all employees to become members of the union within a specific time after hiring (usually 30 to 60 days) and to maintain membership as a condition of employment. An agency shop requires all employees in the negotiating unit who do not join the union to pay a fixed amount equivalent to organization dues on a regular basis as a condition of employment. The money may go to the organization's welfare fund or to a charity. The maintenance-of-membership clause requires union members to maintain their membership during a specific period, such as the duration of the contract.

Financial remuneration—including wages and salaries, shift differentials, overtime rates, holiday pay, cost-of-living adjustment, longevity, and merit increases—receives considerable attention. Nonfinancial remuneration—including insurance, retirement plans, employee services such as free lunches and parking, vacations, holidays, leaves, and educational assistance—also receives considerable attention. The union usually strives to have rewards made on the basis of seniority. Guidelines for discipline, grievance procedures, and professional standards are also negotiated. After acceptance of the contract by the union members through a ratification vote, the contract is signed by employee and employer representatives and becomes binding.

Contract Administration

Implementation of the agreement, the final phase of the unionization process, interprets and enforces the agreement developed during negotiations. When one of the parties involved does not abide by the terms of the contract, a grievance may result. Grievances are most commonly filed against management because management has a more active role than the union in the administration of the contract. The grievance procedure is usually addressed in the contract.

Underlying causes of grievances should be identified and corrected so that future grievances will be prevented. Different types of grievances require different reactions from managers and union leaders. A legitimate grievance results when one party violates the agreement between parties. Managers' ignorance of the agreement and lack of commitment are the major causes. It is not uncommon for first-line managers to function without having read the contract and with the attitude that labor relations are a chore. On the other hand, union stewards are more motivated to understand the agreement and must have an interest in labor relations to obtain their positions. Consequently, most legitimate grievances are against management. It is advisable to develop training programs to familiarize managers with the contract and to set labor relations objectives as priorities for managers.

Imagined grievances occur when a party incorrectly believes that there has been a violation. Employees sometimes imagine a grievance because they do not understand their rights. The steward should correct the misunderstanding before it becomes a formal grievance.

Political grievances occur for reasons other than the concern itself. Management may want to appear supportive to subordinate managers and stewards to union members, so they do not adequately advise the complainant. A cooperative atmosphere between labor and management is the best way to avoid political grievances.

Harassment grievances are fabricated to distress the other side. They are most commonly used by unions in connection with negotiations. Management usually denies the grievances, forcing the union to drop the grievance or request arbitration. If the contract indicates that both sides share arbitration expenses, harassment grievances are usually dropped.

Organizations should have a grievance procedure even if they are not unionized. This allows employees access to management regarding issues of concern to them and conveys management's intent to be fair. Grievances should be handled quickly through the use of a grievance procedure. Grievances may be handled in a centralized or decentralized manner. In a decentralized process, the immediate supervisor tries to resolve as many problems as possible, and grievances rarely progress further. This encourages a close working relationship between manager and staff associates. Unfortunately, there may be inconsistent decisions because of the number of different people involved in the process. In a centralized grievance procedure, the immediate manager denies the validity of the grievance, and it is handled by the next level of management or by a personnel department. Thus decisions are made consistently among units because of the few people involved in the decision making. Unfortunately, cooperation between the manager and staff associate is not fostered.

Arbitration.   Most contracts allow either side to seek arbitration when a grievance is not satisfactorily resolved, but both parties must agree on the arbitrator. The American Arbitration Association and the Federal Mediation and Conciliation Service are primary sources for professional arbitrators. The payment of costs involved is specified in the contract. Commonly, both parties share the costs, but some contracts specify that the loser must pay.

In any case, arbitration is not automatic and must be requested by the dissatisfied party. Both sides select a representative, the grievance is reviewed, fact finding is done, and witnesses are interviewed. Preparation of one's case from the opponent's view encourages one to consider both sides and develop a stronger case. Presenting one's case to a friend who will act as an advocate helps further identify weaknesses in one's presentation and further strengthens the case. Documents should be prepared in triplicate for the hearing so that the arbitrator, opponent, and presenter can each have a copy. Witnesses may be used for the hearing. Their availability should be confirmed. Witnesses should be informed of where and when to attend the hearing and what will be expected of them.

A hearing is similar to courtroom proceedings. The arbitrator makes opening remarks, and the initiating party comments on the purpose of the hearing and outcomes desired. The responding side may respond then or wait until later. Witnesses are presented and cross-examined in an alternating pattern. First, a witness testifies for the initiator, and then one for the responding party testifies and is cross-examined. The initiating party makes closing remarks, followed by the responding party's closing statement, each pointing out evidence to support that side. The arbitrator studies the evidence and makes a decision. The arbitrator may issue a summary judgment shortly after the proceedings or a written decision to both parties within a month. The decision of the arbitrator is enforceable in court.

Decertification

When employees no longer want to be represented by their present union, they can request a decertification election. Management may also request an election if it is in good faith doubt that the union is representing the majority of employees. The decertification election is similar to the certification process. First, a decertification petition must be signed by at least 30% of the bargaining unit to file a show of interest. In reality, more than 50% and probably closer to 75% need to show interest to guarantee a successful election. The petition is filed with the NLRB by the employer. It can be filed on the expiration date of a contract or ideally during the 30-day period before the 90-day period preceding expiration of the contract.

After receiving the decertification petition, the NLRB distributes a notice about it to the union, the petitioners, and the employer. The employer is asked to submit to the NLRB (1) names and addresses of other interested unions, (2) copies of current and recent contracts covering the employees petitioning for decertification, and (3) names and job classifications of all employees in the bargaining unit.

A preelection hearing may be scheduled if there are questions regarding representation. If neither the union nor the employer requests a hearing, an election date and time are set. The selection of the date is extremely important to the success of the election. Campaigning is limited to 24 hours before the election so that the decertification process momentum is not disrupted by a weekend. Wednesday, Thursday, and Friday are preferable days for the election. A day that will ensure maximal turnout, such as payday, is de-sirable. The election should be held within 3 weeks of confirmation of the election by the NLRB.

Decertification campaigns are similar to certification efforts. Managers should have various meetings, including individual meetings, small group meetings, and entire unit meetings, to assure personnel that they are in good hands with management and that they will be better off without a union. However, decertification cannot be accomplished just by holding meetings during the campaign. Management needs to have earned the confidence of the employees over time through the use of good management techniques.

The NLRB conducts the election on the specified date. If the union loses the election, management stops negotiating with the union. If not, the next contract is negotiated.

Key terms used in collective bargaining are defined in Box 5-6.

Box 5-6   KEY TERMS USED IN COLLECTIVE BARGAINING

Agency shop: A business where nonmembers are required to join the union as a condition of employment.

Arbitration: Procedures for using the services of a third party to settle labor disputes.

Arbitrator: The person chosen by agreement of both parties to decide the dispute between them.

Authorization cards: Cards the employees sign to authorize representation by a specific union.

Bargaining agent: A person or group accepted by an employer and chosen by members of the bargaining unit to represent them in collective bargaining.

Bargaining unit: An employee group that the state or National Labor Relations Board recognizes as an appropriate division for collective bargaining.

Certification: The official recognition of a labor organization as the exclusive bargaining agent for employees of a specific bargaining unit.

Collective bargaining: A legal process used by organized employees to negotiate with an employer about wages and related concerns resulting in an employment contract.

Contract violations: Acts that break the terms of a contract.

Deadlock: A stall in negotiations when neither party is willing to compromise about an issue.

Decertification: The withdrawal of official recognition of a union as the exclusive bargaining agent for a bargaining unit.

Grievance: Any complaint by an employer or union concerning an aspect of employment.

Grievance procedures: Steps both sides have agreed to follow to settle disputes.

Mediation: A process for settling labor disputes where a mediator helps the parties reach their own agreements.

Open shop: A business where employees are not required to belong to the bargaining unit.

From Foley M, Center for Labor Relations: *Key terms used in collective bargaining*, Washington, DC, American Nurses Association.

STRIKES
Types of Strikes

Economic strikes. Employees attempt to get their employer to meet their demands by withdrawing their services. An employee cannot be fired for participating in an economic strike but can be replaced.

Unfair labor strikes. This type of strike results from an unfair labor practice by an employer or a union.

Sympathy strikes. Employees of one employer strike in support of another. Workers can refuse to cross picket lines.

Jurisdictional strikes. In this type of strike there is a work stoppage over the assignment of work to two or more unions. Employees may strike because the employer assigned a particular job to another union.

Recognition strikes. This is a work stoppage to force an employer to bargain with a particular organization.

Illegal strikes. This category comprises violent strikes, boycott or secondary strikes, and wildcat or surprise strikes that are not authorized by the union (Dienemann, 1990; Vestal, 1995).

NURSE MANAGERS' ROLE IN COLLECTIVE BARGAINING

Nurse managers should evaluate their management skills and take continuing education courses to improve them. Motivational techniques are particularly important for nurse administrators to possess because they work through others. They must listen carefully to staff concerns and represent staff associates' wishes to top management. Nurse administrators need to know about labor relations.

The director of nursing should not serve as the chief negotiator during collective bargaining because it would put the director in an adversary role. The agency legal representative is usually the negotiator. During negotiations the director of nursing defines what is best for the nursing care of patients. Once the contract has been negotiated, nurse managers must learn the terms of the contract and have copies of the contract available to them. Problems should be solved through problem-solving techniques as they arise.

ADVANTAGES AND DISADVANTAGES OF COLLECTIVE BARGAINING

There are advantages and disadvantages to collective bargaining. Some equalization of power between administrators and staff associates can be obtained because of the staff associates' strength in numbers. Professionalism can be promoted. Nurses can gain control of practice. Grievance procedures become viable, and staffing for systematic and equitable distribution of work can be established. Unfair treatment of employees can be reduced. The quality of services can be influenced. Economic security can be increased. Unfortunately, an adversary relationship may develop between administration and staff associates, and strikes may not be prevented. Unionization is considered unprofessional by many nurses. Unions can interfere with the management of the organizations. Leadership for unions may be difficult to obtain because many professional nurses have little experience in positions of authority. Women tend to view employment as a job instead of a career, minimizing interest in leadership

Box 5-7	ADVANTAGES AND DISADVANTAGES OF COLLECTIVE BARGAINING

Advantages	Disadvantages
Equalization of power	Adversary relationship
Viable grievance procedures	Strikes may not be prevented
Equitable distribution of work	Leadership may be difficult to obtain
Professionalism promoted	Unprofessional behavior
Nurses control practice	Interference with management

positions, and if the bargaining unit and the professional association are the same, top administrators may have to drop membership in the professional organization, further depleting the leadership (Box 5-7).

CHAPTER SUMMARY

Chapter 5 covered the following:
Power, Authority, and Politics
    Sources of Power
        Reward
        Coercive power
        Legitimate power
        Referent power
        Expert power
        Information
        Connection
    Sources of Personal Power
    Sources of Interpersonal Power
        Connection power
        Information power
        Group decision-making power
    Sources of Position Power
        Centrality
        Criticality
        Flexibility
        Relevance
        Visibility
    Informal Sources of Power
    Power Relations
    Kinds of Power
    Authority
    Power and Gender
    Empowerment
    Empowered Delegation
    Politics
        Stages of political development
        Levels of political participation
        Communicating with legislators
        Organizing political meetings
        The legislative process
Negotiation
    Negotiation Process
Labor Relations
    Why Employees Join Unions
    Labor Law

        Unfair labor practices by management
        Unfair labor practices by unions
    Unionization
        Organizing Phase
        Recognition Phase
        Contract Negotiation Phase
        Contract Administration
            Arbitration
        Decertification
    Strikes
        Types of Strikes
            Economic strikes
            Unfair labor strikes
            Sympathy strikes
            Jurisdictional strikes
            Recognition strikes
            Illegal strikes
Nurse Managers' Role in Collective Bargaining
Advantages and Disadvantages of Collective Bargaining

REFERENCES

ANA House of Delegates Conference materials, June 1999.

Block P: *The empowered manager,* San Francisco, 1987, Jossey-Bass.

Cohen SS, Mason DJ, Kovner C et al.: Stages of nursing political development: where we've been and where we ought to go, *Nurs Outlook* 44:259-266, Nov-Dec 1996.

Cummings S: Atilla the Hun versus Atilla the hen: gender socialization of the American nurse, *Nurs Adm Q* 19(2):19-29, 1995.

Davis CK, Oakley D, Sochalski JA: Leadership for expanding nursing influence on health policy, *JONA* 12:15-21, Jan 1982.

Decker PJ, Sullivan EJ: *Nursing administration,* Norwalk, Conn, 1992, Appleton & Lange.

Dienemann J: *Nursing administration: strategic perspectives and application,* Norwalk, Conn, 1990, Appleton & Lange.

Fisher R, Ury W: *Getting to yes,* Boston, 1981, Houghton-Mifflin.

Gillies DA: *Nursing management: a systems approach,* Philadelphia, 1994, WB Saunders.

Grohar-Murray ME, DiCroce HR: *Leadership and management in nursing,* Stamford, Conn, 1997, Appleton & Lange.

Hein EC: *Contemporary leadership behavior,* Philadelphia, 1998, Lippincott.

Kalisch BJ, Kalisch PA: *Politics of nursing,* Philadelphia, 1982, JB Lippincott.

Loveridge CE, Cummings SH: *Nursing management in the new paradigm,* Gaithersburg, Md, 1996, Aspen.

Management Science Associates: *Positive employee relations and union free management,* Independence, Mo, 1997, Management Science Associates.

Marquis BL, Huston CJ: *Leadership roles and management functions in nursing,* Philadelphia, 1996, Lippincott.

Marquis BL, Huston CJ: *Management decision making for nurses: 124 case studies,* Philadelphia, 1998, Lippincott-Raven.

May R: *Power and innocence,* New York, 1972, WW Norton and Company.

McCrory JL: Personal communication, 1999.

Mishra AK: Organizational response to crisis: the role of mutual trust and top management teams, doctoral dissertation, Ann Arbor, 1992, University of Michigan.

National Labor Relations Act, 1935.

Negotiating self-taught, Stamford, Conn, 1984, Learning International.

Spreitzer GM: When organizations dare: the dynamics of individual empowerment in the workplace, doctoral dissertation, Ann Arbor, 1992, University of Michigan.

Tappen RM: *Nursing leadership and management: concepts and practice,* Philadelphia, 1995, FA Davis.

Vestal KW: *Nursing management: concepts and issues,* ed 2, Philadelphia, 1995, JB Lippincott.

Vroom VH, Jago AG: Decision making as social process: normative and descriptive models of leader behavior, *Decision Sciences* 5:743-769, Oct 1974.

Vroom VH, Yetton PG: *Leadership and decision making,* Pittsburgh, 1973, University of Pittsburgh Press.

Whetten DA, Cameron KS: *Developing management skills,* Reading, Mass, 1998, Addison-Wesley.

Yoder-Wise PS: *Leading and managing in nursing,* St. Louis, 1999, Mosby.

BIBLIOGRAPHY

Autry JA, Mitchell S: *Real power: business lessons from the Tao Te Ching,* New York, 1998, Riverhead Books.

Betts VT: Nursing's agenda for health care reform: policy, politics, and power through professional leadership, *Nurs Adm Q* 20(3):1-8, 1996.

Boston C: Breaking down the walls without tearing down the house . . . patient focused care, *JONA* 24:5-6, March 1994.

Brosnan J, Roper JM: The reality of political ethical conflicts, *JONA* 27(9):42-45, Sept 1997.

Dixit AK, Nalebuff BJ: *Thinking strategically: the competitive edge in business, politics, and everyday life,* New York, 1991, WW Norton and Company.

Ellis JR, Hartley CL: *Managing and coordinating nursing care,* Philadelphia, 1995, JB Lippincott.

Huber D: *Leadership and nursing care management,* Philadelphia, 1996, WB Saunders.

Parsons LC: Delegation skills and nurse job satisfaction, *Nurs Econ* 16:18-26, Jan-Feb 1998.

Pfeffer J: *Managing with power,* Boston, 1992, Harvard Business School Press.

Prince SB: Shared governance: sharing power and opportunity, *JONA* 27:28-35, March 1997.

Skelton R: Nursing and empowerment: concepts and strategies, *J Adv Nurs* 19:415-423, March 1994.

Wilson B, Laschinger HKS: Staff nurse perception of job empowerment and organizational commitment: a test of Kanter's theory of structural power in organizations, *JONA* 24(suppl 45):39-47, April 1994.

Wyatt D: Negotiation strategies for men and women, *Nurs Manage* 30(1):22-25, Jan 1999.

Wywialowski EF: *Managing client care,* ed 2, St. Louis, 1997, Mosby.

Zander KS: Negotiating outcomes with patients and families, *Semin Nurse Managers* 4(3):172-177, Sept 1996.

CASE STUDY

Everyone on your unit wants a raise, but you have a limited amount of money to use. Describe how you will apply principled negotiations to the situation.

CASE STUDY

In the hospital where you work, patients' length of stay is greatly reduced and the patient census is down. Nurses' time has been cut back. Nurses are increasingly dissatisfied, and there is some talk of unionizing. As a manager what can you do to reduce the felt need to unionize?

Critical Thinking Activities for this chapter begin on page 483.

CHAPTER 6

CONFLICT MANAGE-MENT

Chapter Overview

Chapter 6 presents sources of conflict, types of conflict, reactions to conflict, escalation techniques, stages of conflict, approaches to conflict management, deescalation tactics, and strategies for managing intrapersonal, interpersonal, group, intergroup, and organizational conflict. Nominal group technique, role negotiations, and decision charting are discussed in detail.

MAJOR CONCEPTS AND DEFINITIONS	
Conflict	clash, fight, battle, struggle
Role ambiguity	person does not know what is expected
Role overload	person is unable to accomplish what is expected within the allotted time frame
Nominal group technique	a group participation method for making decisions
Role negotiations	the process of preventing role conflicts, role ambiguities, and role overload

CONFLICT THEORY

Conflict, which is closely related to power and political issues, is inevitable and can be constructive or destructive. It may offer an individual personal gain, provide prestige to the winner, be an incentive for creativity, and serve as a powerful motivator. Indeed, there seems to be an optimal level of conflict or anxiety necessary for effective functioning. Conflict that is managed instead of avoided, ignored, or suppressed can be used effectively. If conflict goes beyond the invigorating stage, it becomes debilitating. Conflict is a warning to management that something is amiss, and it should stimulate a search for new solutions through problem solving, the clarification of objectives, the establishment of group norms, and the determination of group boundaries. However, eliminating conflict is not necessary. If managers learn the sources and types of conflict and how to manage them, they can minimize stress on individuals and the organization and maximize effectiveness (Box 6-1).

Sources of Conflict

Cultural differences may contribute to differing attitudes, values, beliefs, and behaviors. Conflict can arise because the individuals involved do not have the same facts. They define the problem differently, have different pieces of information, place more or less importance on various aspects, or have divergent views of their own power and authority. Varying goals and objectives or contrasting procedural strategies for accomplishing mutually acceptable goals produce conflict. Variations in personal value systems or in perceptions of ethical responsibilities can lead to divergence in choices of both goals and methods, thus producing conflict.

When people work together in a complex organization, there are numerous sources of conflict. Conflict increases with both the number of organizational levels and the number of specialties. It is greater as the degree of association increases and when some parties are dependent on others. Competition for scarce resources, ambiguous jurisdictions, and the need for consensus all contribute to conflict. Communication barriers impede understanding, and separations in time and space foster factionalism rather than mutual cooperation. Although standardized policies, rules, and procedures regulate behavior, make relationships more predictable, and decrease the number of arbitrary decisions, they impose added controls over the individual. Men and women who value autonomy are likely to resist such control. Clearly, the sources of

Box 6-1   MODEL FOR MANAGING CONFLICT

Determine the basis of the conflict.	Parties dependent on others
Intrapersonal	Competition for scarce resources
Interpersonal	Ambiguous jurisdictions
Group	Need for consensus
Intergroup	Communication barriers
Organizational	Separation in time and space
Analyze the sources of the conflict.	Accumulation of unresolved conflict
Cultural differences	Consider alternative approaches to conflict management.
Different facts	Avoiding
Separate pieces of information	Accommodating
Different perceptions of the event	Compromising
Defining the problem differently	Collaborating
Divergent views of power and authority	Competing
Role conflicts	Choose the most appropriate approach.
Number of organizational levels	Implement the conflict management strategy.
Degree of association	Evaluate the results.

conflict are endless, and the number of conflicts increases with the number of unresolved differences.

Types of Conflict

Structurally based conflict is either vertical or horizontal. Differences between managers and staff associates (vertical conflict) are often related to inadequate communication, opposing interests, and lack of shared perceptions and attitudes. In vertical situations, managers often attempt to control staff associates' behavior, and the staff associates resist, often causing managers to apply their position power through impersonal bureaucratic rules. Line-staff conflict, which is usually horizontal, is commonly a struggle between domains related to activities, expertise, and authority and is often related to interdepartmental strife.

Interdepartmental differences are related to the degree of interdependence between departments. Interdependence demands collaboration, and the latter provides the occasion for conflict. The need for consensus, the work sequence, and common use of shared facilities or services are areas of interdependence aggravated by differing departmental goals. Both the personalities and the status of the individuals involved affect attitudes such as trust and cooperation, which are just as important as the communication and interaction structures.

There are several types of role conflict (Box 6-2). *Intrasender* conflict originates in the sender who gives conflicting instructions or expects conflicting or mutually exclusive behavioral responses. For example, the same supervisor may demand a higher quality of nursing care, refuse to allow the head nurse to fire incompetent help, and, in an effort to cut costs, refuse to increase an inadequate staff or to permit overtime.

Intersender conflict arises when an individual receives conflicting messages from two or more sources. For example, management may implement an incentive plan to stimulate production and peer pressures may discourage rate busting. In university settings, the dean may expect department chairpersons to function as administrators, and the faculty may expect them to act as their advocates. The matrix organization that imposes project management

| Box 6-2 | **TYPES OF CONFLICT** |

Intrasender	Person-role	Intergroup
Intersender	Interperson	Role ambiguity
Interrole	Intragroup	Role overload

on a functional structure creates intersender role conflict. Any time one is responsible to more than one person, one can anticipate intersender role conflict.

Interrole conflict can occur when an individual belongs to more than one group. Simultaneous, multiple roles within the same organization or the conflicting expectations that result from being a member of more than one organization are sources of such conflict. For example, a person may be expected to attend two different committee meetings at the same time. Job expectations can easily interfere with one's family life. The individual has to develop a system of trade-offs to determine how to behave at certain times.

Person-role conflict is the result of disparity between internal and external roles. An individual has perceived roles and expectations based on one's values and perceptions of oneself. When one's values, needs, or capabilities are incompatible with the role requirement, person-role conflict is created. Behavioral expectations that exceed one's current level of knowledge and skill are also stressful. If the nurse believes that people are important but must process patients through a large clinic in a relatively impersonal manner, the nurse is bound to suffer person-role conflict.

Interperson conflict is common between people whose positions require interaction with other persons who fill various roles in the same organization or other organizations. Interperson conflict is usually not personal but rather the result of each person's acting as a protagonist for that person's department. For example, the director of nursing competes with other departmental heads for resources. Occasionally the conflict arising from the

nature of the roles involved is complicated by personal animosity.

Intragroup conflict occurs when the group faces a new problem, when new values are imposed on the group from outside, or when one's extragroup role conflicts with one's intragroup role. In an academic setting, pressures to have baccalaureate nursing students prepared by faculty with master's degrees and graduate students prepared by faculty with doctoral degrees produces intragroup conflict. Faculty members are caught in a conflict over their teaching responsibilities, continuation of their own education, and fulfillment of expectations for community service and scholarly work. A group facing a new problem may require a change in role relationships that requires role negotiations. When intragroup conflict becomes intense, two new groups may form and give rise to intergroup conflict.

Intergroup conflict is common where two groups have different goals and can achieve their goals only at the other's expense. The conflict may be between groups on the same level or between groups on different levels within an organization. Competition between groups also produces conflict. Resolution may be reached by the dominance of one group over the other, by a compromise that rarely satisfies either group, or by an integration of goals attained when each group recognizes the role of the other group in the system. Intergroup conflict need not be dysfunctional. It can stimulate creativity, innovation, and progress. A conflict-free organization suggests stasis, a situation that offers little challenge for group members.

Role ambiguity, a condition in which individuals do not know what is expected of them, frequently occurs in organizations. Inadequate job descriptions, incomplete explanations of assigned tasks, rapid technological change, and the increasing complexity of organizations contribute to role ambiguity and produce uncertainty and frustration.

If individuals cannot meet the expectations placed on them, they will experience *role overload.* This does not involve a questioning of the legitimacy of the request or of what is expected. Rather, the person is simply unable to accomplish so much within a limited time period. As a result, quality is sacrificed for quantity, the ego is threatened, and frustration develops.

Reactions to Conflict

Numerous psychological mechanisms exist for coping with one's own behavioral reactions to conflict, but such stress contributes to somatic reactions, for example, cardiovascular diseases and gastric disorders. Box 6-3 lists some common reactions to conflict.

Sublimation is one of the most constructive psychological mechanisms whereby unacceptable feelings are repressed and channeled into socially acceptable activities. Energy from hostility and anger that would be destructive if expressed directly is diverted with positive results into other activities such as jogging, tennis, or community service. *Vigorous physical activity* often reduces interpersonal aggression.

People who are displeased with the results of their behavior may *increase their efforts.* Working longer and harder is likely to increase productivity. Flight into activity, a defense mechanism whereby a person keeps busy to avoid thinking about problems, provides some temporary relief but does not solve the problems.

Identification is the practice of enhancing one's self-esteem by imitating another's behavior. The values and beliefs of the other person are internalized, and both achievements and suffering are experienced vicariously. This illustrates the adage, "If you can't beat them, join them." An individual may compensate for a real or imagined inadequacy in one area by substituting a high degree of proficiency in another area. For example, one who lacks social skills may excel academically.

Goals may be *reinterpreted* to attain an unmet goal, or the goal may be lowered or another goal *substituted.* A person promoted to vice president with little hope of becoming president may decide that the vice presidency is a satisfactory position. A rejected job applicant may find another job the applicant enjoys more.

Rationalization provides acceptable explanations for undesirable beliefs or behaviors. Managers may find reasons to fire someone they do not like or pad the expense account because "everyone does it."

Attention getting may involve seeking highly visible jobs, engaging in loud or excessive talking, wearing bright or sexy clothing and unusual hair styles, or driving flashy cars. These displays are destructive only if they divert attention from problem solving.

When individuals repress unacceptable behaviors and values and substitute the opposite attitudes and behaviors, they are using a coping mechanism called *reaction formation.* For example, an employee who was denied a merit pay increase may defend the manager and vigorously support the related policies.

Another mechanism people use to cope with stress is *flight into fantasy.* Flight into fantasy allows one to think about something else. For example, the nurse's aide may daydream about being the charge nurse. Although daydreaming, watching television, and going to the movies are constructive forms of

---

Box 6-3 **REACTIONS TO CONFLICT**		
Sublimation	Rationalization	Displacement
Vigorous physical exercise	Attention getting	Fixation
Increased efforts	Reaction formation	Withdrawal
Identification	Flight into fantasy	Repression
Reinterpreting goals	Projection	Conversion
Substituting goals		

relaxation, engaging in excessive fantasy interferes with one's productivity.

People may protect themselves from their undesirable feelings and traits by attributing them to others. This defense mechanism is called *projection.* For example, a student who is unable to answer a test question may claim that the question is unclear. An unsuccessful person who wants to block another's success claims that the colleague is hostile and uncooperative. Projection is a destructive way to meet needs.

Displacement redirects emotions toward ideas, people, or objects other than the source of the emotions. For example, after the director corrects the head nurse, the nurse manager may displace aggression by snapping at the staff. Some individuals reacting to conflict may resort to negativism, picking apart every idea and action and putting everything in the worst light.

Fixation is the maintenance of a certain maladaptive behavior even though it is obvious that it is not effective in this situation. One who depends on this escape mechanism will make the same mistake repeatedly.

Withdrawal removes one from the area of frustration. For example, a staff nurse who is frustrated by hospital working conditions may go into teaching. This mechanism can be constructive if the person withdraws from a dangerous situation.

Repression pushes painful information and memories into the subconscious, but the material is not truly forgotten. An individual may revert to earlier, even childish behavior. When regressing, staff members may transfer their attitudes toward their parents to their manager and expect the manager to act like a parent. Some people may even have temper tantrums. Regression moves one away from the present and is rarely constructive.

An individual may unconsciously convert an emotional conflict into physical symptoms, for example, the common tension headache. Paralysis of an arm to avoid writing a report or losing one's voice to avoid discussing an unpleasant topic are extreme forms of the coping mechanism called *conversion.*

Everyone uses psychological mechanisms. They are our unconscious defenses against impaired self-esteem, anxiety and guilt, and other threatening or uncomfortable feelings. Defense mechanisms serve a purpose. They become harmful only when excessive.

Escalation-of-Conflict Tactics

Competition escalates conflict. One tries to outdo the other and often vice versa. When we feel we are righteous, we often stop listening. Then we lose an opportunity to learn. Labeling like calling someone lazy escalates the conflict. Identifying the behavior and the negative outcomes can assist with problem solving. For example, "You are often late. That means you do not get the change-of-shift report in a timely way, and patients do not get the care they deserve at the beginning of the shift. People have to tell you what you missed, and we all seem to get off to a bad start." Dealing with personalities escalates conflict and is not appropriate. We should separate the person from the problem. Issue expansion includes issues from other times. We should stay focused. Bickering often makes conflict worse unless we identify the problem causing the discomfort and take a problem-solving approach. Coalition formation gets other people involved and is a power strategy. Constricting others and making threats escalate conflict. One of the most difficult situations to handle is intentional hurt. That may lead to revenge (Box 6-4).

Stages of Conflict

Conflict may be divided into four progressive stages (Box 6-5): latent, perceived, felt, and manifest. *La-*

Box 6-4	**ESCALATION-OF-CONFLICT TACTICS**

Competition	Bickering
Righteousness	Coalition formation
Stop listening	Threats
Labeling	Constricting others
Dealing with personalities	Intentional hurt
Issue expansion	

tent conflict is a phase of anticipation in which antecedent conditions such as scarcity of resources
predict conflict behavior. When change is required,
the manager anticipates differences of opinion
about the desirability of the change, how it should
be implemented, and how the consequences should
be handled.

Perceived conflict, which may or may not be discussed, indicates a cognitive awareness of a stressful
situation. One's personal perceptions can contribute to either an accurate or inaccurate assessment of
the situation and affect the amount of threat and
potential loss the individual anticipates. Conflicts
can be perceived when antecedent conditions do
not exist, as when individuals have a limited knowledge of the facts or do not know others' opinions
and values. For instance, a manager may think there
are limited resources or that someone else wants to
use the same materials when, in fact, there is plenty
for everyone or no one else is interested anyway.
Personal perceptions also can help to avoid conflict.
A suppression mechanism may be used to ignore
conflict that involves low potential loss or is only
minimally threatening. An attention-focus mechanism helps the individual select which conditions to
change and which to ignore.

Affective states such as stress, tension, anxiety,
anger, and hostility are present during the *felt conflict.* Feelings and attitudes may create or avoid conflict. Trust, for example, is a significant factor in the
development of a manifest conflict. If the individuals involved possess trusting attitudes, they share information and control and recognize their mutual
vulnerability. In the absence of trust, individuals
may withhold information so it cannot be used
against them or distort communications to their
advantage. They may scheme to increase their control over others and strive to decrease others' control over them. Clearly, trusting attitudes may prevent potential conflict, and the lack of them may
actually create conflict. Two self-serving individuals
are more likely to have manifest conflict than a
dominant and submissive pair.

The personalization or depersonalization of
the situation affects the evolution of conflict. When
the situation is personalized, the individual is
threatened or judged negatively. With a depersonalized approach, the behavior rather than the individual is identified as creating the problem. "You are
wrong" is personalized, whereas "your views are
very different from mine" is depersonalized. Personalized comments increase anxiety; a depersonalized approach is conducive to problem solving.

Manifest conflict is overt behavior resulting
from the latent, perceived, and felt conflict. It can be
either constructive or destructive to problem solving. Unfortunately, aggression, competition, and
other defenses are learned unconsciously, whereas
problem solving requires a more deliberate, conscious effort.

CONFLICT MANAGEMENT
Approaches to Managing Conflict

Some common approaches to handling conflict are
avoiding, accommodating, compromising, collaborating, and competing (Box 6-6). Avoiding creates
lose-lose situations through unassertive and uncooperative means. The conflict is simply not addressed. This approach may be appropriate when
the other party is more powerful, the issue is unimportant, one has no chance of meeting the goals, or
the cost of dealing with the conflict is higher than
the benefit of the resolution. It may also be used
when it is more appropriate for others to solve a
problem, when more information is needed, or
when one wishes to reduce tension and gain com-
posure. Withdrawing from a conflict does not re-

APPROACHES TO CONFLICT RESOLUTION

> Avoiding—unassertive and uncooperative
> Accommodating—cooperative but unassertive
> Compromising—assertive and cooperative
> Collaborating—assertive and cooperative
> Competing—assertive but uncooperative

solve it, and the individual who retreats frequently harbors a gnawing anger over a situation that drains energy needed for more constructive purposes.

Accommodating is cooperative but unassertive. It is self-sacrificing—the opposite of competing. One neglects one's own needs to meet the goals of the other party. It is appropriate when the opponent is right, the opponent is more powerful, or the issue is more important to someone else. It can be used when preserving harmony is important or when collecting social credits is necessary for later, more important issues. By complimenting one's opponent and accentuating points of agreement, one may smooth out an agreement on minor issues, but the real problems still have to be dealt with.

Compromising moderates both assertiveness and cooperation. It addresses a problem more effectively than avoidance but less than collaboration. Compromisers are willing to yield less than accommodaters but more than competitors as they seek expedient, mutually acceptable answers. Because both parties feel that they sacrifice something, they are only partially satisfied, and a lose-lose atmosphere results. Compromising is useful for reaching expedient answers for limited periods when the goals are only moderately important and the parties have equivalent power.

Collaborating is assertive and cooperative. It is a win-win strategy. It contributes to effective problem solving because both parties try to find mutually satisfying solutions. This method integrates insights from different perspectives with the commitment developed through participation and the resolution of hard feelings. Problems are identified, alternatives explored, and ramifications considered until

difficulties are resolved. Unfortunately, it may take more time than the results are worth. Generally this is a most effective method of conflict resolution. It should be used for important issues and can be used to find creative solutions to interpersonal problems.

Competing is a power-oriented mode that is assertive but uncooperative. In competition one is aggressive and pursues one's own goals at another's expense. This creates a win-lose situation. Nevertheless, it is appropriate when a quick or unpopular decision is needed, when the person is very knowledgeable about the situation and able to make a sound decision, or when one must protect oneself from other aggressive people. If this strategy is used too often, colleagues may become afraid to admit mistakes and may simply say what they think the aggressor wants to hear. A manager can always fall back on authority and give orders to a subordinate, but because the resolution is forced, it almost certainly will be unsatisfactory (Thomas and Kilmann, 1974).

A foundation of mutual trust must underlie any attempt to understand alternative views and to actively seek solutions that will allow each party to achieve its goals. This trust creates an atmosphere conducive to successful conflict resolution.

Deescalation-of-Conflict Tactics

Listening is a good way to deescalate conflict. It shows that you care about the person by taking your precious time to listen to them. The other person may be able to talk through the problem and solve it particularly if you ask questions that lead her through problem solving, such as the following: What is the problem? What are your options? What will happen if you do that? What do you think is the best way to handle this situation? What are you going to do? Showing tact and concern for others is important. Appealing to deescalation by saying something like "I don't want to fight about this" can help. Goodwill gestures like "Let's get a cup of coffee and discuss this" and allowing the airing of feelings are good. Our feelings often dissipate after we talk about how we are feeling. We usually feel better after talking about our feelings. Negative inquiry is

Box
6-7 **DEESCALATION-OF-CONFLICT TACTICS**

Listening
Showing tact and concern for others
Appealing to deescalation
Goodwill gestures
Airing feelings
Negative inquiry
Metacommunications
Responding to all levels of communication
Fractionalization
Position paper
Problem solving
Establishing outside criteria

an assertive technique of asking for more information and trying to resolve the problem. When we are criticized, we tend to get defensive, which escalates the conflict. Then the other person has to work harder to get us to understand where we went wrong. When we ask for more information, the criticizer may end up defending the accused.

Using metacommunications, one discusses the communication as it is occurring. "I am trying to talk to you, and you are walking away from me." It is important to respond to all levels of communications, the facts and the feelings. "I know that it is my weekend to work, but I am angry that I have to work." Once again, expressing the feelings helps dissipate them. Focusing on the facts helps with reality testing and problem solving. Fractionalization breaks the problem down into more manageable components. Position papers help move people from opposite poles to a more middle-of-the-road stance. People will often follow flat statements with qualifiers. Problem solving is a very effective deescalator. When all else fails, establishment of outside criteria may be used (Box 6-7).

Strategies for Management of Conflict

There are three ways of dealing with conflict: the *win-lose, lose-lose,* or *win-win* strategy (Box 6-8).

Win-lose methods include the use of position power, mental or physical power, failure to respond, majority rule, and railroading a minority position over the majority. *Lose-lose* strategies include compromise, bribes for accomplishing disagreeable tasks, arbitration by a neutral third party, and resortion to the use of general rules instead of considering the merits of individual cases. In win-lose and lose-lose strategies, the parties often personalize the issues by focusing on each other instead of on the problem. Intent on their personal differences, they avoid the more important matter of how to mutually solve their problem. Solutions are emphasized instead of goals and values. Rather than identifying mutual needs, planning activities for resolution, and solving the problem, the parties involved look at the issue from their own point of view and strive for total victory.

By contrast, *win-win* strategies focus on goals. They emphasize consensus and integrative approaches to decision making. The consensus process demands a focus on the problem (instead of on each other), on the collection of facts, on the acceptance of the useful aspects of conflict, and on the avoidance of averaging and self-oriented behavior. Thus the group decision is often better than the best individual decision.

Problem-solving strategies include identifying both the problem and each party's needs, exploring alternatives, choosing the most acceptable alternative, planning, defining roles, implementing, and evaluating the decision.

Intrapersonal Conflict

Intrapersonal conflict occurs within the person and usually involves a struggle over values, desires, or incompatible activities. The conflict is internalized. One should set personal goals and priorities and do problem solving. Being self-aware and working to resolve the conflict as soon as possible are important for the manager to remain physically and psychologically well. The manager should help associates be self-aware and do problem solving too (Douglas, 1996; Marquis and Huston, 1996; Wywialowski, 1997).

Box 6-8	STRATEGIES FOR CONFLICT RESOLUTION		

WIN-LOSE	**LOSE-LOSE**	**WIN-WIN**
Position power	Compromise	Consensus
Mental or physical power	Bribes	Problem solving
Failure to respond	Arbitration	Collaborating
Majority rule	General rules	
Railroading		
Competing		

Interpersonal Conflict

Interpersonal conflict is inevitable, but the manager can lessen its impact by coaching staff associates in assertive communication and fair fighting. Engaging in a fair fight demands that individuals with a complaint first ask their opponent for a meeting. Once a time and place are agreed on, both parties should determine whether or not their manager should be present. Moreover, a fair fight demands that both parties know the purpose of the meeting so neither will be caught off guard—each can be prepared. The encounter should begin with a statement of the problem. The manager, if present, should act as a mediator, asking the complainer to explain the perceived problem to the opponent. The opponent then should relate her understanding of how the complainer perceives the problem. After each has spoken, each can clarify any differences over the statement of the problem. Next, the opponent describes her perception of the problem; this description then should be followed by the complainer's repeating her understanding of how the opponent perceives the problem. Again, there is a pause for clarification.

A clear statement of the problem helps shed light on the negative effects of each person's behavior. This feedback process, which requires each party to repeat what the other has just said, forces each to listen carefully. Were it not for such interaction, one might be so busy thinking of what one is going to say next that one fails to hear what is being said. Feedback does not imply parroting, because an understanding of meaning is more important than

sheer memorization of words. Differences often begin to disappear when both parties really hear each other for the first time.

By exploring the alternatives to the problem and the ramifications of their options, the parties can identify and request changes in each other's behavior and respond to the other's requests. The discussion should close with an agreement on whether to change and the establishment of the accompanying conditions. A follow-up engagement should be set to discuss the success or failure of the agreement (Bach and Goldberg, 1974).

Helpful strategies for mediating interpersonal conflict include the following (Loveridge and Cummings, 1996):

- Do not blame anyone for the problem.

- Focus on the issues, not the personalities.

- Protect each party's self-respect.

- Facilitate open and complete discussion of the issues.

- Give equal time to each party.

- Encourage the expression of both positive and negative feelings.

- Encourage each party to listen actively and try to understand the other person's point of view.

- Help develop alternative solutions.

- Summarize key points and plans.

- Later follow up on the plans and give positive reinforcement as appropriate.

- Facilitate further problem solving as necessary.

Interpersonal conflict can result from sexual harassment. The employer is vicariously liable for harassment. The only defense the employer will have is an effective antiharassment policy in place. In-service classes about sexual harassment are appropriate.

Awareness of sexual harassment in the workplace was heightened in 1991 during the Senate confirmation hearing for Judge Clarence Thomas's appointment to the U.S. Supreme Court. Thousands of sexual harassment complaints are filed each year in the United States. Women seem more likely to be sexually harassed than men, often by male co-workers. There seems to be a high prevalence of sexual harassment in the hospital setting. Nurses are often harassed by physicians, patients, and co-workers. Harassment may include repeated requests for dates, sexual teasing, sexual jokes, suggestive looks or gestures, actual touching and fondling, or trapping and leaning over a worker. That can lead to low morale, inefficiency, and decreased productivity resulting from embarrassment and anger related to sexual harassment. Women often do nothing but try to avoid the harasser because of guilt from thinking one must have done something to cause the other's behavior or fear of retaliation.

Sexual harassment is a legal issue that should be confronted immediately. Be assertive and confront the issue. "I want to be very clear that I will not tolerate this sexual harassment. I do not want you telling me dirty jokes, brushing against me, and asking me out with an offer of serving me breakfast in bed." Then listen to the harasser's response, hope for an apology, and accept it, making your position clear. "I accept your apology, but I will follow the sexual harassment policies and report this to my supervisor. I will take action on any further harassment. Sexual harassment is illegal." That way you have made your position clear and implied legal action. File a report. If a situation occurs again, confront the behavior immediately and follow the policies of the agency (Douglas, 1996).

Deborah Swiss (1996) discusses resolving the harassment dilemma in *Women Breaking Through: Overcoming the Final 10 Obstacles at Work.* The women interviewed advised other women to trust their instincts. If they feel harassed, they probably are. Then they have to assess their risk/reward situation, decide how to stop the harassment, and decide whether to deal with it informally or to file a formal complaint. Women are advised to choose an option to stop harassment that feels right to them. One may be able to handle the harassment privately by dealing directly with the offending individual or may need to go public. One may write a letter to the harasser, even if it is never sent. That will help organize thoughts for a confrontation. Role-playing how to approach the offender with a friend will help build confidence. If one wants to be less direct, one can send a highlighted version of the company's sexual harassment statement to the offender. Copies of the policy can be posted on bulletin boards. One can send a clear, anonymous, generic message. Or one may have an intermediary help confront the harasser directly.

It is advisable to record the dates and details of the harassment—noting in particular incidents that can be substantiated by others—if only for one's private files. If harassment continues, one will have historical documentation to take formal action. Otherwise, one may read the account later to find assurance that nothing was done to encourage the harassment and to help relieve self-blame and embarrassment.

If the risk is not too high, a direct approach can be assertive. Allowing the harasser to save face when the harassment has stopped will decrease the likelihood of damage to one's career. If the offender harasses women, makes explicit threats if sexual favors are not granted, or uses physical contact, a formal complaint is appropriate. It is advisable to have contingency plans like the following: If confronting the harasser doesn't work, I will discuss the situation with my boss. If my boss isn't responsive, I will discuss the situation with the personnel officer or other appropriate official.

Women are encouraged to discuss the harassment with a friend. Otherwise the harassment may be an emotional drain that causes a decrease in self-confidence.

Group Conflict

Team development can help prevent and resolve conflict. Planning, goal setting, and rating goals represent the first step in team development. The statement of the core mission of the team is developed by brainstorming and sharing individual mission statements.

The *nominal group technique* is very effective for developing team-performance goals and priorities (Box 6-9). First, individual group members list on separate pieces of paper what they think team-performance goals should be. The group leader helps keep the group problem centered by presenting the question and prevents interruptions of thoughts by asking participants to work silently and independently. This step allows time for thinking, avoids status and conformity pressures, prevents focusing on a particular idea because of a vocal person, and helps avoid choosing between ideas prematurely.

Second, during a round-robin session, each person in turn states one team-performance goal, which is then written on a chalkboard or paper for all to see. It is probable that equalization of participation and sharing of all ideas foster group creativity. By citing one goal, each member is encouraged to participate equally. By the second round, each member has participated and the precedent is set,

and thus competition from aggressive or high-status members is minimized.

If all of an individual's listed goals have been cited, that individual passes and other members continue to offer listed goals in turn until all are exhausted. Ideas are not repeated. However, "hitchhiking" may occur. An idea listed by one member may stimulate another member to have an idea not previously listed. That idea can be added to the member's list and cited during the round-robin session.

It is common for many of an individual's ideas about a problem to remain unspoken because of fear of self-disclosure and embarrassment. When one person states several ideas at once, those ideas tend to be associated with that person. However, with the round-robin method, it is difficult to remember who presented what ideas and full disclosure is encouraged.

The written list can be the basis of recorded minutes and serve as a source of information from which the group continues to work. During this step the group leader should see that ideas are recorded as rapidly as possible and in the words used by the contributor. The entire list should be made visible to all group members. Tearing completed sheets from a flip chart and taping them on the walls works well, and it is an early reward in that the group can see the array of ideas generated. The written ideas are more objective and less personal than oral comments because the personality and position of the contributors are separated from the written statement. The group leader should encourage the simple listing of ideas by explaining that a discussion period will follow. Discussion of the ideas, arguments about them, and side conversations while the list is being made should not be allowed.

The third step is a serial discussion for clarification. During this step each listed idea is discussed in order. This provides an opportunity to clarify ideas, state differences of opinion, provide the logic behind ideas, and prevent undue focusing on any one idea. The group leader's responsibility is to clarify the purpose of this step and to pace the group. Arguments can be curtailed by stating that

Box 6-9   NOMINAL GROUP TECHNIQUE

Listing ideas on paper
Round-robin session
Serial discussion for clarification
Preliminary vote
Analysis of votes
Discussion of preliminary vote
Revote

both points of view have been noted and then moving on to the next point. It is better not to ask the contributors to clarify their own items, because such a request can put them on the spot. Instead, the group members can be asked what the items mean to them. The contributor can clarify when appropriate. This method helps reduce identification of items with specific individuals.

The preliminary vote on item importance is the fourth step. In the nominal group process individuals make independent judgments, express their judgments mathematically by ranking items, use the mean value of the independent judgments for the group's decision, talk over the results, and revote (Delbecq, Van de Ven, and Gustafson, 1975).

Alternative ways to determine a group decision are consensus, majority rule, and independent listing. When using consensus, group members may distort their judgments to maintain group cohesion, and consequently a regression toward the mean may occur. A showing of hands for majority rule is subject to social pressure, and minority positions do not count. Consequently, it may not truly reflect group preference. Independent listing, however, overcomes status, personality, and conformity pressures but does not indicate degree of importance. For example, an item listing might look like the one shown in Box 6-10. An analysis of the votes in Box 6-10 suggests that items 1, 4, 5, and 6 are considered the most important by frequency. Information about degree of importance can be ob-

tained by having the items ranked. Ranking of the list might look like the one shown in Box 6-11. Using a scale of 5 as most important and 1 as least important, an analysis of the votes reveals that items 6, 4, 1, 5, and 8 are considered most important in descending order from 6 to 8. This method is more likely to reflect the true group preference.

The group leader asks each individual to select a specific number of most important items from the list. Individuals seem most able to accurately list five to nine items. Each member is asked to take that specific number of 3×5 index cards, identify that number of items from the list, place the item number in the upper left-hand corner, and write some identifying words in the middle of the card (Figure 6-1). Then the participants are asked to spread out the cards, choose the item they consider most important, and put the high number in the lower right-hand corner of the card and underline it. If five items are being selected, 5 would be the high number. For nine items, 9 would be the high number. That card is turned over, the remaining cards are assessed, and a 1 is put in the lower right-hand corner and underlined for the least important card. That card is turned over, and the next most important item is selected and rated as one less than the highest number: for instance, 8 for nine items or 4 for five items. Then the next-to-the-lowest item is chosen and marked as 2, and so on, until the middle item is left and numbered. This process encourages careful decisions.

Box 6-10 — ANALYSIS BY FREQUENCY

Item	Votes
1	5
2	1
3	2
4	5
5	5
6	5
7	1
8	2

Box 6-11 — ANALYSIS BY RANKING

Item	Votes	Totals
1	1-2-5-5-1	14
2	2	2
3	3-2	5
4	4-3-2-4-2	15
5	1-2-1-3-1	8
6	5-5-4-5-4	23
7	1	1
8	3-3	6

When the card ranking is complete, the group leader collects and shuffles the cards and records the votes on the written list of items.

The fifth step is an analysis of the preliminary vote. Inconsistent voting patterns can be examined, and items receiving many or few votes can be discussed. The sixth step, discussion, will probably allow for corrections of misinformation, misunderstandings, and unequal information, thereby offering a more accurate indication of preferences than voting only.

The final step is the revote, which determines the outcome of the process, documents the group judgment, and closes the nominal group process.

Role negotiations—the process of preventing role conflicts, role ambiguities, and role overload—become important once priorities have been set. During this process group members clarify each individual's role on the team and help resolve any disagreements over the team members' roles. Members initially send one written message to each team member indicating that for them to act, they need the other team member to do more, less, or to continue her previous performance (Figure 6-2). *To*

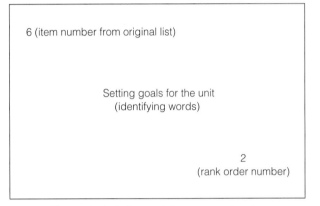

Figure 6-1 Index card illustrating rank order.

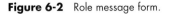

Figure 6-2 Role message form.

whom and *from whom* are essential parts of the message. The number of role messages sent to any one individual should be limited to prevent an information overload. The message must clearly state how the sender wants the receiver to behave and how a change will help the sender. Each role message must indicate the need for more, less, or the same of some activity. More than one message in the "same" category indicates support for the other person.

Receivers respond by indicating what they can or cannot do, explaining why, and offering alternative solutions, for example, "I can't do *x*, but I can do *y*, which should help solve your problem," or "If I do *x*, I would like you to do *y*." Receivers analyze the role messages they receive in the "do more, do less, and do the same" categories according to who sent the message and their response to that mes-

sage. Do the receivers know what is expected of them? Do different people want them to do more and less of the same activity at the same time? Do the receivers have time to meet all the demands made of them? Role definition helps identify role ambiguity, role conflict, and role overload. After roles are negotiated, a contract (Figure 6-3) is written that defines the problem, identifies what each involved person will do, and sets a date for a follow-up check.

Negotiating involves good communication skills. One can identify needs, ideas, and information by using open-ended probes to clarify. Closed probes can be used to pinpoint specifications and to confirm understanding. One should indicate one's intent ("I support your idea") when one offers ideas of information. It is preferable to present reasons before conclusions, because they seem to be heard

---

ROLE CONTRACT

1. Problem:

2. Person **x** agrees to:

3. Person **y** agrees to:

4. Others agree to:

We agree that a follow-up check will be done by _____.
                                                    (date)

                                              Signatures

                                              _____
                                              x

                                              _____
                                              y

                                              _____
                                              others

Figure 6-3 Role contract.

better that way, and the speaker is more likely to be considered reasonable. To build on ideas, one should acknowledge the connection ("Bill's comment made me think of . . .") and then add value. To criticize constructively, merits should be stated before concerns. One should then ask for ways to retain merits and eliminate concerns. One should confront counterproductive tactics by confirming the behavior and expressing its impact. ("That seemed like a personal attack. Is that what you intended? I feel angry when I am treated that way.") To break an impasse, one can indicate one's desire to continue and then initiate a change of pace. ("Let's go get a cup of coffee and then try to solve this problem.")

To come to an agreement, the purpose of the meeting and a review of the situation should be discussed. Identify the needs and restrictions, examine ideas from both points of view, and determine the best alternative. The discussion can be closed by summarizing the agreement and confirming the next steps (*Negotiating Self-Taught*, 1984).

Decision charting is the next major phase of team development and is concerned with who should be involved in decision making and with the nature of that involvement. To determine who should be involved in decision making, one should assess who has the information necessary to make a sound decision and who is responsible for implementing that decision. The latter needs to understand the decision and be committed to it.

People can be involved in decision making in a variety of ways. Some are directly involved because they have the necessary information and are responsible for implementing the decision. The involvement of some may be limited to input or consultation. Others need to be informed about the decision, and someone must be responsible for managing the overall decision-making process.

A decision chart helps one visualize the decision-making process (Figure 6-4). Decisions to be made are listed down the side of the page, and the involved people across the top in a grid pattern. Placing an M in a square indicates who manages the process; D indicates who is directly involved; C indicates who should be consulted; and I indicates who should be informed. Anyone who is expected to implement the decision obviously must be informed (Rubin, Plovnick, and Fry, 1975, 1978).

Intergroup Conflict

Intergroup conflict is common and can be dysfunctional. As with interpersonal conflict, intergroup resistance may result from low trust, poor communications, and false assumptions. People resist what they perceive as threatening. Intergroup actions may threaten territorial rights and contribute to role overload and conflict. By preventing win-lose situations, emphasizing the organization's goals and effectiveness, rotating personnel among groups to facilitate understanding, and increasing interaction

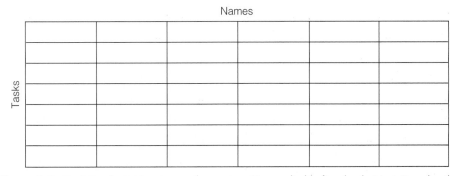

Figure 6-4 Decision chart. M, manages the process; C, consulted before the decision; D, makes the decision; I, informed of the decision.

and communication between groups, one can help reduce intergroup conflict.

When a group recognizes its need to solve some intergroup conflict, it must first decide how to begin. A study of the organizational chart will determine who should be involved. Who should represent the group—a person or a committee? Someone who is already friendly with members of the other group? Someone with strong or moderate feelings about the position? What is the group's position, and how much negotiation is acceptable? It helps to emphasize common goals and discuss constraints. The same process used in interpersonal conflict should be used in group conflict situations: setting and rating goals, negotiating roles, and making decisions.

Organizational Conflict

Organizations in conflict display the collective symptoms of their members. Personnel feel frustration at work. If they do not think their skills are being used, they experience a loss of self-esteem and a sense of powerlessness, both of which lead to withdrawal from the situation instead of an attempt to solve the problems. Group members also engage in backbiting and blame others for the problems. Subgroup formations are common. Members of the organization identify the same task and group maintenance problems but act contrary to the information, thereby increasing their frustrations. However, personnel do not have the same frustrations or exhibit the same dysfunctional behavior outside the organization.

Organizational factors that increase conflict include the number of organizational levels, number of specialties, degree of association, and some parties' dependency on others. The higher the number of levels and specialties, the more opportunities for conflict. More need to associate with others and greater dependency of one on another increase the risk of conflict. Competition for scarce resources, ambiguous jurisdictions, and need for consensus increase conflict. Communication barriers, including separation in time and space and differing values, increase conflict. An accumulation of unresolved conflict increases the challenge for conflict management.

A manager may sooth a party during organizational conflict to facilitate the process and then deal with the underlying problem later. Managers should encourage personnel to confront each other and work their problems out themselves. Appropriate behavior change should be expected and may require sensitivity training, team development, and educational tools. The manager should assess things such as the organizational structure, titles, job descriptions, policies, and procedures as related to the apparent conflict. Responsibility charting can help clarify jurisdictional conflicts. A consultant may be appointed to assess the situation and make recommendations (Marquis and Huston, 1996).

The consultant must analyze the organization's structure, the leadership and authority of the institution, the communication patterns, the amount of intergroup cooperation and competition, the group's norms and goals, the group's problem-solving and decision-making processes, and various individual roles and functions within the group. Organizational research can help provide the information necessary to solve the problem.

After data have been collected and analyzed, the consultant offers feedback. Members of the organization can publicly vote on whether or not they agree with the consultant's views. A public vote facilitates ownership of ideas. If there is disagreement, the consultant helps the group clarify the reasons for the differences and modifies the statement until it reflects the group's thinking.

The consultant then asks all members to write a few sentences about how they contribute to the situation so that they can recognize their own part in the problem. Individuals are likely to maintain the status quo for fear of serious consequences if they confront the issues. The consultant shares her theory with the group, helps develop an awareness of dysfunctional behavior, helps individuals cope with their feelings, encourages fantasy and reality testing, and coaches group members toward new behaviors.

Prevention of Conflict

Careful development of an organization's structure, strategic and comprehensive planning, management and organizational development, and careful selection and placement of personnel help prevent organizational conflict. The same strategies also prevent intergroup, group, and interpersonal conflict. Although conflict can be reduced, it cannot be totally avoided. Conflict can be constructive or destructive. By capitalizing on the positive aspects, the negative features can seem more bearable.

CHAPTER SUMMARY

Chapter 6 covered the following:
Conflict Theory
　　Sources of Conflict
　　Types of Conflict
　　Reactions to Conflict
　　Escalation-of-Conflict Tactics
　　Stages of Conflict
Conflict Management
　　Approaches to Managing Conflict
　　Deescalation-of-Conflict Tactics
　　Strategies for Management of Conflict
　　Intrapersonal Conflict
　　Interpersonal Conflict
　　Group Conflict
　　Intergroup Conflict
　　Organizational Conflict
　　Prevention of Conflict

REFERENCES

Bach GR, Goldberg H: *Creative aggression: the art of assertive living,* New York, 1974, Avon Books.

Delbecq AL, Van de Ven AH, Gustafson DH: *Group techniques for program planning: a guide to nominal group and Delphi processes,* Glenview, Ill, 1975, Scott Foresman.

Douglas LM: *The effective nurse,* ed 5, St. Louis, 1996, Mosby.

Loveridge CE, Cummings SH: *Nursing management in the new paradigm,* Gaithersburg, Md, 1996, Aspen.

Marquis BL, Huston CJ: *Leadership roles and management functions in nursing,* Philadelphia, 1996, Lippincott.

Negotiating self-taught, Stamford, Conn, 1984, Learning International.

Rubin IM, Plovnick MS, Fry RE: *Improving the coordination of care: a program for health team development,* Cambridge, Mass, 1975, Ballinger.

Rubin IM, Plovnick MS, Fry RE: *Managing human resources in health care organizations: an applied approach,* Reston, Va, 1978, Reston.

Swiss DJ: *Women breaking through: overcoming the final 10 obstacles at work,* Princeton, NJ, 1996, Peterson's/Pacesetter Books.

Thomas KW, Kilmann RH: *Thomas-Kilmann conflict mode instrument,* Sterling Forest, Tuxedo, NY, 1974, XICOM.

Wywialowski EF: *Managing client care,* ed 2, St. Louis, 1997, Mosby.

BIBLIOGRAPHY

Baker KM: Improving staff nurse conflict resolution skills, *Nurs Econ* 13:295-298, Sept-Oct 1995.

Dove MA: Conflict: process and resolution, *Nurs Manage,* pp 30-32, April 1998.

Forte PS: The high cost of conflict, *Nurs Econ* 15:119-123, May-June 1997.

Hayes PM: Team building: bringing RNs and NAs together, *Nurs Manage* 25:52-54, May 1994.

Karrass CL: *Negotiate to close,* New York, 1987, Simon & Schuster.

Kusbell E, Rub S: Dealing with conflict: the Margaret Chapman case, *JONA* 26:34-40, Feb 1996.

Likert R, Likert JG: *New ways of managing conflict,* New York, 1984, McGraw-Hill.

Lowenstein AJ, Glanville C: Cultural diversity and conflict in the health care workplace, *Nurs Econ* 13:203-209, July-Aug 1995.

Martin K, Wimberly D, O'Keefe K: Resolving conflict in a multicultural nursing department, *Nurs Manage* 25:49-51, Jan 1994.

McElhaney R: Conflict management in nursing administration, *Nurs Manage,* pp 49-50, March 1996.

Megel ME, Elrod MEB, Rausch AK: Conflicts experienced by quality assurance/improvement professionals: a Delphi study, *J Nurs Care Qual* 10(2):75-82, 1996.

Sherer JL: Resolving conflict the right way, *Hosp Health Netw,* pp 52-55, April 20, 1994.

CASE STUDY

Two staff nurses on the team want the same weekend off. You need someone to work. How are you going to go about resolving the conflict?

Critical Thinking Activities for this chapter begin on page 487.

CHAPTER 7

THEORIES OF LEADERSHIP

Chapter Overview

Chapter 7 discusses several theories of leadership and the development of management thought.

MAJOR CONCEPTS AND DEFINITIONS	
Lead	to show, mark the way, guide the course
Transaction	the negotiation of business
Transformation	a change in the nature of someone or something
Charisma	an inspirational quality that some leaders possess
Situational	appropriate to the requirements of different situations
Contingency	the uncertainty of an event's occurrence
Management	act of planning, organizing, staffing, directing, and controlling
Scientific management	focused on the best way to do a task
Classic organization	focused on planning, organizing, and controlling of the organization as a whole
Human relations	focused on the effect individuals have on the success of the organization
Behavioral science	focused on scientific validation

THEORIES OF LEADERSHIP

Theories of leadership are numerous. The following survey covers the alternatives, beginning with the oldest notion and advancing to ideas currently in vogue. By familiarizing themselves with them, nurses can select and adapt the most suitable approach for dealing with different situations. As a role model, the nursing leader can reduce the autocratic atmosphere and, hence, some of the role conflicts.

Leaders need to do the right things, are challenged by change, focus on purposes, and have a future time frame. They ask why and use strategies on their journeys to human potential. On the other hand, managers do things right, are challenged by continuity, and focus on structures and procedures in a present time frame. They ask who, what, when, where, and how as they use schedules to get to destinations and evaluate human performance (Box 7-1).

Great Man Theory

The great man theory argues that a few people are born with the necessary characteristics to be great. Leaders are well rounded and simultaneously display both instrumental and supportive leadership behavior. Instrumental activities include planning, organizing, and controlling the activities of subordinates to accomplish the organization's goals. Obtaining and allocating resources such as people, equipment, materials, funds, and space are particularly important. Supportive leadership is socially oriented and allows for participation and consultation from subordinates for decisions that affect them. People who use both instrumental and supportive leadership behaviors are considered "great men" and supposedly are effective leaders in any situation. Many find this theory unattractive because of its premise that leaders are born and not made, which suggests that leadership cannot be developed.

Box 7-1   COMPARISON OF LEADERSHIP AND MANAGEMENT

	Leadership	Management
Motto	Do the right things	Do things right
Challenge	Change	Continuity
Focus	Purposes	Structures and procedures
Time frame	Future	Present
Methods	Strategies	Schedules
Questions	Why?	Who, what, when, where, and how?
Outcomes	Journeys	Destinations
Human	Potential	Performance

Charismatic Theory

People may be leaders because they are charismatic, but relatively little is known about this intangible characteristic. What constitutes charisma? Most agree that it is an inspirational quality possessed by some people that makes others feel better in their presence. The charismatic leader inspires others by obtaining emotional commitment from followers and by arousing strong feelings of loyalty and enthusiasm. Under charismatic leadership one may overcome obstacles not thought possible. However, because charisma is so elusive, some may sense it while others do not.

Gary Yukl (1994) has reported findings from Robert House's, Bernard Bass's, and Jay Conger and Rabindra Kanungo's research about charisma. House found that followers of charismatic leaders trust the leader's beliefs; have similar beliefs; exhibit affection for, obedience to, and unquestioning acceptance of the leader; and are emotionally involved in and believe they can contribute to the mission. He found that charismatic leaders have a strong conviction in their own beliefs, high self-confidence, and a need for power. They are likely to set an example by their behavior, communicate high expectations to followers and express confidence in them, and arouse motives for the group's mission.

Conger and Kanungo's research approached charisma as an attributional phenomenon. They found that charisma is more likely attributed to a leader who advocates a vision discrepant from the status quo, emerges during a crisis, accurately assesses the situation, communicates self-confidence, uses personal power, makes self-sacrifices, and uses unconventional strategies.

Bass proposed that charismatic leaders perceive themselves as having supernatural purpose and destiny and that followers may idolize and worship them as spiritual figures or superhumans. This blind obedience can lead to bad outcomes such as group suicide. Transformational leaders use charisma for good.

Trait Theory

Until the mid-1940s, the trait theory was the basis for most leadership research. Early work in this area maintained that traits are inherited, but later theories suggested that traits could be obtained through learning and experience. Researchers identified the leadership traits as energy, drive, enthusiasm, ambition, aggressiveness, decisiveness, self-assurance, self-confidence, friendliness, affection, honesty, fairness, loyalty, dependability, technical mastery, and teaching skill. Asking themselves what traits leaders possess, various researchers arrived at different conclusions but identified some common leadership traits:

1. Leaders need to be more intelligent than the group they lead. However, a highly intelligent person may not find leadership responsibilities challenging enough, may prefer to work with abstract ideas and research, and may have difficulty relating to the group.
2. Leaders must possess initiative, the ability to perceive and start courses of action not considered by others.
3. Creativity is an asset. Having originality—the ability to think of new solutions to problems and ideas of new ways to be productive—is helpful.
4. Emotional maturity with integrity—a sense of purpose and direction, persistence, dependability, and objectivity—is another important trait. Mature leaders do what they say they will and are consistent in their actions. They often work long hours, apply themselves intensely, and spread enthusiasm to followers. Energy, drive, and good health are necessary to endure the long hours, overcome obstacles, and sustain continuous achievement. Self-assurance is self-confidence. It is hoped that leaders perceive themselves as effective problem solvers who can successfully handle the difficulties that confront them.
5. Communication skills are important. The leader needs to understand others and speak and write clearly.
6. Persuasion often is used by leaders to gain the consent of followers. The leader may make suggestions, supply supportive data, ask penetrating questions, make compromises, and request action to persuade others.
7. Leaders need to be perceptive enough to distinguish their allies from their opponents and to place their subordinates in suitable positions.
8. Leaders participate in social activities. They can socialize with all kinds of people and adapt to various groups. Approachable, friendly, and helpful, they gain the confidence and loyalty of others in such a way that makes people willing to cooperate.

The authoritarian leader maintains strong control, does the planning, makes the decisions, and gives the orders. Autocratic leaders tend to be directive, critical, and punitive. They may make decisions that are not in the best interest of the group. They give themselves a higher status than the group members, which reduces open communications and trust. They tend to get good quantity and quality of output but little autonomy, creativity, or self-motivation. This can be appropriate for an emergency situation when the leader knows what to do, but it does not develop people (Box 7-2).

Democratic leaders maintain less control, ask questions and make suggestions rather than issue

Box 7-2 COMPARISON OF AUTOCRATIC, DEMOCRATIC, AND LAISSEZ-FAIRE LEADERSHIP

Autocratic	Democratic	Laissez-faire
Strong control	Less control	No control
Gives orders	Offers suggestions	Nondirective
Does decision making	Makes suggestions	Abdicates decision making
Leader does planning	Group does planning	No planning
Directive	Participative	Uninvolved
Fosters dependency	Fosters independence	Fosters chaos

orders, and get the group involved in planning, problem solving, and decision making. The participation tends to increase motivation and creativity. It works when people have knowledge and skills and work well together over time. It can be cumbersome. It is often less efficient than autocratic control.

Laissez-faire is very permissive, nondirective, passive, and inactive. Members may work independently and possibly at cross-purposes because there is no planning or coordination and little cooperation. Chaos is likely to develop unless an informal leader emerges. This style can work with very mature, autonomous workers, but it is more likely to be inefficient and unproductive.

The trait theory expanded knowledge about leadership, but it was not without its flaws. Few if any traits are identified in all trait theory research. They are not mutually exclusive, and there is considerable overlap between categories or definitions of the characteristics. It is not clear which traits are most important, which traits are needed to acquire leadership, and which traits are needed to maintain it. Trait theory does not view personality as an integrated whole, does not deal with subordinates, and avoids environmental influences and situational factors.

Ohio State Leadership Studies researchers compiled a list of about 1800 examples of leadership behavior that factored out two dimensions: consideration and initiating structure. Consideration involves behaving in a friendly and supportive way, looking out for others' welfare, showing concern, treating others as equals, taking time to listen, consulting others on important matters, being willing to accept suggestions, and doing personal favors.

Initiating structure is the way the leader structures roles to attain the goals. It includes assigning tasks, defining procedures, setting deadlines, maintaining standards, suggesting new approaches, and coordinating activities.

Researchers at the University of Michigan focused on identification of relationships between leader behavior, group process, and group performance. They found that three types of leadership behavior marked the difference between effective and ineffective leaders: (1) task-oriented behavior, (2) relationship-oriented behavior, and (3) participative leadership. Task-oriented behavior includes planning, scheduling, and coordinating activities. Relationship-oriented behavior includes acting friendly and considerate, showing trust and confidence, expressing appreciation, and providing recognition. Participative leadership uses group meetings to enlist associate participation in decision making, improve communications, promote cooperation, and facilitate conflict resolution.

Situational Theory

Situational theories became popular during the 1950s. These theories suggest that the traits required of a leader differ according to varying situations. Among the variables that determine the effectiveness of leadership style are factors such as the personality of the leader; the performance requirements of both the leader and followers; the attitudes, needs, and expectations of the leader and followers; the degree of interpersonal contact possible; time pressures; physical environment; organizational structure; the nature of the organization; the state of the organization's development; and the influence of the leader outside the group. A person may be a leader in one situation and a follower in another or a leader at one time and a follower at others because the type of leadership needed depends on the situation.

Contingency Theory

During the 1960s Fred Fiedler introduced the contingency model of leadership. Refuting the ideal leadership style theory, he argued that a leadership style will be effective or ineffective depending on the situation. He identified three aspects of a situation that structure the leader's role: (1) leader-member relations, (2) task structure, and (3) position power.

Leader-member relations involve the amount of confidence and loyalty the followers have with regard to their leader. Leadership is assessed by a group-atmosphere scale (Box 7-3). Fiedler also used

Box 7-3

GROUP-ATMOSPHERE SCALE

Describe the atmosphere of your group by checking the following items:

	8	7	6	5	4	3	2	1	
1. Friendly	:	:	:	:	:	:	:	:	Unfriendly
2. Accepting	:	:	:	:	:	:	:	:	Rejecting
3. Satisfying	:	:	:	:	:	:	:	:	Frustrating
4. Enthusiastic	:	:	:	:	:	:	:	:	Unenthusiastic
5. Productive	:	:	:	:	:	:	:	:	Nonproductive
6. Warm	:	:	:	:	:	:	:	:	Cold
7. Cooperative	:	:	:	:	:	:	:	:	Uncooperative
8. Supportive	:	:	:	:	:	:	:	:	Hostile
9. Interesting	:	:	:	:	:	:	:	:	Boring
10. Successful	:	:	:	:	:	:	:	:	Unsuccessful

From Fiedler FE: *A theory of leadership effectiveness*, New York, 1967, McGraw-Hill, p. 269.

a sociometric index of the least-preferred co-worker (LPC) score. Followers were asked to think of everyone with whom they have ever worked and to rate the least-preferred co-worker on an eight-point bipolar adjective scale, which includes adjectives such as friendly and cooperative. A high score describes the person in favorable terms, and a low score is a negative rating. Although the LPC scores are difficult to interpret and it is hard to say what they measure, Fiedler suggests that high scorers are relationship oriented and low scorers are mostly task oriented.

Task structure is high if it is easy to define and measure a task. The structure is low if it is difficult to define the task and to measure progress toward its completion. Fiedler used four criteria to determine the degree of task structure: (1) goal clarity: extent to which a goal is understood by followers; (2) extent to which a decision can be verified: knowing who is responsible for what; (3) multiplicity of goal paths: number of solutions; and (4) specificity of solution: number of correct an-

swers. Technical nursing, which focuses on procedures, may have a high task structure, but situations involving human relations and value judgments may have numerous solutions with no specific correct answer and consequently have a low task structure.

Position power refers to the authority inherent in a position, the power to use rewards and punishment, and the organization's support of one's decisions. Directors of nursing, managers, and sometimes patient care coordinators have high position power with the right to hire and fire, promote, and adjust salaries. People with low position power may be elected, function in an acting position, or be subject to removal by peers or subordinates. Elected committee chairpersons have low position power. Team leaders and staff nurses usually have low position power. Given the critical conditions, Fiedler argues that one can predict the most productive leadership style (Table 7-1).

If a task is structured but the leader is disliked and therefore needs to be diplomatic, or if the task

Table 7-1   Summary of Fiedler Investigations of Leadership

| | Group Situation | | | |
Condition	Leader-Member Relations	Task Structure	Position Power	Leadership Style Correlating With Productivity
1	Good	Structured	Strong	Directive
2	Good	Structured	Weak	Directive
3	Good	Unstructured	Strong	Directive
4	Good	Unstructured	Weak	Permissive
5	Moderately poor	Structured	Strong	Permissive
6	Moderately poor	Structured	Weak	No data
7	Moderately poor	Unstructured	Strong	No relationship found
8	Moderately poor	Unstructured	Weak	Directive

From Donnelly JH Jr, Gibson JL, Ivancevich JM: *Fundamentals of management functions, behavior, models,* Dallas, 1981, Business Publications, © 1981 by Business Publications, Inc.

is ambiguous and the leader is liked and therefore seeks the cooperation of the workers, the considerate, accepting leadership style probably will be most productive. When a disliked leader faces ambiguous tasks, a directive style is more productive. The most productive leadership style is contingent on the situational variables.

Empirical evidence does not supply conclusive evidence for the contingency model. It is difficult to say what the psychologically distant manager and psychologically closer manager measures are really recording. Correlations were used for predicted direction even when they were not statistically significant. The model is primarily academic in that it has not been used in management development for improving group performance and organizational effectiveness, and Fiedler's complex, three-dimensional contingency model has contributed to leadership theories (Fiedler, 1967; Fiedler and Chemers, 1974; Fiedler, Chemers, and Mahar, 1976).

Path-Goal Theory

House derived the path-goal theory from the expectancy theory. The expectancy theory argues that people act as they do because they expect their behavior to produce satisfactory results. In the path-

goal relationship, the leader facilitates task accomplishment by minimizing obstructions to the goals and by rewarding followers for completing their tasks. The leader helps staff associates assess needs, explores alternatives, helps associates make the most beneficial decisions, rewards personnel for task achievement, and provides additional opportunities for satisfying goal accomplishment.

House noted that studies done during the 1950s revealed that leaders who structured activities for staff associates generally had more productive work groups and got higher performance evaluations from superiors. Structure includes planning, organizing, directing, and controlling through activities such as clarifying expectations of staff associates, scheduling work, making assignments, determining procedures, and setting standards. Structured activity can increase motivation by reducing role ambiguity and allowing for externally imposed controls. In contrast, considerate leaders had more satisfied workers. They created an atmosphere of friendliness, warmth, and support by tending to the personal welfare of their subordinates. Leader consideration seems particularly important for routine jobs. People who perform a variety of tasks may find their jobs more satisfying and have less need for social support.

House recognized that individual differences will affect the staff associates' perception of leader behavior. For instance, experienced staff associates may prefer a task-oriented style, whereas less mature, less experienced, and consequently less secure individuals may prefer a considerate leader. Staff associates with a high need for achievement probably will prefer a task-oriented leader, but people with a high need for affiliation will prefer a considerate leader. The path-goal theory introduced staff associates as a variable (House, 1971).

Situational Leadership Theory

The situational leadership theory predicts the most appropriate leadership style from the level of maturity of the followers. Paul Hersey and Kenneth Blanchard illustrate this theory in a four-quadrant model (Figure 7-1). A horizontal continuum registers low emphasis on the accomplishment of tasks

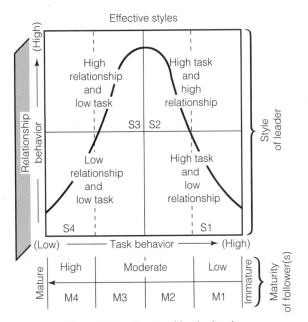

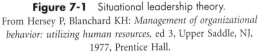

Figure 7-1 Situational leadership theory.
From Hersey P, Blanchard KH: *Management of organizational behavior: utilizing human resources,* ed 3, Upper Saddle, NJ, 1977, Prentice Hall.

on the left side of the model to high emphasis on task behavior on the right side. The vertical continuum depicts low emphasis on interpersonal relationships at the bottom of the model to high emphasis on relationships at the top. The lower left quadrant therefore represents a laissez-faire type of leadership style with little concern for production or relationships. The lower right quadrant represents an autocratic leadership style with considerable concern for production but little concern for relationships. The upper right quadrant designates a high concern for both tasks and relationships. The upper left quadrant represents a leadership style that stresses relationships but shows little concern for tasks.

The maturity level of the group or individual is depicted on a continuum from high maturity on the left to low maturity on the right under the four quadrants. The maturity levels are superimposed on the quadrants with dashed lines. The best leadership style for given levels of maturity is shown by a curvilinear line in the four quadrants. To determine the most appropriate leadership style, one must assess the maturity level of the individual or group, plot it on the maturity continuum, and project a line at a right angle from that point until it intersects with the curvilinear line. The quadrant in which the intersection occurs depicts the most appropriate leadership style. With increased maturity less structure and emotional support are needed. In contrast, high-task and low-relationship style is considered best for below-average maturity. The leadership styles in quadrants 2 and 3 are recommended for the average group or individual.

This model is consistent with Chris Argyris's immaturity-maturity continuum, which indicates that as people mature, they progress from a passive to an active state and from dependence to independence. With maturity they pass from a need for structure and little relationship through a decreasing need for structure and increasing need for relationship to little need for either. The progression is not always smooth. Stress may cause members of the group to regress, and leaders must adjust their behavior accordingly. The situational leadership theory therefore emphasizes the importance of the maturity level of the group, and the leader needs to adapt leadership styles accordingly.

Transactional Leadership

Transactional leadership is an exchange posture that identifies needs of followers and provides rewards to meet those needs in exchange for expected performance. It is a contract for mutual benefits that has contingent rewards. The leader is a caretaker who sets goals for employees, focuses on day-to-day operations, and uses management by exception. It is a competitive, task-focused approach that takes place in a hierarchy.

Transformational Leadership

Transformational leadership promotes employee development, attends to needs and motives of followers, inspires through optimism, influences changes in perception, provides intellectual stimulation, and encourages follower creativity. The leader is a role model who uses individualized consideration, provides a sense of direction, and en-courages self-management. It is a cooperative, process-focused networking. Box 7-4 summarizes the key points of several views of transactional and transformational leadership.

Bass (1985) has described transformational leaders in terms of charisma, inspirational leadership, individualized consideration, and intellectual stimulation.

Warren Bennis and Burt Nanus (1985) indicate that leaders do the right things, whereas managers do things right. Leaders focus on effectiveness; managers deal with efficiency. Bennis and Nanus identify four strategies for taking charge: (1) attention through vision, (2) meaning through communication, (3) trust through positioning, and (4) deployment of self. The leader's vision should be clear, attractive, and attainable. Communication through stories, allegories, fables, parables, analogies, and so on helps give meaning to the vision. The leader's position must be clear because associates are more likely to be trusting when they know the leader's view of the organization. Open communications, honesty, and consistency are important to building trust. Leaders are continuous learners and use the organization as a learning environment.

Box 7-4 COMPARISON OF TRANSACTIONAL AND TRANSFORMATIONAL LEADERSHIP

Transactional	Transformational
Hierarchy	Networking
Competitive	Cooperative
Task focus	Process focus
Exchange posture	Promote employee development
Identify needs of followers	Attend to needs and motives of followers
Provide rewards to meet needs	Inspire through optimism
Exchange for expected performance	Influence change in perception
Contract for mutual benefits	Provide intellectual stimulation
Contingent rewards	Encouragement of follower creativity
Caretaker	Role model
Set goals for employees	Individualize consideration
Focus on day-to-day operations	Provide sense of direction
Management by exception	Encouragement of self-management

They deploy themselves as they foster a learning environment.

James Kouzes and Barry Posner (1987, 1990) identify five basic practices and ten specific behaviors that leadership involves: (1) challenging the process by searching for opportunities and experimenting and taking risks, (2) inspiring a shared vision by envisioning the future and enlisting others, (3) enabling others to act by fostering collaboration and strengthening others, (4) modeling the way by setting an example and planning small wins, and (5) encouraging the heart by recognizing individual contributions and celebrating accomplishments.

Bass and Bruce Avolio (1993) indicate that transformational leaders change the organization by realigning the organization's culture with the new vision and revision of assumptions, values, and norms. They identify four components that characterize transformational leaders: (1) idealized influence, (2) inspirational motivation, (3) intellectual stimulation, and (4) individualized consideration. They believe that organizations should maintain a base of effective transactional qualities while moving in the direction of transformational qualities.

William Hitt (1993) defines leadership as affecting people so that they will strive willingly toward group goals. He identifies five types of knowledge needed by a leader: (1) knowing oneself, (2) knowing the job, (3) knowing the organization, (4) knowing the business, and (5) knowing the world. He also identifies six core functions of leaders: (1) valuing, (2) visioning, (3) coaching, (4) empowering, (5) team building, and (6) promoting quality. He lists the attributes essential for leadership as identity, independence, authenticity, responsibility, courage, and integrity.

Integrative Leadership Model

From a review of leadership theories, obviously there is no one best leadership style. Leaders are rarely totally people or task oriented. Leader, followers, situation—all influence leadership effectiveness. Consequently, an integration of leadership theories seems appropriate. Leaders need to be aware of their own behavior and influence on oth-

ers, individual differences of followers, group characteristics, motivation, task structures, environmental factors, and situational variables and adjust their leadership style accordingly. Leadership requires adaptive behavior.

DEVELOPMENT OF MANAGEMENT THOUGHT

A familiarity with the development of management thought can be useful to nursing leaders in creating their own management styles. No single management theory is sufficient in itself to guide the nursing leader's every action. But through an eclectic approach, drawing from the best and most applicable theories in each situation, nurse administrators can create individual management styles to meet their particular needs.

Scientific Management

Theories of management do not remain static. Since the introduction of the earliest principles of scientific management nearly a century ago, management thought has been marked by constant change.

Taylor. Frederick Taylor (1856-1915) is generally recognized as the father of scientific management. Through the use of stopwatch studies, he applied the principles of observation, measurement, and scientific comparison to determine the most efficient way to accomplish a task. Taylor conducted time-and-motion studies to time workers, analyze their movements, and set work standards. He usually found that the same result could be obtained in less time with fewer or shorter motions. When the most efficient way to complete a task was determined, workers were trained to follow that method. The most productive workers were hired, and even when they were paid an incentive wage, labor costs per unit were reduced.

Taylor, an engineer in steel manufacture, applied his pioneering experience in scientific management to the service of Bethlehem Steel in 1898 and later became an independent business consultant. Identifying the responsibilities of management and separating them from the functions of the workers, Taylor threw aside rule-of-thumb judgments and developed a systematic approach to determine the most efficient means of production. He considered management's function to be planning. Working conditions and methods had to be standardized to maximize production. It was management's responsibility to select and train workers rather than allow them to choose their own jobs and methods and train themselves. An incentive plan whereby workers were paid according to their rates of production was introduced to minimize worker dissent and reduce resistance to improved methods, increase production, and produce higher profits. Taylor's scientific management reduced wasted efforts, set standards for performance, encouraged specialization, and stressed the selection of qualified workers who could be developed for a particular job. His *Shop Management* (1903) and *The Principles of Scientific Management* (1911) spread his ideas throughout Europe and the United States.

Gilbreth. Frank Gilbreth (1868-1924) and Lillian Gilbreth (1878-1972) also did pioneering work in time-and-motion studies. They emphasized the benefits of job simplification and the establishment of work standards, as well as the effects of the incentive wage plans and fatigue on work performance. As an apprentice bricklayer, Frank Gilbreth was instructed differently by each workman on how to lay bricks. To add to his confusion, the men used one set of motions to teach him, another for a slow pace, and still another for a fast pace. Wondering what methods would be most efficient, the young bricklayer started studying the workers' motions. Gilbreth reduced the number of motions required to lay a brick from 18 to 4 by developing a new way to stack bricks; developed an adjustable stand to eliminate excessive stooping, bending, and walking back and forth; and prescribed a mortar consistency that prevented excessive tapping on the brick with a trowel. His system of "speed work" eliminated haste and also increased work output by cutting out unnecessary motions. Workers could be paid

higher wages because they accomplished more in a shorter time.

The Gilbreths were among the first to use motion-picture films to analyze workers' motions. Because early cameras did not work at a steady speed, Gilbreth developed a microchronometer, a clock with a large hand measuring 1/2000 of a minute. The clock was photographed with the task and used to study motion patterns. A small, blinking electric bulb was attached to the worker's hand so speed and direction of movement could be studied. For his study of hand motions, Gilbreth developed 17 classifications for hand movements, such as "find," "select," "grasp," "position," and "rest," which he labeled "therbligs" (Gilbreth spelled backward with the th transposed). The Gilbreths also developed the flow diagram and the process chart to record their observations. The work process was diagrammed to indicate operations, delays, inspection, transportation, and storage, and the process was then studied to shorten, combine, or eliminate steps. The Gilbreths recommended written instructions to prevent misunderstandings and started a merit-rating system for workers.

Lillian Gilbreth is known as the first lady of management. Her doctoral dissertation, *The Psychology of Management* (1914), was published with the author listed as L.M. Gilbreth, thus obscuring the fact that she was a woman. It was one of the first contributions toward understanding human factors in industry. Her work on the effects of fatigue complemented her husband's efforts. The Gilbreths and their 12 children are the subjects of the popular book *Cheaper by the Dozen*.

Gantt. Henry Gantt (1861-1919), a disciple of Taylor, also was concerned with problems of efficiency. He contributed to scientific management by refining previous work rather than introducing new concepts. The Gantt chart, a forerunner of the PERT chart, depicts the relationship of the work planned or completed on one axis to the amount of time needed or used on the other. Gantt also developed a task and bonus remuneration plan whereby workers received a guaranteed day's wage plus a bonus for production above the standard to stimulate higher performance. Gantt recommended that workers be selected scientifically and provided with detailed instructions for their tasks. He argued for a more humanitarian approach by management, placing emphasis on service rather than profit objectives, recognizing useful nonmonetary incentives such as job security, and encouraging staff development (Gantt, 1910, 1916, 1919).

Classic Organization

Classic administration-organization thinking began to receive attention in 1930. Deductive rather than inductive, it views the organization as a whole rather than focusing solely on production. Managerial activities are classified as planning, organizing, and controlling. The concepts of scalar levels, span of control, authority, responsibility, accountability, line-staff relationships, decentralization, and departmentalization became prevalent.

Fayol. Henri Fayol (1841-1925), known as the "father of the management process school," was a French industrialist concerned with the management of production shops. Fayol studied the functions of managers and concluded that management is universal. All managers, regardless of the type of organization or their level in the organization, have essentially the same tasks: planning, organizing, issuing orders, coordinating, and controlling.

Fayol derived some general principles of administration from his observations. A believer in the division of work, he argued that specialization increases efficiency. Fayol recommended centralization through the use of a scalar chain or levels of authority, responsibility accompanied by authority, and unity of command and direction so that each employee receives orders from only one superior. He believed that although individual interests should be subordinated to agency interest, workers should be allowed to think through and implement plans and should be adequately remunerated for their services. Fayol encouraged development of group harmony through equal treatment and stability of tenure of personnel. A firm believer in order, he advocated "a place for everything and every-

thing in its place." He also urged that management be taught in the colleges (Fayol, 1925).

Weber. Max Weber (1864-1920), a German sociologist, earned the title of "father of organization theory" by his conceptualization of bureaucracy with emphasis on rules instead of individuals and on competence over favoritism as the most efficient basis for organization. He conceptualized a structure of authority that would facilitate the accomplishment of the organizational objectives. The three bases of authority, according to Weber, are (1) traditional authority, which is accepted because it seems things have always been that way, such as the rule of a king in a monarchy; (2) charisma, typified by Abraham Lincoln and Otto von Bismarck; and (3) rational, legal authority, which is considered rational in formal organizations because the person has demonstrated the knowledge, skill, and ability to fulfill the position. Weber recognized that if subordinates do not believe a person is qualified for the position, they may not accept that person's authority.

Favoring a rational, legal basis for authority, he suggested the avoidance of traditional and charismatic leadership through systematic selection of personnel. Administrators are chosen for their competence; their authority is clearly defined; they are given legal means for exercising their authority; and continuity of administration is provided. In Weber's bureaucracy administrators are appointed, not elected. They are career officials who work for fixed salaries and do not own what they administer. Like other personnel, they are subject to strict rules that are applied impersonally and uniformly. All personnel are selected for competence; the division of labor, authority, and responsibility is clearly defined; and positions are organized into a hierarchy.

Mooney. Working independently of Fayol and Weber, James Mooney (1884-1957) formed similar ideas. Mooney believed management to be the technique of directing people and organization the technique of relating functions. Organization is management's responsibility. Mooney enumerated four universal principles of organization: (1) coordination and synchronization of activities for the accomplishment of a goal can be accomplished in part through (2) functional effects, the performance of one's job description, and (3) scalar process organizes (4) authority into a hierarchy. Consequently, people get their right to command from their position in the organization (Mooney and Reily, 1931, 1939).

Urwick.   Lyndall Urwick (1891-1939) integrated the ideas of Fayol and Mooney with those of Taylor. His conceptual framework blended scientific management and classic organization theory into the beginnings of classic management theory. He described the managerial process as planning, coordinating, and controlling, and he popularized such concepts as the balance of authority with responsibility, span of control, unity of command, use of general and special staffs, the proper use of personnel, delegation, and departmentalization.

Human Relations

The human relations movement began in the 1940s with attention focused on the effect individuals have on the success or failure of an organization. Classic organization and management theory concentrates on the physical environment and fails to analyze the human element; human relations theory stresses the social environment. The chief concerns of the human relations movement are individuals, group process, interpersonal relations, leadership, and communication. Instead of concentrating on the organization's structure, managers encourage workers to develop their potential and help them meet their needs for recognition, accomplishment, and sense of belonging.

Barnard.   Chester Barnard (1886-1961) studied the functions of the executive while he was a manager for the New Jersey Bell Telephone System. Barnard saw the manager's responsibilities as defining objectives, acquiring resources, and coordinating activities. Stressing the importance of cooperation between management and labor, he noted that the degree of cooperation depends on nonfinancial inducements, which informal organization can help

provide. Formal channels of communication must be known and should be as short as possible. Barnard said authority depends on acceptance by the followers, and he stressed the role of informal organizations for aiding communication, meeting individuals' needs, and maintaining cohesiveness. Because small units are the building blocks for complex organizations, the worker contributes to the large organization, as well as the basic work unit. Barnard's work, which was done at the end of the classic period before human relations were emphasized, influenced the development of a behavioral focus (Barnard, 1938, 1940).

Follett.   In the 1920s Mary Follett (1868-1933) stressed the importance of coordinating the psychological and sociological aspects of management. Perceiving the organization as a social system and management as a social process, she considered subordination offensive. Follett distinguished between power with others and power over others and indicated that legitimate power is produced by a circular behavior whereby superiors and subordinates mutually influence one another. The law of the situation dictates that a person does not take orders from another person but from the situation. For instance, nurses will work through their lunch break during an emergency. The problem with this idea is that it is difficult for workers to know the total situation. Follett advocated that managers study the total situation to achieve unity because she believed that control would be obtained through cooperation among all of the elements, people, and materials. Her work was a link between the classic and human relations eras (Follett, 1949).

The Hawthorne studies.   The Hawthorne studies, though criticized for poor research methods, stimulated considerable interest in human problems on the job. Conducted at the Chicago Hawthorne plant of Western Electric by researchers from Harvard University under the direction of the psychologist Elton Mayo (1880-1949) and reported by the sociologist Fritz Rothlesberger, the studies investigated the effects of changes in illumination on productivity. Lighting was changed for the experimental group but remained constant for the control group. As the illumination was increased for the experimental group, the production of both groups increased. When it was decreased for the experimental group, production continued to increase for both groups until the level of illumination reached moonlight, at which point there was a significant decrease in output. The researchers concluded that lighting had little effect on production. The effects of the number and length of work breaks, refreshments, length of workdays and workweeks, temperature, and humidity were observed on five volunteers with little or no effects shown. A group piecework incentive plan was studied. The researchers anticipated that fast workers would pressure slow workers to increase their output. However, they found that group norms were set and workers were pressured not to be rate-busters by overproducing or chiselers by underproducing. Workers slacked off when it became apparent that they could meet the rate for the day. Work norms obviously had more influence than wage incentive plans. The Hawthorne studies gave the human relations movement its thrust.

Lewin. In the early 1930s Kurt Lewin (1890-1947), a Jewish psychologist, fled from Germany to the United States, where he revived the study of group dynamics. Lewin maintained that groups have personalities of their own: composites of the members' personalities. He showed that group forces can overcome individual interests. He confirmed the importance of group control over output and coined the terms *life space, space of free movement,* and *field forces* to describe group pressures on individuals.

Lewin advocated democratic supervision. His research indicated that democratic groups in which participants solve their own problems and have the opportunity to consult with the leader are most effective. Autocratic leadership, on the other hand, tends to promote hostility and aggression or apathy and to decrease initiative. Conducting experiments during World War II to change people's eating habits to consumption of more organ meats, he found that only 3% of the women who attended lectures

(autocratic method) changed their behavior, but 32% of the women who participated in a discussion after the lecture (democratic method) started eating more organ meats. Lewin was one of the first to apply Gestalt psychology to the study of individual personality (Lewin, 1951).

Moreno. Jacob Moreno (1892-1974) developed sociometry to analyze group behavior. Claiming that people are either attracted to, repulsed by, or indifferent toward others, he developed the sociogram to chart pairings and rankings of preferences for others. This process of classification can be used to calculate which workers are capable of harmonious interpersonal relationships. With this knowledge, work groups can be organized with a predicted minimum of disruptive tendencies for maximal efficiency and for promotion of high morale. Moreno also contributed to psychodrama (individual therapy), sociodrama (related to social and cultural roles), and role-playing techniques for the analysis of interpersonal relations.

Behavioral Science

During the 1950s advocates of the behavioral sciences became concerned that much scientific, classic, and human relations management theory had been accepted without scientific validation. Behavioral science emphasizes the use of scientific procedures to study the psychological, sociological, and anthropological aspects of human behavior in organizations. Behavioral scientists indicate that management is not strictly a technical process, that it cannot be haphazard, and that it should not be executed through authority. Rather, they stress the importance of maintaining a positive attitude toward people, training managers, fitting supervisory action to the situation, meeting employees' needs, promoting employees' sense of achievement, and obtaining commitment through participation in planning and decision making.

Maslow. Abraham Maslow (1908-1970) initiated the human behavioral school in 1943 with his development of a hierarchy-of-needs theory. He outlined a hierarchical structure for human needs classified into five categories: (1) physiological, (2) safety, (3) belonging, (4) esteem, and (5) self-actualization. The physiological needs are the most important and the most necessary for survival. They include the needs for oxygen, water, food, sleep, sex, and activity. Safety includes freedom from various kinds of danger, threat, and deprivation, such as physical harm, economic distress, ill health, and unnecessary, unexpected occurrences. Belonging needs are composed of affectionate relations with others, acceptance by one's peers, recognition as a group member, and companionship. Esteem comprises self-respect, positive self-evaluation, and regard by others. Self-actualization is composed of self-fulfillment and achievement of one's full capacity. In Maslow's hierarchy physical needs must be met before other needs become prepotent, and so on, and the satisfaction of self-actualization needs is possible only after all other needs are met. Once a need is satisfied, it is no longer a motivator and the next need becomes prepotent. As a need begins to be satisfied, it decreases in importance as a motivator in relation to other needs, some of which are never completely satisfied and never completely cease to motivate.

Maslow's work has been very influential in management and has stimulated subsequent research. Although Maslow's outline is correct in general, human needs are more complex than a simple listing would indicate. Because no two people are alike, needs vary in type and intensity from one person to another. People differ in the amount of gratification needed before the next goal becomes prepotent. For example, some people do well with 6 hours of sleep a day, but others need 10 hours to function. Varying degrees of importance may be placed on the needs dependent on cultural and individual differences. One person may desire recognition, whereas a sense of belonging to a group may be more important to someone else. People do tend to attach importance to what they do not have. It is socially more acceptable to request that physical needs be met than that social or psychological goals receive attention. The process of motivation is complicated by the fact that one's needs change. When one accepts a job, the pay, work hours, and geographical location may be prepotent. Soon after, the social needs and need for achievement and recognition may become prepotent. People also meet their needs in different ways. Some people may get recognition for the quantity and quality of work they produce, whereas others may get even more attention through negative behavior such as inferior work and tardiness. There are some situations that seem to defy Maslow's theory. Although most of us will eat if we are hungry, some people fast to achieve higher-level needs. Maslow's work marked the beginning of behavioral science. Much subsequent work has been based on his theory (Maslow, 1970).

Herzberg. Frederick Herzberg (1923-) and his colleagues used the critical-incident method in 1959 to interview 200 Pittsburgh-area engineers and accountants about job situations that they had found satisfying or dissatisfying. The stories were analyzed according to content and classified according to the job factors each contained. The researchers found that job factors in situations associated with satisfaction were different from job factors in situations associated with dissatisfaction. The motivators or satisfiers identified were achievement, recognition, work itself, responsibility, advancement, and the potential for growth. These job-content factors (factors in the job) can raise the level of performance and meet the higher-order needs. In Maslow's hierarchy-of-needs model, the hygiene factors or dissatisfiers identified were supervision; company policy; working conditions; interpersonal relations with superiors, peers, and subordinates; status; job security; and effect on one's personal life. These job-context factors (surrounding environmental factors) cannot motivate but can lower performance and cause job dissatisfaction. They meet lower-order needs in Maslow's model.

Herzberg's theory is very controversial and has stimulated considerable research, some of which supports the theory and some of which does not. His work has been the subject of much criticism. He studied only two jobs and used only one measure of job attitude. No validity or reliability data were reported. Statements of critical incidents were subject to memory loss and selective perception. The mere fact that one is more likely to blame others than oneself when asked about an unpleasant experience but is willing to assume the responsibility when something good happens could explain Herzberg's findings. No observations or measurement of job behavior were taken. Wrong categories could be identified, and the highly subjective stories could be misclassified. Herzberg did, however, develop a taxonomy of job situations based on research that has contributed to a better understanding of human motivation. His work complements Maslow's (Herzberg, 1977). (See Figures 4-2 and 4-3.)

McGregor. Douglas McGregor (1932-) developed the managerial implications of Maslow's theory. He notes that one's style of management is dependent on one's philosophy of humans and categorizes those assumptions as Theory X and Theory Y. In Theory X the manager's emphasis is on the goal of the organization. The theory assumes that people dislike work and will avoid it; consequently, workers must be directed, controlled, coerced, and threatened so that organizational goals can be met. According to Theory X, most people want to be directed and to avoid responsibility because they have little ambition. They desire security. Managers who accept the assumptions of Theory X will do the thinking and planning with little input from staff associates. They will delegate little, supervise closely, and motivate workers through fear and threats, failing to make use of their potentials.

In Theory Y the emphasis is on the goal of the individual. It is the manager's assumption that people do not inherently dislike work and that work can be a source of satisfaction. Theory Y managers assume that workers have the self-direction and self-control necessary for meeting their objectives and will respond to rewards for the accomplishment of those goals. They believe that under favorable conditions people seek responsibility and display imagination, ingenuity, and creativity. According to Theory Y, human potentials are only partially used. Managers who believe the assumptions of Theory Y will allow participation. They will delegate, give general rather than close supervision, support job enlargement, and use positive incentives such as praise and recognition.

McGregor suggests that when people are unable to satisfy their higher-level needs, they experience personal frustrations resulting in negative behaviors. Some managers have responded to the consequences of the personal frustration with punitive measures without determining the cause. Managers with a human relations orientation have made working conditions pleasant and have provided rewards unrelated to job performance. McGregor believes that both approaches are ineffective and recommends that the work situation be structured so that workers can meet their personal goals while working toward the goals of the organization. He suggests collaboration between the manager and the worker for integration of goals. Table 7-2 shows the relationships between the Maslow, Herzberg, and McGregor theories (McGregor, 1960).

Table 7-2 Relationships Between the Maslow, Herzberg, and McGregor Theories

Maslow	Herzberg	McGregor
Physiological needs	Hygiene factors	Theory X
Safety needs		
Belonging needs		
Esteem needs	Motivators	Theory Y
Self-actualization needs		

Modified from Kelly J: *Organizational behaviour*, rev ed, Homewood, Ill, 1980, Irwin, p. 220. © by Richard D. Irwin.

Ouchi, Pascale, and Athos. William Ouchi published *Theory Z: How American Business Can Meet the Japanese Challenge* in 1981. Richard Pascale and Anthony Athos gave a more extensive discussion of *The Art of Japanese Management: Applications for American Executives* in 1981. Ouchi contrasts Japanese organizations with organizations in the United States. The Japanese organizations have "lifetime employment; slow evaluation and promotion; non-specialized career paths; implicit control mechanisms; collective decision making; collective responsibility; and wholistic concern," whereas the organizations in the United States have "short-term employment; rapid evaluation and promotion; specialized career paths; explicit control mechanisms; individual decision making; individual responsibility; and segmented concern" (pp. 48-49). Pascale and Athos explain that organizations in the United States tend to favor strategy, structure, and systems, whereas the Japanese organizations focus on staff, skills, style, and superordinate goals (Ouchi, 1981; Pascale and Athos, 1981).

Argyris. Chris Argyris (1923-), focusing his research on the coexistence of personal and organizational needs, found that individuals give priority to meeting their own needs. He found that the greater the disparity between individual and organizational needs, the more tension, conflict, dissatisfaction, and subversion result. Argyris recommends that leaders help workers achieve self-actualization by implementing a Theory Y philosophy and maintains that this will help one's personality to grow from passivity and dependence to activity and independence. Incongruency between the mature personality and management based on classic principles makes workers subordinate, dependent, and passive, thereby causing psychological failure and job dissatisfaction. Managers can make jobs more meaningful by taking advantage of people's talents and letting them participate in planning, goal setting, and problem solving (Argyris, 1953, 1957, 1964, 1993; Argyris, Putnam, and Smith, 1985; Argyris and Schon, 1978).

Likert. Rensis Likert's (1903-1981) theory of management is based on his work at the University of Michigan's Institute for Social Research. He identified three types of variables in organizations: (1) causal, (2) intervening, and (3) end result. The causal variables include leadership behavior, organizational structure, policies, and controls. Intervening variables are perceptions, attitudes, and motivations. The end-result variables are measures of profits, costs, and productivity. Likert believed that managers may act in ways harmful to the organization because they evaluate end results to the exclusion of intervening variables. Consequently, he developed a Likert scale questionnaire that includes measures of causal and intervening variables. The Likert scale measures several factors related to leadership behavior process, motivation, managerial influence, communication, decision-making processes, goal setting, and staff development.

Likert also identified four types of management systems: (1) exploitative-authoritative, (2) benevolent-authoritative, (3) consultative, and (4) participative group. He associated the first system with the least effective performance. Managers show little confidence in staff associates and ignore their ideas. Consequently, staff associates do not feel free to discuss their jobs with their managers. Responsibility for the organization's goals is at the top; goals are established through orders. What little communication is used is directed downward, is often inaccurate, and is accepted with suspicion. Although managers do not know about their staff associates' problems, they make decisions without input from below. Policing and punishment are used as control functions by top administration. Allowed no input, the workers strongly resist the organization's goals and develop an informal organization of their own.

In the benevolent-authoritative system, the second type of system, the manager is condescending to staff associates. Staff associates' ideas are sometimes sought, but they do not feel very free to discuss their jobs with their manager. Top and middle management are responsible for setting goals. There is little communication, and it is mostly directed downward after being censored by the manager and is received with some suspicion. Decisions are made at the top with some delegation. Managers do have some knowledge of the staff associates' situation, and staff associates are occasionally consulted for problem solving. Goals are established through orders with some comment invited and moderate resistance received. Rewards and punishment are used as control functions by top administration. There is usually an informal organization resisting the formal one.

In the third system, the consultative system, the manager has substantial confidence in staff associates. Their ideas are usually sought, and they feel free to discuss their work with the manager. Responsibility for setting goals is fairly general. Although there is considerable communication, both upward and downward, it has limited accuracy and is accepted with some caution. Managers are quite familiar with the problems faced by their staff associates. Broad policy is set at the top with delegation; goals are set after discussion; and there is decision making throughout the organization. Control functions are delegated to lower levels, where reward and self-guidance are used. Sometimes an informal organization resists the formal goals.

Participative management, the fourth system, is associated with the most effective performance. Managers have complete confidence in their staff associates. Staff associates' ideas are always sought, and they feel completely free to discuss their jobs with the manager. Goals are set at all levels. There is a great deal of communication—upward, down-ward, and sideways—that is accurate and received with an open mind. Managers are very well informed about the problems faced by their staff associates, and the decision making is well integrated throughout the organization with full involvement of staff associates. Because goals are established through group action, there is little or no resistance to them. There is not an informal organization resisting the goals of the formal organization, because the goals of both are the same. Control is widely shared through the use of self-guidance and problem solving.

Likert was a strong proponent of participative management and supportive relationships. His linking-pin concept is based on studies about the differences between good and poor managers as measured by their level of productivity. Good managers were found to have more influence on their own managers than did poor managers, and their managerial procedures were better received by their staff associates. Consequently, Likert suggested that managers form groups for supportive relationships and that those groups be linked by overlapping groups of managers. This facilitates three-way communications—upward, downward, and sideways. When middle managers have the opportunity for interaction with their manager, workers can have input, and there is a chance for the individual's and the organization's goals to become similar (Figure 7-2) (Likert, 1961).

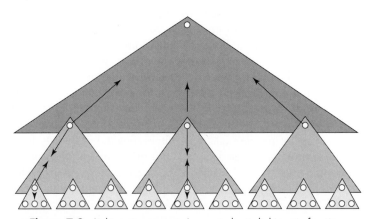

Figure 7-2 Linking-pin concept. Arrows indicate linking-pin function.
From Likert R, Likert JG: *New ways of managing conflict*, New York, 1976, McGraw-Hill.

Blake and Mouton. Robert Blake (1918-) and Jane Mouton (1930-) maintain that there are two critical dimensions of leadership: (1) concern for people and (2) concern for production. They depict these on a 9 × 9 or 81-square managerial grid (Figure 7-3). The two dimensions are independent, so a manager can be high on both, low on both, or high on one and low on the other. The vertical axis represents the manager's concern for people, and the horizontal axis represents concern for production. Each axis is on a 1-to-9 scale, from a minimal concern for people or production to a maximal concern. The five basic styles are located at each corner and in the middle.

The task manager at 9,1 has the highest regard for production and the lowest concern for people.

This manager stresses operating efficiency through controls and views people as tools of production. Workers are paid to do what they are told without questioning.

As reflected on the grid, 1,1 management is impoverished. The manager has a lack of concern for both production and people. This style may be found in some managers who feel they have been repeatedly denied promotion or otherwise mistreated and who have consequently compensated through a low level of involvement with their jobs. The organization man management at 5,5 represents a moderate concern for both people and production but not necessarily at the same time. The manager's emphasis shifts. The country club manager, 1,9, is thought-

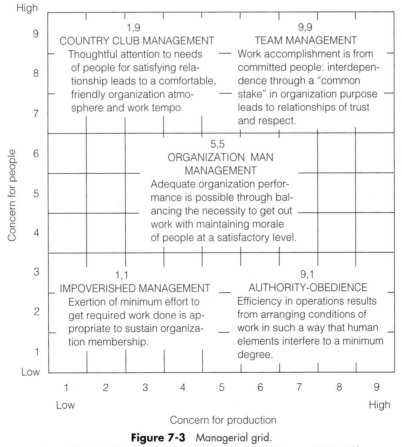

Figure 7-3 Managerial grid.
From Blake RR, Mouton JS: *The new managerial grid,* Houston, 1978, Gulf.

ful and friendly but has little concern for production.

Blake and Mouton consider team management, 9,9, the optimal managerial style. These managers integrate their concern for people and production. Problems are confronted directly, and mutual trust, respect, and interdependence are fostered (Blake and Mouton, 1978).

Fiedler. During the 1960s Fred Fiedler (1922-) introduced the contingency model of leadership effectiveness. He identified three important dimensions of a situation for his contingency model: (1) leader-member relations, (2) task structure, and (3) position power. Leader-member relations are related to the amount of confidence and loyalty followers have in their leader. Task structure is related to the number of correct solutions to a problem. Position power depends on the amount of organizational support available to the leader (Fiedler, 1967; Fiedler and Chemers, 1974; Fiedler, Chemers, and Mahar, 1976).

Hersey and Blanchard. Paul Hersey (1930-) and Kenneth Blanchard (1939-) extended the work of Blake, Mouton, and Fiedler by considering the maturity of the followers in more detail. As the maturity of one's followers increases, the leadership style requires less structure and emotional support. Groups with below-average maturity function best under leaders with high task–low relationship orientations. Groups with average maturity function best under leaders with high task–high relationship or high relationship–low task orientations. The most effective leadership style depends on the maturity of the group (Hersey, 1984; Hersey and Blanchard, 1969, 1982; Hersey and Duldt, 1989).

Drucker. In his prolific writings about management, Peter Drucker (1909-) maintains that the only way for management to justify its existence is through economic results. However, he recognizes noneconomic consequences of managerial decisions, such as job satisfaction, as by-products of the focus on economic performance. He identifies three areas of management: (1) managing a business, (2) managing managers, and (3) managing workers. Activity, decision, and relations analyses are recommended to determine the structure and organization needed. Drucker has studied the advantages and disadvantages of decentralization, supports decentralization, and says managers should create markets and products rather than being passive.

Drucker introduced management by objectives as a way to manage managers. Relying on self-control instead of control from above, managers are directed by objectives of performance rather than by their manager. For management by objectives, the manager develops the framework, and the staff associate supplies the goals, which are agreed on by both. The staff associate gives progress reports to the manager. Objectives are developed for every level of management in the hierarchy and each unit in the organization. The manager checks objectives for compatibility with other units and contribution to the objectives at the next level of the hierarchy. Drucker maintains that it is more productive for workers to set their own norms and measure their own performance than for minimal standards to be set.

For managing the worker, Drucker recommends that jobs be designed to fit the worker, that workers be given more control over their jobs, and that the worker be considered the most vital resource in the agency.

For decades Drucker has been one of the leading thinkers about the study and practice of management through his landmark articles in *Harvard Business Review* and numerous books. He has stressed the importance of managing for the future. He believes it is pointless to predict the future, that the future has already happened, and that we should identify major events that have occurred and identify the predictable effects, such as demographics including the overpopulation of the world with increasing underpopulation of the developed countries. By the late 1990s he was indicating the importance of managing society's knowledge resources (Drucker, 1964, 1974, 1980, 1985, 1992, 1998).

Odiorne. George Odiorne (1920-1992), director of the Bureau of Industrial Relations of the University of Michigan, was previously assistant director of personnel for General Mills, Inc., where he pioneered the installation of a management-by-objectives system. He advocated effective management through personal and agency goals and had written about the executive's responsibilities for implementing a management-by-objectives system. He also recommended training by objectives as an economic strategy for management training (Odiorne, 1965).

Peters. Tom Peters has been provocative during the 1980s and 1990s through seminars and several books. In the book *In Search of Excellence,* he and Robert Waterman (1982) stressed the importance of managing ambiguity and paradox, having a bias for action to get things done, remaining close to the customer to know his needs and anticipate his wants, fostering autonomy and entrepreneurship, reinforcing shared values by celebrating heroes, getting productivity through people, demonstrating values through direct interventions, keeping to what you know instead of widely diversifying, keeping a simple form and lean staff, and maintaining simultaneous loose-tight properties. In 1985 he and Nancy Austin stressed the importance of having a passion and searching for excellence through team-based innovations in *A Passion for Excellence.* In 1987 he did a handbook for management of revolution, *Thriving on Chaos.* He did a guide to economic excellence, *Liberation Management,* in 1992. *The Tom Peters Seminar* (1994) presented the slides and lecture content from a typical 2-day seminar. In *The Circle of Innovation* (1997) Peters continued to discuss how the obsessed transformational leader lives life out loud and presents current trends.

Kotter. John Kotter has reported his research about topics related to leadership in a number of books, including but not limited to *The General Managers* (1982), *Power and Influence* (1985), *The Leadership Factor* (1988), *A Force for Change* (1990), and *Leading Change* (1996). The research is primarily about traits, management, and transactional issues.

Transformational Leadership

Transformational leadership became popular during the 1980s and 1990s with stress on the need for leadership versus management, the importance of values, and a commitment to service.

Bass. In *Leadership and Performance Beyond Expectations* (1985) Bernard Bass identifies the need for charisma, inspirational leadership, individualized consideration, and intellectual stimulation to have transformational leadership instead of just transactional or a contingent reinforcement leadership.

Bennis and Nanus. Warren Bennis has stressed the importance of leading rather than just managing. In *Leaders: The Strategies for Taking Charge* (1985), he and Burt Nanus lead a paradigm shift to transformative leadership. They discuss the need to manage oneself to lead others, attention through vision, meaning through communication, trust through positioning, deployment of self, and empowerment. In his second report based on his study of leadership, *On Becoming a Leader* (1989), Bennis describes how people become leaders, how they lead, and how organizations can encourage or stifle leaders. In *Organizing Genius* (1997) Bennis tells the stories of seven groups and concludes by describing the characteristics of great groups. In *The Leader's Edge* (1989) Nanus discusses four conceptual skills: (1) farsightedness, (2) mastery of interdependence, (3) anticipatory learning, and (4) high integrity; four roles: (1) direction-setter, (2) change agent, (3) spokesperson, and (4) coach; and three action skills: (1) organization design, (2) initiative, and (3) mastery of change.

Kouzes and Posner. In *The Leadership Challenge: How to Get Extraordinary Things Done in Organizations,* James Kouzes and Barry Posner (1987, 1990) identify five practices and ten behaviors to implement those practices: (1) challenging the process by searching for opportunities by (a) confronting and changing the status quo and by (b) experimenting and taking risks and learning from mistakes and successes; (2) inspiring a shared vision by (a) envisioning the future through imagining ideal scenarios and by (b) enlisting others by attracting people to common purposes; (3) enabling others to act by (a) getting people to work together through collaboration and by (b) sharing power and information to strengthen others; (4) modeling the way by (a) leading by example and doing and by (b) building commitment to action through small wins; and (5) encouraging the heart by (a) linking rewards with performance and recognizing contributions and by (b) celebrating accomplishments. In *Credibility* (1993) they identify credibility as the cornerstone of leadership and discuss how leaders encourage initiative, risk taking, and productivity through trust in people and by using principles rather than positions to manage conflict. They elaborate on seven essentials of encouragement: (1) setting clear standards, (2) expecting the best, (3) paying attention, (4) personalizing recognition, (5) telling the story, (6) celebrating together, and (7) setting the example in *Encouraging the Heart* (1999).

Tichy.   Noel Tichy and Stratford Sherman present *Control Your Destiny or Someone Else Will* (1993) as a three-act play: (1) the awakening, (2) the vision, and (3) revolution as a way of life. Tichy and Mary Anne Devanna think that transformational leaders would control the quality of life inside and outside of the workplace. They too present corporate transformation as a three-act drama: (1) recognizing the need for revitalization, (2) creating a new vision, and (3) institutionalizing change in *The Transformational Leader* (1986, 1997). In *The Leadership Engine* (1997) Tichy and Eli Cohen stress the importance of developing leaders at all levels and the necessity of quantum transformation, not just incremental quality improvement.

Blanchard.   Ken Blanchard has written numerous books during the 1980s and 1990s. In *Gung Ho!*

(1998) he and Sheldon Bowles report lessons learned by observing the worthwhile work of squirrels, the control of achieving the goal by beavers, and how the geese cheer each other on.

Greenleaf.   Robert Greenleaf wrote *Servant Leadership* (1977, 1991). He conceptualized the idea of the servant as leader from Hermann Hesse's *The Journey to the East* (1956), in which the servant who does the menial chores also sustained the party's spirits through his extraordinary presence. When the servant left the group, the group fell into disarray and the journey was abandoned. Servant leadership puts serving first, takes a holistic approach, shares decision making, and builds community. Larry Spears has identified 10 characteristics of the servant-leader by studying Greenleaf's work: (1) listening, (2) empathy, (3) healing, (4) awareness, (5) persuasion, (6) conceptualization, (7) foresight, (8) stewardship, (9) commitment to the growth of people, and (10) building community. Spears has edited the following anthologies about servant leadership: *Insights on Leadership: Service, Stewardship, Spirit, and Servant Leadership* (1998) and *Reflections on Leadership: How Robert K. Greenleaf's Theory on Servant Leadership Influenced Today's Top Management Thinkers* (1995). Max DePree, author of *Leadership is an Art* (1989) and *Leadership Jazz* (1992), has been influenced by Greenleaf. He stresses the importance of connecting one's voice and one's touch. The personal transformation can be related to Parker Palmer's works *The Courage to Teach: Exploring the Inner Landscape of a Teacher's Life* (1998) and *To Know as We Are Known/A Spirituality of Education* (1983). He believes that good teaching comes from the identity and integrity of the teacher, not just from good technique, and that inner work can help create communities of learning. M. Scott Peck addresses the new psychology of love, traditional values, and spiritual growth in *The Road Less Traveled* (1978). Ann McGee-Cooper describes a program to bring joy, energy, and balance back into one's life in *You Don't Have to Go Home From Work Exhausted* (1990, 1992). Peter Vaill believes that executive development is spiritual development and uses a metaphor, *Managing as a Performing Art*

(1989), to discuss his ideas. Peter Block wrote *The Empowered Manager: Positive Political Skills at Work* (1987) but found that the rhetoric about visionary leadership, customer-driven service, and quality improvement addresses only cosmetic changes. Then he wrote *Stewardship: Choosing Service Over Self-Interest* (1993). Stewards hold themselves responsible and accountable. They lead by serving. Stephen Covey's books *The 7 Habits of Highly Effective People* (1989), *Principle-Centered Leadership* (1990), and *First Things First* (Covey, Merrill, and Merrill, 1994) teach how to manage relationships instead of just manage time around priorities. Joseph Jaworski describes his personal transformation in *Synchronicity: The Inner Path of Leadership* (Jaworski and Flowers, 1996, 1998).

Learning Organizations

Senge. Peter Senge discusses five disciplines—(1) systems thinking, (2) personal mastery, (3) mental models, (4) shared vision, and (5) team learning—in his book *The Fifth Discipline: The Art and Practice of the Learning Organization* (1990) and discusses tools and strategies to build a learning organization in *The Fifth Discipline Fieldbook* (Senge, Kleiner, Roberts et al., 1994). They address participation as a basis of learning to prevent organizational learning disabilities instead of participation as an entitlement.

Senge's beliefs about systems thinking have been influenced by many people and books. In *Belonging to the Universe* Fritjol Capra, David Steindl-Rast, and Thomas Matus (1991) explain changes from seeing things as structures to seeing them as processes, from linear thinking to systems thinking. For example, a tree is not just a structure. It is a photosynthesis process that unites sun and earth. Margaret Wheatley (1992) observes nature and concludes in *Leadership and the New Science* that everything is a bundle of potentiality and that order emerges from chaos. Now the new science describes the nature of people's lives better than mechanical models. David Meadows, Dennis Meadows, and Jorgen Randers indicate the global limits have already been exceeded in some areas in *Beyond the Limits* (1992). So it does not make sense to continue toward the same kind of growth. Robert Schaffer recommends a simple and direct approach to small, tangible steps toward strategic breakthroughs, looking for projects that do not take additional resources, and choosing indicators that show results within a few months in *The Breakthrough Strategy* (1988).

There are a number of books about simulations, use of computer technology, and mapping techniques. In *Improving Performance* Geary Rummler and Allen Brache (1995) address improving process relationships to form a link between individuals and the organization strategy. The book is a practical guide for a holistic view of the organizational skeleton, process levels, and interdependencies. Christopher Meyer indicates that *Fast Cycle Time* (1993) is achieved by aligning the organization to learn faster rather than merely work faster. Sometimes we have to slow down to speed up. In *Creating the Corporate Future: Plan or Be Planned for,* Russell Ackoff (1981) describes interactive planning as a participative, systems approach to corporate development.

The Path of Least Resistance (1989) and *Creating* (1991), both by Robert Fritz, provide exercises and ideas for developing personal mastery and creativity. Argyris influenced thought on mental models and has been studying learning in organizations for a long time. He has published *Organizational Learning: A Theory of Action Perspective* (Argyris and Schon, 1978), *Action Science* (Argyris, Putnam, and Smith, 1985), and *Knowledge for Action* (1993), among other books. Edgar Schein describes how culture emerges and changes through birth and early growth, midlife, maturity, and possibly destruction in *Organizational Culture and Leadership* (1985, 1997).

In *Creating Shared Vision* Marjorie Parker (1990) tells a story of how a Norwegian aluminum company had each employee sketch his personal vision of the organization and link it with other images. The vision statement was a garden mural with each plant having metaphorical meaning.

Team learning is influenced by conversations. *The Abilene Paradox* by Jerry Harvey (1988) is a metaphor of how groups can agree to take action that contradicts individual members' beliefs of what is right and end up where no one wanted to go. *You Just Don't Understand: Women and Men in Conversation* by Deborah Tannen (1990) addresses the differing communication styles of men and women and was the seminal work for *Men Are From Mars, Women Are From Venus* (Gray, 1992). Men tend to be problem solvers, whereas women want to make connections.

Although Henry Sims published *The Thinking Organization: Dynamics of Organizational Social Cognition* in 1986, Senge's *The Fifth Discipline* (1990) was the path breaking book on learning organizations. The book is based on science, psychology, and spiritual wisdom. The field book contains success stories, essays, ideas, and exercises for individuals and teams.

Daniel Goleman's *Working With Emotional Intelligence* (1998) applies the concepts from his *Emotional Intelligence* (1997) in the workplace. In his emotional competence framework he identifies self-awareness, self-regulation, and motivation as important to personal competence and empathy and social skills as important to social competence. He stresses the importance of teaching emotional competence and gives guidelines for training, including how to assess the job, assess the individual, deliver assessments with care, gauge readiness, motivate, make change self-directed, focus on clear and manageable goals, prevent relapse, give performance feedback, encourage practice, arrange support, provide models, encourage, reinforce change, and evaluate. Emotional intelligence is more important than intelligence quotient (IQ) or technical expertise for success in organizations.

DIVERSITY AMONG LEADERS
Diversity

Diversity should be defined in a broad and inclusive way to prevent widespread opposition. Employees should understand that everyone's diversity is valued. Diversity can affect individuals' values, perceptions of self and others, and opportunities at work. Primary dimensions include age, ethnicity, gender,

mental and physical abilities, race, and sexual orientation. Secondary dimensions include communication style, education, family status, first language, geographical location, income, military experience, organizational role, religion, work experience, and work style. Organizations should value primary and secondary diversity. At first, organizations focus on expectations, norms, and operating assumptions. As the organization moves up the continuum of diversity implementation, diversity in styles, communications, and problem solving gains greater acceptance. In *Implementing Diversity* Marilyn Loden (1996) identifies five segments of a diversity adoption curve: innovators, change agents, pragmatists, skeptics, and traditionalists. Adoption is speeded up by compatibility, high relative advantage, observability, simplicity, and testability. Adoption is slowed down by complexity, incompatibility, little or no relative advantage, little observability, and little or no testability. The different concerns and needs of all segments of the diversity should be considered in a plan to ensure a rapid and successful adoption. It seems to be the diversity mind-set that separates effective facilitators from those who merely pay lip service to the need to implement diversity. The valuing diversity mind-set includes valuing that diversity benefits all and is good for individuals, as well as the company. Diversity must be inclusive, requires investment of time and human resources, and requires a long-term culture change. Building support among those who are willing to adopt change while minimizing involvement of resistant people helps minimize backlash. Building a business case of the strategic and financial arguments for valuing diversity will help strengthen the adoption. While excellent training will not ensure cultural change, inappropriate training can do harm to diversity efforts. Focusing on the common needs for inclusion, opportunity, and respect can help close the gaps among diverse employee groups. Administrative support is the single most important factor for predicting implementation success.

Segmentation helps adoption occur more quickly with less confusion and less conflict. Innovators generally look for opportunities to create. Change agents are among the first to try out new ideas and are interested in self-learning. Pragmatists are suspicious about the practicality of change and tend to wait rather than move quickly. They want to know that something is "good for the people." Skeptics are predisposed to delay implementation of change. They start considering change when they find themselves out of synch with mainstream values. Traditionalists tend to totally avoid involvement. They need ongoing repetitive endorsements from leaders about the strategic importance and adoption of change as less painful than continued resistance. The timing and content of training should be different for different segments. Loden identifies best practices across organizations as follows: (1) setting the context for change, (2) providing ongoing communication, (3) focusing on data-driven change, (4) providing awareness and skill-based training, (5) encouraging ongoing learning, (6) multicultural mentoring, (7) providing flexible benefits and scheduling, (8) linking rewards to effective diversity management, and (9) building common ground.

Gender differences.   There are differences in male and female leadership styles. Women tend to be more democratic and participative by sharing power and information, encouraging consultation, and enhancing group members' self-worth. They use their interpersonal skills, charisma, and networking to influence others toward the accomplishment of goals. Men tend to be more direct and autocratic. They use the organization's formal authority structure and their positions as their power base. With the organizational trends from competitive individualism, secrecy, and control toward trust, teamwork, and information sharing, women seem well equipped for leadership beyond the nineties.

In the classic book *The Managerial Woman,* Margaret Hennig and Anne Jardim (1966, 1977) discuss why women are at a comparative disadvantage to men for advancement in companies; how they are socialized to be a nurse, not a doctor, or a secretary, not a boss; and how "queen bees," women who have made it to the top, do not want to share their power with other women. It and *Games*

Mother Never Taught You: Corporate Gamesmanship for Women by Betty Harragan (1977) describe games that still exist, making it difficult for women to advance in business. Harragan elaborates on a football metaphor to explain how women need to act. JoAnn Ashley (1976) speaks specifically to *Hospitals, Paternalism, and the Role of the Nurse.* In *Breaking Into the Boardroom: What Every Woman Needs to Know,* Jinex Melia (1986) indicates that it is women keeping women out of the boardroom. Melia says that men stab each other in the back for gain, but women do it just to do it.

With the help of Equal Opportunity Employment legislation, women have been able to make an impact in business. Ann Morrison, Randall White, and Ellen Van Velsor (1987) did a 3-year study to determine success or derailment factors in *Breaking the Glass Ceiling: Can Women Reach the Top of America's Largest Corporations?,* a transparent barrier that few women have been able to break. They found that men and women did not score differently on most factors measured. The few statistically significant sex differences that emerged were as follows (p. 50):

> Executive men are more likely than executive women to feel equal to the demands for time and energy.
>
> Executive men feel more in tune with their surroundings and are more likely than executive women to perceive things as their peers do.
>
> Executive men are more comfortable than executive women in an environment where conformity to intellectual authority is desirable and the criteria for excellence are clearly specified (called "achievement via conformance").
>
> Executive women are more likely than executive men to move in new and original directions.
>
> Executive women are more likely than executive men to behave as individuals and to personalize their experiences.

Many of the 76 executive women said they needed to take risks but be consistently outstanding; be tough but not macho; be ambitious but not expect equal treatment; and take responsibility and follow others' advice (pp. 57-70). The six lessons learned were as follows: (1) learn the ropes, (2) take control of your career, (3) build confidence, (4) rely on others, (5) go for "the bottom line," and (6) integrate life and work (pp. 74-122).

In *On Our Own Terms* Liane Enkelis, Karen Olsen, and Marion Lewenstein (1995) present 14 portraits of women business leaders who have broken the glass ceiling.

To know how women manage differently from men, Sally Helgesen needed to know how men manage. She referred to Henry Mitzberg's 1968 dissertation, which was published in 1973 as *The Nature of Managerial Work*. Mitzberg followed five male executives through their days and found that they worked at a relentless pace without breaks. Their days were filled with interruptions, discontinuity, and fragmentation. They had little time for activities not directly related to their work. They had a preference for live action encounters and maintained a complex network of relationships with people outside the organization. They immersed themselves in their jobs, had little time for reflection, had difficulty sharing information, and identified with the job.

Helgesen (1990) did diary studies on four women, two of whom are entrepreneurs. She found that women worked at a steady pace with small breaks throughout the day. The pace was steady and fast but not frantic. The subjects did not view unscheduled tasks as interruptions. They made time for activities not directly related to their work. They did not sacrifice important family time or restrict their reading to work-related items. They preferred live action but did schedule time to read the mail. They too maintained a complex network of relationships with people outside the organization. They focused on the ecology of leadership, scheduled time to share information, and saw their identities as complex and multifaceted. Men have been socialized to work sun up to sun down, whereas women know their work is never done. Women's work is cyclical and unending. They are process oriented and get pleasure from doing the work instead

of getting it done. Women repeatedly used the metaphor of voice. They lead with voice. She found that the most successful women executives knew they had complex identities with various roles in both public and private life.

In *Everyday Revolutionaries* Helgesen (1998) addresses how the entry of women into the workforce since 1970 has changed how businesses are managed, how families are structured, how communities are organized, how services are conceived and marketed, and how children are raised. Entry of women into the public arena has been occurring at the same time as rapid economic and technological change. The postindustrial economy has been influenced by women who are pioneers in new ways of learning and who improvise their own lives instead of just conform to the needs of large organizations.

Rosabeth Kanter's *Men and Women of the Corporation* (1977, 1993) hypothesized that large numbers of women in the workforce would overcome the problem of sexual discrimination. However, many women are clustered at entry-level and mid-level positions. Not many women have reached the top or broken sexual stereotypes. For *Reach for the Top* Nancy Nichols (1977, 1994) interviewed women who described themselves as transformational. They did interactive leadership by encouraging participation, sharing power and information, enhancing people's self-worth, and getting others excited about their work (pp. 13-23).

Arlie Hochschild and others (1989) interviewed 50 families, including artisans, students, and professionals, in Berkeley, California, in the late 1970s. The results were published in *The Second Shift*, indicating that men who shared the load at home felt just as pressed as their wives. However, the majority of the men did not share the load at home. As women have moved into the economy, there has been a speedup at work and at home. Consequently, women talk of being overly tired, sick, and emotionally drained. Women who do all the work at home and have a job become known as supermoms. Yet the black woman who works to support her family is known as a matriarch instead of a supermom.

In *Backlash: The Undeclared War Against Women*, Susan Faludi (1991) chronicled the resentment of women's accomplishments that is characterized by antagonism and scapegoating. Some angry white men believe that women's growing presence in the workforce is depriving them of well-paying jobs and job security.

America's Competitive Secret: Utilizing Women as a Management Strategy reports the results of Judy Rosener's (1995) telephone interview with executive men across the country. A content analysis revealed four working relationships: supervising women, working with women as peers, competing with women, and working for women. The major issues of concern for the men were loss of power and control, loss of male identity and self-esteem, and increasing discomfort or sexual static. Women have some of the same career aspirations and receive challenging assignments, but taking time off for family reasons continues to be a problem for them. The men thought that women bring attention to detail, compassion, different perspectives, sensitivity, and a willingness to work hard to the job. Black men felt differently about working with women. They are sympathetic about the underutilization of women in the workforce but also think women have taken jobs away from them. There is a need for corporations to increase gender awareness through specific training, including role playing, videos, case studies, and skill development. The female underutilization is worldwide. The number of Japanese women with career aspirations is quite small, and there is an increase in Japanese women requesting to be assigned abroad. American and British women, especially married women, feel underutilized. Some believe that women are the greatest undeveloped natural resource in the world.

In *Career Strategies for the Working Woman*, Adele Scheele (1994) discusses discovering one's self at work, building relationships with management, clients, and colleagues, and triggering one's ambition. She recommends that one provide bosses with what they need, study leaders in the organization, read profiles and biographies of achievers, de-velop one's own talents into expertise, make one's self visible, and work in a safe environment by joining professional and civic organizations.

Pamela Gilberd (1996) gives *The Eleven Commandments of Wildly Successful Women* as follows:

1. Create your own definition of success by finding your passion so you can love your work, believing that you deserve success, asking yourself the right questions, expanding your view of the world, knowing your priorities and values, integrating your career and your personal goals, learning how to get back on track, and giving your own definition of success the test of time.
2. Take responsibility for your career by adopting an entrepreneurial attitude, describing what you want, keeping the big picture in mind, using transitions to evaluate your work choices, being willing to change gears, and creating your own solutions.
3. Change your thinking and change your life by using the power of belief to create success, adopting a "why not?" attitude, choosing to deal with your circumstances, remembering the importance of flexibility, stretching your comfort zone, and practicing optimism.
4. When the odds are against you, defy the odds by seeing yourself as a player, taking the first step, refusing to believe conventional wisdom, doing what you know best, getting support when you need it, knowing when you need help and asking for it, and being willing to learn.
5. Fantasize about your future but create your game plan by creating a vision from your dreams, knowing your destination, creating your own luck, making preparation part of planning, and using action plans to make your dreams come true.
6. Get ready, get set, risk by knowing your tolerance for risk, understanding the risk and its consequences, looking at the long term, not being afraid of the imposter syndrome, calling on your past experience, trusting your intuition, having a fall-back plan, and using networking.

7. When someone says "you can't," say "watch me" by addressing your obstacles, keeping your sense of humor, ignoring the naysayers, following your passion with conviction, and remembering your past successes.

8. Become financially savvy by understanding the big financial picture, taking charge of learning what you need to know, making sure you get paid what you are worth, researching and writing your own business plan, and setting solid financial goals.

9. See mistakes as road signs, not road blocks, by assuming that mistakes are useful teachers, avoiding the really big mistakes, learning to recognize warning signs, and moving on after a mistake.

10. Enjoy your work and your life by defining and enriching your creative side, nurturing your own growth, starting anew when you have outgrown your work, and creating incentives and teamwork.

11. Give back to keep the cycle of success going by sharing what you know to help others succeed, believing that each person makes a difference, learning to be a good mentor, and participating in organizations that further others' success.

In *Seven Secrets of Successful Women,* Donna Brooks and Lynn Brooks (1997) indicate that successful people (1) realize the importance of a mentor/advocate/cheerleader/coach, (2) know how to increase their visibility, (3) know how to develop an effective network, (4) have learned to communicate effectively, (5) know how to balance work and home, (6) know when to take smart risks, and (7) understand the politics of the organization. The second part of the book discusses gender differences at length. In *Success on Our Own Terms* Virginia O'Brien, Virginia O'Brien, and Lynn Martin (1998) say a key to success is finding a culture that matches your values.

Advancing Women in Business—the Catalyst Guide by Catalyst (1998) indicates that efforts to maximize women's talents will probably be successful only if an organization takes a comprehensive, problem-solving approach. Both internal and external benchmarking of women's advancement should be done. Internal research allows companies to establish the current status of women in the organization by reviewing recruitment, retention, and advancement data; develop short- and long-term goals for improvement after the baseline has been determined; and evaluate the effectiveness of the initiatives that were generated from the benchmarking by measuring and reporting the progress toward specific goals.

Racial differences. William Wilson (in Grusky, 1994) identifies three stages of race relations in the United States: (1) plantation economy and racial-caste oppression, (2) industrial expansion, class conflict, and racial oppression, and (3) progressive transition from racial inequalities to class irregularities. Racial diversity is visible and subject to stereotyping, in which the person is viewed as a member of a group and the images others have about that group are ascribed to the person, and prejudice, when predetermined negative attitudes toward people are based on a group identity. Taylor Cox and Ruby Beale (1997) identify numerous ways of *Developing Competency to Manage Diversity,* including providing awareness training; providing opportunities for in-house trainers; creating interorganizational relationships with organizations with different dominant groups; providing some support for on- and off-site dialogue meetings; providing a reading list on diversity; sponsoring cultural diversity celebrations; sponsoring events to facilitate mentor-protégé matchups; providing overseas assignments; allowing time for travel or sponsoring travel for career development; providing financial support for college courses about diversity, foreign language courses, and national conferences on diversity; sponsoring cultural social events; creating diversity task forces; sponsoring educational activities and diversity roundtables; integrating cultural diversity issues into staff meetings; and helping employees obtain requested job assignments.

The working environment is often lonely and unfriendly for nontraditional managers. Sometimes people of color and women have information withheld from them to sabotage them. They may have trouble finding role models and mentors. They may lack organizational savvy, take comfort in working with their own kind, have difficulty balancing career and family, get a backlash from threatened white males, have infighting from the oppressed group, and have to deal with prejudice. Agencies should give management training. Helping new managers get acquainted with key workers so they will feel comfortable dealing with them later is important (Morrison, 1992).

Sexual orientation differences.   Lesbian, gay, and bisexual development is more invisible than some other minorities. They are less likely to be considered to have mental illness than earlier but still have risk of loss of employment, housing, and family relationships (Trickett, Watts, and Birman, 1994).

Disabilities.   Many disabilities are visible and affect people at different chronological ages with a variety of physical disabilities. The disability culture is built on a kinship based on identification of shared understandings of life experiences (Trickett, Watts, and Birman, 1994).

FOLLOWERSHIP

We need great followers, as well as great leaders. Leaders contribute only about 20% percent to the success of organizations. Followers do the remaining 80%. We spend more time reporting to others than having them report to us. Some leaders have been such good followers that their peers have asked them to take on leadership responsibilities. In *Leadership Is an Art,* DePree suggests that leadership and followership involve intimacy and personal covenants that people at work make with each other.

Effective followers view themselves as equals of the leaders and work for common good. Conformist followers believe they must always please the boss, and alienated followers tend to snipe at leaders. Less effective followers have a limited world view, mainly considering their own needs and rarely considering the pressures the leader has. Excellent followers work cooperatively with leaders rather than as adversaries.

Effective followers do not always agree with the leader but are likely to use the following guidelines: When disagreeing with the leader, discuss the disagreement privately rather than in a public forum. Do not approach the leader during a crisis or deadline. Present the situation as a joint problem, not as the leader's stupid idea. Go to the meeting with potential solutions. Take the leader's point of view into consideration when brainstorming alternatives. Do not go to the leader while angry, because that is likely to escalate conflict.

In *The Power of Followership* Robert Kelley (1992) recommends that followers ask themselves the following six questions to choose their battles wisely (pp. 177-182):

1. What is at stake for the organization?
2. What will happen if you fail to act?
3. Does the leader have both the expertise and the legitimate authority to issue this order?
4. Are human costs and societal values being overlooked?
5. What role are you being asked to play?
6. What is at stake for you personally?

Followers do maintain independent and critical thinking. They are vigilant about unchecked leaders. Kelley also outlines 10 steps to a courageous conscience as follows (pp. 185-197):

1. Be proactive. . . .
2. Gather your facts. . . .
3. Before taking a stand, seek wise counsel. . . .
4. Build your fortitude. . . .
5. Work within the system. . . .
6. Frame your position so it will be heard. . . .
7. Educate others on how your view serves their best interests. . . .
8. Take collective action. . . .
9. If you meet leader resistance, seek higher authority. . . .
10. Have the financial and emotional cushions to exercise other alternatives. . . .

Janice Ellis and Celia Hartley (1995) suggest the following to be a good follower (pp. 22-23):

1. Invest yourself. . . .
2. Clearly identify your responsibilities as a follower. . . .

3. Clearly identify your expectations of the leader. . . .
4. Support your leader and your group. . . .
5. Challenge your leader and your group. . . .
6. Follow channels of communications and responsibilities. . . .

IMPLICATIONS FOR NURSING ADMINISTRATION

Surveying the development of management thought, one can see that there has been a trend from autocratic to democratic management and from a focus on efficiency to a greater regard for the well-being of personnel. Although the focus has changed, elements from each era maintain their validity and can be used by the nurse administrator. For example, Taylor's time studies and the Gilbreths' motion studies in the scientific era are illustrations of how the nurse can study complexity of care to predict staffing needs and study efficiency of nursing care. An adaption of Gantt's chart can be used to visualize the time element of planning and controlling.

Nurse administrators should be aware of their managerial tasks as defined by Fayol: planning, organizing, directing, coordinating, and controlling. His definition of management can help clarify the manager's role, and his principles of management can help direct one's actions. Assistance with the organizing function can be obtained from Weber's conceptualization of bureaucracy and authority and Urwick's popularization of such concepts as balancing authority with responsibility, unity of direction, unity of command, and span of control.

To a large extent the social environment results from organization and management. The work of Barnard, Follett, Mayo, and Lewin during the human relations era should remind the nurse administrator of the importance of developing workers to their potential and meeting their needs for recognition, accomplishment, and sense of belonging. It is hoped that nurse administrators will consider the results of Lewin's research about autocratic and democratic leadership when determining their own style. They can use Moreno's sociometry to study the group behavior of workers.

Much has been learned about management from the behavioral science studies. The nurse can apply Maslow's hierarchy-of-needs theory to the care of individual patients, to functions of individual workers, or to groups of people. The importance of achievement, recognition, responsibility, and advancement as motivators and satisfiers is stressed in Herzberg's two-factor theory. The research of McGregor, Argyris, Likert, Blake, and Mouton supports the benefits of positive attitudes toward people, development of workers, satisfaction of their needs, and commitment through participation. Fiedler indicates that a leadership style may or may not be effective, depending on the situation. Nurse administrators can use his work in assessing their work situation to determine the most effective style or choosing the work situation according to what fits their style best. The leader can also incorporate Drucker's and Odiorne's work on management by objectives for the planning, directing, and controlling phases of the management process.

By studying the development of management thought, nurse administrators can define their management role, develop their philosophy of management, learn tools and techniques for implementation of their responsibilities, and gain an increased understanding of how to work with others to accomplish goals.

CHAPTER SUMMARY

Chapter 7 covered the following:
Theories of Leadership
    Great Man Theory
    Charismatic Theory
    Trait Theory
    Situational Theory
    Contingency Theory
    Path-Goal Theory
    Situational Leadership Theory
    Transactional Leadership
    Transformational Leadership
    Integrative Leadership Model

REFERENCES

Ackoff RL: *Creating the corporate future: plan or be planned for,* New York, 1981, John Wiley & Sons.

Argyris C: *Executive leadership,* New York, 1953, Harper & Bros.

Argyris C: *Personality and organization,* New York, 1957, Harper & Bros.

Argyris C: *Integrating the individual and the organization,* New York, 1964, John Wiley & Sons.

Argyris C: *Knowledge for action,* San Francisco, 1993, Jossey-Bass.

Argyris C, Putnam R, Smith DM: *Action science,* San Francisco, 1985, Jossey-Bass.

Argyris C, Schon DA: *Organizational learning: a theory of action perspective,* Reading, Mass, 1978, Addison-Wesley.

Ashley JA: *Hospitals, paternalism, and the role of the nurse,* New York, 1976, Teachers College Press.

Barnard CI: *The functions of the executive,* Cambridge, Mass, 1938, Harvard University Press.

Barnard CI: *The nature of leadership,* Cambridge, Mass, 1940, Harvard University Press.

Bass BM: *Leadership and performance beyond expectations,* New York, 1985, Free Press.

Bass BM, Avolio BJ: Transformational leadership and organizational culture, *Publ Adm Q* 17:112-121, Spring 1993.

Bennis W: *On becoming a leader,* Reading, Mass, 1989, Addison-Wesley.

Bennis W: *Organizing genius,* Reading, Mass, 1997, Perseus Books.

Bennis W, Nanus B: *Leaders: the strategies for taking charge,* New York, 1985, 1997, Harper & Row.

Blake RR, Mouton JS: *The new managerial grid,* Houston, 1978, Gulf.

Blanchard K, Bowles S: *Gung Ho!* New York, 1998, William Morrow and Co.

Block P: *The empowered manager: positive political skills at work,* San Francisco, 1987, Jossey-Bass.

Block P: *Stewardship: choosing service over self-interest,* San Francisco, 1993, Berrett-Koehler.

Brooks DL, Brooks LM: *Seven secrets of successful women,* New York, 1997, McGraw-Hill.

Capra F, Steindl-Rast D, Madison T: *Belonging to the universe,* San Francisco, 1991, Harper.

Catalyst: *Advancing women in business—the catalyst guide,* San Francisco, 1998, Jossey-Bass.

Conger J, Kanungo R: *Charismatic leadership in organizations,* Newbury Park, Calif, 1998, Sage.

Covey SR: *The 7 habits of highly effective people,* New York, 1989, Simon & Schuster.

Covey SR: *Principle-centered leadership,* New York, 1990, Summit Books.

Covey SR, Merrill AR, Merrill RR: *First things first,* New York, 1994, Simon & Schuster.

Cox T, Beale RL: *Developing competency to manage diversity,* San Francisco, 1997, Berrett-Koehler.

DePree M: *Leadership is an art,* New York, 1989, Dell.

DePree M: *Leadership jazz,* New York, 1992, Doubleday.

Donnelly JH Jr, Gibson JL, Ivancevich JM: *Fundamentals of management functions, behavior, models,* Dallas, 1981, Business Publications.

Drucker P: *Managing for results: economic tasks and risk-taking decisions,* New York, 1964, Harper & Row.

Drucker P: *Innovation and entrepreneurship: practice and principles,* New York, 1985, Harper & Row.

Drucker PF: *Management: tasks, responsibilities, practices,* New York, 1974, Harper & Row.

Drucker PF: *Managing in turbulent times,* New York, 1980, Harper & Row.

Drucker PF: *Managing for the future: the 1990s and beyond,* New York, 1992, Truman Talley Books/Plume.

Drucker PF: *On the profession of management,* Boston, 1998, Harvard Business School.

Ellis JR, Hartley CL: *Managing and coordinating nursing care,* Philadelphia, 1995, JB Lippincott.

Enkelis L, Olsen K, Lewenstein M: *On our own terms,* San Francisco, 1995, Berrett-Koehler.

Faludi S: *Backlash: the undeclared war against women,* New York, 1991, Anchor Books/Doubleday.

Fayol H: *Administration industrielle et generale,* Paris, 1925, Dunod.

Fiedler FE: *A theory of leadership effectiveness,* New York, 1967, McGraw-Hill.

Fiedler FE, Chemers MM: *Leadership and effective management,* Glenview, Ill, 1974, Scott, Foresman, and Co.

Fiedler FE, Chemers MM, Mahar L: *Improving leadership effectiveness: the leader match concept,* New York, 1976, John Wiley & Sons.

Follett MP: *Freedom and coordination,* London, 1949, Management Publications Trust.

Fritz R: *The path of least resistance,* New York, 1989, Fawcett Columbine.

Fritz R: *Creating,* New York, 1991, Fawcett Columbine.

Gantt HL: *Industrial leadership,* New Haven, Conn, 1916, Yale University Press.

Gantt HL: *Organizing for work,* New York, 1919, Harcourt, Brace and Howe.

Gilberd P: *The eleven commandments of wildly successful women,* Tappan, NJ, 1996, Macmillan Spectrum.

Gilbreth FB: *Bricklaying system,* New York, 1909, Myron C Clark.

Gilbreth FB: *Motion study,* New York, 1911, D Van Nostrand.

Gilbreth LM: *The psychology of management,* New York, 1914, Sturgis and Walton.

Gilbreth FB, Carey EG, McKay D: *Cheaper by the dozen,* New York, 1984, Bantam Books.

Gilbreth FB, Gilbreth LM: *Applied motion study,* New York, 1917, Sturgis and Walton.

Gilbreth FB, Gilbreth LM: *Fatigue study,* ed 2, New York, 1919, Macmillan.

Goleman D: *Emotional intelligence,* New York, 1997, Bantam Books.

Goleman D: *Working with emotional intelligence,* New York, 1998, Bantam Books.

Gray J: *Men are from Mars, women are from Venus,* New York, 1992, HarperCollins.

Greenleaf RK: *Servant leadership,* New York, 1977, 1991, Paulist Press.

Harragan BL: *Games Mother never taught you: corporate gamesmanship for women,* New York, 1977, Warner Books.

Harvey JB: *The Abilene paradox,* San Diego, Calif, 1988, University Associates.

Helgesen S: *The female advantage: women's ways of leadership,* New York, 1990, Bantam Doubleday Dell.

Helgesen S: *Everyday revolutionaries,* New York, 1998, Doubleday.

Hennig MM, Jardim A: *The managerial woman,* Garden City, NY, 1966, 1977, Anchor Press/Doubleday.

Hersey P: *The situational leader,* New York, 1984, Warner Books.

Hersey P, Blanchard KH: *Management of organizational behavior: utilizing human resources,* Parmus, NJ, 1969, 1982, Prentice Hall.

Hersey P, Duldt BW: *Situational leadership in nursing,* Norwalk, Conn, 1989, Appleton & Lange.

Herzberg F: One more time: how do you motivate employees? In Carroll L, Paine R, Miner A, editors: *The management process,* ed 2, New York, 1977, Macmillan.

Herzberg F, Mausner B, Snyderman BB: *The motivation to work,* ed 2, New York, 1959, John Wiley & Sons.

Hesse H: *The journey to the east,* New York, 1956, Noonday Press.

Hitt WD: The model leader: a fully functioning person, *Leadership Organ Development J* 14(7):4-11, 1993.

Hochschild A: *The second shift,* New York, 1989, Viking Penguin.

House RJ: A path-goal theory of leader effectiveness, *Adm Sci Q* 16:321-339, 1971.

Jaworski J, Flowers BS: *Synchronicity: the inner path of leadership,* San Francisco, 1996, 1998, Berrett-Koehler.

Kanter RM: *Men and women of the corporation,* New York, 1977, 1993, Basic Books.

Kelley R: *The power of followership,* New York, 1992, Doubleday Currency.

Kelly J: *Organizational behaviour,* rev ed, Homewood, Ill, 1980, Irwin.

Kotter JP: *The general managers,* New York, 1982, Free Press.

Kotter JP: *Power and influence,* New York, 1985, Free Press.

Kotter JP: *The leadership factor,* New York, 1988, Free Press.

Kotter JP: *A force for change,* New York, 1990, Free Press.

Kotter JP: *Leading change,* Boston, 1996, Harvard Business School Press.

Kouzes JM, Posner BZ: *The leadership challenge: how to get extraordinary things done in organizations,* San Francisco, 1987, 1990, Jossey-Bass.

Kouzes JM, Posner BZ: *Credibility,* San Francisco, 1993, Jossey-Bass.

Kouzes JM, Posner BZ: *Encouraging the heart,* San Francisco, 1999, Jossey-Bass.

Lewin K: *Field theory in social sciences,* New York, 1951, Harper & Row.

Likert R: *New patterns of management,* New York, 1961, McGraw-Hill.

Likert R, Likert JG: *New ways of managing conflict,* New York, 1976, McGraw-Hill.

Loden M: *Implementing diversity,* Chicago, 1996, Irwin.

Maslow A: *Motivation and personality,* ed 2, New York, 1970, Harper & Row.

McGee-Cooper A, Trammel D, Lau B: *You don't have to go home from work exhausted,* New York, 1990, 1992, Bantam Books.

McGregor D: *The human side of enterprise,* New York, 1960, McGraw-Hill.

Meadows DH, Meadows D, Randers J: *Beyond the limits,* Past Hills, Vt, 1992, Chelsea Green.

Melia J: *Breaking into the boardroom: what every woman needs to know,* New York, 1986, GP Putnam's Sons.

Meyer C: *Fast cycle time,* New York, 1993, Free Press/Macmillan.

Mintzberg H: *The nature of managerial work,* New York, 1973, Harper & Row.

Mooney JD, Reiley AC: *Onward industry!* New York, 1931, Harper & Bros.

Mooney JD, Reiley AC: *The principles of organization,* New York, 1939, Harper & Bros.

Morrison AM: *The new leaders,* San Francisco, 1992, Jossey-Bass.

Morrison AM et al.: *Breaking the glass ceiling: can women reach the top of America's largest corporations?* Reading, Mass, 1987, Addison-Wesley.

Nanus B: *The leader's edge,* Chicago, 1989, Contemporary Books.

Nichols NA: *Reach for the top,* Boston, 1977, 1994, Harvard College.

O'Brien V, O'Brien V, Martin L: *Success on our own terms,* New York, 1998, John Wiley & Sons.

Odiorne GS: *Management by objectives,* New York, 1965, Pitman.

Ouchi WG: *Theory Z: how American business can meet the Japanese challenge,* New York, 1981, Avon Books.

Palmer PJ: *To know as we are known/a spirituality of education,* New York, 1983, HarperCollins.

Palmer PJ: *The courage to teach: exploring the inner landscape of a teacher's life,* San Francisco, 1998, Jossey-Bass.

Parker M: *Creating shared vision,* Oslo, 1990, Norwegian Center for Leadership Development.

Pascale RT, Athos AG: *The art of Japanese management: applications for American executives,* New York, 1981, Warner Books.

Peck MS: *The road less traveled,* New York, 1978, Simon & Schuster.

Peters T: *Thriving on chaos,* New York, 1987, Harper & Row.

Peters T: *Liberation management,* New York, 1992, Fawcett Columbine.

Peters T: *The Tom Peters Seminar,* New York, 1994, Vintage Books.

Peters T: *The circle of innovation,* New York, 1997, Alfred A Knopf.

Peters T, Austin N: *A passion for excellence,* New York, 1985, Warner Books.

Peters T, Waterman RH: *In search of excellence,* New York, 1982, Harper & Row.

Rosener JB: *America's competitive secret: utilizing women as a management strategy,* New York, 1995, Oxford University Press.

Rummler G, Brache AP: *Improving performance,* San Francisco, 1995, Jossey-Bass.

Schaffer RH: *The breakthrough strategy,* New York, 1988, Harper Business.

Scheele A: *Career strategies for the working woman,* New York, 1994, Simon & Schuster.

Schein EH: *Organizational culture and leadership,* San Francisco, 1985, 1997, Jossey-Bass.

Senge PM: *The fifth discipline: the art and practice of the learning organization,* New York, 1990, Doubleday.

Senge PM et al.: *The fifth discipline fieldbook,* New York, 1994, Doubleday.

Sims HP: *The thinking organization: dynamics of organizational social cognition,* San Francisco, 1986, Jossey-Bass.

Spears LC, editor: *Reflections on leadership: how Robert K. Greenleaf's theory on servant leadership influenced today's top management thinkers,* New York, 1995, John Wiley & Sons.

Spears LC, editor: *Insights on leadership: service, stewardship, spirit, and servant leadership,* New York, 1998, John Wiley & Sons.

Tannen D: *You just don't understand: women and men in conversation,* New York, 1990, Ballantine Books.

Taylor FW: *Shop management,* New York, 1903, Harper & Bros.

Taylor FW: *The principles of scientific management,* New York, 1911, Harper & Bros.

Tichy NM, Cohen E: *The leadership engine,* New York, 1997, HarperCollins.

Tichy NM, Devanna MA: *The transformational leader,* New York, 1986, 1997, John Wiley & Sons.

Tichy NM, Sherman S: *Control your destiny or someone else will,* New York, 1993, Doubleday.

Trickett EJ, Watts RJ, Birman D: *Human diversity: perspectives on people in context,* San Francisco, 1994, Jossey-Bass.

Urwick L: *The elements of administration,* New York, 1944, Harper & Bros.

Vaill PB: *Managing as a performing art,* San Francisco, 1989, Jossey-Bass.

Wheatley M: *Leadership and the new science,* San Francisco, 1992, Berrett-Koehler.

Wilson WJ: The declining significance of race: blacks and changing American institutions. In Grusky DB: *Social stratification,* pp. 520-531, Boulder, Colo, 1994, Westview Press.

Yukl GA: *Leadership in organizations,* ed 3, Gaithersburg, Md, 1994, Aspen.

BIBLIOGRAPHY

Adams JD, editor: *Transforming work,* Alexandria, Va, 1984, Miles River Press.

Adams JD, editor: *Transforming leadership: from vision to results,* Alexandria, Va, 1986, Miles River Press.

Agor WH, editor: *Intuition in organizations,* Newbury Park, Calif, 1989, Sage.

Allen DW: How nurses become leaders: perception and beliefs about leadership development, *JONA* 28:115-120, Sept 1998.

Baker AM: *Transformational nursing leadership: a vision for the future,* Baltimore, 1990, Williams & Wilkins.

Ballein KM: Entrepreneurial leadership characteristics of SNEs emerge as their role develops, *Nurs Adm Q* 22(2):60-69, 1998.

Barnum BS, Kerfoot KM: *The nurse as executive,* ed 4, Githersburg, Md, 1995, Aspen.

Benton DA: *Lions don't need to roar: using the leadership power of professional presence to stand out, fit in and move ahead,* New York, 1992, Warner Books.

Blake RR, Mouton JS: *Executive achievement: making it at the top,* New York, 1986, McGraw-Hill.

Blake RR, Mouton JS, Tapper M: *Grid approaches for managerial leadership in nursing,* St. Louis, 1981, Mosby.

Burns JM: *Leadership,* New York, 1978, Harper & Row.

Byham WC: *Zapp! The lightening of empowerment,* New York, 1988, Harmony Books.

Chappell T: *The soul of a business: managing for profit and the common good,* New York, 1993, Bantam Books.

Cohen AR, Bradford D: *Influence without authority,* New York, 1990, John Wiley & Sons.

Curtin L: How—and how not—to be a transformational leader, *Nurs Manage* 28(2):7-8, Feb 1997.

De Vries RE, Roe RA, Taillieu TCB: Need for supervision: its impact on leadership effectiveness, *J Applied Behavioral Science* 34:486-501, Dec 1998.

Denton DK: *Horizontal management: beyond total customer satisfaction,* New York, 1991, Lexington Books.

Donnelly JH Jr, Gibson JL, Ivancevich JM: *Fundamentals of management: functions, behavior, models,* Dallas, 1981, 1990, Business.

Douglas LM: *The effective nurse: leader and manager,* St. Louis, 1992, Mosby–Year Book.

Dunham-Taylor J, Fisher E, Kinion E: Experiences, events, people: do they influence the leadership style of nurse executives? *JONA* 23:30-34, July/Aug 1993.

Flarey DL: Reinventing leadership, *JONA* 26:9-10, Oct 1996.

Frenier CR: *Business and the feminine principle,* Boston, 1997, Butterworth-Heinemann.

Fullam C, Lando AR, Johansen ML et al.: The triad of empowerment: leadership, environment, and professional traits, *Nurs Econ* 16:254-257, Sept-Oct 1998.

Gardner JW: *On leadership,* New York, 1990, Free Press.

George CS: *The history of management thought,* Englewood Cliffs, NJ, 1972, Prentice Hall.

Glynn P et al.: The interconnectedness of nurses' lives, *JONA* 26:36-42, May 1996.

Goode CJ, Belgen MA: Development and evaluation of a research-based management intervention: a recognition protocol, *JONA* 32:61-66, April 1993.

Hansen HE, Woods CQ, Boyle DK et al.: Nurse manager personal traits and leadership characteristics, *Nurs Adm Q* 19(4):23-35, 1995.

Hardy VS, Forrer J: A comprehensive quality management approach, *Nurs Manage* 27(1):35-39, Jan 1996.

Heider J: *The tao of leadership,* New York, 1985, Bantam Books.

Herman SM, Korenich M: *Authentic management: a gestalt orientation to organizations and their development,* Reading, Mass, 1977, Addison-Wesley.

Houser HF: Charisma and leadership in organizations, *Personnel Psychol* 46:419-421, Summer 1993.

Ingersoll GL et al.: The effect of a professional practice model on staff nurse perception of work groups and nurse leaders, *JONA* 26:52-59, May 1996.

Jamison K: *The nibble theory and the kernel of power: a book about leadership, self-empowerment and personal growth,* New York, 1984, Paulist Press.

Jeffries EN: *The heart of leadership: influencing by design,* Dubuque, Iowa, 1993, Kendall/Hunt.

Kelly J: *Organizational behaviour,* Homewood, Ill, 1980, Irwin.

Klakovich MD: Connective leadership for the 21st century: a historical perspective and future directions, *Adv Nurs Sci* 16(4):42-54, 1994.

Koerner JEG, Bunkers SS: Transformation leadership: the power of symbol, *Nurs Adm Q* 17(1): 1-9, 1992.

Kohles MK, Baker WG, Donaho BA: *Transformational leadership: renewing fundamental values and achieving new relationships in health care,* Chicago, 1995, American Hospital.

Krejci JW, Malin S: Impact of leadership development on competencies, *Nurs Econ* 15:235-241, Sept-Oct 1997.

Lebo F: *Mastering the diversity challenge: easy on-the-job applications for measurable results,* Delray Beach, Fla, 1996, St. Lucie Press.

Liebig JE: *Merchants of vision: people bringing new purposes and values to business,* San Francisco, 1994, Berrett-Koehler.

Longenecker PD: Managing nurse managers, *Nurs Manage* 29:35-37, March 1998.

Lynch D, Kordis PL: *Strategy of the dolphin: scoring a win in a chaotic world,* New York, 1988, Ballantine Books.

Manion J, Sieg MJ, Watson P: Managerial partnerships: the wave of the future, *JONA* 28:47-55, April 1998.

Mark BA: The emerging role of the nurse manager, *JONA* 24:48-55, Jan 1994.

McCall MW, Lombardo MM, Morrison AM: *The lessons of experience,* Lexington, Ky, 1988, Lexington Books.

Moore BW et al.: Patient care leadership within an emerging integrated delivery network, *Nurs Adm Q* 20(2):54-64, 1996.

Morf M: *The work/life dichotomy: prospects for reintegrating people and jobs,* New York, 1989, Quorum Books.

Morrison AM: *The new leaders: guidelines on leadership diversity in America,* San Francisco, 1992, Jossey-Bass.

Morrison RS, Jones L, Fuller B: The relationship between leadership style and empowerment on job satisfaction of nurses, *JONA* 27:27-34, May 1997.

Osborne D, Gaebler T: *Reinventing government: how the entrepreneurial spirit is transforming the public sector,* Reading, Mass, 1992, Addison-Wesley.

Parachin VM: Ten essential leadership skills, *Am Salesman* 43:3-6, Nov 1998.

Pascarella P: *The new achievers: creating a modern work ethic,* New York, 1984, Free Press.

Pascarella P, Frohman MA: *The purpose-driven organization: unleashing the power of direction and commitment,* San Francisco, 1989, Jossey-Bass.

Peale NV: *The power of positive thinking,* New York, 1952, Fawcett Crest.

Pearce T: *Leading out loud: the authentic speaker, the credible leader,* San Francisco, 1995, Jossey-Bass.

Perra BM: The leader in you, *Nurs Manage* 30:35-39, Jan 1999.

Pillai R: Context and charisma: the role of organic structure, collectivism, and crisis in the emergence of charismatic leadership, *Academy Manage J Best Papers Proceedings 1995*:332-338, 1995.

Pitcher P: *The drama of leadership,* New York, 1997, John Wiley & Sons.

Prenkert F, Ehnfors M: A measure of organizational effectiveness in nursing management in relation to transactional and transformational leadership: a study in a Swedish county hospital, *J Nurs Manage* 5:279-287, Sept 1997.

Ray M, Rinzler A: *The new paradigm in business: emerging strategies for leadership and organizational change,* New York, 1993, GP Putnam/JP Parcher.

Renesch J, editor: *New traditions in business,* San Francisco, 1992, Berrett-Koehler.

Renesch J, editor: *Leadership in the new era: visionary approaches to the biggest crisis of our time,* San Francisco, 1994, New Leaders Press.

Richardson RJ, Thayer SK: *The charisma factor: how to develop your natural leadership ability,* Englewood Cliffs, NJ, 1993, Prentice Hall.

Roberts W: *Leadership secrets of Attila the hun,* New York, 1985, Warner Books.

Rowan R: *The intuitive manager,* New York, 1986, Berkley Books.

Schafe AW: *Women's reality: an emerging female system in a white male society,* San Francisco, 1981, 1985, Harper & Row.

Schweitzer A: *The age of charisma,* Chicago, 1984, Nelson-Hall.

Seligman MEP: *Learned optimism,* New York, 1990, Alfred A. Knopf.

Sergiovanni TJ: *Moral leadership: getting to the heart of school improvement,* San Francisco, 1992, Jossey-Bass.

Stahl DA: Leadership in these changing times, *Nurs Manage* 29:16-18, April 1998.

Stogdill RM, Coons AE: *Leader behavior: its description and measurement,* Columbus, Ohio, 1957, College of Administrative Science.

Taccetta-Chapnick M: Transformational leadership, *Nurs Adm Q* 21:60-66, Fall 1996.

Terry RT: *Authentic leadership: courage in action,* San Francisco, 1993, Jossey-Bass.

Tyrrell RA: Visioning: an important management tool, *Nurs Econ* 12:93-95, March-April 1994.

Vogt JF, Murrell KL: *Empowerment in organizations: how to spark exceptional performance,* San Diego, 1990, Pfeiffer & Co.

White J: *A few good women: breaking the barriers to top management,* Englewood Cliffs, NJ, 1992, Prentice Hall.

Wigens L: The conflict between "new nursing" and "scientific management" as perceived by surgical nurses, *J Adv Nurs* 25:1116-1122, June 1997.

CASE STUDY

You are a new patient care coordinator. The previous one was very autocratic. How will you begin changing from the autocratic atmosphere to a participative style?

CASE STUDY

You have just accepted the nursing leadership role in a long-term care facility. Identify the management process and list the activities you will need to do to plan, organize, staff, direct, and evaluate.

Critical Thinking Activities for this chapter begin on page 489.

Two

MANAGEMENT

CHAPTER 8

STRATEGIC AND OPERATIONAL PLANNING

Chapter Overview

Chapter 8 illustrates the planning process, history of strategic planning, strategic planning process, vision, values, mission, philosophy, goals, objectives, strategies, policies, and procedures.

MAJOR CONCEPTS AND DEFINITIONS	
Strategic planning	long-range planning usually extending 3 to 5 years into the future
Operational planning	short-range planning that deals with day-to-day maintenance activities
Belief	conviction that certain things are true
Vision	mental image of something not actually visible
Value	the worth, usefulness, or importance of something
Mission/purpose	an aim to be accomplished; mission statement
Philosophy	statement of beliefs and values that directs behavior
Goal	the end to be accomplished
Objective	something aimed at or striven for; things done to achieve the goal
Policy	a governing plan for accomplishing goals and objectives
Procedure	chronological sequence of steps within a process
Protocols	documents of agreement
Business plan	plan for new ventures like new products or services

PLANNING PROCESS

There are two major types of organizational planning: long-range, or strategic, planning and short-range, or operational, planning. Strategic planning extends 3 to 5 years into the future. It begins with in-depth analysis of the internal environment's strengths and weaknesses and the external opportunities and threats so that realistic goals can be set for the preferred future. It determines the direction of the organization, allocates resources, assigns responsibilities, and determines time frames. Strategic planning goals are more generic and less specific than operational planning.

Nurse managers are more likely to be involved in the operational planning. Operational planning is done in conjunction with budgeting, usually a few months before the new fiscal year. It develops the departmental maintenance and improvement goals for the coming year.

History of Strategic Planning

Private business started using strategic planning in the mid-1950s when the demand for products began to level off and decline and substitute products became available from foreign competitors. The health care industry started during the mid-1970s when the federal government established restricted payment regulations. Third-party payers also developed restrictions, and payment shifted from the federal government to individuals and other payers. This increased price sensitivity and competition. Alternative delivery systems such as preferred provider arrangements, health maintenance organizations, self-help and wellness programs, and ambulatory services proliferated. As chief executive officers looked at job redesign to increase productivity while cutting costs, mergers, acquisitions, joint ventures, and informal networking increased.

High-cost technology responded to the competitive environment, with greater acuity of care in acute-care settings, tertiary settings, and homes. At the same time the population was aging, increasing numbers of the population were under- and uninsured. Quality of life and ethics also became important issues. Consequently, strategic planning became prevalent in health care settings and literature during the 1980s.

During the 1990s trends moved from individual specialist providers to team primary care providers; from reliance on physician care to use of physician extenders; from hospital episodical care to ambulatory care; from institutional care to alternative care; from individual-based treatments to population-based treatments; from curative, uncoordinated care to preventive, integrated care; from acute care to chronic care; from technological orientation to humanistic orientation; from younger population to older population; from content mastery to process mastery; from being governed professionally to being governed managerially; from competitive to cooperative; from cost unaware to cost aware; from fee for service to capitation; from paper health records to computerized health records; and from no data on best practices to emerging data about best practices (Box 8-1).

Purpose of Strategic Planning

Strategic planning clarifies beliefs and values: What are the organization's strengths and weaknesses? What are the potential opportunities and threats? Where is the organization going? How is it going to get there? It gives direction to the organization, improves efficiency, weeds out poor or underused programs, eliminates duplication of efforts, concentrates resources on important services, improves communications and coordination of activities, provides a mind-expanding opportunity, allows adaptation to the changing environment, sets realistic and attainable yet challenging goals, and helps ensure goal achievement.

Leaders need vision that is realistic and feasible. Development of a strategic vision involves analysis of the agency's environment, capabilities,

| Box 8-1 | **TRENDS DURING THE 1990S** |

Moving From	Moving To
Individual provider	Team provider
Physician's needs	Payer's/customer's needs
Specialties	Primary care
Reliance on physician care	Use of physician extenders
Hospital episodic care	Ambulatory continuum of care
Institutional care	Alternative care
Individual-based treatment	Population-based treatment
Curative care	Preventive care
Acute care	Chronic care
Technologically oriented	Humanistically oriented
Younger population	Older population
Content mastery	Process mastery
Governed professionally	Governed managerially
Competitive	Cooperative
Cost unaware	Cost aware
Fee for service	Capitation
Paper health record	Computerized health record
No data on best practices	Emerging data on best practices

and resources; development and articulation of a conceptual image; clarification of values; development of a mission statement; identification of goals and objectives; and identification of strategies for reaching the goals. The strategic vision should be clear, cohesive, consistent, and flexible (Box 8-2).

Strategic Planning Process

It is important that top-level administrators are committed to strategic planning. Otherwise such planning may be viewed as mere busy work. Managers need to be taught the importance of long-range planning and the way to do it.

<table>
<tbody>
<tr><td>

Box 8-2

STRATEGIC PLANNING PROCESS

External assessment
    Opportunities and threats
Internal assessment
    Strengths and weaknesses
Priority strategic issues and programs
Vision
Values
Mission
Philosophy
Goals
    Strategic
        Organization
    Operational
        Division
        Unit
Objectives
Strategies
    Timelines
    Plans
Policies
Procedures
Implementation
Evaluation
    Production/operations
    Finance
    Marketing

</td></tr>
</tbody>
</table>

An external assessment looks at opportunities and threats, whereas an internal assessment checks for strengths and weaknesses. A situation audit, or environmental assessment, analyzes the past, current, and future forces that affect the organization. Expectations of outside interests such as opinion leaders, governmental officials, insurance companies, and consumers are sought. Expectations of inside interests such as doctors, staff, administrators, and patients are collected.

The management team can use a grid to visualize the situation audit. (See Worksheet 8-1 on p. 492.) The past, present, and future are represented on the horizontal axis. Criteria for areas such as clients, competition, market share, environment, demographics, economics, laws, politics, technol-

ogy, resources and facilities, finances, and human resources are represented on the vertical axis.

A SWOT (strengths, weaknesses, opportunities, and threats) analysis worksheet is also helpful. Each quadrant of a paper is labeled as one of the four categories, and appropriate factors are listed in each quadrant for a bird's-eye view of the situation audit. (See Worksheet 8-2 on p. 493.) Internal strengths or weaknesses may include management development, qualifications of staff, medical staff expertise, abundance or scarcity of staff, financial situation, cash flow position, marketing efforts, market share, facilities, location, and quality of services.

Opportunities include nurse and physician recruitment, referral patterns, new programs, new markets, diversification, population growth, improved technology, and new facilities.

Threats may be shortage of nurses, decrease in patient satisfaction, decrease in insured patients, increase in accounts receivable, decrease in demand for services, competition, regulations, litigation, legislative changes, unionization, and loss of accreditation.

After the situation audit is done, the management team reviews the philosophy, identifies vision and values, writes a purpose or mission statement, identifies organizational goals and objectives, plans strategies to accomplish the objectives, identifies required resources, determines priorities, sets time frames, and determines accountability.

Business plans are plans for new ventures such as new products or services that meet many of the standards for strategic plans (Box 8-3). They integrate strategic, operational, and financial planning. The cover page notes the name of the company, the business plan and year, and names and phone numbers of the contact person(s). The executive summary, which is about two pages long, is a brief overview of the entire plan. The table of contents should identify at least each major section of the report. The introduction describes the nature of the organization and identifies philosophy, goals, objectives, and projected outcomes. The market analysis identifies the product, price, place, and promotions for the new product or service. The analysis of the competition describes the competition and identi-

Box 8-3	BUSINESS PLAN

Cover page
Executive summary
Table of contents
Introduction
    Description of the business
Analysis of the market
Analysis of the competition
Product or service development
Operational plan
Marketing plan
Organizational plan
Development schedule
Financial plan

Box 8-4	LEVELS OF PLANNING

Strategic planning   Top-level management
Intermediate planning   Middle-level management
Operational planning   Lower-level management

Box 8-5	PLANNING TOOLS

Vision
Values
Mission
Philosophy
Goals
Objectives
Policies
Procedures

fies the competitive edge. Product development identifies the resources needed and a time frame for the development of the new product or service and presents a quality control plan. The operational plan identifies the desired location and the needed facilities, equipment, and personnel. The marketing plan describes the mission, goals, strategies, staffing, and financial plans for marketing. The organizational plan presents an organizational chart with job descriptions and short résumés. The development schedule identifies tasks and timelines. The financial plan identifies developmental costs and projects income goals and expenditures (Burton and McBride, 1991; Swansburg, 1996).

Top-level managers such as chief executive officers, presidents, and division heads do strategic planning for 3 to 5 years. Middle-level managers such as supervisors and clinical specialists do intermediate planning for 6 months to 2 years. Lower-level managers such as managers of nursing units, team leaders, case managers, and primary care nurses do operational planning of 1 week to 1 year (Douglas, 1996) (Box 8-4).

VISION

Vision is a mental image or the power of imagination to see something that is not actually visible.

When doing strategic planning, the vision should be the preferred future (Boxes 8-5 and 8-6).

VALUES

Value is the worth, usefulness, or importance of something. Leadership, management, and personnel should determine what their values are and keep their plans and actions consistent with their values. A values statement is a planning tool (Box 8-7).

PURPOSE OR MISSION STATEMENT

Organizations exist for a purpose. Clarification of the mission or purpose is a high priority for planning. Most nursing services exist to provide high-quality nursing care to clients. Some also encourage teaching and research. Each specialty area, with its own specific purposes, contributes to the overall purpose of the institution. For example, the purpose of the in-service education department is to orient staff to the job and to provide educational programs to improve the quality of the staff work.

Box 8-6 SAMPLE VISION

GENERAL HOSPITAL VISION STATEMENT

The vision for General Hospital is to be the preeminent health care provider in the region by doing the following:

Being the premier full-service, integrated health care delivery network that provides a continuum of health services,

Creating an environment that exceeds the expectations of our customers,

Developing creative solutions to the challenges facing us,

Providing economically viable, cost-effective services to our customers, and

Working in partnership with other leading health care organizations

Box 8-7 SAMPLE VALUES STATEMENT

The guiding values for General Hospital are as follows:

Quality,

Compassion,

Fairness,

Integrity,

Innovation, and

Fiscal responsibility.

Box 8-8 SAMPLE MISSION STATEMENT

The mission of General Hospital is to deliver comprehensive health care services to promote physical and mental health; to prevent disease, injury, and disability; and to promote healing of the body, mind, and spirit. Related instruction, public service programs, and research will facilitate high-quality health care.

goals, and objectives should be examined periodically for consistency. Box 8-8 provides an example of a mission statement.

The burn unit exists to provide good-quality nursing service to patients with burns.

The mission or purpose influences philosophy, goals, and objectives. For example, if a progressive care unit exists to help patients adjust to their diseases, it should be staffed with professional nurses particularly skilled in teaching and counseling. If, however, the unit's purpose is to cut hospital and patient expenses, it may be a minimal care unit with reduced services given by nonprofessional workers. The relationships between the mission, philosophy,

PHILOSOPHY

The philosophy articulates a vision and provides a statement of beliefs and values that direct one's practice. It should be written, included in appropriate documents, and reviewed periodically. If the philosophy is stated in vague, abstract terms that are not easily understood, it is useless. Conflicting philosophies between overlapping units cause confusion and should be avoided. Workers are most likely to interpret the philosophy from the pronouncements and actions of the leaders in the institution. Therefore conformity of action to belief is important.

When developing or reevaluating a philosophy, the manager should consider theory, education, practice, research, and nursing's role in the total organization. Gaye Poteet and Alice Hill (1988) identify three approaches that can be used to incorporate nursing theory into the philosophy. An eclectic approach would select ideas from various nursing theories and incorporate them into the philosophy statements, a theory might be adopted and integrated into the philosophy, or another might be referred to throughout. Attaching an explanation of the theory to the philosophy would also be useful.

Myra Levine and Dorothea Orem focus on nursing therapeutics. Dorothy Johnson and Sister Callista Roy emphasize the client. Imogene King, Margaret Newman, Ida Orlando, Josephine Patterson, Loretta Zderad, Joyce Travelbee, and Ernestine Wiedebach discuss interaction. Martha Rogers focuses on the environment and interactions of human beings (Marriner-Tomey and Alligood, 1998).

It is appropriate to comment on skill levels needed, advanced preparation for certain positions, need for continuing education, provision of educational opportunities for students, and specific practice modalities. Value of applying research findings to practice, supporting research efforts, and nursing's role in the overall organization could also be clarified in the philosophy (Box 8-9).

GOALS AND OBJECTIVES

Goals and objectives state actions for achieving the mission and philosophy. In fact, if the mission or purpose and philosophy are to be more than good intentions, they must be translated into explicit goals. The more quantitative the goal, the more likely its achievement is to receive attention and the less likely it is to be distorted. Goals are central to the whole management process—planning, organizing, staffing, directing, and controlling. Planning defines the goals. The institution is organized and staffed to accomplish the goals. Direction stimulates personnel toward accomplishment of the objec-

| Box 8-9 | SAMPLE PHILOSOPHY |

PHILOSOPHY OF GENERAL HOSPITAL

General Hospital is committed to assessing and meeting the physical, emotional, spiritual, environmental, social, and rehabilitative health needs of the citizens in the region. The worth, dignity, and autonomy of individuals (customers, employees, and others) are recognized, as is each individual's right to self-direction and responsibility for one's own life. Individual uniqueness will be considered when assessing needs and delivering quality care. Educational pursuits, research, and public service programs will be used toward innovations and improvement of health care in the region. General Hospital personnel will work in collaboration with customers and in partnership with other organizations to provide cost-effective services.

---

tives, and control compares the results with the objectives to evaluate accomplishments.

Goals and objectives may address services rendered, economics, use of resources—people, funds, and facilities—innovations, and social responsibilities. Objectives are selective rather than global, are multiple, and cover a wide range of activities. The immediate, short-term, and long-term goals should be balanced, interdependent, and ranked in order of importance. It is common to have more short-term than long-term goals.

Classic theory contends that the board of directors and top administration should determine institutional goals. Behavioral scientists are interested in having workers involved in setting goals and identifying real versus stated goals. The real goals can be identified by observing the day-by-day decisions and actions. Service interest, profit motives, governmental regulations, union representation, and personal goals all influence decision making.

It is appropriate for the board of directors and top administrators to set institutional goals and objectives; for the vice president for nursing, directors

---

<table>
<tr><td>
Box 8-10

SAMPLE GOAL AND OBJECTIVES

Goal

Develop and implement staff development programs to meet the need for increased knowledge

Objective

To develop and implement at least 12 staff development programs by the end of the fiscal year

Strategies

Continue to develop, implement, and evaluate continuing education programs for personnel

Evaluate, revise, and implement the orientation program for new personnel

Develop, implement, and evaluate in-service programs regarding new products
</td></tr>
</table>

of nurses, and patient care coordinators to set the goals and objectives for the nursing service; for the staff associates to determine the unit goals and objectives; and for the nurses to determine their goals and objectives with their immediate manager. The overlap created by the vice president's and director's working on institutional and nursing service goals and the patient care coordinator's contributing to nursing service and her unit's goals helps facilitate continuity and compatibility of goals. Participation in the determination of goals and objectives increases commitment, transforming them from stated to real goals. Because goals are dynamic, they change over time. They should be reviewed periodically so that they can be changed in an evolutionary rather than a radical manner. Goals should be specific rather than vague and challenging yet reachable. Necessary support elements should be available (Box 8-10).

Goals help focus attention on what is important and are broader statements than objectives. Objectives are more specific ways to reach the goal. It is recommended that objectives be achievable, specific, measurable, and outcome oriented, starting with "to" followed by a verb. Each objective should be about a single result with a target date. Strategies identify how the organization will attain the vision. The development of long- and short-term objectives is appropriate. A form with four columns (one for goals/objectives, one for strategies/actions, one for target dates and person(s) responsible, and one for accomplishments) can be a helpful planning tool (Swansburg and Swansburg, 1999; Yoder-Wise, 1999) (Box 8-11).

Policies

Policies and procedures are means for accomplishing goals and objectives. Policies explain how goals will be achieved and serve as guides that define the general course and scope of activities permissible for goal accomplishment. They serve as a basis for future decisions and actions, help coordinate plans, control performance, and increase consistency of action by increasing the probability that different managers will make similar decisions when independently facing similar situations. Consequently, morale is increased when personnel perceive that they are being treated equally. Policies also serve as a means by which authority can be delegated.

Policies should be comprehensive in scope, stable, and flexible so they can be applied to different conditions that are not so diverse that they require separate sets of policies. Consistency is important because inconsistency introduces uncertainty and contributes to feelings of bias, preferential treatment, and unfairness. Fairness is an important characteristic that is attributed to the application of the policy. Policies should be written and understandable.

Policies can be implied or expressed. Implied policies are not directly voiced or written but are established by patterns of decisions. They may have either favorable or unfavorable effects and represent an interpretation of observed behavior. Courteous treatment of clients may be implied versus expressed. The presence or absence of workers who are over 50 or 55 years of age, minority members, women, or pregnant women may lead to an inter-

Box 8-11	PLANNING TOOL

Goals/Objectives	Strategies/Actions	Target Dates/Person(s) Responsible	Accomplishments
1. To develop and implement at least 12 staff development programs by the end of the fiscal year	A. Develop class regarding performance appraisal for middle managers.	January 2000 Nurse manager educator	Collect materials first week; write lesson plans second week; develop course teaching tools third week; print course packet fourth week
	B. Implement performance appraisal class for middle managers.	February 2000 Nurse manager educator	Class taught February
	C. Evaluate class regarding performance appraisal.	February 2000 Nurse manager educator	Pass out evaluation form at end of class; tabulate data within week

pretation of implied policies. Sometimes policies are implied simply because no one has ever bothered to state them. At other times they may deliberately be only implied because they are illegal or reflect questionable ethics. Sometimes implied policy conflicts with expressed policy. These double standards should be prevented.

Expressed policies may be oral or written. Oral policies are more flexible than written ones and can be easily adjusted to changing circumstances. However, they are less desirable than written ones because they may not be known.

The process of writing policies reveals discrepancies and omissions and causes the manager to think critically about the policy, thus contributing to clarity. Once written, they are readily available to all in the same form; their meaning cannot be changed by word of mouth; misunderstandings can be referred to the written words; the chance of misinterpretation is decreased; policy statements can be sent to all affected by them; they can be referred to whoever wishes to check the policy; and they can be used for orientation purposes. Written policies in-

dicate the integrity of the organization's intention and generate confidence in management.

A disadvantage of written policies is the reluctance to revise them when they become outdated. However, even oral policies become obsolete. Managers should review policies periodically, and if that fails, personnel can appeal for a revision.

Policies can emerge in several ways — originated, appealed, or imposed (Box 8-12). The originated, or internal, policies are usually developed by top management to guide subordinates in their functions. Strategy for originated policy flows from the objectives of the organization as defined by top management and may be broad in scope, allowing staff associates to develop supplemental policies, or well defined with little room for interpretation. All of the lower managerial decisions should implement the broader policy defined by top management.

Sometimes policies are generated at the operating and first-line manager levels and imposed upward. The extent to which this happens is influenced by the organizational atmosphere and

Originated
Appealed
Imposed

adequacy of policies generated by top management. At times policies may be formulated simultaneously from both directions.

When staff associates do not know how to solve a problem, disagree with a previous decision, or otherwise want a question reviewed, they appeal to the manager for a decision. As appeals are taken up the hierarchy and decisions are made, precedents known as appealed policy develop and guide future managerial actions.

Policies developed from appeals are likely to be incomplete, uncoordinated, and unclear. Unintended precedents can be set when decisions are made for a given situation without consideration for possible effects on other dimensions of the organization. This aimless formation of policy makes it difficult to know what policies exist. Sometimes managers dislike facing issues until forced to do so and consequently delay policy making until precedents have been set. Appealed policies can be foresighted and consistent, especially when the manager knows that the decision constitutes policy. Nevertheless, when a number of policies are being appealed, it is time to assess policies for gaps and needs for updating and clarification so originated policies can dominate. One can expect health care agencies to require policies about patient care assignments, noting physicians' orders, administration of medications, patient safety, charting, and infection control.

Imposed, or external, policies are thrust on an organization by external forces such as government or labor unions. Policies of the organization must conform to local, state, and federal laws. Collective bargaining and union contracts direct labor policies. Professional and social groups—such as the American Nurses Association, the National League

for Nursing, and church, school, and charitable organizations—mold policy.

The planning process involves defining, communicating, applying, and maintaining policies. The development of a policy can originate anywhere in an organization and should involve personnel who will be affected by the policy. They have valuable information for sound policy formation and can ensure that the policy will be implemented. Before writing a policy, one must consider whether there are specific, recurring problems, how frequently they occur, whether they are temporary or permanent in nature, and whether a policy statement would clarify thinking and promote efficiency.

When policies are written, the purpose, philosophy, goals, and objectives should serve as guides. Policies should be consistent and help solve or prevent specific problems. Clear, concise statements that establish areas of authority and perhaps include reference to supporting policies minimize exceptions. Managers need sufficient guidance with accompanying freedom for action. It is advisable to have the policy statement reviewed and approved by superiors and the affected managers before the policy is formalized.

Policies are of no use if no one knows of their existence. Oral communication is appropriate to introduce and explain new policies. It is appropriate to send a letter of purpose and a copy of policies to personnel affected by them. The written policies can then be referred to later. Policies should be written in a specific, concise, and complete manner and stored in a policy manual that is easily accessible to all personnel to whom the policies apply. The manual will be well organized if policies are classified, noted in the table of contents, and indexed by topic. Policies should be easily replaceable with revised ones.

Once a policy has been stated and approved, it is applied. Policy formation is a continuous process; the policy is continually reappraised and restated as necessary (Figure 8-1). Continuing surveillance to determine that the policy is understood and applied is important. Periodic analysis and evaluation of existing policies can suggest the

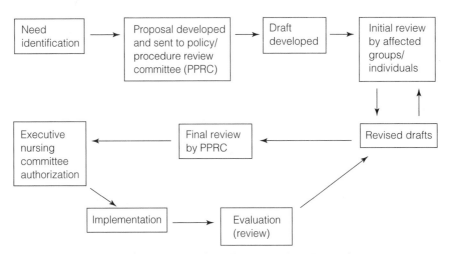

Figure 8-1 Flowchart for policies/procedures/protocols.

need for revision. Personnel should be encouraged to help formulate, review, and revise policies. Boxes 8-13 through 8-17 present sample policies for generating and reviewing nursing policies, procedures, and protocols.

Procedures

Procedures supply a more specific guide to action than policy does. They help achieve a high degree of regularity by enumerating the chronological sequence of steps. Procedures are intradepartmental or interdepartmental and consequently do not affect the entire organization to the extent that policy statements do.

Procedure manuals provide a basis for orientation and staff development and are a ready reference for all personnel. They standardize procedures and equipment and can provide a basis for evaluation. Good procedures can result in time and labor savings. Box 8-18 presents a sample procedure for taking a blood pressure measurement.

Improvement in operating procedures increases productivity and reduces cost. Waste in performing work can be decreased by applying work simplification that strives to make each part of a procedure productive. First, one decides what work requires simplification by identifying problem areas. Next, the work selected is analyzed carefully and in detail. Charts that depict the components of

the work and the work flow are useful for motion or procedural analysis.

A questioning attitude helps determine why work is done, by whom, when, where, and how. What is the purpose of the procedure? Does it need to be done? Can it be eliminated? For example, are "closed" and "surgical" beds really necessary, or could "open" beds be used for all purposes? Who does the work? Can someone else do it better, or can it be assigned to someone with less skill? Is there duplication of efforts? Can two or more activities be combined? Will changing the time sequence improve the procedure? Can transportation be reduced by changing the location? Once these questions have been answered, work should be simplified by rearranging, combining, or eliminating components. Then the improved methods must be communicated so they can be implemented.

Writing procedures demands a consistent format that considers the definition; purpose; materials needed and how to locate, requisition, and dispose of them; steps in the procedure; expected results; precautions; legal implications; nurse, patient, and physician responsibilities; and appropriate charting. Each step in the procedure leading to the accomplishment of a goal should be necessary and in proper relationship to the other steps. Balance between flexibility and stability should be maintained. As with the policy manual, the proce-

Text continued on p. 192.

Box 8-13 PROCESS FOR GENERATION OF POLICY/PROCEDURE/PROTOCOL

Issue Date July 1989	*PROCESS FOR GENERATION OF A* *NURSING POLICY/PROCEDURE/* *PROTOCOL*	**Policy No.** A/O QA.08
Review Dates Annually		**Subject** Quality Assurance

POLICY

Written policies, procedures, and protocols that reflect optimal standards of nursing practice will guide the provision of nursing care.

SCOPE

This policy applies to all of Nursing Services.

PURPOSE

To provide a consistent format for the writing and processing of policies/procedures/protocols (P/P/P): to identify resources for creating, reviewing, and changing P/P/P for Indiana University Hospitals Nursing Services; to eliminate duplication of efforts and ensure current and consistent practice.

PROCESS

1. A written P/P/P may be initiated by any nurse with approval of the unit director or associate director when appropriate. A self-study packet is available to assist with this process.

2. A proposal for all new P/P/Ps will be sent to the Nursing Service Policy/Procedure Review Committee (PPRC). (See attached form.) The proposal includes the topic/title, patients affected by the procedure, why it is needed, resource persons who will be used to write or consult, and appropriate signature(s). In some cases a proposal may not be necessary, but the intent to write a P/P/P should be communicated to the PPRC. The committee will then serve as a resource for format, other resources, and for distribution. Exceptions for the initial proposal might be direction from the Executive Nursing Council or the hospital system.

3. Approval/disapproval to write will then be communicated to the initiating individual(s) by the PPRC after considering the possible overall need, already existent P/P/P, and additional resources. A member of the PPRC will be assigned to each approved proposal to ensure consistency of format. (See attached format guidelines.)

Associated Director of Hospitals for Nursing	Date
Sonna Ehrlich	7/11/89

Used with permission from Indiana Hospitals.

Box 8-14

PROPOSAL FOR POLICY/PROCEDURE

PROPOSAL FOR POLICY/PROCEDURE

This form is submitted to the Policy/Procedure Committee of Nursing Services to request a written Policy/ Procedure designed to implement policy and maintain policy standards in regard to the following nursing care:

Topic: _____

Patients affected by the policy/procedure: _____

Explanation of the policy/procedure: _____

_____

Problems that arise as a result of not having a written policy/procedure: _____

_____

Resources that you will use to write and document the validity of this policy/procedure: _____

Name _____

Unit director _____

Associate director _____

****

For Use by Policy/Procedure Committee

Date received: _____

Approval for writing of policy/procedure: Yes   No

Contacts within Nursing Services and Medicine that must be made for coordination of the writing of this procedure: _____

_____

Committee member assigned to supervise project: _____

Guidelines for Procedure Format

Title
Policy statement
Scope
Purpose (optional)
Assessment and planning
   Nursing considerations
   Cautions
   Resources
Implementation
   Sequence of interventions/rationale
   Cautions
Evaluation
Documentation
Authorization signature
Reference:
Written by:
Date of revision(s):
Date of review(s):

Used with permission from Indiana Hospitals.

Box 8-15　REVIEW PROCESS FOR POLICIES/PROCEDURES/PROTOCOLS

Issue Date November 1987	*PROCESS FOR GENERATION OF A* *NURSING POLICY/PROCEDURE/* *PROTOCOL*	Policy No. A/O QA.07
Review Dates Annually		**Subject** Quality Assurance

POLICY

All policies, procedures, and protocols (P/P/P) will be reviewed annually and revised as necessary.

SCOPE

This policy applies to all Nursing service policies, procedures, and protocols.

PROCESS

1. Reviews of P/P/P will be conducted in quarterly periods (Jan-Mar, Apr-Jun, Jul-Sept, Oct-Dec).

2. Before the beginning of the upcoming quarter, the Policy/Procedure Review Committee (PPRC) will receive notice of which P/P/Ps are due for review. Members of the PPRC will be assigned accountability for the review of specific P/P/Ps.

3. The accountable PPRC member will review the P/P/P and will solicit feedback from appropriate content experts, using the appropriate Policy or Procedure Review Questionnaire. (See attached.)

4. The content experts will complete the Review Questionnaire after obtaining input from most affected groups or individuals. The completed questionnaire and a draft of the revised P/P/P will be returned to the accountable PPRC member by the deadline date indicated.

5. On receipt of the questionnaire and draft, the accountable PPRC member will submit the final draft of the revised P/P/P to the PPRC.

6. Upon approval by the PPRC, the final draft will be submitted to the Executive Nursing Council for authorization and signature.

7. Revised P/P/P will then be distributed to all holders of Nursing Service Policy/Procedure Manuals.

8. Requests to review P/P/Ps can be made at any time during the year to the PPRC. (See attached flowchart.)

Date of Revision(s): 7/89
Date of Review(s): 7/90

Associated Director of Hospitals for Nursing	Date
Sonna Ehrlich	7/21/89

Used with permission from Indiana Hospitals.

Box 8-16   **PROCEDURE REVIEW QUESTIONNAIRE**

PROCEDURE REVIEW QUESTIONNAIRE

Name of Procedure _____

Date of review _____

Reviewer(s) _____

| (Name) | (Title) | (Service/Unit) |

| (Name) | (Title) | (Service/Unit) |

(Note: The reviewer may wish to carry out the procedure exactly as written before addressing the questions below.)
Please circle the number that most accurately reflects your response to the following.

Where procedure differs from practice, please note discrepancies on separate sheet of paper. Please write recommended revision on separate sheet of paper and return to _____ by _____.

	Yes	No	Uncertain	Comments
1. Does the procedure accurately reflect all equipment/materials necessary to carry out the procedure				
a) safely?				
b) competently	1	2	3	
2. Does the procedure reflect equipment used at IUHs?	1	2	3	
3. Is the sequence of steps correct?	1	2	3	
4. Is the sequence of steps complete?	1	2	3	
5. Are the contraindications, if any, clearly identified?	1	2	3	
6. Does the scientific rationale provide a meaningful reason for each intervention?	1	2	3	
7. Does the procedure reflect results of current research and state-of-the-art clinical nursing practice?	1	2	3	
8. Does the procedure reflect current clinical practice at IUHs?	1	2	3	
9. Is the procedure in conflict with any other hospital or Nursing Services' policies/procedures? If so, please list.	1	3	3	

Additional Comments:

RECOMMENDED ACTION

_____ The procedure is correct as written. Recommend adoption of procedure.

_____ Discrepancies noted. Recommended revision attached.

_____ Recommend procedure not be adopted.

12/84

Box 8-17   **POLICY REVIEW FORM**

POLICY REVIEW FORM

Name of policy _____

Date of review _____

Reviewer _____

                        (Name)   (Service)

INSTRUCTIONS: Please circle the number that most accurately reflects your response to the following questions. Please check at the bottom your recommended action.

	Yes	No	Comments
1. Is there a need for the policy?	1	2	
2. Is the policy relevant to this institution and staff?	1	2	
3. Is the policy consistent with Indiana University Hospitals Nursing Services philosophy?	1	2	
4. Is the policy in conflict with any other hospital or nursing policies?	1	2	
5. Does the policy create any inequities between hospital staff or patients?	1	2	
6. Is the policy reasonable (i.e., can compliance be enforced)?	1	2	
7. Is the policy clearly written so that anyone unfamiliar with the subject can understand it?	1	2	
8. Is the information accurate?	1	2	
9. Is the policy complete (i.e., does it include the scope, purpose, and any related information)?	1	2	

ADDITIONAL COMMENTS

RECOMMENDED ACTION:

_____ No action required   _____ Revision required   _____ Remove from manual
      Approved as written   (Changes attached)   (Justification attached)

Courtesy Indiana Hospitals.

Box 8-18   **PROCEDURE**

PROCEDURE

Blood Pressure Measurement

A. Definition: Amount of pressure exerted against the arterial wall as the blood is forced by the pumping action of the heart

B. Purpose: To determine the changes in the arterial walls, the condition of the heart, and the volume of the blood

C. Materials needed
  1. Stethoscope
  2. Mercury sphygmomanometer
  3. Cuffs (12 to 14 cm for adults; 18 to 20 cm for large adults; 2.5 to 9.5 cm for children)

D. Location of materials
  1. Stethoscope, sphygmomanometer, and cuffs are located at the nursing stations.
  2. Materials do not need to be requisitioned.

E. Steps in procedure

Steps in procedure	Key points
1. Collect equipment and check to see that it is in working order.	Be sure that all connections are right. Examine rubber bladder and pressure bulbs for leaks. Check that the edge of the meniscus of the mercury manometer is at the zero mark.
2. Cleanse earpieces of stethoscope with a Zephiran or alcohol sponge.	
3. Wash your hands.	
4. Enter patient's room and verify name.	Assess environmental conditions that may influence pressure.
5. Explain procedure to patient.	It is very important to gain the cooperation of the patient because distress will alter the reading of the blood pressure. Identify other factors that may affect the blood pressure reading (such as exercise, eating, weight, changes in posture, full bladder).
6. Position patient in a relaxed, reclining, or sitting position with the arm flexed, palm up, and with the whole forearm supported at heart level (fourth intercostal space) on a smooth surface.	If arm is placed above the level of the heart, the reading will be falsely low; if placed below the level of the heart, the reading will be falsely high. Quiet must be maintained to allow hearing the blood pressure sounds.
7. Position yourself no more than 3 ft away from the sphygmomanometer with the meniscus of the mercury model at eye level.	
8. Select correct cuff size.	Average adult size is 12 to 14 cm; large adult, 18 to 20 cm; child, 2.5 to 9.5 cm.
9. Measure length of bladder to fit two thirds distance between shoulder and elbow. It should be 20% wider than the diameter of the arm, or 40% wider than its circumference.	If cuff is too narrow, pressure reading will be abnormally high; if too wide, the reading will be falsely low.

10. Palpate brachial artery in the medial surface of the arm and place the center of the bladder directly over the brachial artery 2.5 cm above the antecubital space.

11. Apply cuff snugly and smoothly.

> If cuff is wrapped too loosely, the results will be falsely high.

12. Palpate radial pulse by placing index and middle finger on radial pulse. Inflate cuff rapidly until radial pulsation disappears. Identify this reading as the palpatory systolic reading.

13. Wait 30 to 60 sec before reinflation of cuff to 30 cm above the palpatory systolic reading.

> This waiting period is necessary to allow time for the release of blood trapped in the veins. Failure to do so may prevent recognition of auscultatory gap (sound initially appears at a high level, fades completely, and reappears 10 to 40 mm later), accounting for falsely low systolic pressure.

14. Position stethoscope with ear tips forward.

15. Place diaphragm or bell of stethoscope over brachial artery in antecubital fossa with as little pressure as possible and with no space between skin and stethoscope.

> Heavy pressure distorts the artery, and sounds are heard below the diastolic pressure.

16. Tighten screw on bulb and inflate cuff rapidly to 30 mm above palpatory systolic pressure.

> Column of mercury (Hg) must be in a vertical position. If it is tilted, results will be falsely high. The edge of the mercury meniscus should be exactly at zero.

17. Deflate cuff 2 to 4 mm Hg per heartbeat to zero levels.

> Deflating too slowly will cause a falsely high reading.

18. Note reading at the meniscus on the mercury column at which the first two regular tapping sounds (Korotkoff phase I) are heard. This is the systolic pressure.

> If sounds are difficult to hear, raise the arm a few seconds to drain venous blood before inflating cuff; inflate cuff, then lower the arm, deflate, and listen for sounds; or have patient open and close fist 10 times after the systolic level has been obtained.

19. Deflate cuff at an even rate of 2 to 4 mm while the sounds change from faint and clear tapping sounds (Korotkoff phase I), to a swishing quality (Korotkoff phase II), to crisper and louder sounds (Korotkoff phase III), to abrupt muffling of sound (Korotkoff phase IV), to the point at which sounds disappear (Korotkoff phase V).

> The best index of diastolic pressure in adults is the point at which the sounds disappear. The onset of muffling (fourth phase) is the best index of diastolic pressure in children.

20. Expel any air in cuff and remove from patient's arm.

21. Return equipment to nursing station.

A. Charting

1. Chart systolic pressure over diastolic pressure on graphic sheet at foot of patient's bed.

2. Chart systolic pressure over diastolic pressure on flowchart in patient's chart. If sounds were heard to zero, chart systolic, fourth phase (muffling sound), and disappearance of sound (for example, 148/72/0 or 10/60/50).

3. Specify position of patient: "L" (lying), "ST" (standing), "SIT" (sitting), "RA" (right arm), or "LA" (left arm).

dure manual should be easily accessible, well organized with a table of contents, and indexed. Each procedure should be easily replaceable with a revised one. Because there is a tendency to add new procedures instead of revising existing ones, it is important to review and revise the procedure manual periodically.

In reviewing, one should check the effectiveness and workability with personnel to determine whether the procedure has been followed. Procedures should be realistic and written in simple language that is easy to understand. Changes should be dated and provided to all appropriate personnel.

Before spending valuable time writing procedures, one must consider whether a procedure is actually needed. With preservice and on-the-job preparation, is there really a need to have on each unit procedures on how to feed a patient and how to make a bed? Goals can be reached in a variety of ways, and consequently nursing students are taught principles rather than procedures. There are textbooks with bedside nursing procedures, and many disposable products with directions are available. It seems most important for the procedure manual to contain information that may vary from institution to institution. Not all parts of the procedure format may be necessary for each procedure. New personnel and float nurses can serve as valuable resources for nursing managers to consult when they are determining what content is important for the procedure manual.

The planning process is a critical element of management. It must be learned by nurse administrators, because it will not happen by accident. Planning is largely conceptual, but its results are clearly visible. The statement of the purpose or mission, philosophy, goals, objectives, policies, and procedures are all consequences of planning. They set the stage for smooth operations.

CHAPTER SUMMARY

Chapter 8 covered the following:
Planning Process
    History of Strategic Planning
    Purpose of Strategic Planning
    Strategic Planning Process
Vision
Values
Purpose or Mission Statement
Philosophy
Goals and Objectives
    Policies
    Procedures

REFERENCES

Burton EJ, McBride WB: *Total business planning : a step-by-step guide with forms,* New York, 1991, John Wiley & Sons.
Douglas LM: *The effective nurse leader and manager,* St. Louis, 1996, Mosby.
Marriner-Tomey A, Alligood MR: *Nursing theorists and their work,* St. Louis, 1998, Mosby.
Poteet GW, Hill AS: Identifying the components of a nursing philosophy, *J Nurs Adm* 18:29-33, Oct 1988.
Swansburg RC: *Management and leadership for nurse managers,* ed 2, Boston, 1996, Jones & Bartlett.
Swansburg RC, Swansburg RJ: *Introductory management and leadership for nurses,* ed 2, Boston, 1999, Jones & Bartlett.
Yoder-Wise PS: *Leading and managing in nursing,* ed 2, St. Louis, 1999, Mosby.

BIBLIOGRAPHY

Bombard CF: Strategic planning: a practical approach, *JONA* 23:41-45, July-Aug 1993.
Brooks BA, Rosenberg S: Incorporating nursing theory into a nursing department strategic plan, *Nurs Adm Q* 20:81-86, Fall 1995.
Bryant L, Dobal M, Johnson E: Strategic planning: collaboration and empowerment, *Nurs Connections* 3:31-36, Fall 1990.
Certo SC, Peter JP: *Strategic management: concepts and applications,* ed 2, New York, 1991, McGraw-Hill.
Dienemann J: *Nursing administration: strategic perspectives and application,* Norwalk, Conn, 1990, Appleton & Lange.
Dobson P, Starkey K: *The strategic management blueprint,* Oxford, UK, 1993, Blackwell.
Fogg CD: *Team-based strategic planning: a complete guide to structuring, facilitating, and implementing the process,* New York, 1994, AMACOM.

Georgantzas NC, Acar W: *Scenario-driven planning: learning to manage strategic uncertainty,* Westport, Conn, 1995, Quorum Books.

Gillies DA: *Nursing management: a systems approach,* Philadelphia, 1994, WB Saunders.

Marquis BL, Huston CJ: *Leadership roles and management functions in nursing: theory and application,* Philadelphia, 1996, Lippincott.

Martin M: Achieving the right balance with strategic planning, *Nurs Manage* 29:30-31, May 1998.

McCabe LR: Simplify and energize policy development, *Nurs Manage* 29:43-45, Oct 1998.

Popcorn F, Marigold LYS: *Clicking: 16 trends to future fit your life, your work, and your business,* New York, 1996, HarperCollins.

Stahl DA: Health care networks: opportunities and threats for subacute care, *Nurs Manage* 28: 28-29, July 1997.

Stoffels JD: *Strategic issues management: a comprehensive guide to environmental scanning,* New York, 1994, Pergamon.

CASE STUDY

Lake View Hospital is a 98-bed general hospital. Its organizational chart is shown in the Appendix. It is one of two hospitals serving an industrial community with a population of about 90,000. Patients are being discharged earlier, so there is an increasing vacancy rate on the medical-surgical units. At the same time there is an increasing demand for geriatric services and ambulatory care. Demands for home health have also increased.

Critical Thinking Activities for this chapter begin on page 491.

CHAPTER 9

FINANCIAL MANAGE- MENT, COST CONTAIN- MENT, AND MARKETING

CHAPTER OBJECTIVES

- Define capitation.
- Identify at least three prerequisites to budgeting.
- Describe at least four types of budgets.
- List at least three advantages and three disadvantages of budgeting.
- Discuss at least five strategies for cost containment.
- Explain fixed and variable costs as they relate to break-even points.
- List at least three factors to consider when costing out nursing services.
- Identify at least five factors that should be considered when making a marketing audit and ask a question to evaluate each of those factors.
- Describe the four p's of the marketing mix.
- Describe the Boston consulting group's grid of potential growth and profitability possibilities for identifying marketing strategies.
- Identify the four stages in the life cycle of a product.
- Identify at least three ways to do pricing.
- List at least four promotion tools.

Chapter Overview

Chapter 9 discusses history of health care financing, budgetary leadership and management, budgets, cost containment, costing out nursing services, personal finances, and marketing.

MAJOR CONCEPTS AND DEFINITIONS	
Accounting	a system that accumulates bookkeeping entries into summaries of the financial situation of the agency
Budget	a plan for the allocation of resources and a control for ensuring that results comply with the plans
Cost containment	to hold back costs within fixed limits
Economics	production, distribution, and consumption of wealth
Costing out	calculating the cost of specific items
Marketing	the analysis, planning, implementation, and control of programs for exchanges of values with target markets to achieve organizational objectives
Exchange	resource dependency
Publics	distinct groups of people or organizations that have an actual or potential interest in or impact on an organization
Market	potential arena for trading resources
Image	sum of a person's beliefs, ideas, and impressions about an object or person
Audit	identification, collection, and evaluation of information that needs examination to evaluate market relations
Segmentation	subsets of the total market
Marketing mix	product, price, place, and promotions
Life cycle	introduction, growth, maturity, and market decline stages of a product
Break-even calculations	direct and indirect costs equal income
Direct costs	specific costs of program
Indirect costs	generalized costs such as maintenance and administration allocated to the program
Variable costs	costs that vary in direct proportion to volume
Fixed costs	costs unrelated to volume
Semifixed costs	costs that are fixed within a range of activity
Semivariable costs	costs that are fixed at zero output and increase with volume

HISTORY OF HEALTH CARE FINANCING

During the 1930s most health care was privately financed. Insurance plans increased during the 1950s. During that time cost-based pricing was used. The price of service was based on direct costs (such as salaries, benefits, and supplies) and indirect costs or overhead costs (including services like accounting, administration, housekeeping, and medical records, and depreciation, interest expenses, repayment of debt, return on investments, bad debts, and other uncollectible accounts). The more treatments and services provided, the more income to the health care providers. This retrospective approach increased hospital profits, increased health care costs, and in turn increased insurance rates.

Medicare was developed during the 1960s and brought average pricing to the health care market by establishing the average price it would pay. That lead to competitive-based pricing, which forced providers to achieve the marketplace average or lose money.

Health costs have been increasing because of the aging population with increased health care needs, increased use of expensive technology, new and expensive treatment modalities, and administrative costs. Previously, third-party payers paid hospitals for services. The employers paid the insurance premiums. The insurance companies paid the bill, and the customers felt little effect. During the 1980s insurance companies raised their premiums dramatically to meet the rising costs, making it difficult for employers to pay the premiums. Consequently customers are required to pay larger portions of the costs as deductibles and are becoming increasingly aware of the high costs of health care and the need to be selective.

A prospective reimbursement system encourages the implementation of cost-effective health care services. The Tax Equity Fiscal Responsibility Act of 1982 added case-mix into Medicare based on diagnostic-related groups (DRGs). A prospective payment system based on 467 DRG categories that provided pretreatment diagnosis billing categories for most U.S. hospitals reimbursed by Medicare was signed into law as HR 1900 (P.L. 98-21) by President Reagan. It used a prospective rather than the traditional retrospective time frame. Reimbursement is by case or costs related to treatment of specific DRGs rather than per diem or total hospital costs divided by patient days. The payment unit is the diagnosis rather than patient day. Rates are determined from local, regional, and national rural and urban costs instead of the hospital's own costs. There are incentive payments when the length of stay is lower than average and disincentives when costs exceed the standard so that hospitals profit from cost containment. Previously hospitals were reimbursed for costs retrospectively and had little incentive to contain costs. The prospective payment system applies to all Medicare-participating hospitals except long-term care, rehabilitation, children's, and psychiatric care hospitals.

The results of DRGs include a decrease in number of patients in acute care settings caused by early discharge, an increase in the acuteness of illness among hospitalized patients, an increase in the use of ambulatory and home care facilities, and a focus on cost-effectiveness.

Managed care became widespread during the 1980s. Coordination of high-cost health care services became a goal of health care insurance companies. Since 1988 there has been rapid growth of case management or utilization review organizations that monitor the delivery of care and are gatekeepers to providers of care. Clinical pathways use outcome criteria as indicators of quality. Cooperation between health care providers is necessary to reach the expected outcomes in the most efficient manner.

Insurance companies have developed policies to control costs that direct beneficiaries away from providers that have charges above the marketplace average. By 2000 insurance companies were demanding discounted services. Insurance companies were contracting amounts discounted or deducted from patient care revenues that health care providers must write off.

The exclusive provider arrangement provides insurance coverage only for services provided by a contracted professional or institution except in the event of an emergency or while out of a geographical area.

Health maintenance organizations (HMOs) provide comprehensive health care services to enrollees for a fixed periodic payment. Capitation is the fixed rate paid to the provider per member per month for a specified amount of health care services. Actuarial services provide statistical analysis of demographical, financial, and utilization trends to predict health plan premiums or costs. The clients choose their physician from a medical group roster. The primary care physician is a gatekeeper who assesses the patient and determines if referral to a specialist or hospitalization is necessary. The incentive is to keep patients healthy and to reduce physician, diagnostic, and hospital services. Under capitation, the financial risk for provision of care is transferred from the payer to the health care delivery system. Visits to a physician or services are expenses, not revenue to the provider. Hospitals have incentives to lower hospitalizations, decrease the length of stay, and minimize the variance of stays between patients with like diagnosis. Consequently, hospital utilization has dropped drastically, and hospitals have many empty beds. Hospitals may subcontract some services like dialysis to others for less cost. Because hospitals have large fixed costs in physical facilities, the trend of the 1980s and 1990s to give care outside of the hospital may be reversed. Hospitals may get involved with services like home health care and hospice that were provided outside of the hospital. Hospital administrators may become health care system managers.

Preferred provider organizations (PPOs) negotiate a special, usually reduced, rate for insurance-plan beneficiaries usually on a fee-for-service basis with incentives of lowered rates for consumers when they use the preferred providers.

Individual provider arrangements (IPAs) allow health care providers to provide medical services in their offices for managed care or prepaid plans. This was one of the first alternative delivery prepaid plans with a set of benefits provided by a group of providers within a specific geographical area. Dur-ing the 1940s Kaiser Permanent was one of the first employers to provide such a plan.

Now managed competition exists between pre-paid providers such as HMOs, PPOs, and IPAs and leads to early discharge of patients, early retirement of the better paid senior nurses, narrow differentials between associate degree (AD), bachelor of science (BS), and master of science (MS) prepared nurses, slower wage growth rates, substitution of RNs with less trained, more poorly paid unlicensed personnel, substitution of physicians and psychologists with greater use of advanced practice nurses, use of RNs as utilization reviewers, and mergers or resized agencies.

Supply and demand leads to demand-based pricing. Higher prices are paid for products or services that are in high demand. Reduced demand leads to lower prices. This makes entrepreneurial activities important both within the organization and to external markets. Entrepreneurs take risks for profits. Strategic planning is needed to determine which activities can be in the most demand and make the most profits. For example, a hospital may provide food service instead of outsourcing that service and open the cafeteria to the public community for profit.

It is appropriate for entrepreneurs to prepare a business plan for their new ventures. They need to identify the new product or service; analyze the competition and identify the competitive edge; identify the resources needed, such as facilities, equipment, and personnel; identify the time frame needed to develop the product or service; and develop a quality control plan. Financial forecasting to predict the future from past and present information should be done along with benefit-to-cost analysis (the number of dollars returned for each dollar invested) and break-even analysis to determine the price. Planning the marketing from determining the purchase cost (price), identifying the product or service (product), determining the market (place), and planning advertising and determining the medium for the least expense (promotions) are important. (See discussion of the four *p*'s of the marketing mix later in this chapter.) Entrepreneurs are leaders (Douglass, 1996; Ellis and Hartley, 1995; Hein, 1998; Loveridge and Cummings, 1996; Marquis and Huston, 1996; Marrelli, 1993; Swansburg, 1996).

BUDGETARY LEADERSHIP AND MANAGEMENT

Budgetary leaders inspire proactive fiscal planning, determine resource needs, guide visioning of justification for resources, negotiate for needed resources, analyze expenses, anticipate, recognize, and creatively deal with budgetary problems, create a financially savvy work environment, involve group members in fiscal planning, and help groups find innovative ways to be more cost effective (Box 9-1). The fiscal manager coordinates fiscal planning, plans the budget, organizes the justification, implements the budget process, determines resource requirements within the constraints, coordinates expenses and budget control, documents needs to other administrative levels, organizes needed resources, explains budgeting to others, and

evaluates technology (Huber, 1996; Marquis and Huston, 1996).

BUDGETS

A budget is a plan for the allocation of resources and a control for ensuring that results comply with the plans. Results are expressed in quantitative terms. Although budgets are usually associated with financial statements, such as revenues and expenses, they also may be nonfinancial statements covering output, materials, and equipment. Budgets help coordinate the efforts of the agency by determining what resources will be used by whom, when, and for what purpose. They are frequently prepared for each organizational unit and for each function within the unit.

Planning is done for a specific time period, usually a fiscal year, but may be subdivided into monthly, quarterly, or semiannual periods. The budgeting period is determined by the desired frequency of checks and should complete a normal cycle of activity. Budget periods that coincide with

---

Box 9-1   BUDGETARY LEADERSHIP AND MANAGEMENT

Leader	Manager
Inspires proactive versus reactive fiscal planning	Coordinates fiscal planning to be consistent with organizational goals and objectives
Determines resource needs	Plans the budget
Guides visioning of justification for resources	Organizes the budget justification
Negotiates for needed resources	Implements the budget process
Locates new sources of resources	Determines resource requirements within constraints
Analyzes expenses	Coordinates expenses and budget control
Anticipates, recognizes, and creatively deals with budgetary problems	Documents needs to other administrative levels
Creates a financially savvy work environment	Organizes needed resources
Involves group members in fiscal planning	Explains budgeting to others
Helps groups find innovative ways to be more cost effective	Evaluates technology

Modified from Huber D: *Leadership and nursing case management*, Philadelphia, 1996, Saunders; and Marquis BL, Huston CJ: *Leadership roles and management functions in nursing: theory and application*, Philadelphia, 1996, Lippincott.

other control devices—such as managerial reports, balance sheets, and profit-and-loss statements—are helpful.

The extent to which accurate forecasts can be made must be considered. If the budget forecasts too far in advance, its usefulness is diminished. On the other hand, factors such as seasonal fluctuations make it impossible to predict long-range needs from short budget periods. Managers therefore necessarily revise budgets as more information becomes available. Top management and the board of directors also may prepare long-term budgets of 3, 5, or more years, but these are not used as direct operating budgets.

PREREQUISITES TO BUDGETING

Some conditions are necessary for the development and implementation of a budgetary program. First, there is the need for a sound organizational structure with clear lines of authority and responsibility. All employees know their responsibilities and the person to whom they are responsible; they have the authority to do what they are responsible for and are held accountable for their actions. Organization charts and job descriptions are available, and goals and objectives are set for areas of responsibilities. Budgets are then developed to conform to the pattern of authority and responsibility.

Nonmonetary statistical data—such as number of admissions, average length of stay, percentage of occupancy, and number of patient days—are used for planning and control of the budgetary process. Someone must be responsible for collecting and reporting statistical data.

Charts of accounts are designed to be consistent with the organizational plan. Revenues and expenses are reported by responsibility areas, thus providing historical data that are valuable for planning and providing budgetary control for evaluation as performance can be compared with plans. Nurse managers focus their attention on the principle of management by exception by noting what is not going as planned so they can take necessary action.

Managerial support is essential for a budgetary program. Although budgeting is done at the departmental level, it must be valued by top administration. Managers must be willing to devote their time and energy to the budgeting process. They are most likely to do that when they are familiar, through budget education, with the principles of budgeting and its usefulness for planning and controlling.

Formal budgeting policies and procedures should be available in a budget manual, in which objectives of the budgetary program are defined, authority and responsibility for budgeting are clarified, and instructions for budget development are discussed in detail. Samples of standardized forms are available. A calendar of the budgeting activities with the schedule for each stage of the program is presented. Procedures for review, revision, and approval of budgets are discussed in detail.

APPLIED ECONOMICS

Economic goods are goods or services purchased by consumers from suppliers to provide a benefit to the consumer. Goods and services are acquired through exchange, generally of money. *Wealth* is the value of the consumer's resources. *Income* is additional resources gained over time. Consumers do not have the wealth to buy everything they want, so they must make choices about what to purchase.

Utility is the benefit consumers get from the purchase of goods and services. It helps determine how much the consumer is willing to pay. *Marginal utility* is the additional utility gained by consuming one more unit. Marginal utility is not the same for all consumers or for additional units. The person who likes chocolate is more willing to pay for a chocolate candy bar than a person who does not like chocolate but may not be as willing to buy a second or third chocolate bar. People try to maximize their total utility. To do that, a mix of goods should be consumed so that the last unit has the same marginal utility per dollar spent.

Supply and demand influence costs. *Supply* is the amount of goods or service that suppliers are willing to provide at a given price. *Demand* is the amount of goods or service the consumers are willing to buy at that price. For an equilibrium price, the quantity offered and the quantity demanded are the same. As supply goes up and demand goes down, the price is likely to go down. As the supply goes down and the demand goes up, the price is likely to go up.

Elasticity of demand is the degree to which the demand for a good or service decreases in response to a price increase and increases in response to a price decrease. The demand for health care is generally inelastic.

Economies of scale indicate that the cost of providing goods or services falls as quantity increases and fixed costs are shared with the larger volume. Large volumes can eventually lead to decreasing returns to scale as more personnel and supplies are needed.

Incentives encourage action. Managers may use them to encourage good use of scarce resources. Health insurance deductibles are incentives to encourage desirable behavior.

Market efficiency is the optimal allocation and use of goods and services resulting from supply and demand.

Redistribution of resources may be done to improve equality.

Market failure occurs when the free market does not operate efficiently and may result from lack of information, lack of direct patient payment, monopoly, government intervention and induced inefficiency, and other externalities.

ACCOUNTING

Accounting is a system that accumulates bookkeeping entries into summaries of the financial situation of an enterprise. The fundamental equation of accounting is

$$\text{Assets} = \text{Liabilities} + \text{Fund balance}$$

Assets are the valuable resources owned by the agency. *Liabilities* are what the agency owes. *Fund balance* is the agency's assets. The *balance sheet* is a financial statement that shows the financial position of the agency and a specific time. The *income statement,* or statement of revenues and expenses, shows

the financial results of the agency's activities for a specified period. *Depreciation* is the allocation of a portion of the cost of an asset with a multiyear life over the years the asset will be used. A *journal* is a book or computer file recording the financial events of the agency in chronological order. *Ledgers* are sets of individual accounts to which information from the journal is transferred or posted so that the balance in any account can be determined and reported. *Fund accounting* is an optional accounting system used by not-for-profit agencies to establish a complete, distinct set of accounting records for separate accounts of agency assets. These assets may be restricted and unrestricted funds set aside for specific purposes such as endowments, renovations, or buildings (Finkler and Kovner, 1999).

Several terms must be understood to interpret financial accounting reports. *Entity* is a definable organizational unit. The accountant considers only *transactions* between one entity and another. Transactions that occur within the entity or do not involve it are not considered. If each department is an entity, performance can be compared between departments. However, if the agency as a whole is the entity, the transfer of resources from one department to another is not taken into account. Accounts deal only with transactions, definable changes in the financial situation of an entity: income, expenditure, depreciation. *Cost valuation* values goods at their cost minus any depreciation. *Double entry* compares the assets, what is owed to or owned by the entity, with the liabilities, what is owed by the entity to others. Accountants are to balance total assets with the total liabilities and net worth. The double entry makes it possible to know where the entity stands financially at any given time. *Accrual* allows one to determine the overall assets and liabilities by entering transactions on the accounting records at the time a commitment is made rather than waiting until it is billed or paid. *Matching* is the principle of matching revenues with expenses during a budget period.

There are several standard accounting practices. *Consistency* means that categories of transactions may not be changed during or between reporting periods without noting the changes and providing comparable figures. *Materiality* means that transactions can be combined for accounting purposes unless one transaction has a significant impact by itself. *Conservatism* is the act of understating revenue and overstating expenses to provide a margin of safety. *Industry practices* are specific to industries. Special fund accounts designated by donors and a separate account for charitable care provided are examples of industry practices.

TYPES OF BUDGETS
Operating, or Revenue-and-Expense, Budgets

The operating budget provides an overview of an agency's functions by projecting the planned operations, usually for the upcoming year. The operating table reveals an input-output analysis of expected revenues and expenses. Among the factors that nurse managers might include in their operating budgets are personnel salaries, employee benefits, insurance, medical-surgical supplies, office supplies, rent, heat, light, housekeeping, laundry service, drugs and pharmaceuticals, repairs and maintenance, depreciation, in-service education, travel to professional meetings, educational leaves, books, periodicals, subscriptions, dues and membership fees, legal fees, and recreation, such as Christmas parties and retirement teas.

Both controllable and noncontrollable expenses are projected. The manager determines the number of personnel needed and the level of skills required of each. Wage levels and quality of materials used are other controllable expenses. Indirect expenses, such as rent, lighting, and depreciation of equipment, are noncontrollable. The noncontrollable expenses and the probability of rises in material prices or labor costs during the budgetary period demand that an operating budget include some cushion funds to provide for changes beyond the agency's control.

The operating budget deals primarily with salaries, supplies, and contractual services. Nonfinancial factors, such as time, materials, and space, can

be translated into dollar values. Work hours, nurse-patient interaction hours, units of materials, equipment hours, and floor space also can be assigned dollar values.

Personnel Budgets

Personnel budgets estimate the cost of direct labor necessary to meet the agency's objectives. They determine the recruitment, hiring, assignment, layoff, and discharge of personnel. The nurse manager decides on the type of nursing care necessary to meet the nursing needs of the estimated patient population. How many aides, orderlies, LPNs, and RNs are needed during what shifts, in what months, and in what areas? The current staffing patterns, number of unfilled positions, and last year's reports can provide a base for examination and proposals. Patient occupancy and the general complexity of cases affect staffing patterns. Seasonal fluctuations must be considered. Personnel budgets also are affected by personnel policies such as salary related to position and number of days allowed for educational and personal leave. Overtime costs should be compared with the cost of new positions. Employee turnover, recruitment, and orientation costs must be considered.

Capital Expenditure Budgets

Capital expenditure budgets are related to long-range planning. Capital expenditures include physical changes such as replacement or expansion of the plant, major equipment, and inventories. These items are usually major investments and reduce the flexibility in budgeting because it takes a long time to recover the costs. For instance, a patient may be charged per treatment or per day for use of equipment, but it may take many months or even years to recover the cost of the equipment.

The hospital administrator usually establishes the ceiling for capital expenses. Under this budget the nurse manager must establish priorities if requests exceed availability of funds. When filling out request forms for capital items, it is advisable to include names of manufacturers and suppliers, trade-in credits, and estimates of purchase, delivery, installation, and maintenance costs. Written justification for each item should be given.

Inventories are helpful in budgeting. If supplies are checked routinely, use and replacement figures are available for projection of future needs. Central supply services enhance budgetary control, and storage space facilitates inventory maintenance. Stocked supply shelves on each unit with replacement service twice a day can provide a simplified recording system. Disposable equipment and supplies need careful evaluation to determine whether they are more economical than nondisposables.

Cash Budgets

Cash budgets are planned to make adequate funds available as needed and to use any extra funds profitably. They ensure that the agency has enough, but not too much, cash on hand during the budgetary period. This is necessary because income does not always coincide with expenditures. The manager must anticipate fluctuations in resource needs caused by such factors as seasonal variations. If managers have insufficient cash on hand, they will not be able to purchase needed resources. At the other extreme, if too much cash is available, interest or other earnings that money could generate are lost. Budgeting cash requirements may not significantly affect profits, but it does ensure a liquid position and is a sign of prudent management. Using a cash budget, the nurse manager estimates the amount of money to be collected from clients and other sources and allocates that cash to expenditures. If the budget is well planned, it will provide cash as needed and produce interest on excess funds (Box 9-2).

Flexible Budgets

Some costs are fixed and do not change with the volume of business. Other costs vary proportionately with changes in volume. Some variable expenses are unpredictable and can be determined

---

Box 9-2 TYPES OF BUDGETS

Operating budget (daily revenues and expenses to operate the health care institution)
  Revenues (income, return on investments and property)
  Expenses (costs)
    Personnel (employed people)
    Supplies (stock, materials—office supplies, pharmaceuticals, medical-surgical supplies)
    Other expenses (spending such as travel, training, dues, rentals, repairs, depreciation)
Capital expenditure budget (capital often defined as something that costs more than $500 and is used more than once)
Cash budget (for money available for immediate use)

---

only after change has begun: thus the need for flexible budgets, to show the effects of changes in volume of business on expense items. Periodic budget reviews help managers compensate for changes. Relationships between the volume of business and variable costs may be predicted by a historical analysis of costs and development of standard costs.

Historical approach to budgeting. The historical approach is most effective for calculating the relationship between volume of business and variable costs when a company manufactures a few products and each product contributes a relatively stable percentage to the total sales volume. Using the historical approach, the nurse manager may observe that there are more fractures during skiing season. Consequently, more casting materials are used at that time, and there is a need for increased staffing on the orthopedic ward. A supervising community health nurse in a small college town may note that there is less use of family planning services during the summer months and again during December when students leave for vacations. Consequently, there is less need for contraceptive devices and staffing during these months. There may be an increased demand for immunizations just before elementary schools open in the fall. By plotting on a graph the high and low volumes, the nurse manager can predict the expected costs for each level between the extreme volumes. This historical perspective helps determine the amount of supplies to stock and staffing patterns.

Standard cost.   Standard cost may be developed to predict what labor and supplies should cost. Multiplying the standard cost by the volume predicts the variable cost. Supervising community health nurses can predict the standard number of clinic visits and the number of birth control pills that will be required for each family planning client who has chosen birth control pills as a method of contraception. Multiplying the number of pills needed by each client by the number of clients using birth control pills, nurse managers can predict the inventory needed and the cost. They also can predict the number of clinic visits needed and plan staffing.

ZERO-BASED BUDGETING

Many budgeting procedures allocate funds to departments on the basis of their previous year's expenditures. Then the department managers decide how the funds will be used. This procedure usually allows for enrichment and enlargement of programs but seldom for decreases in or deletion of programs. Obsolescence is seldom examined, and this leads to increased costs.

With zero-based budgeting, no program is taken for granted. Each program or service must be justified each time funds are requested. Managers decide what will be done, what will not be done, and how much of an activity will be implemented. A decision package is prepared. The package includes a list of the activities that make up a program, the total cost, a description of what level of service can be performed at various levels of funding, and the ramifications of including them in or excluding them from the budget. The manager may identify the activity, state the purpose, list related activities, outline alternative ways of performing activities, and give the cost of the resources needed.

After decision packages are developed, they are ranked in order of decreasing benefits to the agency. They can be divided into high-, medium-, and low-priority categories and reviewed in order of rank for funding. Resources are allocated based on the priority of the decision package. The cost of each package is added to the cost of approved packages until the agreed-on spending level is reached. Lower ranked packages are then excluded.

A major advantage to zero-based budgeting is that it forces managers to set priorities and justify resources. Unfortunately the process is time-consuming.

PERIODIC BUDGETARY REVIEW

Managers should review the budget at periodic intervals, compare actual with projected performances, and make necessary changes. However, if changes are too frequent or too great, the original budget becomes useless. One way to minimize variance between the annual budget and the revised budget is to anticipate such factors as increased labor costs and the inflationary cost of materials. When discrepancies are found between actual performance and the budget, management must determine the cause of variation to make appropriate adjustments for future plans. A variance may not be reason for changing the budget. It may be a symptom that alerts management to the need for further investigation and explanation. What may demand change is not the budget but the situation.

ADVANTAGES AND DISADVANTAGES
Advantages and Disadvantages of Flexible Budgets

The major advantage of flexible budgets is the study and analysis necessary to prepare one. Fixed and variable costs and their effect on the total cost are analyzed. Unfortunately, flexible budgets are very costly to prepare and very time-consuming. It is difficult to predict short-term variations in volume, and it is unlikely that the information can result in savings of variable expenses.

Advantages of Budgeting

Budgets plan for detailed program activities. They help fix accountability by assignment of responsibility and authority. They state goals for all units, offer a standard of performance, and stress the continuous nature of the planning and control process. Budgets encourage managers to make a careful analysis of operations and to base decisions on careful consideration. Consequently, hasty judgments are minimized. Weaknesses in the organization can be revealed and corrective measures taken. Staffing, equipment, and supply needs can be projected and waste minimized. Financial matters can be handled in an orderly fashion, and agency activities can be coordinated and balanced.

Disadvantages of Budgeting

Budgets convert all aspects of organizational performance into monetary values for a single comparable unit of measurement. Consequently, only those aspects that are easy to measure may be considered, and equally important factors, such as organizational development and research efforts, may be ignored. Symptoms may be treated as causes. Reasons for the symptoms should be explored; a decrease in revenue from the family planning clinic may be related to the way people are treated at the clinic, a new competitive service in the neighborhood, or other factors. The budget may become an end in itself instead of the means to an end. Budgetary goals may supersede agency goals and gain autocratic control of the organization. There is a danger of overbudgeting; the budget becomes cumbersome, meaningless, and expensive. Forecasting is required but uncertain because budgetary control is subject to human judgment, interpretation, and evaluation. Skill and experience are required for successful budgetary control. Budget planning is time-consuming and expensive.

BUDGETING PROCESS

Identifying financial planning responsibilities is needed before beginning budget preparation. The governing board, administrator, budget director, steering committee, and department heads are often involved in the budgetary process. The governing board is responsible for the general planning function. It selects the budget steering committee, determines the budgetary objectives, and reviews and approves the master budget. The administrator is responsible for the formulation and execution of the budget by correlating the governing board's goals with the guidelines for budget preparation and supervising the budget preparation. The budget director, who is responsible for the budgeting procedures and reporting, establishes a completion timetable, has forms prepared, and supervises data collection and budget preparation. The budget director serves as the chairperson of the steering committee, which approves the budget before it is submitted to the governing board. Department heads prepare and review goals and objectives and prepare the budgets for their departments.

The first step in the budget process is the establishment of operational goals and policies for the entire agency. The governing board should approve a long-range plan of 3 to 5 years that reflects the community's future health needs and other community health care providers' activities. Because the situation changes over time, flexibility is built into the plan. Then operational goals must be translated into quantifiable management objectives for the organizational units. The department heads use the organizational goals as a framework for the development of departmental goals. A formal plan for budget preparation and review, including assignment of responsibilities and timetables, must be prepared. Historical, financial, and statistical data must be collected monthly so that seasonal fluctuation can be observed. Preparing and coordinating departmental budgets are important. During this phase, units of service, staffing patterns, salary and nonsalary expenses, and revenues are forecasted so that preliminary rate setting can be done. Next, departmental budgets are revised, and the master budget is prepared. At this point, operating, payroll, nonsalary, capital, and cash budgets can be incorporated into the master budget. Then the financial feasibility of the master budget is tested, and the final document is approved and distributed to all involved parties.

During the budget period, there should be periodic performance reporting by responsibility centers.

COST CONTAINMENT

The goal of cost containment is to keep costs within acceptable limits for volume, inflation, and other parameters. It involves cost awareness, monitoring, management, and incentives to prevent, reduce, and control costs.

Cost Awareness

Cost awareness focuses the employee's attention on costs. It increases organizational awareness of what costs are, the process available for containing them, how they can be managed, and by whom. Delegating budget planning and control to the unit level increases awareness. Managers should be provided a course about budgeting and be oriented to the agency budgeting process before being assigned the responsibility. They should have a budget manual that contains budget forms, budget calendar, and budget periods.

Cost Fairs

Cost fairs in frequented areas such as the cafeteria increase awareness by displaying frequently disappearing items that are labeled with the cost per unit and by posting lists of estimated costs of inventory losses. Staff development programs, unit conferences, and poster contests help increase awareness. Tagging supply items and posting a computer printout of unit charges for supplies and services are revealing. Reviewing a patient's itemized bill during a conference can also be effective.

Cost Monitoring

Cost monitoring focuses on how much will be spent where, when, and why. It identifies, reports, and monitors costs. Staffing costs should be identi-

fied. Recruitment, turnover, absenteeism, and sick time are analyzed, and inventories are controlled. A central supply exchange chart prevents hoarding of supplies and allows identification of lost items.

Cost Management

Cost management focuses on what can be done by whom to contain costs. Programs, plans, objectives, and strategies are important. Responsibility and accountability for the control should be established. A committee can identify long- and short-range plans and strategies. A suggestion box can be used, as can contests for the idea that saves the most money.

Money has been saved by means such as forming a staff pool to maximize flexibility in staffing for census fluctuations, cross-training personnel, closing units for cleaning or remodeling and encouraging staff vacations when census is low, balancing the workload among shifts to minimize peaks and valleys in assigned tasks, reducing shift overlap, charting by exception, tape-recording shift reports, revising forms, improving drug ordering and delivery systems, controlling central supplies, not controlling oral analgesics, modifying food services, allowing volunteers to discharge and transport patients, reducing the amount of time nurses spend in nonnursing functions, and using guest relations personnel, a discharge holding area, outpatient clinics, progressive care, and ambulatory care.

Cost Incentives

Cost incentives motivate cost containment and reward desired behavior. Contests for the best money-saving ideas, perfect attendance, and nurse of the month help recognize personnel efforts.

Cost Avoidance

Cost avoidance means not buying supplies, technology, or services. Supply and equipment costs should be carefully analyzed. Costs and effectiveness of disposable versus reusable items are compared. The receipt, storage, and delivery of disposables and labor and processing costs of reusable items are part of the analysis. The least expensive and most effective supplies, equipment, and services should be identified, and expensive and less effective items avoided.

Cost Reduction

Cost reduction means spending less for goods and services. The amount of reduction depends on the size of the agency, previous efficiency, skill of managers, and cooperation of employees. Safety programs that reduce the costs of worker's compensation and absenteeism programs that reduce sick time, absenteeism, and turnover reduce costs. Healthy living programs such as exercise activities, heart wise foods in the cafeteria, and cease-smoking classes may help keep workers healthy and thus reduce sick time, absenteeism, and health care costs. Volume buying (getting a cheaper price because of the economies of scale), conservation of supplies, and careful handling of equipment to reduce cost of repairs help reduce costs. Costs can also be reduced through inventory control.

Inventory control. The manager needs to determine the most economical level of inventory because supplies represent a significant cost factor. The purchasing, order, storage, and costs of long and short stock must all be considered to determine the most economical level of inventory. The purchasing cost is the price paid per item. Cost may be related to the size of the order with cost per item decreasing as the size of the order increases. Purchasing cost equals PD, where P is the cost or price per unit and D is the number of units purchased.

The order costs involve writing specifications, soliciting and analyzing bids, writing orders, receiving the supplies, accounting for the materials, and paying the bills. The order cost may be relatively large the first time an item is purchased or relatively small for routine purchasing processes. The order cost varies with the number of orders placed. The more orders per year, the greater the annual costs will be. Annual order cost equals (D/Q)O, where D is the number of units purchased, Q is the order size, and O is the average cost of placing a single order.

The carrying cost is the expense involved with holding inventories. It involves expenses such as storage, insurance, and security. To keep carrying costs down, small orders should be placed frequently; this approach is in direct conflict with keeping the purchasing and order costs low. Carrying cost equals

$$HQ + \frac{IPQ}{2}$$

where H is the cost of storage per item and Q is the order size. The opportunity cost element is

$$\frac{IPQ}{2}$$

where I represents the highest obtainable rate of return at the current interest rate, P is price per unit, and Q is the order size.

The short or stock-out costs involved with holding an insufficient amount of inventory must be considered. The manager considers the consequences of running out of stock. Not only is a sale lost, but client satisfaction may also suffer. Although this expense is difficult to measure, it is a real cost.

Total cost is expressed as follows:

$$TC = PD + \frac{DO}{Q} + \left(\frac{HQ + IPQ}{2}\right) + L + S$$

where:

$$TC = \text{Total cost}$$
$$PD = \text{Purchase cost}$$
$$\frac{DO}{Q} = \text{Order cost}$$
$$HQ + \frac{IPQ}{2} = \text{Carrying cost}$$
$$L = \text{Overstocked cost}$$
$$S = \text{Stock−out cost}$$

The economical order quantity is expressed as follows:

$$EOQ = \sqrt{\frac{2DP}{C}}$$

where:

> EOQ = Economical order quantity
> D = Usage in units or demand
> P = Order cost
> C = Annual cost of carrying one unit in inventory

A large order size is merited when there is a large demand, high order cost, and low carrying cost. However, a small order size is desired when there is little demand for the item, the order cost is small, and the carrying cost is high.

A high inventory turnover is desired. Low inventory turnover may be caused by poor purchasing policies, overstocking, or a decrease in demand for the item. The inventory turnover can be calculated as follows:

$$\text{Inventory turnover} = \frac{\text{Total cost of supplies}}{\text{Inventories}}$$

To determine when to reorder, the manager needs to know the average daily usage and the lead time required to receive the supplies. The manager needs to keep the average daily usage multiplied by the number of days it takes to receive the goods to not run out of stock.

Some managers use the ABC method for maintaining inventories. *A* refers to a small number of items that account for a large percentage of the budget and are carefully monitored; *B* refers to moderate-cost items that receive some monitoring; and *C* refers to a bulk of inexpensive, expendable items such as rubber bands that receive little monitoring.

Cost Control

Cost control is effective use of available resources through careful forecasting, planning, budget preparing, reporting, and monitoring. Cost-effectiveness compares costs and identifies the most beneficial outcomes to costs by specifying programs; identifying goals; analyzing alternatives; comparing costs per program, unit of service, and amount of service needed; assessing effect of the outcome; and determining cost outcome and cost-effectiveness. Patient classification systems can be used to predict the appropriate staffing levels. Time management can help control costs. Making meetings worthwhile, reducing repetitious paperwork, improving communication systems, and streamlining the system help save time. Activities to promote retention of personnel, such as a good orientation program, careful placement and mentoring of new personnel, and helping people feel welcome and appreciated can reduce recruitment, orientation, and development expenses. Careful selection of supplies and equipment and in-servicing to teach personnel how to use them can save frustration and damage. Proper charging of supplies and use of equipment through things such as bar codes and charge slips could help the health care system recover millions of dollars lost from supplies that were not charged to patients. Delegation of appropriate tasks to unlicensed personnel can save more expensive nurses' time for activities requiring more knowledge and skill. Teaching how to delegate, supervise, and develop teams may help control costs in the long run.

Cost-Effectiveness and Cost-Benefit Analysis

Cost-effectiveness is a method of economic evaluation that ranks programs by the cost of achieving the objective. It is measured in nonmonetary units like fewer readmissions to the hospital or fewer unwed teenage pregnancies. Cost-benefit analysis is a procedure that determines cost of installing and operating a program and converts that into a dollar amount. It also converts all benefits of the program into a dollar amount. A ratio reflects the relationship of costs to benefits. Cost-benefit analysis is measured in monetary units that facilitate a conclusion regarding whether the program savings outweigh the costs. If the benefit-to-cost ratio is equal to or greater than 1, the investment is considered good. If the ratio is less than 1, it is not advisable to pursue the venture because the number of dollars returned is less than the number invested. It often involves estimating the value of saving a life and adjusting the outcome for quality that is measured as quality-adjusted life-years (QALYS). Each incre-

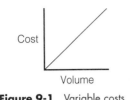

Figure 9-1 Variable costs.

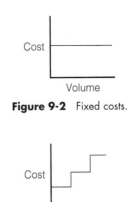

Figure 9-2 Fixed costs.

Figure 9-3 Semifixed costs.

ment of variable costs may not yield a comparable increment in work output. For example, one additional employee decreases the service volume for a time as the work increment of each employee decreases. An additional employee may even cause a decrease in output for the group as communication problems and interpersonal conflict increase. Break-even analysis is used to calculate the break-even point for each program (Gillies, 1994; Loveridge and Cummings, 1996; Rocchiccioli and Tilbury, 1998; Sullivan and Decker, 1999).

Break-even calculations. A *ProForma Income Statement* is a projection of the operations and activities of the business. The ProForma Income and ProForma Cash Flow Statements are used to develop the ProForma Balance Sheet. That reflects the revenue to be generated and cost to be incurred over a period of time. It can be used to help calculate break-even points. Full costs equal all direct costs that can be traced to a source plus indirect costs such as maintenance, administration, and the building that are allocated to the source. Cost finding is an attempt to find the full cost and to allocate indirect costs. Indirect costs allocated may include housekeeping calculated by square feet, utilities by square feet, laboratory by number of tests, and dietary services by number of meals served.

The cost-volume-profit relationships can be visualized on a break-even chart. The manager considers variable, fixed, semifixed, and semivariable costs when doing a break-even analysis. Variable costs vary in direct proportion to volume (Figure 9-1). Two disposable syringes probably cost twice as much as one. Fixed costs are relatively fixed in total regardless of changes in volume (Figure 9-2). A nurse receives a certain salary regardless of the number of injections the nurse gives. Sunk costs are fixed costs that cannot be recovered even if the ser-

vice is not provided. Semifixed costs are fixed within a range of activity (Figure 9-3). One nurse can give just so many injections per shift, and beyond that a second nurse will need to be hired. Semivariable costs are fixed at zero output and increase with volume (Figure 9-4). The break-even point is depicted on a break-even chart where revenues equal expenditures (Figure 9-5). The formula for break-even analysis is

$$R = FC + VC + P,$$

where:

R = Total revenue
FC = Fixed cost
VC = Variable cost
P = Profit

Average cost is the full cost divided by the volume of service units. The average cost decreases as the volume of patients increases because more patients share the fixed costs.

Mixed costs contain both the variable and fixed cost elements.

Marginal costs are the extra costs created by providing care to one more service unit. It is the difference in the total costs before and after adding one more service unit. Decisions about changes should be decided on the basis of marginal costs versus average or full costs.

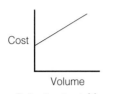

Figure 9-4   Semivariable costs.

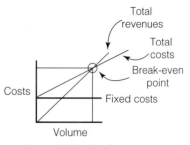

Figure 9-5   Break-even costs.

Cost estimation is the prediction of costs. It is a complicated process that involves dividing historical costs into fixed and variable components and adjusting historical costs for inflation to predict future costs.

To adjust cost for *inflation*, the historical cost is multiplied by the current value of the appropriate price index divided by the value of that index when the cost was incurred.

Regression analysis considers costs as the dependent variable and service units as the independent variable. The coefficient of the independent variable represents the variable costs, and the constant term of the regression represents fixed costs.

Contribution margin is the price minus the variable costs per service unit and represents the additional financial benefit for each additional service unit (Finkler and Kovner, 1999).

Strategic Cost Decisions

Taking a strategic approach to cost containment involves a comprehensive view of costs of the organization without being limited to direct, measurable costs. Albert Einstein said, "Not everything that counts can be counted, and not everything that can be counted counts" (Brinker, 1996, p. D4-1). This approach uses a total cost perspective that includes a broad range of tangible and intangible operating and strategic costs. A cost audit is important in the creation of a cost management strategy. The audit provides an assessment of the organization's cost position, compares it with competitors, and evaluates it for future profitability. This allows an assessment of the organization's current cost management processes.

Some accounting personnel may need to learn about management information needs. Defining what reports are needed is important. Managers and staff need to be supported in cost containment efforts with data that are focused rather than be overwhelmed with data that bury the critical data. Report formats should be clear and simple. Accountants' capabilities should be matched with the needs of management and staff.

Managers need to change their view of cost reductions from a negative exercise to something that can be creative and exciting. Then they should involve employees in the challenging and exciting process. Effective management communication is needed to increase employee awareness for and understanding of cost management. Having more employees involved in the task can create the greatest leverage. Brainstorming can be done with employees at all levels, who can then contribute to cost reduction. Short presentations about what actions are necessary, what employees can do, and rewards for results are key ingredients. Personal talks, videotaped presentations, newsletters, bulletin boards, staff meetings, and the grapevine can be used for communications. Meetings and discussions with employees can help alleviate fears and uncertainties about cost management.

Many ideas do not need simultaneous development and implementation. Factors such as what can be implemented quickly, cheaply, and with the greatest results should be considered. Short-term successes can be celebrated on the way to long-term improvements as management-employee attitudes and relationships change. Cost-reduction successes should be rewarded. Recognition is a reward for most types of agency achievement. It can be formal, like an employee-of-the-month program or public recognition in the form of a photograph and article in the newsletter or other media, or informal, like a pat on the back or a simple thank you. Employees may quickly forget positive comments but remember any negative ones, so small token awards like company pens or other items with the agency logo that may be used to hand out to customers can be used as a physical reminder of the manager's appreciation. Status rewards like employee of the month can be used to create role models and heroes. Money can be rewarded for proposing cost-reducing ideas, usually within a suggestion plan. An effective cost management strategy can take a long time to fully implement. Persistence is a quality of good cost cutters. The long-run commitment to successful cost management strategies helps give the organization the competitive edge.

Cost cutting often involves workforce reduction. Increasing the number of cuts may become increasingly less effective as muscle gets cut with fat. Attrition and early retirement are preferable to layoffs. Unfortunately, negative side effects can offset direct savings. High performers may become insecure and accept other positions, morale and productivity may drop, employees may stop suggesting ways to reduce costs, and absenteeism and grievances are likely to increase (Richardson, 1988). Silent sabotage may occur in the form of increased employee theft; the water cooler gang or company gossip in a public place; huddle and chatter, which is gossip about what happened or might happen, causing hours of nonproductive time; stay-and-quit syndrome, where employees lose their enthusiasm and refuse to go the extra mile; or the deviators, who divert business by not providing good service (Morin, 1995). Restructuring work relationships, cross-skills utilization, and gaining greater employee involvement may offer significant effects through increased productivity.

Across-the-board cuts may lead to customer complaints, inability to do the work, or lost time because of shortages of parts and maintenance that consequently greatly increase costs. Focused cuts are more useful. Some managers focus on controlling direct expenditures and cut nickel-and-dime items like free coffee. That can lead to greater losses as employees spend time complaining about the lost privilege instead of getting the work done.

Soft items that lead indirectly to cost reductions are sometimes the first expenditures to be cut. Sometimes it is necessary to spend money to make or save money. Staff development, travel to new experiences, staff meeting on company time, seed money, and maintenance can lead indirectly to cost savings.

Capital or technology-intensive approaches may lead to cost reductions but may also lead to higher overall costs and can involve painful implementation (Richardson, 1988). Activity-based cost management should be used with caution because a high percentage of the cost in health care organizations is indirect, and the indirect costs are not distributed evenly among units. Activity-based costing software packages translate financial information onto a management tool by aligning costs with the activities and by assigning costs directly to nursing practice. They can help differentiate value-added from non–value-added activities (Cokins, 1996; Storfjell and Jessup, 1996). Developing learning organizations, maximizing employee satisfaction, and simplifying and improving performance measures can be cost management strategies (Brinker, 1996; Ostrenga et al., 1992; Tomasko, 1996).

COSTING OUT NURSING SERVICES

The traditional model's equation follows:

$$NT \times (ANHS + BAI + ICA) = TNC \text{ per DRG}$$

where:

NT = Amount of nursing time per intensity level for a DRG
$ANHS$ = Average nursing hourly salary
BAI = Benefits across the institution
ICA = Indirect cost amount
TNC = Total nursing cost

The McCloskey model's equation (Huber, 1996; McCloskey, 1989) follows:

$$\text{NT/NI} \times (\text{ANHS} + \text{BAI} + \text{EC} + \text{ICA}) = \text{TNC}$$

where:

NT = Amount of nursing time
NI = Nursing intervention (instead of intensity level for a DRG)
ANHS = Average nursing hourly salary
BAI = Benefits across the institution
EC = Equipment cost (not in traditional model)
ICA = Indirect cost amount
TNC = Total nursing cost (instead of cost per DRG)

In general, the key problems related to costing out nursing are a lack of comparability of data used, multiple definitions of costs, and neglect of variables that affect nursing care. We need a forum where administrators, researchers, educators, and staff can share ideas about cost-effectiveness. We need models to describe the relationships between cost, quality, and price of nursing functions. We need to continue to compare methods for costing out nursing care and to identify data sets needed to cost out nursing and relate that to the minimum data set identified by Harriette Werley and others. Levels of care, expected outcomes, and cost of care can be related to pricing of nursing care. Nurses must be concerned about maintaining cost-effective, high-quality health care (Johnson, 1989).

PERSONAL FINANCES

This discussion of personal finances will help you understand broader economic and financial principles by applying them to your personal situation.

Assess Personal Finances

To assess your personal finances, ask the following:

Assets. How much do you have?

Debts. How much do you owe?

Income. How much do you earn?

Expenditures. How much do you spend?

Savings. Are you saving enough?

After using Worksheets 9-1 and 9-2 on pp. 495 and 496 to assess your assets and liabilities and cash flow, consider making changes in your personal finances by trying to find places to spend less and save more and looking for patterns of spending that could indicate trouble.

Money Makes Money

Make sure your money is earning interest whenever possible. You also need cash on hand or assets located where they can be converted into cash. Banks, savings and loans, and credit unions offer a variety of accounts that pay interest and are insured by the federal government, including money-market deposit accounts, savings accounts, and interest-paying checking accounts. Interest rates vary. There may be a fee if your balance falls below a minimum level. There may also be annual fees, monthly maintenance charges, and per-check charges.

Financial Goals

Using Worksheet 9-3 on p. 497, set and prioritize financial goals. Evaluate if your goals are realistic. Achieving your goals depends on the following:

• How soon you want to achieve them

• How much you can save

• How much risk you are willing to take

• What rate of return that risk will bring

There is no risk of losing your money in federally insured savings accounts within the insured limit of $100,000, but savings accounts pay a low interest. Money-market funds and certificates of deposit usually pay a little more than savings accounts with virtually no risk. Bonds pay more interest but have some market risk. When interest rates rise, the market value of stocks rises and the market value of bonds falls. Stocks have brought investors double-

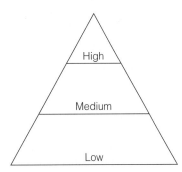

Figure 9-6 Pyramid of risk.

Box 9-3 **LOW-, MEDIUM-, AND HIGH-RISK INVESTMENTS**

LOW-RISK SAVINGS AND INVESTMENTS

Certificates of deposit
Interest-paying checking accounts
Money-market funds
Savings accounts
Savings bonds
Treasury bills and bonds

MEDIUM-RISK INVESTMENTS

Growth and income mutual funds
High-quality bond mutual funds
High-quality municipal and corporate bonds
Income mutual funds
Income stocks
Long-term growth stocks
Long-term growth stock mutual funds
Rental real estate
Tax-deferred annuities
Utility stocks

HIGH-RISK INVESTMENTS

Aggressive growth stock mutual funds
Collectibles
Emerging technology company stocks
Gold and other precious metals
High-yield bonds
High-yield mutual finds
Mutual funds investing in emerging technology firms
Oil and gas partnerships
Stocks of small companies listed in the over-the-counter market

digit annual returns over time. Your attitude toward risk will influence which investment you choose. If you cannot meet your goals in the time frame you set, you may need to (1) delay one or more goals, (2) set aside more money for savings, or (3) take more risk in the hope that your savings will grow faster.

Investment Strategies

The objectives of investment strategies are to preserve capital and to make it grow at a rate faster than inflation. To do that, you need to allocate and diversify your funds. A large portion of your investments and savings should be at low risk. Fewer should be in higher-risk ventures. Spread your risk (Figure 9-6). Box 9-3 lists some low-, medium-, and high-risk investments.

It takes discipline to save money. Savings should be treated as a fixed income, just another bill to pay each month. Payroll deductions can save your money before you get your check, and automatic bank payments can make deposits into mutual funds or savings plans. Planning for college and retirement requires big savings plans. Assets can be protected through insurance—health, disability, auto, home, and life.

It is important to get good financial advice. A lawyer can help with estate planning and wills. A tax adviser can help minimize taxes on various financial transactions. A stockbroker and an independent insurance agent can make valuable recommendations (Young, 1988).

MARKETING

Marketing is the analysis, planning, implementation, and control of carefully formulated programs designed to bring about voluntary exchanges of values with target markets for the purpose of achieving organizational objectives. It relies heavily on designing the organization's offering in terms of the target markets' needs and desires and on using effective pricing, communication, and distribution to inform, motivate, and service the markets (Kotler, 1982, p. 6).

Social Marketing

Social marketing is a fast-growing segment of non-profit marketing in this age of rapid population growth and economic, social, and environmental problems. Firms should consider consumer short-run wants and long-run welfare and make decisions that are best for consumers and society in the long run. Social marketing applies generic marketing to change social behavior of a target audience or to the well-being of society in general. For example, health care agencies market antismoking campaigns, nutrition education, exercise programs, immunizations, cancer detection, healthy hearts, safe sexual practices, and occupational safety. Marketing can be aimed at one-time or continuing behavior, high or low involvement, and individual or group behavior. Continuing, high-involvement behavior of groups is the most difficult to change. Social marketing may try to influence nonexistent or negative demand and may target relatively nonliterate audiences. It often deals with hard-to-research, sensitive issues or relatively invisible benefits while waiting for long-term change. If one is lucky, sustaining the new behavior becomes an issue. All companies have four basic social responsibilities: (1) economic—to be profitable, (2) legal—to obey the law and do what is legally correct, (3) ethical—to do what is right, just, and fair, and (4) philanthropical—to be a good citizen and contribute resources to improve the quality of life in the community (Kotler and Andreasen, 1991; Kotler and Armstrong, 1996; Kotler and Roberto, 1989; Pride and Ferrell 1997; Yoder-Wise, 1999).

Trends in Marketing

Technology has caused changes in marketing. Before the industrial revolution peddlers carried products to the door. They took large pots and pans to communities with many children and smaller pots to retirement communities. Technology can now be used for a large-scale, individualized approach to large markets. The industrial revolution mass-produced products, created a faceless society, and led to marketing designed from economic sciences and consumer models that were based on rational behavior. Target groups were defined for marketing when people wanted the same things. With cultures that value self-fulfillment and enjoyment of life more than being part of a group, consumption pressure aimed at the masses may not work. The new pattern has people wanting different things with less loyalty to brands. As people want goods and services tailored to them, individual ordering emerges along with the mass markets. A modular product range can give customers a large choice while requiring the production of only a limited number of variants. There may be just a few colors, styles, and sizes, but that gives numerous possibilities of combinations. This creates an abundance of diversity that people can search out with the media to put all kinds of options together, thus creating a fast, interactive means that is available 24 hours a day (Box 9-4). People do not easily change their habits, so electronics do not supersede everything but offer additional possibilities as people mail what they faxed or copy and distribute what they e-mailed. Agencies used to use generic, thematic one-sided bombardment advertising based on market research, generic models, and reported behaviors (which may not be actual behaviors) to manage target groups. Agencies are now more likely to use dialogue to listen and react to actual behaviors by using media and marketing databases to manage personal client relationships (Postma, 1999).

Popcorn and Marigold's Cultural Trends

Leaders need to consider trends to create long-term competitive advantages. Faith Popcorn and Lys Marigold (1996) identify 16 trends.

SOS (save our society) is a renewed social conscience with respect to ethics, education, and the environment. People are joining groups to promote social responsibility. Marketers can encourage their agencies to do socially responsible marketing.

Being alive is a desire for more years of quality living. People are increasingly taking more responsibility for their own health because they know lifestyles of eating the wrong foods, smoking, drinking, abusing drugs, breathing bad air, and having unsafe sex can kill them. It is time to market healthier products and services.

Down aging is feeling and acting younger than one is. People buy adult toys, dress young, take adventure vacations, and get plastic surgery. Senior citizens can make good volunteers for social causes.

Cashing out is when men and women question the price they pay for high-powered jobs and choose a simpler way of life.

Cocooning is the stay-at-home trend where one is protected from the harsh, unpredictable outside world. With technology one can shop,

bank, be entertained, and get an education right from home.

Anchoring is the trend to seek out our spiritual roots and take comfort from the past to secure the future. As people return to church, that may be a good place for social programs.

Clanning is the tendency to join groups with similar beliefs where one can be validated by consensus.

99 Lives is juggling many roles and responsibilities. People resort to fax, car phones, and fast food restaurants to cope. Cluster marketing or one-stop shopping such as a launderette with a copy machine, fax, and exercise bike may meet several needs.

Egonomics is the desire for personalized service. High tech needs to be high touch.

Small indulgences allow people to find an emotional fix by rewarding themselves with affordable luxuries in response to stress. Some may eat ice cream on the weekend to reward themselves for eating well all week or take a weekend trip when unable to afford a luxury vacation. Marketers should note ways people feel deprived and watch for small indulgences that give an emotional lift.

Fantasy adventure is an emotional escape from daily tensions through risk-free adventures like fantasy parks, food, and travel.

Female think is a trend toward more familial caring and sharing from the goal-oriented, hierarchical model.

Mancipation allows men to be individuals instead of strictly business.

Vigilante consumers are those who demand quality products and services. Agencies should focus on customer-centered, high-quality products and services.

Icon toppling is the questioning and sometimes rejection of our monuments of business and government.

Pleasure revenge is a counterreaction to following rules and regulations without the desirable results. It is the pursuit of pleasure through indulgences like smoking, drinking, overeating fatty foods, and not exercising (Kotler and Armstrong, 1996; Popcorn and Marigold, 1996).

| Box 9-4 | **TRENDS IN MARKETING** |

From	To
Masses	Individual
Generic	Specific
Limited choice	Abundance
Print	Electronic
Passive	Interactive
Plenty of time	Fast, faster, fastest
9 AM-5 PM	24-hour service
Agency calls out to market	Agency listens and reacts
One-sided bombardment	Dialogue
Market research	Marketing databases
Generic models	Marketing databases
Generic, thematic advertising	Media
Reported behaviors	Actual behaviors
Management of target groups	Management of personal client relationships

Leadership and Management of Strategic Planning for Marketing

Top-level administrators define the agency mission, which is a statement of the purpose, and set goals and objectives, which will be detailed in each unit. An analysis of strengths, weaknesses, opportunities, and threats is desirable. Administrators also design the agency portfolio, which is the collection of products and services the agency provides (Box 9-5). Market opportunities can be explored using a market expansion grid (Box 9-6).

Agencies have the following market opportunities: (1) market penetration when using existing products in existing markets, (2) market development by taking existing products into new markets, (3) product development by taking new products into existing markets, and (4) diversification by taking new products to new markets.

The marketing unit managers are responsible for developing marketing plans from the agency strategic plan, implementing the plans, evaluating the results, and taking corrective actions (Kotler and Armstrong, 1996; Pride and Ferrell, 1987, 1997).

Market Research

Market research is the research process applied to marketing. It involves the following: (1) defining the problem and research questions, (2) designing the research project, (3) collecting data, (4) analyzing data, and (5) interpreting and reporting the findings. It should furnish unbiased information to help avoid the false assumptions and misunderstanding that can lead to poor marketing (Box 9-7).

The first step is to define the problem and state the research questions. The problem may be failure to reach a goal. The research questions may identify the information needed to solve the problem. Refining an indefinite problem into a precise, researchable statement is challenging.

The research project should be designed to be reliable and valid. Reliability is repeatability. Validity is measuring what one intends to measure. The hypothesis is an informed guess about the problem and is tested. An exploratory study has a tentative hypothesis that needs to be made more specific. A descriptive study is intended to give an accurate portrayal of the characteristics of the situation and may use statistics and predictive tools. Causal studies assume that one variable causes another and tests that the independent variable causes a change in the dependent variable.

Box 9-5

LEADERSHIP AND MANAGEMENT OF STRATEGIC PLANNING FOR MARKETING

CORPORATE-LEVEL LEADERSHIP

Define agency mission.

Set agency goals and objectives.

Design agency portfolio.

MARKETING UNIT MANAGEMENT

Develop marketing plans from the strategic plan.

Implement the plans.

Evaluate results.

Take corrective actions.

Box 9-6

MARKET EXPANSION GRID

	Existing Products	New Products
Existing markets	1. Market penetration	3. Product development
New markets	2. Market development	4. Diversification

MARKETING RESEARCH

Defining problem and research questions
Designing the research project
    Reliability
    Validity
    Hypothesis
    Exploratory studies
    Descriptive studies
    Causal studies
Collecting data
    Primary data
    Secondary data
    Survey methods
      Interviews
        Mail
        Telephone
        E-mail
        Personal interviews
        On-site computer
      Questionnaires
      Observations
    Sampling
      Random
      Stratified
      Area
      Quota
Analyzing data
Interpreting and reporting findings

Primary and secondary data may be collected. Primary data are collected directly from the subjects. Secondary data are reports and other information from internal or external sources that may be used to study the problem. There are several ways to collect data. Mail surveys are questionnaires sent to subjects. They are appropriate when subjects are scattered over a large geographical area and the funds are limited. The interviewer records telephone surveys. Computer-assisted telephone interviewing can be done with the interviewer typing the answers to the questions into the computer during the interview. They have better response rates than mail surveys because it takes less effort to answer by telephone, but they are limited to people with tele-

phones. E-mail surveys are an alternative to both mailed and telephone surveys but are limited to people with e-mail. Personal interviews may be in-home, door-to-door interviews, focus interviews with several people at one time, or interviews of people in public places. On-site computer interviewing can be done in public places by putting the questionnaire on the computer, teaching the subjects how to answer the questions on the computer, and letting them self-pace themselves through the questionnaire. For observations researchers observe overt behavior and record it along with notes about the physical conditions and events.

Sampling is the selection of subjects from the total population. The population is all subjects of interest to the researcher. A sample is a limited number of subjects from the population, who can be selected in a number of ways. Random sampling is usually considered the best method of sampling and gives all subjects an equal opportunity to be in the sample. Stratified sampling divides the population into groups and does a probability sample of each group. Area sampling selects subjects from a specific area. Quota samples are not probability samples because not everyone has an equal chance to be in the sample. Variables are unique, such as who wears eyeglasses or has had a specific procedure done. Controls are usually limited to two or three variables like age, sex, and education to facilitate representativeness of categories of respondents.

Data are analyzed, often using statistical interpretation, and then interpreted and reported. The report is usually prepared as a formal written document but may also involve verbal presentations (Kotler and Armstrong, 1996; Pride and Ferrell, 1997).

Marketing Concepts

Exchange. Marketing is based on resource dependency or exchange. Organizations offer satisfactions such as goods, services, or benefits to markets that in return provide needed resources such as goods, services, time, money, or energy (Box 9-8). Exchange involves four conditions: (1) there are at least two parties, (2) each party offers something

Box 9-8   EXCHANGE MODEL

Seller has something of value, like products, services, and ideas, for the buyer.

Buyer has something of value, like money, credit, services, and products, for the seller.

Data from Pride WM, Ferrell OC: *Marketing: concepts and strategies*, Boston, 1997, Houghton Mifflin.

that the other considers valuable, (3) each party is capable of communication and delivery, and (4) each party is free to accept or reject the offer (Kotler, 1982, p. 37).

Publics.   "A public is a distinct group of people and/or organizations that has an actual or a potential interest and/or impact on an organization" (Kotler, 1982, p. 47). Input publics supply resources and constraints and consist of suppliers, donors, and regulatory publics. Those inputs are then managed by the organization's internal publics, such as the board of directors, management, staff, and volunteers, to accomplish the organization's mission. Intermediary publics are used to promote and distribute goods and services to consumers. The consuming publics, such as patients, clients, and students, consume the output of the organization. Reciprocal publics are interested in the agency, and the agency is interested in them. Patients are an example. Sought publics are desired by the agency but are not necessarily interested in the agency. For instance, wealthy people who are potential donors could be a sought public. Unwelcome publics are interested in the agency, but the agency is not interested in them. One unwelcome public consists of emergency room patients for nonemergency care. Publics are related to each other, as well as to the agency, and they influence each other's attitudes and behaviors. Publics are groups that have actual or potential interests in or impact on the agency.

Market.   "A market is a potential arena for the trading of resources." It is "a distinct group of people and/or organizations that [has] resources which they want to exchange, or might conceivably be willing to exchange, for distinct benefits" (Kotler, 1982, p. 50). A market is composed of actual or potential buyers and is a place where people negotiate to transfer goods or services. The health care agency goes to the labor market to obtain employees, to the professional market to obtain physicians, and to the financial market to obtain capital.

Image.   "An image is the sum of beliefs, ideas, and impressions that a person has of an 'object' " (Kotler, 1982, p. 57). Publics with a positive image of an organization will be drawn to it, whereas those with a negative image will avoid or disparage it.

There are two opposite theories about image formation. Object-determined theory maintains that people perceive the reality of the object. They experience the object and process the sensory data in a similar way despite different backgrounds. Therefore when people see a building in a beautiful setting, they perceive it as a beautiful hospital. Person-determined theory maintains that people have different degrees of contact with an object; they selectively perceive different aspects of the object, and through individual ways of processing the sensory data, they experience selective distortion. In this case some people may perceive the hospital as beautiful and others may not.

Image is a function of deeds and communications. Good deeds about which others are not told and talk without action are not enough. A strong, favorable image develops from satisfied publics that tell others their opinions.

Buyer decision process.   Both individuals and organizations follow similar processes when making buying decisions. First, the problem or need is identified. Second, specifications needed to solve the problem are identified, and then there is a search for products, services, or ideas to meet the need. Alternatives are evaluated, a purchase decision is made, and then the product, service, or idea is reevaluated on performance (Kotler and Armstrong, 1996; Pride and Ferrell, 1997) (Figure 9-7).

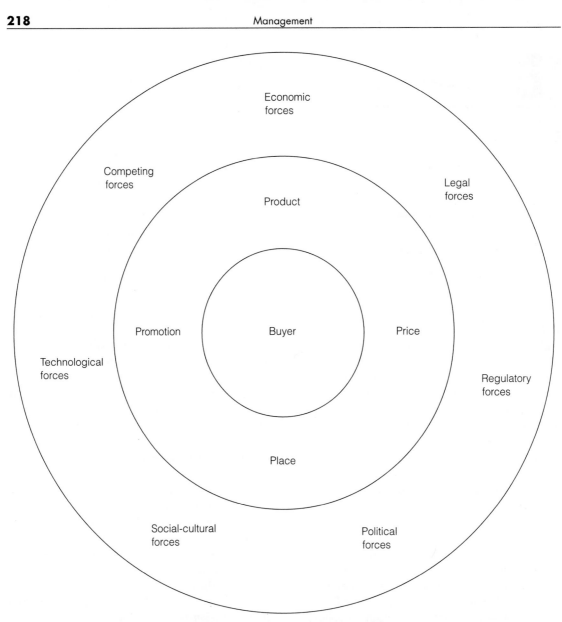

Figure 9-7 Marketing environment model.

Marketing Process

Marketing involves informing the market of services provided and fitting services to the market needs. It has evolved through different philosophies (Box 9-9).

Mass marketing occurs when the seller mass produces, distributes, and promotes one product or service to all customers. *Product-variety marketing* exists when the seller provides variety to the customers by having two or more products with different features. *Target marketing* involves the seller's identifying market segments, selecting specific target markets, and then developing products or services and marketing mixes specific to each target market (Box 9-10).

The marketing process involves several steps.

PHILOSOPHIES OF MARKETING

Mass marketing

Product-variety marketing

Target marketing

MARKETING PROCESS

Market segmentation
　Identify bases for segmenting the market
　Develop profiles of segments
Market targeting
　Develop measures of segment attractiveness
　Select the target segment(s)
Market positioning
　Develop positioning for each target segment
　Develop marketing mix for each target segment
Implement
Evaluate and control

Data from Kotler P, Armstrong G: *Principles of marketing*, ed 7, Upper Saddle River, NJ, 1996, Prentice Hall.

Market segmentation. An audit can be used to identify the bases for segmenting the market and to develop profiles of the segments. Marketing involves informing the market of services provided and fitting services to market needs. It is a complex process that generally includes the audit, market segmentation, marketing mix, implementation, and evaluation and control.

The marketing audit involves identification, collection, and evaluation of information that needs to be examined to evaluate market relations. Identifying the market and market segments is required. How large is the area to be served? Is it rural, urban, or both? How many potential customers are there? What are their ages, occupations, income levels, and interests? How many are aware of the organization's services? Are there seasonal differences? How satisfied are the clients with the services offered now?

The *organization* should be assessed. What is the mission of the organization? What are its philosophy, goals, objectives, and priorities? What are the services provided? What are the strengths and weaknesses? How do its services compare with those of others? What conditions of the industry affect the organization? What internal and external controls affect it?

As *services* are further analyzed, one should note distinctive superiorities. What services are heavily used? Why? What services are underused? Why? Are there voids? If so, can they be filled? How can needed materials, supplies, and personnel be obtained? Who pays for the services?

Who are the *competitors?* How many are there? Are their numbers increasing or decreasing? Who are the principal competitors? What areas do they serve? How do their size and strength compare? How do their charges compare?

What is the profile of present and future *clients* for the services? Are client profiles different between services? What is the frequency of client usage of the services?

What are the perceptions of the *nursing market?* What are the internal perceptions of nurse recruitment? Focus groups can be formed to discuss reasons why nurses decided to work at the institution, the positive and negative aspects of the job, and ways working conditions can be improved. Interviews with directors of nursing education programs can be used to learn how the institution is perceived, where graduates of that school are going and why, and how personnel at the health care agency can influence those decisions.

What is the organization's pricing philosophy? How are *prices* determined? How are prices viewed by the staff, clients, and competitors?

In what *location* is the service provided? How accessible is it to clients? How far will clients have to travel to obtain the service? Will personnel travel to provide a service? If so, how far? Will the agency charge for travel expenses?

What is the purpose of *promotion?* Is it reaching the intended publics? Is it effective?

What media are being used? What media reach whom?

Many *assessment* tools can be used to collect data for the audit. Questionnaires administered by mail, telephone, or interview, in-depth interviews, and observations are common. A consumer panel can be used to discuss relevant issues. A mediator helps keep a representative group of consumers discussing a specific topic in focus groups. Nominal groups aim at generating consensus about a particular issue. Records can be reviewed, and scientific research designs can be planned and implemented to collect data.

A *sampling plan* is important. Who will be surveyed? What will the sample size be? Large samples are more reliable than small samples. How will the sample be chosen? A random sample is the most reliable.

Statistical techniques such as frequency distributions, means, standard deviations, regression analysis, correlation analysis, factor analysis, discriminant analysis, and cluster analysis can be useful. Statistical techniques are technical; therefore statistical consultation is often advisable.

Profiles can be developed based on demographical, geographical, psychographical, and product-related variables. Demographical variables can include age, sex, education, income, occupation, race, ethnicity, religion, family size, and family life cycle. Geographical variables include country, region, urban, suburban, rural, city size, county size, state size, climate, and market density. Psychographical variables include personality, social class, lifestyle, benefits sought, readiness state (unaware, aware, informed, interested, desirous, intending to buy), rate of adoption (innovator, early adopter, early majority adopter, late majority adopter, laggard), user status (nonuser, ex-user, potential user, first-time user, regular user), user rate (light, medium, and heavy user), loyalty status (none, medium, strong, absolute), and attitude toward the product (enthusiastic, positive, indifferent, negative, hostile). Product-related variables include benefit expectations, price sensitivity, brand loyalty, and volume usage (Kotler and Armstrong, 1996; Pride and Ferrell, 1997).

Box 9-11 **TARGET SEGMENT SELECTION PROCESS**

Identify targeting strategy.

Determine segmentation variables to use.

Develop market segment profiles.

Evaluate market segments.

Select target market segments.

Data from Pride WM, Ferrell OC: *Marketing: concepts and strategies*, Boston, 1997, Houghton Mifflin.

Market targeting. Targeting involves developing measures of segment attractiveness and selecting the target segment(s) to enter. Segmentation identifies subsets of the total market that have similar characteristics (Box 9-11).

There are three major marketing strategies related to segments:

- Differentiated marketing aims directly and differentially at several specific segments.
- Concentrated marketing aims at a specific segment.
- Undifferentiated marketing ignores segments and deals with all as one market.

Market positioning. The product position is the way customers describe the important attributes of the product or service. Leaders need to choose and implement a positioning strategy for a competitive advantage, which often involves offering a greater value for a lower price or justifying the higher price for more benefits. The difference promoted should be important, superior, distinctive, affordable, and profitable. The difference should be communicated and made visible to the buyer.

Marketing mix. A marketing mix is developed for each target segment. It involves the four *p*'s: product, price, place, and promotions (Box 9-12).

Product is something provided for consumption to satisfy a need or want. The inventory of ser-

**Box
9-12   MARKETING MIX**

Product

Price

Place

Promotions

vices and analysis of costs, benefits, and target markets indicate which products are overused, underused, and cost-effective and which are perceived as strong or weak. This information should be used to determine the appropriate product mix.

A product line is composed of similar services that are clustered to manage process, quality, costs, and marketing more efficiently. Product line analysis is a method of analyzing products in terms of inputs and outputs and is built on total cost accounting principles. Because determination of actual cost per case is important, all costs for an admission are tracked. All hospital fixed overhead costs are allocated to patients and product lines. All costs from admission to discharge are determined and compared with the reimbursement per case. Length of stay by product line is important. When the patient's length of stay is too long, the total cost may surpass the reimbursement per case even if the daily expense is reasonable.

Product line analysis shows the relationship of inputs to outputs, gives profit and loss information for a product line, attaches all costs to a product line, increases personnel's cost awareness, facilitates planning, promotes efficiency, encourages better review and control of resources, and promotes better decision making.

A Boston consulting group developed a classification system of potential growth and profitability to identify marketing strategies for products (Figure 9-8). They created a grid with growth potential measured on the vertical axis and profitability along the horizontal axis. Low growth potential and profitability are represented at the lower left corner; the

factor becomes higher toward the top and the right of the grid. Products with low profitability and low growth potential are labeled dogs. They drain the organization and should be divested if possible. Products in the upper left quadrant have low profitability and high growth potential. They are labeled question marks. Aggressive marketing to increase volume and therefore profitability is possible but risky. Cash cows, with high profitability but low growth potential, are in the lower right quadrant. That product may be maintained to use the profits to finance other ventures or to cover other losses. In the upper right quadrant are the rising stars, which have both high profitability and high growth potential. Promotional money should be put here to increase volume and profitability. After increasing growth, rising stars typically become cash cows.

Products have life cycles. The stages of the life cycle are as follows (Figure 9-9):

The introduction stage is the beginning of a new product when the customer's response to the product and its growth potential are relatively unknown.

The growth stage occurs when the number of customers and the size of the market are increased.

The maturity stage is the peak market of the product. Competition enters the market to obtain a share. Marketing strategies during the maturity stage are designed to get and keep the agency's share of the market.

The last stage is the market decline stage, when the market decreases because of new ideas, products, technology, or changes in customer needs.

Question marks occur during the introductory stage, when the future is risky but there is high growth potential. Rising stars form the growth stage, when profitability and growth potential are high. Cash cows are seen during the maturity stage, when there is high profitability but low growth potential. Dogs occur during the decline stage, with the declining growth and profitability (Strasen, 1987).

A fad is a fashion that peaks early and declines rapidly (Figure 9-10, *A*). A fashion is a currently popular style (Figure 9-10, *B*). Style is a basic mode of expression that is distinctive (Figure 9-10, *C*). For example, clothes may be casual or formal; art may

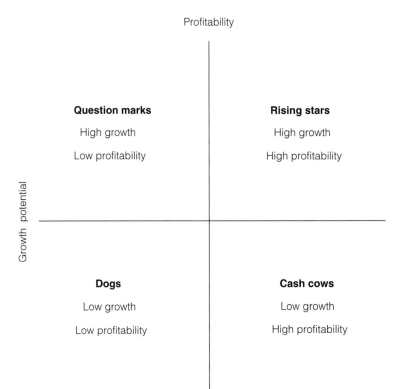

Figure 9-8   Boston consulting firm's grid.

be abstract or realistic. A style may last for decades, coming in and out of vogue with periods of renewed interest (Kotler P et al., 1996; Kotter and Armstrong, 1996).

Price is another major consideration. Because physicians rather than patients usually determine the services used and health care bills are usually paid by third-party payers, nondollar costs such as time and convenience must be considered. Minimization of nondollar costs should benefit the health care agency and the consumer.

There are several pricing goals:

- *Profit-maximizing pricing* tries to set the maximum price that the demand for the product or service will bear.

- *Market-share pricing* sacrifices short-term profits for long-term market domination and attempts to identify the price that maximizes the agency's share of the market.

- *Market-skimming pricing* places a high price and high profitability on a product or service when it is in high demand with no competition.

- *Current-revenue pricing* tries to maximize the current revenue.

- *Target-profit pricing* attains a satisfactory profit.

- *Promotional, loss-leader pricing* sets the price lower than the cost or competition to introduce customers to the new product or service. Profits are regained when the customers purchase other products.

- *Prestige pricing* sets unusually high prices to convey the image of quality or prestige.

Pricing factors include cost of product, demand for product, and competition. When considering the *cost of products or services,* one can use *mark-up*

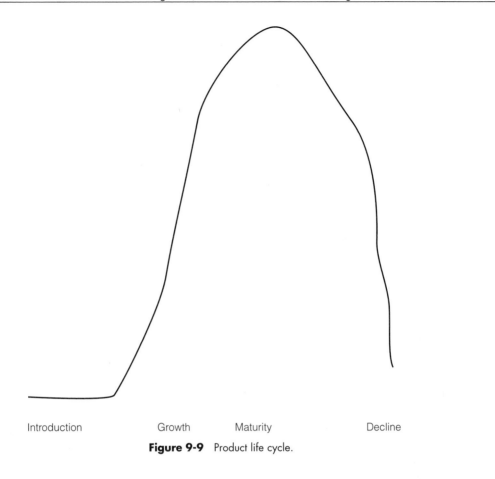

Introduction   Growth   Maturity   Decline

Figure 9-9 Product life cycle.

pricing by adding a certain percentage to the cost, *cost-plus pricing* by adding a fixed amount to the cost, and *target pricing* by setting the price so it yields a specific profit at a particular demand level. When considering the *demand* for the product or service, one can use *perceived-value pricing* by setting the price according to the customer's perception of the value of the product or service or *price-discrimination pricing* by varying the price from one customer or place to another. There might be a sliding pay scale according to the patient's income. One hospital in a corporation might charge more or less than others because of the client's income in general or the facility's location in a rich or poor neighborhood. When considering *competition, going-rate pricing* uses the collective wisdom of the marketplace. In *sealed-bid pricing* the lowest bid gets the business (Strasen, 1987).

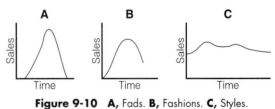

Figure 9-10 **A,** Fads. **B,** Fashions. **C,** Styles.

Place involves the physical location, appearance of the location, its accessibility and availability, resource utilization, the expertise and courtesy of staff, referral mechanisms, and distribution. The goal is to provide the service to the consumer with efficient distribution and minimal inconvenience.

Marketing promotion informs potential consumers of the existence and availability of products and services and persuades them of the benefits to them. Tailoring services to consumer desires is important. Marketing promotion leads to awareness, understanding, interest, decision, utilization, satisfaction, reutilization, and recommendation.

Promotion tools include the following: (1) advertising, which is any paid form of promotion; (2) personal selling, which is an oral presentation by a seller to a buyer; (3) sales promotions, which are short-term incentives for purchasing products or services; and (4) publicity, which is promotion that is not paid for by the agency. *Advertising* includes ads in newspapers, magazines, and journals, direct mail, flyers, billboard advertising, telephone directories, radio, and television. Printed materials can be used—for instance, calendars, matches, pens, telephone stickers, newsletters, and booklets about such topics as diet, exercise, poison control, and first aid. *Personal selling* includes fund-raising, lobbying, and sales calls such as presentations to community groups about health promotion, chemical dependency, weight control, exercise, birth control, and child care. *Sales promotions* include introductory offers, free samples, coupons, discounts, incentives, free lectures, and special credit cards. The best form of *publicity* is the word of mouth of satisfied customers. Other types are public service announcements, public relations campaigns, speakers bureaus, interviews, health fairs, and screening programs (Strasen, 1987).

Promotion has been revolutionized by technology. Personal computers and multimedia applications are readily available and make graphics, moving pictures, and sound possible. Multimedia notebooks are portable compact computers that are so small they can be taken anywhere they are needed and used without a connecting lead. They are very convenient for traveling representatives. A Personal Digital Assistant is fitted with an optical that allows one to write and draw on an electronic slate rather than typing on a keyboard. Television facilitates visual communications. Teletex is a popular form of interactivity that allows choices to be made numerically by a standard remote control. People can get information about things

such as the weather, traffic updates, airport arrivals, and stock indices. Then interests expressed by the choices can simultaneously be marketed by teletex. Travel arrangements can be booked when interest is expressed in a travel program. Direct-response television is interactive by using a commercial to get customers to call a specific number. Most calls are made within 10 minutes of the advertisement. TV videotex is an electronic information service that allows one to choose a teletex page from a menu. One needs to dial a telephone number to get access to a specific page that lists a variety of services. Near Video-on Demand allows customers to view films as they "go by" on a regular basis. The customer pays for what is viewed. The investment costs for Near Video-on Demand are considerably less than Video-on Demand, which is equivalent to a video shop at home (Postma, 1999).

Computers can make databases easily accessible and retrievable. They can then be used for marketing decisions. Electronic bulletin boards are computer network systems that link many computers by phone lines or satellite. They allow marketers to interact with data sources and clients almost instantaneously. Bulletin boards can permit customers to exchange ideas for problem solving, learn from each other, and give the agency new insights into marketing products and services. The Internet is a collection of computers connected by phone lines that enables people to communicate around the world through e-mail, newsgroups, chat rooms, and more. It links companies with customers around the world by computer networks. Although the Internet has been in existence for a few decades, the World Wide Web was not developed until 1992. It organizes information available on the Internet into interconnected pages that may include text, graphics, sound, and video. Software packages that facilitate navigating the Web have made the Web a multimedia communication tool (Pride and Ferrell, 1997). Fax machines, sales-automation software, personal newspapers, videoconferencing, cable television, and the Internet have revolutionized marketing (Kotler, 1999; Kotler and Kotler, 1996).

Implementation

Implementation can be done incrementally or as an entire package. Designing and implementing a marketing program are expensive projects and require personnel with expertise in marketing. Outside consultants can be hired when qualified people are not available within the organization. Dealing with local political conflicts, reaching communities that are out of touch with their own real demands, and sorting real demands from surface expectations are challenging tasks.

Domestic marketing focuses on the market in the country of origin. While there may not be an international marketing plan, sometimes international distributors or foreign companies purchase products or services, creating limited exporting. International marketing includes plans for marketing between countries. Global marketing involves strategies for marketing around the world (Box 9-13).

Dealing with international and global markets is even more challenging than domestic marketing. There are different political climates; different histories; cultural differences; different business customs; different laws, legal systems, and regulations; different technological forces; different stages of economic development; different economic forces; and different local geography. Rather than dealing with one set of market conditions, marketers must address differences for each country and for each market within each country (Cateora and Graham, 1999; Pride and Ferrell, 1997).

Box 9-13   LEVELS OF GLOBAL MARKETING

Domestic marketing

Limited exporting

International marketing

Global marketing

Data from Pride WM, Ferrell OC: *Marketing: concepts and strategies*, Boston, 1997, Houghton Mifflin.

Evaluation and control.   The last phase of the marketing process is evaluation and control. It involves identifying goals and objectives, measuring planned and actual results, determining reason for variance between planned and actual results, correcting action based on causal analysis, and revising goals. Evaluation can be done more or less often—daily through weekly, monthly, yearly, or on a more extended basis—to determine whether implementation is accomplishing desired results.

Health care marketing and ethics.   Historically, many professionals have argued that marketing health care could sacrifice quality for volume, could shift decision-making power to the public that was not qualified to make the decisions, would lower standards of professions, could be harmful to professional image, and was thus unethical. Now many professional groups are marketing to increase awareness of services without sacrificing standards. Some say marketing has increased sensitivity to client needs. Others recommend marketing to recruit nurses. The American Marketing Association's Academy for Health Services Marketing has developed professional ethics for health care marketing. They include respecting the primacy of the client welfare and confidentiality of the relationships; providing communications to inform, not to deceive; being competitive and making fair comparisons; and being vigilant in the application of the standards. Marketing public relations has helped marketing campaigns be successful (Dienemann, 1990; Harris, 1998; Sullivan and Decker, 1999; Swansburg, 1996).

CHAPTER SUMMARY

Chapter 9 covered the following:
History of Health Care Financing
Budgetary Leadership and Management
Budgets
Prerequisites to Budgeting
Applied Economics
Accounting

REFERENCES

Brinker BJ: *Performance measurement: emerging practices in cost management,* Boston, 1996, Warren, Gorham & Lamont.

Cateora PR, Graham JL: *International marketing,* Boston, 1999, Irwin\McGraw-Hill.

Cokins G: *Activity-based cost management: making it work,* Chicago, 1996, Irwin.

Dienemann J: *Nursing administration: strategic perspectives and application,* Norwalk, Conn, 1990, Appleton & Lange.

Douglass LM: *The effective nurse: leader and manager,* ed 5, St. Louis, 1996, Mosby.

Ellis JR, Hartley CL: *Managing and coordinating nursing care,* Philadelphia, 1995, Lippincott.

Finkler SA, Kovner CT: *Financial management for nurse managers and executives,* ed 2, Philadelphia, 1999, Saunders.

Gillies DA: *Nursing management: a systems approach,* ed 3, Philadelphia, 1994, Saunders.

Harris TL: *Value-added public relations: the secret weapon of integrated marketing,* Chicago, 1998, NCT/Contemporary Publishing Group.

Hein EC: *Contemporary leadership behavior: selected readings,* ed 5, Philadelphia, 1998, Lippincott.

Huber D: *Leadership and nursing care management,* Philadelphia, 1996, Saunders.

Johnson M: Perspectives on costing nursing, *Nurs Adm Q* 14:65-71, Fall 1989.

Kotler P: *Marketing for nonprofit organizations,* Englewood Cliffs, NJ, 1982, Prentice Hall.

Kotler P: *Kotler on marketing: how to create, win and dominate markets,* New York, 1999, Free Press.

Kotler P, Andreasen A: *Strategic marketing for nonprofit organizations,* Englewood Cliffs, NJ, 1991, Prentice Hall.

Kotler P, Armstrong G: *Principles of marketing,* ed 7, Upper Saddle River, NJ, 1996, Prentice Hall.

Kotler P, Kotler P: *Marketing management: analysis, planning, implementation, and control,* Upper Saddle River, NJ, 1996, Prentice Hall.

Kotler P, Roberto EL: *Social marketing: strategies for changing public behavior,* New York, 1989, Free Press.

Kotler P et al.: *Marketing management: an Asian perspective,* Singapore, 1996, Prentice Hall.

Loveridge CE, Cummings SH: *Nursing management in the new paradigm.* Gaithersburg, Md, 1996, Aspen.

Marquis BL, Huston CJ: *Leadership roles and management functions in nursing: theory and application,* Philadelphia, 1996, Lippincott.

Marrelli TM: *The nurse manager's survival guide: practical answers to everyday problems,* St. Louis, 1997, Mosby.

McCloskey JC: Implications of costing out nursing for reimbursement, *Nurs Manage* 20(1):245-253, 1989.

Morin WJ: *Silent sabotage: rescuing our careers, our companies, and our lives from the creeping paralysis of anger and bitterness,* New York, 1995, American Management Association.

Ostrenga MR et al.: *The Ernst & Young guide to total cost management,* New York, 1992, John Wiley & Sons.

Popcorn F, Marigold L: *Clicking: 16 trends to future fit your life, your work, and your business,* New York, 1996, HarperCollins.

Postma P: *The new marketing era: marketing to the imagination in a technology-driven world,* New York, 1999, McGraw-Hill.

Pride WM, Ferrell OC: *Marketing: basic concepts and decision,* Boston, 1987, Houghton Mifflin.

Pride WM, Ferrell OC: *Marketing: concepts and strategies,* Boston, 1997, Houghton Mifflin.

Richardson PR: *Cost containment: the ultimate advantage,* New York, 1988, Free Press.

Rocchiccioli JT, Tilbury MS: *Clinical leadership in nursing,* Philadelphia, 1998, Saunders.

Storfjell JL, Jessup S: Bridging the gap between finance and clinical operations with activity-based cost management, *JONA* 26:12-17, Dec 1996.

Strasen L: *Key business skills for nurse managers,* Philadelphia, 1987, Lippincott.

Sullivan EJ, Decker PJ: *Nursing administration: a micro/macro approach for effective nurse executives,* Norwalk, Conn, 1999, Appleton & Lange.

Swansburg RC: *Management and leadership for nurse managers,* ed 2, Boston, 1996, Jones & Bartlett.

Tomasko RM: *Go for growth! Five paths to profit and success—choose the right one for you and your company,* New York, 1996, John Wiley & Sons.

Yoder-Wise PS: *Leading and managing in nursing,* ed 2, St. Louis, 1999, Mosby.

Young A: *Personal finance,* Washington, DC, 1988, Conrad and Associates.

BIBLIOGRAPHY

Aydlotte JHC: From nurse to marketing entrepreneur, *Seminars Nurse Managers* 6(1):26-29, 1998.

Barrett MW: Downsizing: doing it rationally, *Nurs Manage* 26:24-29, May 1995.

Berman HJ, Kukla SF, Weeks LE: *The financial management of hospitals,* ed 8, Ann Arbor, Mich, 1994, Health Administration Press.

Blaney DR, Hobson CJ: *Cost-effective nursing practice: guidelines for nurse managers,* Philadelphia, 1988, Lippincott.

Bryce HJ: *Financial and strategic management for nonprofit organizations,* ed 2, Englewood Cliffs, NJ, 1992, Prentice Hall.

Cavouras CA, McKinley J: Variable budgeting for staffing: analysis and evaluation, *Nurs Manage* 28:34-38, May 1997.

Clark LL: Incorporating OASIS into the Visiting Nurses Association, *Outcomes-Management-for-Nursing-Practice* 2:24-28, Jan-March 1998.

Cleverley WO: *Essentials of health care finance,* ed 3, Rockville, Md, 1992, Aspen.

Cotton TW: Financial management: the changes ahead, *Long Term Care Manage* 46:16-20, May 1997.

De Groot HA, Burke LJ, George VM: Implementing the differentiated pay structure model, *JONA* 28:28-38, May 1998.

de-la-Cuesta C: Marketing: a process in health visiting, *J Adv Nurs* 19:347-353, Feb 1994.

Dinnemann JA, Wintz L: Designing a marketing plan that works, *JONA* 22:23-28, Jan 1992.

Drayton P: Learning from the private sector, *American City County* 113:6, May 1998.

Dreisbach AM: A structured approach to expert financial management: a financial development plan for nurse managers, *Nurs Econ* 12:131-139, June 1994.

Evans DG: Financial services can offer golden opportunities, *Am Agent Broker* 69:22-26+, July 1997.

Feldstein PJ: *Health care economics,* ed 4, New York, 1993, Delmar.

Felteau AL: Tools and techniques to effect budget neutrality, *Nurs Adm Q* 17:59-64, Summer 1993.

Finkler SA, Graft CM: *Budgeting concepts for nurses,* ed 2, Philadelphia, 1992, Saunders.

Finkler SA, Kovner CT: *Financial management for nurse managers and executives,* Philadelphia, 1993, Saunders.

Finkler SA et al.: Innovation in nursing: a benefit/cost analysis, *Nurs Econ* 12:18-27, Jan-Feb 1994.

Gibson SJ et al.: CNS-directed case management: cost and quality in harmony, *JONA* 24:45-51, June 1994.

Grimaldi PL: Building capitation rates, *Nurs Manage* 26:12-15, May 1995.

Grimaldi PL: Detecting financially mismanaged care, *Nurs Manage* 26:12-14, June 1995.

Grimaldi PL: Medical loss ratios under scrutiny, *Nurs Manage* 27:14+, June 1996.

Grimaldi PL: Medicare marketing guidelines for managed care, *Nurs Manage* 28:22-24, April 1997.

Hargreaves WA et al.: *Cost-out methods for mental health,* San Diego, 1998, Academic Press.

Hlusko DL, Pahoulis E, Branson L: Cut training costs with computer-based tutorials, *Nurs Manage* 29:31-33, Nov 1998.

Huggins D, Lehman K: Reducing costs through case management, *Nurs Manage* 28:34-38, Dec 1997.

Jacobs P: *The economics of health and medical care,* ed 4, Rockville, Md, 1996, Aspen.

Jones RJ: Financial management: moving toward managed care, *Seminars Nurs Managers* 5:5-6, March 1997.

Koch MW, Fairly TM: *Integrated quality management: the key to improving nursing care quality,* St. Louis, 1993, Mosby.

Macknick FJ: Two takes on facility marketing, *Nurs Homes* 47:70-73, Oct 1998.

Mason JE: Superb customer service comes from within, *Nurs Manage* 29:31, Sept 1998.

McCarthy EJ: *Basic marketing,* ed 12, Homewood, Ill, 1996, Irwin.

McHugh ML: Cost-effectiveness of clustered unit vs unclustered nurse floating, *Nurs Econ* 15:294-300, Nov-Dec 1997.

Morton LW: Medicaid enrollment choice into managed care health plans, *Med Care Res Rev* 55:211-238, June 1998.

Nowicki M: *The financial management of hospitals and healthcare organizations,* Chicago, 1999, Health Administration Press; Washington, DC, AUPHA Press; and Westchester, Ill, Healthcare Financial Management Association.

Pelfrey S: Managing financial data, *Seminars Nurse Managers* 5:25-30, March 1997.

Person MM: *The zero-base hospital: survival and success in America's evolving healthcare system,* Chicago, 1997, Health Administration Press.

Phillips M, Spaulding R, O'Neal L: Determining appropriate funding for advanced practice nurses, *Nurs Econ* 13:12-17, Jan-Feb 1995.

Price JL: *The study of turnover,* Ames, Iowa, 1977, Iowa State University Press.

Price J, Mueller CW: *Absenteeism and turnover of hospital employees,* Greenwich, Conn, 1986, JAI Press.

Siegel JG, Shim JK, Hartman SW: *The McGraw-Hill pocket guide to business finance: 201 decision-making tools for managers,* New York, 1992, McGraw-Hill.

Smith HL, Mabon SA, Piland NF: Nursing department strategy, planning, and performance in rural hospitals, *JONA* 23:23-33, April 1993.

Soule TRR, Dobson JM: SEPPD and HPPD: more effective control of nursing care costs, *Nurs Econ* 10:205-209, May-June 1992.

Strum AC: *The new rules of healthcare marketing: 23 strategies for success,* Chicago, 1998, Health Administration Press.

Swansburg RC, Swansburg RJ: *Introductory management and leadership for nurses: an interactive text,* Boston, 1999, Jones & Bartlett.

Tappen RM: *Nursing leadership and management: concepts and practice,* ed 3, Philadelphia, 1995, FA Davis.

Ward LA, Augustine LJ, Villano LM: Nursing: an economic entity and profitable enterprise, *Nurs Adm Q* 19:41-44, Spring 1995.

Worthy CH: Clinical ladders: can we afford them? *Nurs Manage* 27:33-34, Sept 1996.

Wywialowski EF: *Managing client care,* ed 2, St. Louis, 1997, Mosby.

Zachry BR, Gilbert RL, Gregg M: Director of nursing finance: controlling health care costs, *Nurs Manage* 26:49-53, Nov 1995.

Zimmet M: Nurses drive pps payment: communication with business office is critical, *Contemp Long Term Care* 22:31-32, Jan 1999.

CASE STUDY

Write the scenario for this case study yourself using yourself as the main character. Using Worksheets 9-1, 9-2, and 9-3 on pp. 495-497, assess assets and liabilities, calculate personal cash flow, and assess your financial goal priorities.

CASE STUDY

A school of nursing started a nurse practitioner program 1 year ago. Because of the high demand for the program, twice as many students are being admitted the second year of admissions as the first year. Using Worksheet 9-4, plot the program in the life cycle and the Boston group's profitability and growth opportunity classifications.

CASE STUDY

Services are changing from having physicians do physical examinations to having nurse practitioners do them. Consequently, there is less use of large gloves and an increased use of smaller gloves. What factors should you consider when determining how many gloves to order how often?

Critical Thinking Activities for this chapter begin on page 494.

CHAPTER 10

ORGANIZA-TIONAL CONCEPTS AND STRUCTURES

CHAPTER OBJECTIVES

- Describe the relationships between span of management, flat or tall structures, and decentralization or centralization.
- Describe ways a manager can facilitate adjustments to mergers and acquisitions.
- Differentiate between line and staff authority.
- Identify at least three principles of organization.
- Describe disadvantages of the bureaucratic structure.
- Identify at least three adhocracy organizational models.
- Describe the corporate model.

Chapter Overview

Chapter 10 outlines factors affecting organizational structures, organizational concepts, and types of organizational structures, including health care networks.

MAJOR CONCEPTS AND DEFINITIONS	
Organizational chart	a drawing that shows how the parts of an organization are linked
Span of management	the number and diversity of people who report to a manager
Centralize	to concentrate power or authority
Decentralize	to distribute power and authority among more places
Merger	the combination of two or more companies into one company
Line authority	the formal chain of command
Staff authority	advisory or service oriented in nature
Organization	consolidated group of elements; systematized whole
Structure	formation or pattern of arrangement
Hierarchy	a group of persons arranged by rank, grade, or class
Bureaucracy	administration through departments and subdivisions managed by officials following an inflexible routine
Adaptive	able to change to make suitable to new or changed circumstances
Matrix	the formation of cells in the organizational structure
Corporation	a group

FACTORS AFFECTING ORGANIZATIONAL STRUCTURES

Organizational structures are affected by the economic, political, social, and technological pressures in society and follow changes in vertical and horizontal integration, geographical dispersion, and unit volume. The structure delimits responsibilities, communication channels, and the decision-making environment. The organizational structure should facilitate the vision, values, mission, philosophy, goals, objectives, strategies, policies, and procedures.

Organizational structures are changing from simple, hierarchical structures with formal channels of communication, functional fiefdoms, and division of labor with division and simplification of work to complex, flat organizations with cross-

functional teams, free access to information, and no boundaries that empower employees and enrich work through multiple tasks (Gore, Murray, and Richardson, 1992; Martin, 1995; Swansburg, 1996) (Box 10-1).

It used to be that only experts could perform complex tasks, information was located in one place, and decision making was centralized with managers. Plans got revised periodically. Field personnel needed an office and had to find out where things were. The best contact was a personal contact. Now generalists can do expert tasks, everyone makes decisions, and the organization is simultaneously centralized and decentralized. Information is simultaneously in many places, and plans can be revised instantaneously. Field workers can work anywhere and can make effective contacts through

Box 10-1　**TRENDS AFFECTING ORGANIZATIONAL STRUCTURES**

From	To
Hierarchical management	Flat organizations with cross-functional teams
Formal channels of communication	Free access to information
Functional fiefdoms	Organization without boundaries
Division of labor	Empowerment of employees
Division and simplification of work	Enrichment of work through multiple tasks and expanded knowledge
Simple	Complex

Box 10-2　**TECHNOLOGICAL INFLUENCES**

Old Ways	New Ways
Information was in only one place.	Information is simultaneously in many places.
Only experts could perform complex tasks.	Generalists can do expert tasks.
The organization was centralized or decentralized.	The organization is simultaneously centralized and decentralized.
Managers made the decisions.	Everyone makes decisions.
Field personnel needed offices.	Field personnel can work anywhere.
Best contact was a personal contact.	Best contact is an effective contact by any of numerous modes.
Field personnel had to find out where things were.	Things tell where they are.
Plans got revised periodically.	Plans get revised instantaneously.

Modified from Wall DK, Proyect MM: *Critical pathway implementation guide: a methodology for managing critical pathways*, Chicago, 1997, Precept Press.

numerous means. Things tell where they are (Box 10-2).

Leaders evaluate the organizational structure, encourage employees to follow the chain of command, counsel employees who do not follow the chain of command, model responsibility and accountability, help staff see how their roles fit into the structure, encourage upward communications, facilitate the informal group, explain the organizational culture, and support advisory personnel. Managers are knowledgeable about the structure, maintain and clarify unity of command, establish a span of control, provide organizational charts, follow the chain of command, use the informal organization, are knowledgeable

about the culture, and use advisory personnel (Box 10-3).

ORGANIZATIONAL CHARTS

An organizational chart is a drawing that shows how the parts of an organization are linked. It depicts the formal organizational relationships, areas of responsibility, persons to whom one is accountable, and channels of communication.

Managers should consider actual working relationships when drawing an organizational chart. The formal organization may not be functioning as was outlined on an older chart. Rather, an alternate structure may have emerged that operates very effectively. It is essential, then, that the manager knows what is happening in actual practice. The process of drawing the chart demands a review of current practices, discovery of relationships not previously examined, and clarification of vague associations.

The organizational chart may be used for outlining administrative control, for policy making and planning (including organizational change) to evaluate strengths and weaknesses of the current structure, and for showing relationships with other departments and agencies. It can also be used to orient new personnel or to present the agency's structural design to others. The visual diagram of a chart is a more effective means of communicating the agency's organizational structure than is a written description.

Organizational charts are not used by all managers. Autocratic managers who wish to control and manipulate others may feel that their power would be diminished if staff associates understood the working environment. Adaptive structures are more difficult to chart because they are more fluid and subject to change.

Charts become outdated as changes are made. On charts the informal structure has not been diagramed, the formal structure may be difficult to define, and duties and responsibilities are not described. Charts may foster rigidity in relationships

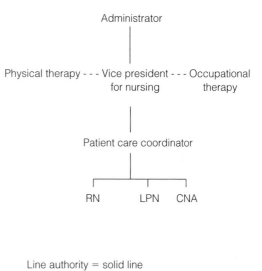

Line authority = solid line

Staff authority = dashed line

Figure 10-1 Line-staff relationships.

and communications. People may be sensitive about their relative status in the organization and may not want their positions revealed. It can be expensive to develop, disseminate, and store the charts.

Vertical charts, depicting the chief executive at the top with formal lines of authority down the hierarchy, are most common, but other modifications are available (Figures 10-1 and 10-2). A left-to-

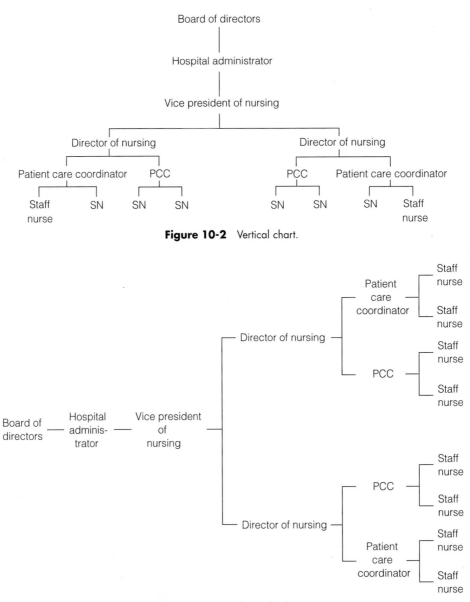

Figure 10-2 Vertical chart.

Figure 10-3 Left-to-right chart.

right, or horizontal, chart depicts the chief executive at the left with lower echelons to the right (Figure 10-3). It follows the normal reading habit, shows relative length of formal lines of authority, helps simplify the lines of authority and responsibility, and can reveal problems within the structure. A concentric, or circular, chart shows the chief executive in the center with successive echelons in concentric circles (Figure 10-4). It helps depict the outward flow of formal authority from the top executive and supposedly reduces status implications.

The informal structure can be superimposed on the formal structure or charted through the use of sociograms. Sociograms analyze data on the choice of, communication between, and interaction between members of a small group. Personnel may be

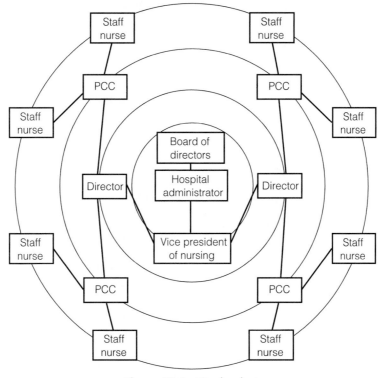

Figure 10-4 Circular chart.

ADVANTAGES AND DISADVANTAGES OF ORGANIZATIONAL CHARTS

Box 10-4

Advantages	Disadvantages
Contributes to sound organizational structure	Becomes obsolete quickly
Maps lines of decision-making authority	Shows only formal relationships
Shows formal lines of communication	Does not show informal communications
Shows how people fit into the organization	May show how things are supposed to be rather than how they are
Helps employees understand their assignments	May help confuse authority and status

asked with whom they prefer to work, or their interactions may be observed and charted. The person with the most relationships is often the leader. Members of the primary group are those most accepted by other group members. Managers should use this information to increase production, because work groups based on sociograms are generally more productive than those arbitrarily designed.

Advantages of organizational charts are that they can contribute to sound organizational structures, map lines of decision-making authority, show formal lines of communication, and help employees understand their assignments, especially in relation to others (Box 10-4). Unfortunately, organizational charts can become obsolete quickly, show only formal relationships, do not show informal communications, may show how things are supposed to be rather than how they are, and may contribute to confusion about authority and status (Marquis and Huston, 1996; Marquis and Huston, 1998).

Chain of Command

The chain of command is the formal line of authority and communications. In hierarchies authority and communications flow from the top down and authority and responsibility are aligned. In the newer structures the chain of command is flatter, with communications flowing in all directions, and authority and responsibility delegated to the lowest operational level possible (Marquis and Huston, 1996, 1998; Swansburg and Swansburg, 1999).

Centrality

Centrality indicates the location of a position in an organization where frequent communication occurs. It is determined by organizational distance. Employees with small organizational distance are able to receive more information than those more peripherally located. Middle managers tend to have a broad view of the organization because of the centrality for receiving upward, downward, and horizontal communications (Marquis and Huston, 1996, 1998).

Unity of Command

Unity of command is represented by the vertical solid line between positions on an organizational chart. It indicates one person has one boss. This is still supported in some structures, as with primary nursing. However, health care professionals are getting increasingly involved with matrix organizations, where they answer to more than one person (Marquis and Huston, 1996, 1998; Swansburg and Swansburg, 1999).

Authority

Authority is the official power to act. It is the power to direct the work of others (Marquis and Huston, 1996, 1998).

Responsibility

Responsibility is a duty or an assignment. A person needs the authority necessary to accomplish the assignment (Marquis and Huston, 1996, 1998).

Accountability

Accountability is a moral responsibility. A manager may delegate responsibility but always remains accountable (Marquis and Huston, 1996, 1998).

Span of Management

Span of management has been of concern since biblical times. Exodus 18:13-26 is an account of how Moses had to deal with the problem of leading the Israelites out of Egypt. His father-in-law, Jethro, observed Moses counseling people all day long, while others had to wait long periods of time to tell Moses their problems. Jethro suggested that he delegate authority by selecting rulers of thousands, hundreds, fifties, and tens who would teach the people laws and leave Moses free to deal only with the exceptions.

Initial work with span of management was quantitative and attempted to devise formulas for determining the most desirable number of people reporting to a manager. General Hamilton, a British officer in World War I, concluded that managers at the lower levels could direct more people than those at higher levels. He thought an effective span of control was three to six others, especially at upper levels. Henri Fayol, a French industrialist and early writer about scientific management, used a similar philosophy to develop a hierarchy.

Hamilton's principle has been elaborated on by A.V. Graicunas, a Lithuanian management consultant whose mathematical analysis of potential relationships illustrates the complex social processes between managers and their staff associates and between the staff; the complexity especially increases with each additional staff associate. Graicunas demonstrated that as the number of staff associates responsible to a manager increases arithmetically, the number of potential interactions increases geometrically. The geometrical interactions can be classified as direct single relationships, direct group relationships, and cross-relationships. If a manager has two staff associates, x and y, the manager may have two direct single relationships, one with x and one with y. The manager may speak to either in the presence of the other, forming two group relationships. Two cross-relationships exist between x and y and between y and x. Consequently, there are six possible interactions between one manager and two staff associates—two direct, two group, and two cross. If a third staff associate is added, one direct relationship, seven group relationships, and four cross-relationships are added, making eighteen potential interactions.

Graicunas's formula is

$$R = n\left(\frac{2^n}{2} + n - 1\right).$$

R equals all types of relationships, and n equals the number of subordinates. The results are presented in Table 10-1.

Table 10-1 Variable Number of Associates and Resulting Number of Potential Relationships

Number of Associates	Number of Relationships
1	1
2	6
3	18
4	44
5	100
6	222
7	490
8	1,080
9	2,376
10	5,210
11	11,374
12	24,708
13	53,404
14	114,872
18	2,359,602

Graicunas's formula calculates the number of potential relationships. It does not deal with the actual frequency or the importance of the various relationships. In reality, the number of relationships with which a manager must deal is probably not so great. One might question whether the relationship in which the manager speaks to x in y's presence is different from speaking to y in x's presence. Graicunas considers them different psychological situations. It is unlikely that people will engage in all of the relationships that are theoretically possible. Nevertheless, Graicunas's formula illustrates how complex a situation can become as additional staff associates report to a manager.

The optimal span of management depends on many considerations that affect the time requirements for management. Managers' competence and qualifications and those of their staff's affect their time requirements. Some managers, because of their education and personal qualities, can work with more people than others. The better prepared staff associates are for their jobs, the less time managers must devote to teaching, clarifying responsibilities, and correcting mistakes.

Rapidly changing technology, procedures, and policies increase training problems and the need for problem solving. Availability of expert advice and services to managers can free their time and widen their span of management. However, a larger personal staff does not necessarily allow a broadening of the span of control because of the supervision required for those assistants. It may be more economical to increase the responsibilities of lower-level management. The greater the clarity of delegated authority, the less time it will take for managers to explain responsibilities and tasks. There will be less need for them to make decisions staff associates can make. If staff associates' tasks are not clearly defined, are unaccompanied by the necessary authority, or are beyond their competence, there will be an increase in time required for supervision.

Much of a manager's time is spent explaining plans, giving instructions, and receiving information about problems and progress. Clear and concise communications transmit information quickly and accurately. Much communication can be written. However, some situations cannot be handled with planning documents, policy statements, written reports, memoranda, or other written communications. These require personal contact. Some situations that could be handled by written communications may be better handled by personal contact. These might include delicate situations and instances where attitudes are involved. Personal contacts require considerable time.

If plans are clear, staff associates will know what is expected of them without frequently checking with the manager. If staff associates do their own planning, they will need more supervision. However, clear policies to guide their planning will reduce demands on the manager. Clear and complete policy statements can also simplify managers' decision making and allow expansion of their span of management. Deciding every problem individually requires more time than making policy decisions that anticipate problems.

The demands on the staff associate vary according to the complexity of functions. Standardization reduces time requirements because people know what is expected. Routine work requires less time than innovative work. But we can expect that as the degree of difficulty for performing a task satisfactorily increases, so does the demand on the manager. As the variability of functions increases, the manager must consider more factors and interrelationships; this takes more time. Interdependent functions require more management time than independent functions because of the increased need for coordination. The greater the geographical separation of personnel reporting to the manager, the more limiting the span of control. The greater the nonmanagerial responsibilities, the less time the manager has for management. Managers in flat organizational structures have a broader range of management than those in tall structures, and lower-level managers have a broader range than top management.

Levels of Management

Top-level managers generally make decisions with the help of few guidelines or structures, coordinate internal and external influences, and view the organization as a whole. They include the chief executive officer (CEO), the organization's highest ranking individual, and the top-level nurse manager. The titles vary but could include president, vice-president, or director. Middle-level managers conduct day-to-day operations with some involvement with long-term planning and policy making. Those titles also vary but could include supervisor, unit manager, or head nurse. First-level managers are concerned with a specific unit's work flow. They deal with immediate day-to-day operations problems. Those titles vary and may include case manager, nurse practice coordinator, primary care nurse, team leader, or charge nurse (Marquis and Huston, 1996, 1998; Rocchiccioli and Tilbury, 1998). The trend is to expand the span of top-level management to multiple organizations, of middle-level managers to multiple units, and of lower-level managers to cases across agencies.

Flat Versus Tall Structures

The flat structure is developed along horizontal dimensions according to the number of organizational functions that are identified separately. There are few levels of management. The tall structure is developed along vertical dimensions by use of the scalar process to define relationships between levels in an organization. Because there are advantages and disadvantages to both the flat and tall structures, it is best to maintain a reasonable balance of dimensions. Changes within the organization bring imbalance over time, so the organizational structure should be reviewed periodically.

The flat structure shortens the administrative distance between top and bottom levels in the organization, thereby minimizing distortions through shorter lines of communication. Communications are direct, simple, fast, and clearly apparent to employees. Another advantage of the flat structure is that large groups have a greater variety of skills available and are capable of solving a greater variety of problems. This structure is believed to contribute to high employee morale and help develop capable, self-confident staff. It lends itself to a democratic approach and general management, which are preferred by many people. This minimal social stratification is consistent with an egalitarian political and social philosophy, which is currently popular.

However, a flat structure may be impractical in large organizations. Large groups have more difficulty reaching a consensus and require more coordination. The flat structure places tremendous pressure on each manager because of the large amount of authority and responsibility and the high penalties for failures. Overburdened managers may not have the time to select, evaluate, and teach subordinates or the energy to think and plan. They may have difficulty making and communicating decisions. Socializing with staff associates may reduce their authority.

Tall structures lend themselves to authoritarianism, which is most effective in situations requiring rapid changes and precise coordination. In a tall structure messages from managers are given more attention than those from peers and consequently pass through levels quickly. The narrow range of management allows staff to evaluate decisions frequently. With small groups decision making takes less time, and there is more opportunity for members to participate and to understand the goals. Such interaction facilitates group cohesiveness.

Levels are expensive because of the large number of executives needed with high salaries. Each additional level makes communication more cumbersome. The more levels that communications pass through, the greater the distortion. Therefore a tall structure reduces the understanding between higher and lower levels and increases impersonality.

Decentralization Versus Centralization

Decentralization is the degree to which decision making is diffused throughout the organization. It is relative, for the degree of decentralization is larger when more important decisions affecting more functions are made at lower levels with less supervision. There are several factors to consider when determining the optimal degree of decentralization for an organization. Top management need a positive attitude toward decentralization, and they need competent personnel to whom they can delegate authority. The latter need access to the information necessary for decision making.

The number of people who need to interact to solve a problem should be considered. In general, the larger the organization, the greater the number of complex decisions that must be made, and that can overburden top management and delay decision making. Smaller, decentralized units reduce the number of decisions made by each manager and increase the time available to devote to each problem. Agencies tend to be more centralized during their early, formative years. If the agency gradually expands from within, it is more likely to remain centralized. An organization that grows rapidly through acquisitions is more likely to be decentralized; thus decentralization is more common in organizations with geographical dispersion of operations. Some functions lend themselves more readily to decentralization than do others; production, marketing, personnel, and some purchasing may be readily decentralized. In contrast, finances, accounting, data processing of statistics, and purchase of capital equipment are likely to remain centralized.

The profit center concept has developed from decentralization and has been popular since World War II. It is particularly characteristic of large organizations with multiple product lines. The organization is divided into manageable units called profit centers that are self-contained and have their own management and staff. Each unit competes with others for profits; this arrangement motivates managers to make decisions that will maximize profits. The manager has considerable freedom for making operational decisions. The profit center concept helps give meaning to decentralization by placing the responsibility for profit making on a number of managers instead of just top management.

The advantages of decentralization seem to outweigh the disadvantages. Decentralization increases morale and promotes interpersonal relationships. When people have a voice in governance, they feel more important and are more willing to contribute. This increased motivation provides a feeling of individuality and freedom that in turn encourages creativity and commits the individual to making the system successful. Decentralization fosters informality and democracy in management and brings decision making closer to the action. Thus decisions may be more effective because people who know the situation and have to implement the decision are the ones who make it. Because managers do not have to wait for the approval of their superiors, flexibility is increased, and reaction time is decreased. Fewer people have to exchange information; consequently, communications are swift and effective. Coordination improves, especially for services, production with sales, and costs with income. Products or operations that are minor to the total production receive more adequate attention. Plans can be tried out on an experimental basis in one unit, modified, and proven before used in other units. Risks of losses of personnel or facilities are dispersed.

Decentralization helps determine accountability. It makes weak management visible through semiindependent and often competitive divisions. Operating on the premise that people learn by doing, decentralization develops managers by allowing them to manage. A management pool can be developed that thereby eases the problem of succession. There is usually less conflict between top management and divisions. Decentralization releases top management from the burden of daily administration, freeing them for long-range planning, goal and policy development, and systems integration.

Nevertheless, several problems can also result from decentralization. An organization may not be large enough to merit decentralization, or it may be difficult to divide the organization into self-contained operating units. Top administrators may not desire decentralization. They may feel it would decrease their status, or they may question the abilities of the people to whom they would delegate. They may feel that most people prefer to be dependent on others and do not want decision-making responsibility. An increased awareness of division consciousness and a decrease in company consciousness may develop. Divisions may become individualized and competitive to the extent that they sacrifice the overall objectives for short-range profitability and work against the best interests of the

whole organization. Because of conflicts between divisions, it may be difficult to obtain a majority vote, and compromises may result. If the majority vote is delayed, it may come too late to be effective.

Decentralization involves increased costs. It requires more managers and larger staffs. Managers may be underused. Divisions may not adequately use the specialists housed at headquarters. Functions are likely to be duplicated between divisions and headquarters. Because decentralization develops managers, there are novice managers in the system who will make mistakes. Division managers may not inform top management of their problems. There are problems with control and nonuniform policies. Some restrictions on autonomy remain. Even with decentralization, top management remain responsible for long-range objectives and goals, broad policies, selection of key executives, and approval of major capital expenditures.

Departmentalization. Departmentalization results from span of management, division of work, and need for cooperation. Its primary purpose is to subdivide the organizational structure so that managers can specialize within limited ranges of activity. Organization of the agency influences group behavior and the effectiveness of the group. The objectives of the agency can be met most easily if the group is properly organized. Two common types of departmentalization are input and output. The input, or process, orientation includes function, time, and simple numbers as bases for departmentalization, whereas the output, or goal, orientation includes product, territory, and client divisions.

The input, or process-oriented, structure emphasizes specialization of skills. It reinforces professional skills by uniting people with similar expertise in the same department. For example, the focus may be on cardiac nursing, respiratory nursing, or transplant nursing, depending on the departmentalization. It is possible for professionals to advance within their field of expertise instead of advancing through the administrative hierarchy. Unfortunately, the process-oriented structure emphasizes professional skills over organizational goals. Conflicts increase as communication and cooperation decrease. Input organization provides less favorable training for general administrators than does a goal-oriented structure.

Departmentalization by function groups activities according to similarity of skills or a group of tasks necessary to accomplish a goal. Logical, simple, and commonly used, it facilitates specialization that contributes to economic operations. It groups functions that can be performed by the same specialists with the same type of equipment and facilities. Less demand for one product may be counteracted by a greater demand for another product. Consequently, staff, equipment, and facilities will have optimal utilization. The combination of administrative activities also is economical. One manager is responsible for all related activities; therefore coordination is improved because it is more easily achieved. The agency benefits from a few people with outstanding abilities, for only top management is able to coordinate the major functions. For example, the hospital may be organized by medical, surgical, and pediatric units.

Functional departmentalization also has its disadvantages. As the size of the agency increases, centralization may become excessive, making effective control more difficult. The necessary additional organizational levels may slow communications and delay decision making. It becomes more difficult to measure performance. Functional departmentalization does not provide good training for general managers. They become expert in their particular function, have little opportunity to learn about other functions, and may emphasize their previous function while deemphasizing others when they become general managers.

Time factors are another basis for organization. Acute care settings require coverage 24 hours a day, 7 days a week, whereas preventive services may require coverage for only 8 to 12 hours a day for 5 to 6 days a week at the most.

Grouping by numbers divides undifferentiated labor into manageable units. A certain number of workers is assigned to each manager. This method is common in underdeveloped countries but is disappearing in industrialized areas.

The output, or goal, structure emphasizes service to the client. It collects all the work for a project under one manager and reduces dependence on other units for needed resources. This allows considerable autonomy, and the client, workers, and goals are readily identified. Systems and procedures are highly standardized. Family planning, pregnancy counseling, and school health are examples of services available from some health departments.

Unfortunately, these units may stress their own goals while deemphasizing agency goals. Duplication of equipment and services may develop. Equipment may not be fully utilized, or smaller-scale equipment may be less effective. The grouping of various skills into one unit can reduce the expertise as professional reinforcement is weakened.

A product or group of closely related products may be the basis of organization for autonomous departments. Emphasis is on the product instead of the process. Improvement, expansion, and diversification of the product are possible because one manager is responsible for all activities affecting that specific product. In a large agency this could result in small, flexible units where functional groupings would be too complex. This method identifies profit responsibilities for specific products. Organization on the basis of products has become increasingly popular. It is common for schools of nursing to organize according to the "products" produced—medical nurses, surgical nurses, obstetrical nurses, pediatric nurses, psychiatric nurses, and community health nurses.

Departmentalization by territories is particularly useful for physically dispersed activities where branches provide similar services at each location. This method serves the local clients with greatest efficiency. Managers consider local circumstances that might be overlooked by a central manager. It uses local people who are familiar with local conditions. It reduces delivery time and may reduce transportation costs related to raw materials and finished products. It is particularly useful for production and sales and when perishability is a problem. However, financial management works best if centralized.

Departmentalization by client makes sense when service is important and the welfare of the client is of primary interest. For example, a clinic may have obstetrical, pediatric, and adolescent clinics. Clinics may be open nights and weekends for working people. Schools of nursing may offer night classes for working students. This better uses facilities and is more satisfactory to the client. However, pressure for special consideration and treatment of specific groups may exist, and coordination problems may increase (Galbraith, 1995).

Clusters. Clusters are two or three clinically similar units that share resources such as staff, equipment, and educational materials. Clustering fosters collaboration and consultation between nurses, decreases the isolation of decentralization, and enhances professional marketability by expanding knowledge and skills.

Units forming cluster work groups should develop written agreements describing how the cluster will work, emphasize sharing resources, and arrange for personnel to meet each other through inservices and social events. New staff should know that clustering is an expectation and should be oriented to the cluster units. Staff should be oriented to cluster units before being shared and during nonstressful times. Cross-training facilitates cost-effective, safe, and satisfying nursing services (Ouellette et al., 1989).

Line-Staff Relationships

Line authority. Line organization is the oldest type of structure. It is a chain of command or a manager–staff associate or leader-follower relationship. The manager delegates authority to a staff associate, who in turn delegates authority to the staff. This progression is the basis for the term *line authority.* The command relationship is a direct line between manager and staff associate and is depicted by a solid line on organizational charts. (See Figure 10-1.) The line positions are related to the direct achievement of organizational objectives. This arrangement fosters quick decision making because managers are given complete charge of their areas and at most would need to consult only with their immediate managers. Buck-passing is reduced, and authority relationships are clearly understood. The manager has the right to give orders, demand accountability, and discipline violators.

Staff authority. Staff support line-authority relationships and are advisory or service oriented in nature. Staff authority is depicted by a dashed line on an organizational chart. They handle details, locate required data, and offer counsel on managerial problems. Staff function through influence, for they do not have authority to accept, use, modify, or reject plans. Staff make the line more effective, but organizations can function without staff authority.

The two major categories of staff authority are personal and specialist. The personal category includes the assistant and general staff. The specialist staff is composed of advisory, service, control, and functional personnel.

Assistant staff. A personal staff member may be called an assistant, a staff assistant, or an administrative assistant and is responsible to one line manager. The assistant's chief purpose is to extend the line manager's capacity for completing a large amount of work by doing the more routine tasks that the manager would otherwise have to perform. The duties vary widely from one manager to another but might include such activities as mail answering, data collection for decision making, consolidation of information from various reports, preparation of documents, development of budgets, interpreting plans to others, and substitution for the manager at various meetings and functions.

Personal staff members have no specific functions. Their duties vary with the assignments. They do not act on their own behalf but rather as personal representatives of a manager. The only specific authority they have comes from a manager on a limited basis, usually for a specific job over a brief time span. With delegated authority, the personal staff member can give instructions in the manager's name and make decisions that affect the organization. It is important for assistants and the people with whom they work to know the extent of their influence. Misuses of and misunderstanding about the assistant are all too common. Some feel that the assistant is unnecessary and that the duties should be delegated to other line managers. When the assistant takes over tasks that belong to others, misunderstanding and poor cooperation result. Some assistants give the impression that they are the manager instead of just acting for one.

General staff. The general staff is composed of top administrators. The top administrator makes the decision after receiving input from these key people who together have the necessary expertise to make sound decisions for the agency. This is a coordinated group performing to maximize results. They serve in an advisory capacity by collecting and sharing information and are functional through their supervisory activities. The military has used this concept extensively, but it is relatively uncommon in business. Rotating general staff members to various areas and levels within the organization fosters an understanding of line problems.

Advisory staff. Advisory staff counsel line managers. They study problems, collect and analyze data, offer alternatives, and prepare plans. Their work may be accepted, rejected, or modified by the line manager. Although ideas are heard, they are not always implemented. This puts staff on the defensive, because they must sell their ideas. It is important that they counsel rather than suggest or confirm just what the line manager wants. Chances of an idea's being approved are increased when staff have discussed proposed recommendations with line managers who will be affected by the decision and have received their approval before presenting the plan to the top administrator. Careful evaluation of the plan is important. The better prepared the advice is, the more likely the staff will be heard and their suggestions implemented. If staff work in seclusion, secretly preparing reports without listening to or discussing them with line managers, they are likely to get a suspicious and negative reception from others.

Service staff. Service staff are not advisory. They perform a centralized service that has been separated from the line to prevent duplication and to allow more economical performance and good con-

trol. This includes dietary and laundry services in a hospital. Line managers rely on staff to get the job done. They do not do it themselves.

Control staff. Control staff also do not advise. They control by restraining line authority. They have direct or indirect control over certain line performance. They control directly by acting as an agent for a line manager or indirectly through procedural compliance and interpretation of policies and reports. Quality control personnel and the affirmative action officers are members of the control staff.

Functional staff. Functional authority exists when a specialist is given decision-making authority for specific activities outside the formal chain of command. This authority may be delegated to line, staff, or service managers and may be exercised over line, staff, and service personnel. The functional staff have limited line authority with power to determine standards in their areas of specialization and to enforce them. This authority is usually of an impersonal nature in the form of schedules, inspection reports, and written orders. It breaks the scalar chain and violates the principle that personnel should only be accountable to one superior. Although done in the interest of convenience and efficiency, it should be restricted, because it can damage line authority, destroy departmentalization, and create confusion.

Line-Staff Conflict

Conflict is likely to arise in any situation where two or more people must interact to get results. Line-staff conflicts occur when there is a lack of understanding of the roles and functions of others and when their lines of responsibility, accountability, and authority are not clear. Line and staff have different responsibilities and goals. Line is generalized, whereas staff is specialized. Line managers are likely to be pragmatists who have received their positions through competent service. They may not have much formal education but pride themselves on common sense. Staff managers probably consider themselves experts by virtue of their extensive formal education or experience in their areas of competence, or both. In addition to their differences in responsibilities and backgrounds, they also have different loyalties. Line managers identify with their work group; staff managers are inclined to be loyal to their professional colleagues and the company as a whole.

Line may complain that staff are impractical and too academic. Specialists sometimes are not aware of the total picture. Offered from a specialized, narrow viewpoint, their advice is impractical because it ignores the ramifications of a given situation. Staff managers may be viewed as outside interference who do not understand line or technical problems. Consultation causes delay. Line may accuse staff of not keeping them informed in an effort to keep them off balance and to claim credit for good ideas that turn out well, while blaming line for failures. Line may believe that staff lack responsibility or assume too much authority and run the show.

On the other hand, staff complain that line ignore them, resist staff assistance, or do not use them properly. Line may make decisions in specialized situations without consulting them or may seek their consultation too late. Line are often viewed as cautious, conservative, and resistant to new ideas. They want to do things as they have always done them. Staff may feel that line managers do not give them enough authority in their area of expertise and may be concerned about the way line implement staff's ideas and plans.

Improving Line-Staff Relationships

Certain conditions can be created to foster the integration of line-staff efforts. It is helpful if both line and staff have participated in determining objectives and plans and their implementation. Participation increases everyone's awareness of the overall goals to be accomplished. Each should be briefed on the roles and functions of other team members. The lines of responsibility, accountability, and authority should be clearly established and publicized. A team-effort atmosphere is more likely to prevail in structures that allow line and staff to interact with

open communications and that have a problem-solving focus.

ORGANIZATIONAL STRUCTURE
Formal

Although planning is the key to effective management, the organizational structure furnishes the formal framework in which the management process takes place. The organizational structure should provide an effective work system, a network of communications, and identity to individuals and the organization and should consequently foster job satisfaction. Agencies contain both informal and formal structures.

Informal

The informal organization comprises personal and social relationships that do not appear on the organizational chart. This might include a group that usually takes breaks together, works together on a particular unit, or takes a class together. Informal organization is based on personal relationships rather than on respect for positional authority. It helps members meet personal objectives and provides social satisfaction. People who have little formal status may gain recognition through the informal structure. Informal authority is not commanded through organizational assignment. It comes from the follower's natural respect for a colleague's knowledge and abilities.

Informal structure provides social control of behavior. The control can be either internal or external. If pressure is intended to make a member conform to group expectancies, it is internal. Kidding a member about her dirty shoelaces is an example. On the other hand, an attempt to control the behavior of someone outside the social group, such ás the manager, is external control.

The informal structure also has its own channels of communication, which may disseminate information more broadly and rapidly than the formal communication system. Unfortunately, the "grapevine" may contain rumors that are not authentic. The best way to correct an invalid rumor is for managers to provide accurate information. It is better that they not state that they are correcting the rumor, for in doing so they may strengthen it, and the facts that they give may be seen primarily as a subterfuge to refute the rumor.

The informal organizational structure is important to management. The manager should be aware of its existence, study its operating techniques, prevent antagonism, and use it to meet the agency's objectives.

Principles of Organization

Certain principles of organization help maximize the efficiency of the bureaucratic structure. The organization should have clear lines of authority running from the highest executive to the employee who has the least responsibility and no authority over others. There should be unity of command, with each person having only one boss. All employees should know to whom they report and who reports to them. The authority and responsibility of every individual should be clearly defined in writing. This reduces role ambiguity. Employees should know what is expected of them and what their limitations are. This prevents gaps between responsibilities, avoids overlapping of authority, and helps determine the proper point for decisions. Although many people do not think it is necessary to have their responsibilities in writing, it can be revealing to have them write what they believe their functions are and to note the duplicated efforts and jurisdictional disputes. When someone leaves an agency, it is not uncommon for no one to know exactly what that person did. Under such circumstances it can be difficult to justify replacement and to offer a meaningful orientation.

A clear definition of roles is necessary for effective delegation, but it does not guarantee it. Role clarity allows employees to know what is expected of them, to whom they report, and to whom they should go for help. In contrast, role ambiguity leads to anxiety, frustration, dissatisfaction, negative attitudes, and decreased productivity. Job descriptions increase productivity and satisfaction; however,

they should not be so exact that innovation is discouraged.

Patient care coordinators should delegate responsibility to the lowest level within the organization where there is enough competence and information for effective performance and appropriate decision making. Ordinarily, increased delegation and general rather than close supervision increase effective performance, production, and employee satisfaction.

The employee should be given formal authority commensurate with the responsibility delegated. It is not uncommon for managers to delegate authority and then undermine it by making decisions that were supposedly delegated. For example, if patient care coordinators are responsible for the quality of care given on their wards, they should not have to accept members on their team who have been hired by the director without consulting them. In turn, patient care coordinators should not tell patients that they can have a bath at a certain time without consulting the person assigned to give that bath. Preferably the nurse's aide and the patient will determine when various routines can be performed in accordance with the physician's orders and the manager's rationale.

The delegation of responsibility should be accompanied by accountability. Most effective control systems are probably those that provide feedback directly to the accountable person; this seems to increase motivation and provide direction. When feedback from a manager is given as performance evaluation rather than guidance, it tends to be nonfunctional and only infrequently contributes to improved performance. The delegation of functions with accompanying responsibility and accountability is particularly difficult for managers because they remain responsible for the actions of their staff associates. They are as responsible as their staff associates for their associates' performance. Consequently, the span-of-control principle becomes important.

There is a limit to the amount of coordination that can be achieved by one person, and it depends on several factors. One can coordinate more similar positions than dissimilar positions. The more the positions are interdependent, the more coordination is involved. A decreased span of control is required as the complexity of the staff associate's tasks increases. The stability of the agency should also be considered. If the agency has been functioning in a similar manner for a long time, the problems that arise have probably been solved before, and coordination is less difficult than in a changing situation where many new problems arise. The span of control is not likely to be uniform throughout an organization. Top-level managers of positions that are interdependent and dissimilar will probably have a smaller range of control than lower-level managers who are coordinating people doing similar tasks in a confined area. The span of control should not be so wide that managers do not have time to deal with the human relations aspects, such as giving workers individual attention, communicating information about the agency's policies, and listening to suggestions, grievances, and problems. On the other hand, they need a span of control large enough to keep them busy so they will not interfere with the delegated responsibilities of others.

Three types of divisions are commonly used to define span of control: (1) function or process, (2) product or service, and (3) region. Function is associated with specialization. Specialization may apply both to individuals and to departments or divisions. For example, one nurse may pass medications and give treatments, another may just start IVs, and the nurse's aides may give the baths and change linens. There may be a surgical nursing division with departments for specific types of surgery. It is preferable that if a person is accountable for more than one type of responsibility, they be similar. Efficiency is maximized if employees perform predominantly the tasks they do best and for which their proficiency will consequently continue to increase; they may, however, become bored. It is not uncommon to find individuals within an organization who are assigned several unrelated tasks. Although that may work for some people in given situations, it is not considered good organization, and their replacements are not likely to be successful. It is more viable to hire personnel to fill the or-

ganizational structure than to change the structure to fit personnel.

Having individuals perform the same or similar tasks and having divisions with specific functions can help expand the range of control. Similarly, having departments that provide specific services, such as cardiac intensive care, or produce certain products can influence the structure. Organization by geographical location becomes increasingly viable when operations are scattered. Many agencies use a combination of these methods. For instance, a school of nursing may be organized according to campuses (regional division); according to undergraduate, graduate, and continuing education (product division); according to inpatient, outpatient, medical-surgical, maternal-child, or some other service division; or it may assign individual faculty members to teach according to specialization (functional division).

The organizational structure should be flexible enough to permit expansion and contraction in response to changing conditions, without disrupting the basic design. It should also be kept as simple as possible, because additional levels of authority complicate communications and excessive use of committees may impede progress (Gailbraith, 1995).

The formal organizational structure is defined by executive decision determined by planning. It can be diagrammed to show the relationships between people and their positions. It describes positions, task responsibilities, and relationships. The two basic forms of formal organizational structure are the hierarchical, or bureaucratic, model and the adaptive, or organic, model.

Bureaucratic Structure

A hierarchy or bureaucracy is an organizational design to facilitate large-scale administration by coordinating the work of many personnel. It is associated with subdivision, specialization, technical qualifications, rules and standards, impersonality, and technical efficiency. In Figure 10-5, which illustrates a typical bureaucratic hierarchy, the managers are responsible to the director of nursing. The director in turn must answer to the hospital adminis-

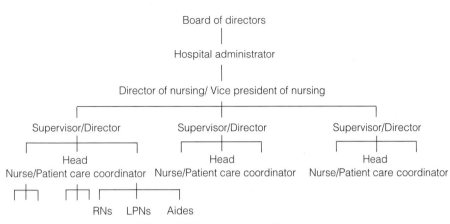

Figure 10-5 Bureaucratic hierarchy.

trator, who is accountable to the board of directors. Managers also have authority over their staff associates, who are accountable to their managers.

Dual management. Dual management separates technical and administrative responsibilities. It has one hierarchy in which technical professionals make technical decisions and control technical matters and another hierarchy in which management makes decisions about issues such as personnel and budget. This dual hierarchy gives equal status to managers and technical professionals. It provides a set of titles and job descriptions for each hierarchy.

Advantages of the bureaucratic structure. The bureaucracy is suited for work requiring large numbers of moderately educated people who perform routine tasks. Orientation is easy because workers do few procedures in a narrowly circumscribed job description. Orders can be transmitted quickly.

Disadvantages of the bureaucratic structure. There are disadvantages to the bureaucratic model. It may be detrimental to healthy personality patterns by predisposing people to the authoritarian leadership style, increasing insistence on the right of authority and status, and fostering a pathological need for control. If managers do not have the technical competence of their staff associates, they may feel insecure and fear their associates. Autocratic

behavior may become a defense mechanism through the use of power and fear strategies over staff members and the enforcement of norms through arbitrary or rigid rules. The use of reward and punishment to get desired behavior may alienate personnel. Self-serving behavior patterns may develop because of competition for the advancement of individual interests. A certain aloofness can result from the specialization that leads to impersonality. Personnel also may develop a ritualistic attachment to routine, develop monotony and alienation, become attached to subgoals, and show resistance to change (Gillies, 1994).

Line and Staff Structure

A line and staff organization develops when a simple line structure is altered to provide support to line authorities. The line functions are command and control. The staff functions are separate from the chain of command, involve specialization, and are supportive to line authorities. Staff do what the executives are too busy to do. It is the function of staff to serve the line organization and to submerge personal interests to champion the executives' long-range objectives. Staff can manage policies and procedures, in-service and continuing education, or quality improvement. (See Figure 10-1.)

Advantages of line and staff structures are that the executive can delegate tasks that the executive does not have the skill or time to do to functional experts. Disadvantages are that executives may get the credit for staff recommendations. Staff may increase their influence by usurping the authority of the executive by making decisions without consulting the executive. The executive may ignore the staff's recommendations.

Functionalized Line and Staff Structure

Staff have some authority over line executives. The staff expert responsible for a specific management function such as staffing, staff development, or quality improvement has authority to command line executives to implement staff plans.

The advantage is that this can increase staff morale. Unfortunately, when the line organization's chain of command is broken, conflict, confusion, and poor communications can result.

Adhocracy Organizational Models

Adhocracy, or organic, models are newer organizational frameworks that are more free form, open, flexible, and fluid than are older bureaucratic models. Boundaries separating internal and external relationships are more easily penetrated. Temporary affiliations such as consultantships are used.

The underlying assumptions, aims, and structures of adaptive frameworks are different from those of the bureaucratic model. They have resulted from behavioral research to facilitate job satisfaction and creativity, as well as efficiency. They give greater recognition to the informal structure and encourage the group to improve its own norms. Adaptive models recognize realities and are designed to meet them. They are less likely to use organizational charts, because the relationships are flexible. Job descriptions are also less meaningful. The models are ambiguous and consequently require being staffed by independent, self-reliant people who have a high tolerance for ambiguity. They lend themselves to participative management. Motivation is derived from system needs, task-related factors, and peer pressure rather than from supervision. Rewards are based on individual and group results rather than subjective evaluations

from managers. Adhocracy comes from ad hoc committee. Adhocracy structures are loosely structured project organizations.

Task forces. Task forces are sometimes used for special projects. The task force has a mission, a leader, and a projected completion date. To be most successful, the project should be short range. There must be a pool from which to select talent, and task force members should be readily reabsorbed by the organization. Personnel are relieved of their usual tasks and given a temporary assignment, usually to investigate, analyze, research, and plan. They are less often used for decisions and actions. The task force allows personnel with special qualifications to combine their expertise and concentrate on a project in a manner that would not be possible while performing their usual duties. Structural flexibility is accomplished by adding members when their potential contribution is high and removing them when their specific talents are no longer required. It can be an efficient problem-solving method and can offer training opportunities for managers. It can unleash creative energies and introduce innovations.

On the other hand, it can be disruptive to the organization. Key personnel may be away from their jobs for unknown lengths of time. As members experience different qualities of supervision by moving from one team to another, they may become more critical of the less capable manager. Assignment to a task force may make employees consider themselves better than their peers. They may feel independent and detached from their usual work groups. It is not uncommon for personnel to be promoted and removed from their original departments after the task force responsibilities are completed. Reabsorbing the task force member back into the organization is sometimes difficult, and that realization is almost certain to increase the employee's anxiety. Or what began as a short-range, problem-solving task force may become an unwanted permanent arrangement.

Project management. Project organizational design is used for large, long-range projects where a number of project groups are developed and administered through the various phases of their existence. This method is useful for one-time projects when the task is unfamiliar and complex; when considerable planning, coordination, high-risk research, and development are involved; and when there is a long lead time between planning and production.

There are several types of project units. The general, or functional, management type is the most common. Project activities are done within functional groups that are managed by department heads. The general manager coordinates the activities. With this type of arrangement there is no strong central project authority, and consequently decisions are likely to be made to the advantage of the strongest functional group rather than in the best interests of the project. Lead time and decision-making time are increased because the coordination and approval of all functional groups are required.

Aggregate management has appointed managers who have their own staff and full authority over their projects. All people involved with a project report directly to the manager, giving the manager a high degree of control over each project. This allows rapid reaction time and reduces lead time. Project management is highly regarded by outside sources, and the people involved tend to be loyal to the project because it is their only job at the time.

There are also disadvantages to aggregate management. The people involved are interested in the technology to do the project, but they do not develop the technology, nor do they develop the essential functional organizations. There tends to be little technical interchange between projects and inefficient use of production elements. Because they are managing just one project each, managers cannot keep all production elements in use at all times. With this management method, production elements are not shared with other projects, and there is consequently duplication of functional activities between projects. There is also a lack of career continuity. Anxiety may increase toward the completion of a project, because project personnel do not know where they will be assigned next. It is difficult to balance workloads as projects begin and

reach completion. Aggregate management is not often used.

The matrix organization combines concepts from both functional and aggregate organizations. It departmentalizes functions and shares authority among functional heads and project managers. The project manager uses people assigned to functional areas to complete the project while they are still assigned to the functional area. Thus the worker has two bosses. Reaction time is quite rapid. Matrix organization seems well received by outside contacts. It does not slow down the development of technology. It facilitates the interchange of technology between projects and provides career continuity because personnel remain in their functional areas. However, conflicts can arise between project and functional managers. Workers have two bosses, and accountability becomes diffuse (Davis and Lawrence, 1977).

In still another design the project manager may monitor the project but serve only in an advisory capacity to the general manager. The project director controls through influence. The director of the project has responsibility without authority. The workers once again report to one boss, the general manager.

Project management offers several advantages. It visualizes projects and focuses on results. It produces good control over the project, shorter development time, improved quality, and lower program costs. This yields higher profit margins and good customer relations. Project management facilitates coordination between functional areas and good mission orientation for people working on the project. It can help elevate morale and develop managers.

There are also numerous disadvantages to project management. It requires changes in patterns of interaction and disrupts the established patterns of hierarchy, span of management, unity of control, resource allocation, departmentalization, priorities, and incentives. Work groups are disrupted, and interfunctional groups develop. Duplication is common. Interdepartmental consensus is used and tends to increase fears of invasion from other departments.

Confusion may arise from authority's ambiguity as new patterns for control develop. Power is one's ability to affect the behavior of others. Authority is power derived from one's position. Influence may be power without authority. Sometimes project managers use authority; at other times they have to use influence. Personnel may report to more than one person with varying patterns of authority. Multiple levels of management are more likely to be problems for project management than functional management. Authority's ambiguity frequently frustrates personnel.

Project managers tend to depend on functional managers for resources. This dependence can create a conflict over those resources. Hence the project may deplete the functional department of premium professional talent, and the competition for talent may disrupt the stability of the organization and interfere with long-range interests by disrupting traditional business. Some professionals complain that incentives for higher-level ego needs are not met. Project personnel are more likely to be anxious about the loss of their jobs, frustrated by make-work assignments between projects, and confused by a lack of role definitions. They are concerned about setbacks in their careers and upset by the apparent lack of concern about their personal development. Conflicts of allegiance result and undermine loyalty to the organization. Shifting personnel can disrupt their training. What is learned may not be transferred from one project to another. Long-range planning suffers when people are more concerned with their temporary projects.

Several factors contribute to the failure of project management. The most common include an initially unsound basis for the project, poor selection of the project manager, lack of agency support, use of inappropriate management techniques, poor role and task definitions, and no projected termination date.

Precautions can be taken to prevent failure. Planning is always essential. The project should be well conceived with its scope outlined and the end results described. Well-qualified managers should be selected, and their roles defined. It is helpful if their executive rank ensures responsiveness from others. They need the authority to control funds, budgeting, and scheduling for the project; to select

subcontractors; and to be able to select, add, or eliminate staff as necessary. They should participate in major managerial activities, especially in policy-making and other decisions related to their projects.

Because functional managers may not wish to take directions from a lesser executive who is suddenly a project manager, top management might select people from high positions of responsibility, assign them impressive titles, support their dealings with functional managers, and have them report to a manager on the same or higher level than the functional managers.

One of the first responsibilities of the project manager is to staff the project. Sometimes several projects compete for the same talent. Functional managers may not be willing to release the requested personnel, or the person may not want to transfer. People may be hesitant to transfer because (1) there is a division of responsibilities between functional and project organizations, (2) the job is less desirable, or (3) they fear unemployment at the end of the project. Management can offer salary increases as incentives. Promotional opportunities may arise from the additional management structure required for the project. Special efforts should be made to relocate people as they are phased out of the project, thus maintaining security. All of these measures, however, are expensive.

Next, the project manager sets time controls. The manager determines what tasks are required from each department to complete the project and what their proper sequence is. Each department itemizes what it needs to know from other departments and then commits itself to an estimate of the time required to do its part. An overall schedule can be developed by use of critical-path scheduling. It should be checked frequently to compare actual progress against the projected deadlines. This network can be the focal point of project implementation. Managers develop information links that serve the project and help them prepare to replan jobs as project dynamics change.

The project manager also needs to determine cost controls. The most sound decisions can be made by dividing the comprehensive cost summary into work packages. Then technical decision makers can offer commitment reports, and the project manager can act on the approximate cost data. After reviewing the detailed estimated costs and current expenses, the manager can switch staff from less productive duties to duties that will reduce costs.

To maintain quality control, the manager defines the project objectives in quality standards, describes performance criteria, and monitors individual and project progress against the standards. It is helpful to reward responsibility and performance and to try to accommodate staff's personal goals while working toward the objectives of the project.

Matrix. Matrix organizational designs try to combine the advantages of project and functional structures. The functional line organization provides support for the project line organization. In a functional organization the functional manager has the authority to determine and rate goals, select personnel, determine pay and promotions, make personnel assignments, and evaluate personnel and the project. Managers are responsible to their superiors but work independently. In a matrix organization the functional manager shares those responsibilities with the project manager, because management by project objectives is important to the matrix organization. Initially, the functional manager may experience a sense of loss in status, authority, and control. Therefore it is important for managers to be able to persuade others by using their personal qualities and knowledge of the program (Figure 10-6). The functional and project managers need each other's cooperation for approvals and sign-offs. The intent in the matrix organization is to have the decision making as far down in the organizational structure as possible. This encourages group consensus. Most decisions are made at the middle-management level, thus freeing top administration for long-range planning. Matrix organizations are more decentralized with fewer levels of decision making and less rigid adherence to formal rules than line and staff or functionalized structures. (See Figure 10-6.)

The matrix organization increases the amount of contact between individuals, and its complexity makes conflict inevitable. Increased communications are essential. Recognizing and dealing with differences are necessary, because collaborative behavior is needed. Team building between departments is encouraged, and consultants are used as connections between parts. Managers need human relations training. Organizational charts showing task responsibilities and levels of responsibility may reduce conflict.

Matrix organizations foster flexibility in dealing with change and uncertainty. They enable managers to balance conflicting objectives by maximizing technical excellence through efficient use of resources. By moving decision making down in the organization, opportunities are provided for personal development and motivation. Commitment is improved, and top management is freed for long-range planning.

Because people are more familiar with bureaucratic structures, there is considerable need to orient personnel to the matrix structure and philosophy. Rigid lines of authority, inflexible boundaries separating jobs and divisions, unambiguous resource allocation to divisions, and specific loyalties that exist in bureaucracies are not appropriate in dynamic organizations with overlapping and sometimes contradictory interests and goals. But because of multiple and often ambiguous roles, some personnel may get frustrated and feel insecure. Matrix structures are increasingly common in health care systems. Because of the generalized education and time spent with patients, nurses are well qualified to coordinate the clinical and nonclinical care for patients. That may involve integrating care from nutritionist, occupational therapist, pharmacist, physician, physiotherapist, and social worker (Davis and Lawrence, 1977) (Box 10-5).

Collegial management. Collegial management restricts monocratic authority by maintaining a division and balance of power among the top management group through collective responsibility. It is most commonly used in Germany and Holland but is also used in Austria, Switzerland, and France. Consequently, it is also referred to as European-style management. The directors usually represent

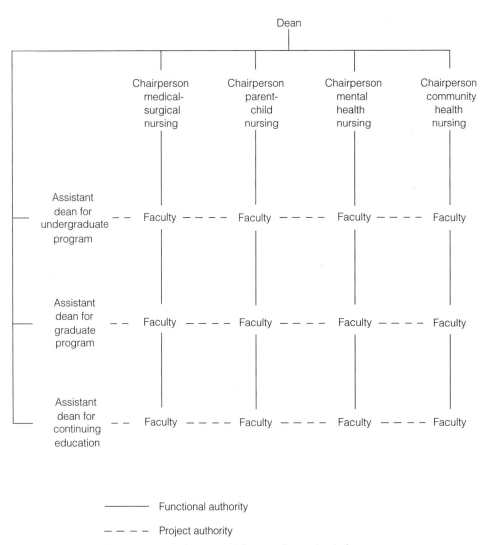

Figure 10-6 Adaptive model: matrix for a school of nursing.

functional areas of the organization. They may or may not have a chairperson. If so, the chairperson may be the first among equals and merely speak for the directors, may coordinate the others, or may be recognized as the general manager or chief executive. The directors may have vice-directors.

The decision-making process varies from one country to another, but in every case it is the board that makes policy decisions. Essentially, the directors need to persuade each other. Although chair-persons may not have strong decision-making powers, they do have strong veto powers.

Collegial management has several strengths. It limits autocratic leadership, breeds democratic management, and ensures representation of each functional area. Because of their collective responsibility, directors are better informed about the other functional areas; this broadens the approach to problem solving. Collegial management prevents precipitous decisions, encourages long-range plan-

Box 10-5	ADVANTAGES AND DISADVANTAGES OF MATRIX

Advantages	Disadvantages
Manages dual demands	Dual authority—1 line, 1 project
Good for complex work	Complicated
Focuses on products and functions	May be viewed as confusing
Good for uncertain environment	Complex structure
Good for nonroutine technologies	Need well-educated personnel
High interdependence between functions	Complex communications
Collaborative management	Advanced interpersonal relationship skills needed
Flexible, efficient use of scarce resources	Group and teamwork skills needed
Adaptive	Role conflicts
Innovative	Role ambiguity
Decisions close to operations	Requires frequent meetings
Fluidity	Time consuming
Improved interpersonal skills and conflict management leading to achievement and job satisfaction	Special learning required in conflict management and interpersonal relationships

Data from Davis and Lawrence, 1977; Decker and Sullivan, 1992; Ellis and Hartley, 1995; Gillies, 1994; Grohar-Murray and DiCroce, 1997; Huber, 1996; Loveridge and Cummings, 1996; Nader and Tushman, 1997; Swansburg, 1996; Swansburg and Swansburg, 1999; Yoder-Wise, 1999.

ning, and fosters objective appraisal of the functions. Camaraderie is possible.

Collegial management also has limitations. The need for consensus can slow decision making. Consensus based on compromise may be an inferior solution. Logrolling results when directors give reciprocal support to programs that are not viable. Collegial management requires considerable, expensive executive time for what may be relatively minor matters or what may be others' functional affairs; this results in a diffusion of responsibility. The management process may even cease at times, especially when policies and programs are to be determined. Differences of opinions may smolder and lead to rudeness and cold wars. Communications are more likely to be vertical than horizontal. Consequently, coordination is a problem. The encouragement of group action may stifle a strong creative director. Because of the inherent problems in collegial management, some organizations are moving toward committee management with an executive to coordinate policy.

Shared governance.   Shared governance was one of the more radical changes during the 1980s. It is an accountability-based governance system for professionals that empowered individuals within the decision-making system and increased nurses' authority and control over their nursing practice. Group professional communications took on an equalitarian structure when joint practice committees were developed to assume power and accountability for decision making. A major resistance has come from nurse managers who were reluctant to change their roles from autocratic decision makers to coaches, consultants, teachers, collaborators, and facilitators of shared decision making. A typical model of shared governance is a committee structure where representative staff nurses belong to nursing committees that are assigned specific management or clinical functions. The committees are typically composed of a staff nurse or administrative chair appointed by an administrator and representatives of staff and administration. The nursing committee chairs and nursing administrators compose the nursing council or cabinet that makes the final decisions on recommendations from the committees.

Participatory management. Participatory management is the foundation for shared governance. However, it allows participation only in decision making over which someone else has the power to make the final decisions. For this model, representative staff nurses are members of forums or committees for designated issues. Managers are also members. Recommendations go to an executive committee, which has staff representation, as well as manager membership. The nurse executive retains the decision-making authority and may or may not agree with committee recommendations.

Self-governance. Self-governance goes beyond participatory management and shared governance to structures that allow nursing staff to govern themselves. These professional practice models place autonomy, authority, and control for services to clients with the professionals providing the care. Representative staff nurses are members of councils with authority for specified functions. The council chairs make up the management committee charged to make the final operational decisions for the organization. Bylaws are developed to specify the authority, responsibility, communication channels, and coordination of the self-governance structure. The councils have the authority to make decisions and are responsible for the results. It is important to clarify what decisions councils will make, what shared decisions will be made by staff and managers, and what decisions will be the responsibility of administration. Councils typically have functional accountability for practice, governance, nursing professional development, peer behavior, and governance with a coordinating council (Marquis and Huston, 1996; Porter-O'Grady and Finnigan, 1984; Yoder-Wise, 1999).

Systems. Systems design is an adaptive organizational model. It has been facilitated by the use of computers. The systems approach can be applied to bureaucracies that are considered closed systems or to adaptive models viewed as open systems. The design develops from the flow of work and information. It considers relationships, time, and decision points.

Mixed model. A mixed model may be the most viable. Bureaucratic design can work very well for routine functions. Adaptive designs may be more useful for research and development. However, the success of any organizational design largely depends on the manager's skills.

Corporate model. A corporation is any group of people who act as one body. Corporations are required to register their articles of incorporation, which specify the purposes and functions of the organization. Corporations may be private or public and proprietary (for-profit) or not-for-profit. A public corporation is subject to government regulations, may issue and trade stock, and is expected to return a profit to the owners of the stock. Most individual investor-owned hospitals are operated for a profit but are privately owned, not public, corporations. However, many hospital management firms are publicly held corporations that manage both for-profit and not-for-profit individual hospitals. Most private corporations are smaller than public corporations.

Corporate growth leads to mergers, buyouts, and other business transactions to increase the value of the business. Large multihospital corporations have emerged within the health care arena. Nurses have opportunities for leadership and management positions in the corporations and may operate their own corporations.

The physician's share of the health care dollar has increased in the newer delivery systems as the hospital's share has decreased and services have moved out of the hospital. The services still tend to be illness based, medically dominated, interventive, and expensive. Decentralization using holding companies with multiple subcorporate entities that provide a range of services is the trend. This trend has created a need to restructure nursing.

For nursing service to be a corporate entity it must be able to sustain its own activities without dependence on other units. Nursing practice must be clearly defined and its contribution to profitability clearly identified. The holding company's mission and purposes must be reflected in the philosophy, purpose, and objectives of the nursing service corporate entity. The relationship to the marketplace and plans to meet market demands should be outlined. Remuneration of nurses should reflect the value of their work in the marketplace.

As nursing becomes increasingly decentralized and incorporated, it is increasingly important to create a network instead of preserving a pyramid. A coordinating council may centralize the activities of individual councils for practice, education, research, and quality assurance. It is an opportunity for the chairpersons of the individual councils to meet together to discuss issues, coordinate councils, and make decisions that affect the entire corporate nursing entity.

The corporate nursing staff should meet at least once a year to (1) review, revise as necessary, and approve as appropriate the nursing staff bylaws; (2) review, discuss, and revise as appropriate the nursing organization's long- and short-range planning process, goals, and objectives; (3) debate issues of concern and vote on them as appropriate; (4) review, discuss, and approve the coordinating council's activities; (5) provide opportunities for informal networking; and (6) provide education sessions (Porter-O'Grady and Finnigan, 1984).

Mergers.   A merger essentially means that an organization will join its assets with another. Economics are forcing health care organizations to seek mergers, cut staff, and emphasize cost-effectiveness over patient care and service quality. There are some multiinstitutional relationships for sharing assets such as a central laundry service, a purchasing department, or a home health agency. However, mergers usually restructure the relationship of one health care organization with another. These activities can stir many feelings among personnel.

It is appropriate for the nurse manager to assess attitudes toward the merger through a questionnaire, personal interviews, or focus groups. Only personnel who are supportive of the merger should be assigned to leadership positions to accommodate it. Managers need to keep staff informed about the changes. Open communications can help minimize pluralistic views about the merger. Staff may need assistance to understand the new organization culture, and managers can help staff understand the unique qualities of the merging agency. Managers should periodically assess how personnel are responding to the merger, identify problems, and do problem solving (Kooi, White, and Smith, 1988).

Health care networks.   Health maintenance organizations (HMOs) are associations of health care professionals and facilities that provide a health care package for a fixed sum of money that was paid in advance for a specific period of time. The HMO contracts with health care professionals and facilities to provide the care. The client cannot usually seek care outside of the contract. Primary care physicians see the client first and decide if a specialist is needed. Consequently, patients are not guaranteed the right to see a specialist for consultation or care unless the primary care physician gatekeeper approves.

Preferred provider organizations (PPOs) are groups of health care professionals and hospitals that contract with an employer, insurance company, or other third party payer to provide health care to a group. The services are not fixed or prepaid and allow more customer choice than an HMO. Consequently, it is more expensive, and customers pay an even greater percentage of fees for services rendered outside those provided by the PPO.

Individual practice associations (IPAs) provide insurance coverage, health care services rates, and bill a fee-for-services.

Physician hospital organizations (PHOs) allow a hospital and the medical staff to have joint managed care contracts. They vary in terms of administration, credentialing, governance, managed care contracting, and structure. The impetus is usually from the hospital, which incorporates a not-for-profit organization with a hospital and a physician board. Medicare fraud, abuse issues, non-profit status, and balance of power between hospitals and

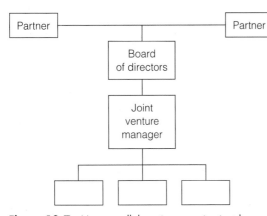

Figure 10-7 Merger collaborative organizational structure.
Modified from Nadler DA, Gerstein MS, Shaw RB et al.: *Organizational architecture: designs for changing organizations*, p. 94, San Francisco, 1992, Jossey-Bass.

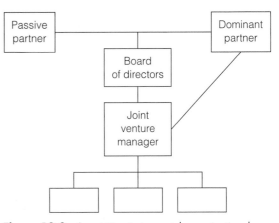

Figure 10-8 Acquisition instrumental organizational structure.
Modified from Nadler DA, Gerstein MS, Shaw RB et al.: *Organizational architecture: designs for changing organizations*, p. 96, San Francisco, 1992, Jossey-Bass.

physicians are issues driving the legal and political perspectives to manage risks and provide what the health care market is demanding. The management skills and infrastructure are critical to the survival of PHOs that will have to develop networks to provide a broader service spectrum to remain competitive. An external focus and customer orientation will be important to success. Care management, risk management, information management, and relationship management are all important components of PHOs to help provide cost-effective care in a timely manner (First Health Associates Consulting Team Web site, accessed June 5, 1999).

Management service organizations (MSOs) provide medical practice management, physician recruitment, information systems, billing and collection systems, quality monitoring, and other services (Pelinet Internet Services, Pelican Coast Publishers Web site, 1997).

Mergers occur when one organization purchases another of approximately the same size. Acquisitions occur when one organization is considerably larger than the other. Both are used to acquire complementary services or products that are connected by common clients and technologies. By increasing the size, they increase organizational power and leverage through products or services, market access, distribution networks, capital access, econo-

mies of scale, technology, people, diversification, name and reputation, and management resources. They gain financial benefits by eliminating employees who have responsibilities that overlap both entities. This makes employees nervous, strains organizational cultures, and often brings out the worst of behaviors. Nurse managers need to resolve their own negative feelings and help employees understand and adjust to the changes (Douglass, 1996) (Figures 10-7 and 10-8).

The objective of integrated health care systems is to keep people healthy and treat them in the lowest cost setting when necessary, thus making primary care and managed care pivotal (Figure 10-9). Efforts are toward improving health care outcomes at reduced health care costs while ensuring patient satisfaction. This requires inventing and managing new health care systems. There is a trend toward a reduction in the numbers of managers and the levels of management, retention and training of workers with multiple skills, data-based decision making, and continuous quality improvement. Hospitals are joining together and linking health promotion, clinics, ambulatory care, acute care, home care, and long-term care into integrated health care (Grohar-Murray and DiCroce, 1997). A moderate rate of integration seems desirable. In cases where the parent moves in quickly and tries to

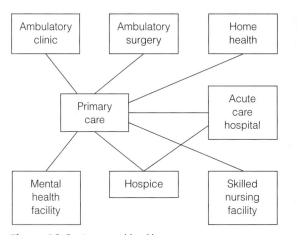

Figure 10-9 Integrated health care system.
Modified from Grohar-Murray ME, DiCroce HR: *Leadership and management in nursing*, p. 144, Stamford, Conn, 1997, Appleton & Lange.

Box 10-6	DEGREES OF INTEGRATION

None

Separate holding

Loosely coupled

Moderate

Coupled

Operationally integrated

Complete

Consolidated

Modified from Nadler DA, Gerstein MS, Shaw RB et al.: *Organizational architecture: designs for changing organizations*, San Francisco, 1992, Jossey-Bass.

integrate in a fast and intense way by imposing its own policies and procedures, the management of the acquired agency often leaves, followed by the technical staff; therefore the parent loses the leverage that was to be gained from the acquisition. If the integration occurs too slowly, people get highly stressed, not knowing what is going to happen to them. This brings out undesirable behaviors, and the best people may accept other positions.

When there is not integration, the parent may adopt a hands-off approach and let the acquiree operate its separate holdings. With the possible exceptions of limited financial controls and reviews of productivity at the board level, the acquiree remains autonomous. In coupled integrations, some of the activities or functions of the acquired agency are integrated with the parent, whereas others are left independent and separate. In loosely coupled acquisitions, a minimum of activities are integrated. Most are left separate and independent. The acquiree functions largely as an independent entity. Moderately coupled integrations have an increasing amount of integration. Operationally integrated organizations still can be identified as entities, but the key procedures and operations are tightly linked to the parent organization. With complete integration, the organizations are consolidated or merged into one (Box 10-6).

Assessment phase. During the assessment phase the organization should assess its strategic plan, its ability to handle the operating requirements for a joint venture, and readiness to manage change. Is the joint venture an appropriate strategic action to address the problem, or are there less complicated alternatives? Is the problem temporary, not meriting a joint venture, or a long-term problem that could best be addressed by integration?

All partners should agree to the long-term goals and compatibility. Convergent objectives are those commonly shared and are probably the primary reason the joint venture is being considered. Compatible objectives are those held by each organization that are unique to it and are compatible with other objectives. Objectives in potential conflict require the most careful assessment. They may be differences in management style, strategies, or whatever presents a potential threat to the viability of the venture. It is better to articulate the potential problems and address them before the joint venture than to be surprised by them later (Box 10-7).

The internal operating and management requirements for the joint venture should be carefully considered. Partners will need to be cooperative and flexible while sharing responsibilities. It can be difficult for some managers to give up power and control. People are likely to resist change. Having a specific plan for the implementation of the change can help manage the change. Is the organization ready to manage change? Is there a deliberate plan of action to minimize disruption during the implementation of change? Is there understanding of the relationship of this venture to the strategic plan? Is there an understanding of the opportunities being sought? Does the other organization provide the resources, skills, or other attributes that are needed? Is the other organization financially sound, trustworthy, and respected? Are the management styles and cultures compatible? Are the people cooperative, flexible, skilled in conflict resolution, and experienced in joint ventures? Are people willing to make a commitment, learn, and make comparable contributions? Do people understand the joint venture's business?

Planning and design phase. After agreeing to integrate, partners need to plan and design the joint venture. The main work in the second phase is to plan the structure, staffing, management style, and support systems. How involved is each partner with the operations? Who makes what decisions? Who reports what to whom? How will the venture be staffed? How do the organizations relate to each other? Chances for success increase when one partner primarily manages the joint venture. The joint venture general manager needs autonomy to act

quickly to achieve the responsiveness required to be successful. When both partners are heavily involved in the operations, it slows down decision making. They need compatible styles and orientations, common understanding of the joint venture's necessities, and skills at conflict management and human relationships. Achieving the necessary relationship takes considerable commitment, time, and effort to make it work. The managers need to be able to handle a lot of ambiguity and uncertainty. A participative style that solicits input from all partners tends to get more commitment to plans than an autocratic style. The venture manager should be positioned as the leader for the venture and as the person who is in control. The venture manager and staff need to establish an independent identity and allegiance to the venture. People from both partner organizations in a collaborative structure may staff the venture. In general, however, staff should not be employed from the passive partner organization, because that can create allegiance problems and managerial interference from the passive partner. Staff should be qualified to do the required tasks, should be viewed as competent, and should be respected. A compensatory reward system should be consistent with the performance criteria and expectations of the venture.

Implementation phase. The implementation focuses on a successful start-up and implementation of the venture. It deals with the organization's culture and major organizational change that typically involves issues of power, anxiety, and control. During change, individuals and groups often compete for power. Change threatens the balance of formal and informal power. As uncertainty increases, so does the political behavior of people wanting to protect their position and gain power. Competition for control emerges. If the venture is expected to be successful, managers may compete for positions and promise appointments to their staff based on networks rather than job requirements. If failure is anticipated, managers may protect themselves, thus keeping commitment, energy, and resources from the venture and contributing to a self-fulfilling prophecy for failure. During organizational change, people are usually concerned about what will happen to them, become anxious, and experience stress. The redistribution of people, material, tasks, and systems during the change usually results in some loss of managerial control and a deterioration of performance. Managers can help shape the political dynamics associated with change by supporting the change and by getting the support of key power groups. Providing anchors to anxious people can help stabilize the organization. Managers can give assurances about what is not going to change, warn people in advance of what changes will occur and the need for the change, and send consistent messages.

Development phase.   Then people in the venture need to be developed. It is important that they have identity with the venture and independence from the partner organizations. The venture should be seen as distinct from the partner organizations. Building allegiance to the venture and severing formal ties to the partner organizations are necessary. People must not think they can just return to the parent organization if the going gets rough. They need commitment to the venture. The strategic plan can help people assess where they fit into future options.

People need to be developed to deal with the characteristics of future organizations. We can expect that organizations will be networks that cooperate with each other to survive in a competitive market. Organizational forms will be fluid and transitory with fuzzy boundaries. Social and technical systems will be used to create high-performance work systems. Teams will be the norm at all levels and will have relative autonomy. Norms and values will dominate over rules and direct supervision and will facilitate the cohesion necessary to achieve coordination and direction. There will be an emphasis on system-level learning and preparing people to understand the broad strategic issues and the specific tasks to accomplish the strategic plan (Nadler, Gerstein, Shaw et al., 1992). John Cotter (1995) reminds us of Pareto's Law, which says that 20% of the factors in most situations account for about 80% of what happens and advises us to pay attention to the 20% of the factors shaping the future that really matter

and to give attention to the 20% of the personnel who will make 80% of what happens happen.

CHAPTER SUMMARY

Chapter 10 covered the following:
Factors Affecting Organizational Structures
Organizational Charts
     Chain of Command
     Centrality
     Unity of Command
     Authority
     Responsibility
     Accountability
     Span of Management
     Levels of Management
     Flat versus Tall Structures
     Decentralization Versus Centralization
         Departmentalization
         Clusters
     Line-Staff Relationships
         Line authority
         Staff authority
         Assistant staff
         General staff
         Advisory staff
         Service staff
         Control staff
         Functional staff
     Line-Staff Conflict
     Improving Line-Staff Relationships
Organizational Structure
     Formal
     Informal
     Principles of Organization
     Bureaucratic Structure
         Dual management
         Advantages of the bureaucratic structure
         Disadvantages of the bureaucratic structure
     Line and Staff Structure
     Functionalized Line and Staff Structure
     Adhocracy Organizational Models
         Task forces
         Project management
         Matrix
         Collegial management

Shared governance
Participatory management
Self-governance
Systems
Mixed model
Corporate model
Mergers
Health care networks
Assessment phase
Planning and design phase
Implementation phase
Development phase

REFERENCES

Cotter JJ: *The 20% solution: using rapid redesign to create tomorrow's organizations today*, New York, 1995, John Wiley & Sons.

Davis SM, Lawrence PR: *Matrix*, Reading, Mass, 1977, Addison-Wesley.

Decker PJ, Sullivan EJ: *Nursing administration: a micro/macro approach for effective nurse executives*, Norwalk, Conn, 1992, Appleton & Lange.

Douglass LM: *The effective nurse: leader and manager*, ed 5, St. Louis, 1996, Mosby.

Ellis JR, Hartley CL: *Managing and coordinating nursing care*, ed 2, Philadelphia, 1995, Lippincott.

First Health Associates Consulting Team: *Positioning your PHO to meet changing market demands* (http://www.fha-inc.com/v1.3_positioning_your_pho.htm), accessed June 5, 1999.

Galbraith JR: *Designing organizations: an executive briefing on strategy, structure, and process*, San Francisco, 1995, Jossey-Bass.

Gillies DA: *Nursing management: a systems approach*, ed 3, Philadelphia, 1994, Saunders.

Gore C, Murray K, Richardson B: *Strategic decision-making*, London, 1992, Cassell.

Grohar-Murray ME, DiCroce HR: *Leadership and management in nursing*, Stamford, Conn, 1997, Appleton & Lange.

Huber D: *Leadership and nursing care management*, Philadelphia, 1996, Saunders.

Kooi D, White RE, Smith HL: Managing organizational mergers, *JONA* 18:10-16, March 1988.

Loveridge CE, Cummings SH: *Nursing management in the new paradigm*, Gaithersburg, Md, 1996, Aspen.

Marquis BL, Huston CJ: *Leadership roles and management functions in nursing: theory and application*, ed 2, Philadelphia, 1996, Lippincott.

Marquis BL, Huston CJ: *Management decision making for nurses: 124 case studies*, Philadelphia, 1998, Lippincott.

Martin J: *The great transition: using the seven disciplines of enterprise engineering to align people, technology, and strategy*, New York, 1995, AMACOM.

Nadler DA, Gerstein MS, Shaw RB et al.: *Organizational architecture: designs for changing organizations*, San Francisco, 1992, Jossey-Bass.

Nadler DA, Tushman ML: *Competing by design: the power of organizational architecture*, New York, 1997, Oxford University Press.

Ouellette JN, Martin LL, Holmes RB et al.: Clustering: decentralization and resource sharing, *Nurs Manage* 20:31-35, June 1989.

Pelinet Internet Services, Pelican Coast Publishers: *HMO* (http://www.medicalsocieties.org/hmo.htm), 1997, accessed June 5, 1999.

Porter-O'Grady T, Finnigan S: *Shared governance for nursing: a creative approach to professional accountability*, Rockville, Md, 1984, Aspen Systems Corporation.

Rocchiccioli JT, Tilbury MS: *Clinical leadership in nursing*, Philadelphia, 1998, Saunders.

Swansburg RC: *Management and leadership for nurse managers*, ed 2, Boston, 1996, Jones & Bartlett.

Swansburg RC, Swansburg RJ: *Introductory management and leadership for nurses: an interactive text*, Boston, 1999, Jones & Bartlett.

Wall DK, Proyect MM: *Critical pathway implementation guide: a methodology for managing critical pathways*, Chicago, 1997, Precept Press.

Yoder-Wise PS: *Leading and managing in nursing*, ed 2, St. Louis, 1999, Mosby.

BIBLIOGRAPHY

Davis AR: Project management: new approaches, *Nurs Manage* 23:62-65, Nov 1992.

Dienemann J: *Nursing administration: strategic perspectives and application*, Norwalk, Conn, 1990, Appleton & Lange.

Eichelberger KM, Bebl S, Lees ML et al.: Administrative support team: a structural innovation, *JONA* 24:42-48, Nov 1994.

Gelinas LS, Manthey M: The impact of organizational re-
    design on nurse executive leadership, *JONA* 27:35-
    42, Oct 1997.
Morrison M: *Professional skills for leadership: foundations
    of a successful career*, St. Louis, 1993, Mosby.
Pinkerton SE: Development of a new organizational
    model, *Nurs Econ* 14:197-204, July-Aug 1996.
Porter-O'Grady T: Whole systems shared governance:
    creating the seamless organization, *Nurs Econ*
    12:187-195, July-Aug 1994.

Smith GB, Danforth DA, Owens PJ: Role restructuring:
    nurse, case manager, and educator, *Nurs Adm Q*
    19(1):21-32, 1994.
Sorrells-Jones J: The challenge of making it real: interdis-
    ciplinary practice in a "seamless" organization, *Nurs
    Adm Q* 21:20-30, Winter 1997.
Stahl DA: Organizational diagnosis: a six-box model,
    Nurs Manage 28:18-20, April 1997.

CASE STUDY

After referring to the case study in the Appendix, identify a possible restructuring of units to maximize hospital profits by serving the changing needs of the community. Consider converting Lake View Hospital's underused medical-surgical units to accommodate the increasing demand for geriatric, home health, and ambulatory care services. Develop a new organizational chart, noting span of management, flat or tall structure, decentralization or centralization, and line authority. Using Worksheet 10-1, list the advantages and disadvantages of the new organization and discuss them with your classmates.

CASE STUDY

Lake View Hospital is adding an ambulatory primary care clinic, hospice, and home care unit to the Director of Nursing Services' responsibilities. The administrative title was changed to chief executive officer and directors to vice presidents for their respective areas. Using the organization chart in the Appendix, make the changes.

Critical Thinking Activities for this chapter begin on page 500.

C H A P T E R *11*

ORGANIZA-
TIONAL
CULTURE
AND
CHANGE

CHAPTER OBJECTIVES

- Describe the interrelationship of values, attitudes, perception, personality, and roles.
- Identify four factors in organizational culture.
- Identify how managers can use heroes.
- Describe a cultural network.
- Identify at least two rituals.
- Define three strategies for effecting change.
- Define at least three types of change.
- Describe the five tracks that must be carefully planned to facilitate complex organizational change.
- Identify the three developmental stages of an organization and discuss what occurs in each stage.

Chapter Overview

Chapter 11 explains individual and organizational culture, diversity, process of change, cultural change, behavioral aspects of organizational change, resistance to change, oscillation, and strategies for change.

MAJOR CONCEPTS AND DEFINITIONS	
Values	basic convictions and beliefs about what is desirable or important
Attitudes	mental states of readiness
Perceptions	consciousness, awareness
Personality	a relatively stable set of characteristics and temperaments
Roles	expected behaviors in given situations
Myers-Briggs Type Indicator	a method of self-examination of one's strengths and weaknesses and how one differs from others
Assumptions	suppositions, presumptions, something taken for granted
Symbols	objects or acts that represent another thing
Language	choice of words and sounds used to express thoughts and feelings
Behaviors	actions or mannerisms
Organizational culture	customary way of thinking and behaving that is shared by members of an organization
Hero	a person honored for outstanding qualities
Cultural network	primary informal means of communication in the organization
Rituals	day-to-day routines
Change	to become different
Change agent	one who helps bring about change
Organizational development	stages of birth, youth, and maturity of organizations

CULTURE OF INDIVIDUALS

Perception is a psychological process that makes sense out of what one sees, hears, smells, tastes, or feels. One's previous experiences and personal value system affect it; thus people may perceive the same situation differently. There are also differences in ability to process data, to remember facts, and to explore alternatives.

Values

Values represent basic convictions about what is right, good, or desirable; as a result, they help an individual decide which mode of conduct is preferable to others. Value systems list an individual's values in order of their relative importance and provide the foundation of attitudes, perceptions, personality, and roles. These values cloud objectivity and rationality by containing interpretations of what is right and wrong and implications that certain behaviors or outcomes are preferred over others. They are relatively stable and enduring and generally influence decisions and behaviors.

Attitudes

Attitudes are mental states of readiness that are organized through experience and exert specific influences on a person's response to the people, objects, and situations to which they are related. Attitudes, like values, are learned from parents, teachers, and peers, but attitudes are less stable than values. They influence decisions and behavior and are close to the core of personality.

In the late 1950s Leon Festinger proposed the theory of cognitive dissonance to explain the linkage between attitudes and behavior. Cognitive dissonance means a perceived inconsistency or incompatibility between attitudes and behavior. Festinger maintained that this inconsistency is uncomfortable and that people will try to reduce the dissonance and consequently the discomfort. People seek a stable state with a minimum of dissonance. For example, if someone thinks she is being paid more than she is worth, she is likely to work harder, but if she thinks she is underpaid, she may slow down and do less (Festinger, 1957).

Perceptions

Perception involves receiving, organizing, and interpreting stimuli. The perceptions then influence behavior and form attitudes. People select various cues that influence their perceptions and consequently often misperceive another person, group, or object.

Selective perception means that people select information that supports their viewpoints. Knowing oneself increases the accuracy of perception of others. People tend to identify their own characteristics in others. Consequently, people who accept themselves are more likely to view others favorably.

A stereotype is a judgment made about people on the basis of their gender or ethnic background that can contribute to selective perception.

A self-fulfilling prophecy occurs when people expect certain behavior, use selective perception to see it, and treat others as if it were so. For example,

if a nurse manager thinks certain ethnic groups are lazy and irresponsible, she may not assign them challenging tasks. That could lead to boredom and demotivation, which reinforce the stereotype, creating a self-fulfilling prophecy.

Cognitive Styles

People gather and process information differently. Myers-Briggs indicates that people gather information through sensing and intuiting and process or evaluate the information through thinking and feeling. Sensing focuses on detail or specific attributes rather than on the relationships between factors. Intuiting emphasizes commonalities and generalizations in relationships between factors. Thinking systematically evaluates information, whereas feeling gives an internal sense of what to do.

Attitudes Toward Change

Tolerance of ambiguity and locus of control influence people's attitudes toward change. Environments are increasingly chaotic, complex, temporary, and overloaded with information. The ability to process information is affected by one's *attitude toward change*. *Tolerance of ambiguity* refers to how a person is threatened by unpredictability or has difficulty coping with complex situations. People who have a tolerance for ambiguity and complexity are more adaptive. Tolerance of ambiguity involves at least three factors: novelty, complexity, and insolubility. *Novelty* is a tolerance of new and unfamiliar information and situations. *Complexity* is tolerance of multiple unrelated pieces. *Insolubility* is tolerance for situations that are difficult to solve because of unavailable information and unidentified alternative solutions.

There are internal and external *loci of control*. An *internal locus of control* means the person feels responsible for the success or failure of a situation. An *external locus of control* means the person feels that someone or something else has caused the results. A person who has an internal locus of control is more adaptable than one with an external locus of control.

Interpersonal Needs

Interpersonal orientations are not the actual behavior but are the tendencies to behave in certain ways. They are influenced by one's basic needs related to relationships with others. People need people and tend to seek compatible relationships with others in social situations. There are at least three basic needs: inclusion, control, and affection. *Inclusion* involves introversion, extraversion, joining and including others, and wanting to be included by others. *Control* is the need to balance influence and power in relationships. There are differences in the need to control others or be controlled by others. People also have a need for *affection,* which is the need for intimacy and the desire for close personal relationships with others (Whetten and Cameron, 1998).

Personality

Personality is a relatively stable set of characteristics, temperaments, and tendencies that is significantly formed by inheritance and by social, cultural, and environmental factors.

Roles

Role theory is a collection of concepts, definitions, and hypotheses that predict how actors will perform in certain roles and under what circumstances given behaviors can be expected. Roles are acts or behaviors expected of a person who occupies a given social position. Positions are locations in social systems, such as nurse or teacher. People who occupy a position collectively share common behaviors. Specific behaviors associated with positions constitute roles. Positions and roles have counterparts or counterroles such as nurse-client, teacher-student, or leader-follower.

Positions may be ascribed or achieved. A person has little or no control over ascribed positions such as age, sex, or birth order in the family. Some degree of control is possible for achieved positions such as marital status, occupation, and social status.

Role structure involves individuals, behaviors, and positions. The individual, or actor, ego, refer-

ent, or self, has a set of attributes that can be described from a variety of viewpoints. An interactionist would look at the interaction of roles, the psychiatrist at personality, and the structuralist at position tasks. Behaviors are actions taken by the role enactor. These acts are learned and influenced by norms. They are often voluntary and goal directed. Prescription refers to what should be done by a person in a certain position. Positions often require specific skills, intelligence, or temperament and may be held based on one's age, sex, and education. Positions often imply titles such as nurse or teacher. People in positions are exchangeable, but the positions are not.

Role socialization is a process of acquiring specific roles and involves role expectations, role learning, and role enactment. Role expectations are beliefs held by others about the specific behaviors inherent in specific positions; they may be general or specific, formal or informal, and extensive or narrow in scope. Some expectations are very clear, whereas others are not. General expectations allow more latitude in the implementation of the role than do specific ones. For example, nurses should be kind and gentle in general. More specifically, nurses use two-way communications skills. Some formal expectations are written, such as codes of ethics and behavioral objectives, whereas informal expectations are communicated indirectly. Expectations for age and sex are extensive in scope in that they transcend other roles. Expectations that apply in only a few positions are narrow in scope. Thus only nurses working in cardiac intensive care units are expected to read and interpret electrocardiograms, and only nurse managers are expected to write a budget.

Role learning involves locating oneself accurately in the social structure. It begins at infancy and early childhood as one prepares to assume adult responsibilities. It involves the development of basic skills such as language, interpersonal competence, and role taking. Role taking is the ability of the person to act out perceptions of how she and others would behave in certain positions. Playing nurse is an example of learning role taking.

Role enactment refers to behaviors and is related to the number of positions one holds, the intensity of involvement in those positions, and the preemptiveness of them. One holds multiple positions at any one time, a situation that sometimes causes conflict and difficulty with role enactment. One may not have enough time to implement each role effectively, and there can be conflicts between various role expectations. A professional nurse who takes a course will have less time for child care. Intensity of involvement is the degree of effort exerted to enact a role. It may vary from noninvolvement to engrossing involvement. For example, a nurse may merely pay for membership in an organization or may become an officer and serve on several committees. Preemptiveness is the amount of time a person spends enacting one role as compared with others.

Role stress or role dissonance is the difference between role enactment and role expectations. The greater the difference, the greater the stress. Role ambiguity results from a lack of clear role expectations. Role shock arises from discrepancies between anticipated and encountered roles. Role conflict is a consequence of contradictory or mutually exclusive roles.

MYERS-BRIGGS TYPE INDICATOR

The Myers-Briggs Type Indicator is a useful method for performing self-examinations to understand one's strengths and weaknesses and how one differs from others. Peter Myers and Isabel Briggs-Myers (1980) have identified four dimensions of psychological type: attitude toward life, perception function, judgment function, and orientation to the outer world. Each of the four dimensions has two categories, thus forming sixteen different types, as shown in Table 11-1.

Introverts like to work alone, think before they act, do not like interruptions, like quiet for concentration, may work on a project for a long time, are interested in ideas, are careful with details, may have difficulty remembering names and faces, and may have trouble communicating.

Extroverts like to be around people, communicate freely, may act without thinking, like variety and action, and may become impatient with slow jobs.

Table 11-1   Myers-Briggs Type Indicator

Dimensions	Contrasting Categories	
Attitude toward life	Introversion	Extroversion
Perception	Sensing	Intuiting
Judgment	Thinking	Feeling
Orientation to outer world	Judging	Perceiving

Sensing types tend to be good at detail work, are not usually inspired, rarely make errors of fact, are patient with routine details, enjoy using skills they know, like established ways of doing things, and work steadily step by step to the end.

Intuitive types like solving new problems, enjoy learning new skills, follow their inspirations, and work in bursts of energy to reach conclusion quickly.

Thinking types value logic, organize ideas into logical sequences, tend to be brief and businesslike, and may seem impersonal.

Feeling types value sentiment, tend to be friendly and agreeable, may undervalue thinking, and are likely to ramble. They are usually stronger in social skills than in executive ability.

Judging types like to plan their work and follow the plan, make decisions quickly, and get things done.

Perceiving types are curious, may start too many projects, and may have trouble finishing them or coming to a conclusion.

Leaders should know their own styles and those of people with whom they work. When leaders are aware of their own limitations, they can consult opposite types to compensate. By knowing their associates' strengths and weaknesses, they can maximize the strengths, minimize the weaknesses, and develop strong teams (Barr and Barr, 1989; Briggs-Myers and Myers, 1980).

DIVERSITY

Diversity is a state of difference and having variety. There is strength in diversity. At the center of diversity is one's personality. Other internal factors include age, gender, race, ethnicity, physical ability, and sexual orientation. External factors include education, work experience, income, religion, marital status, parental status, personal habits, recreational habits, geographical location or living environment, and appearance. Organizational factors include work content field, functional level classification or job roles, division, department, or work environment, seniority, management status, work location, and union affiliation. Respect for diversity comes from finding and acknowledging that good comes from these differences. Multiculturalism refers to maintaining several different cultures. Cross-culturalism refers to mediating between cultures. Transculturalism means bridging significant differences in cultural practice.

Cultural differences are common in several areas, including the following:

1. *Values and norms.* People in the United States may value individual orientation, independence, and direct confrontation of conflict, whereas other cultures may prefer a group orientation, conformity, and harmony.
2. *Beliefs and attitudes.* People in the United States may value egalitarianism, gender equity, and individual control over their own destiny and challenge authority, whereas other cultures may be more hierarchical, respect authority, accept different roles for men and women, and think individuals should accept their destiny.
3. *Mental processes and learning style.* People in the United States may be linear, logical, and sequential with a problem-solving approach, whereas other cultures may be lateral, holistic, simultaneous, and accepting of life difficulties.
4. *Sense of self and space.* The culture in the United States may be informal and use handshakes, whereas other cultures may be more formal and use hugs and bows, as well as handshakes.
5. *Relationships with family and friends.* People in the United States may focus on the nuclear family, value youth, and value responsibility

for self, whereas other cultures may focus on the extended family, respect age, and feel loyalty and responsibility to the family.
6. *Time and time consciousness.* People in the United States may value promptness and be linear and exact with regard to time consciousness, whereas other cultures may use time to enjoy relationships and may be elastic and relatively time conscious.
7. *Communication and language.* People in the United States may use explicit, direct communications with an emphasis on the content, whereas other cultures may use implicit, indirect communications that emphasize contextual meaning found around words.
8. *Food and eating habits.* People in the United States may view eating as a necessity and use fast food, whereas other cultures may view dining as a religious and social experience.
9. *Dress and appearance.* People in the United States may dress for success and accept a wide range of dress codes, whereas other cultures may see dress as a sign of position and prestige. They may follow religious rules.
10. *Work habits and practices.* People in the United States may emphasize tasks, intrinsically value work, and reward workers based on individual achievement, whereas other cultures may put an emphasis on relationships, believe that work is a necessity of life, and reward seniority and relationships.

Ethnocentrism is believing that one's race, culture, or values are superior to those of others. It is the lowest level of *intercultural sensitivity.* There are several stages in the development of intercultural sensitivity. *Denial of differences* is the inability to construe cultural difference. Isolation in homogeneous groups does not allow for noticing and interpreting cultural differences. Separation allows for some awareness of cultural differences but often yields undifferentiated broad categories such as "Asian" or "black." There are only broad categories for different cultures with a relatively benign affect based on ignorance. *Defense against difference* is the recognition of cultural differences accompanied by a negative evaluation of variations from the dominant culture. The greater the variation, the more negative the evaluation. This may be characterized by dualistic thinking of us and them accompanied by overt negative stereotyping and attempts to convert to the dominant culture. *Minimization of difference* is the recognition and acceptance of superficial cultural differences like eating customs. It is assumed that all human beings are essentially the same. There is an emphasis on the similarity of people and basic values. *Acceptance of difference* is recognition and appreciation of cultural differences in both behaviors and values. It emphasizes acquisition of knowledge about cultures, including an increased awareness of one's own culture. *Adaptation to difference* includes a shifting frame of reference to understand and be understood across cultural boundaries, empathy, and communication skills that enable intercultural communication. One is able to consciously shift perspective into an alternative cultural worldview and act in culturally appropriate ways. *Integration of difference* is the internalization of bicultural frames of reference. It is the acceptance of an identity that is not based entirely in one culture (Gardenswartz and Rowe, 1995; Loden, Rosener, and Rosener, 1991; Stewart and Bennett, 1991).

MANAGEMENT OF CULTURAL DIVERSITY

The leader or manager needs to help staff with cultural diversity through awareness building, discrimination control, and prejudice reduction. The organizational mission and goal statements should address diversity. People who want to deal with diversity issues should be supported and open communications encouraged. Development and implementation of a culture audit including focus groups, interviews, and questionnaires help describe the culture. Homogeneous groups who are provided a safe problem-solving environment can make recommendations for solving problems. Long-term contact between culturally and ethnically diverse people can increase awareness. Working with diverse groups may require more time and effort because of the conflict management needed

before a mature group emerges. The importance of cultural diversity should be apparent in the organizational philosophy and goals. Orientation programs, seminars, role-playing, skill building, and workshops can be used to facilitate intercultural sensitivity. Informal networks for coaching, tutoring, mentoring, and role modeling can help develop people. Leaders should be role models for integration of differences. People should be aware that foreign or minority staff may not consider themselves of lesser status than the majority and that some of the majority may have felt they were part of an oppressed group at some time. People with different lifestyles should not be treated as if they need interventions because they may be happy with their choices. Emotional outbursts may not be anger but may be a communication style. Managers should take time to get to know the staff and help give them a perception of dignity and value. Managers should recognize and value diversity.

All managers should participate in discrimination control. Discrimination is the mistreatment of people based on irrelevant factors such as race, sex, age, or handicap. Active recruitment, selection, retention, and promotion of women and minorities, monitoring their progress, affirmative action committees to monitor fairness of policies and the implementation of them, and advisory groups representing minorities can help control discrimination. Managers and staff can be inserviced about the appropriate actions to take when aware of discriminatory behavior. Open discussions between representatives of conflicting groups may help minimize discrimination and should focus on the strengths each group brings to the situation to help reach the organizational goals. Clearly written policies and equal support and resources of career development for all employees can help reduce the risk of reverse discrimination, which occurs when a person of a particular ethnic group is chosen over someone else who has better credentials. People need to be aware that physical features do not always denote a specific race or ethnic group. Jamaicans and Puerto Ricans are not African blacks, and Hispanics may have Asian features. Managers should implement standards of performance and ensure fairness.

Prejudice reduction is more difficult than awareness building or discrimination control. Prejudice is an internal, abstract perception. Organizations can attempt to control the manifestations of prejudice. People who observe and report prejudice can help reduce it. Discouraging racial and gender comments usually decreases the number of racial and gender comments made (Rocchiccioli and Tilbury, 1998; Tappen, 1995; Yoder-Wise, 1999).

ORGANIZATIONAL CULTURE

Organizational culture is the customary way of thinking and behaving that is shared by all members of the organization and must be learned and adopted by newcomers before they can be accepted into the agency. Culture is learned, shared, and transmitted. It is a combination of assumptions, values, symbols, language, and behaviors that manifest the organization's norms and values. Objective aspects exist outside the minds of members of the organization and include such artifacts as pictures of leaders, monuments, stories, ceremonies, and rituals. Subjective aspects are related to assumptions and mind-sets such as shared assumptions, values, meanings, and understandings of how things will be done.

Values are the basic beliefs of the organization. Agencies with strong cultures have a complex system of values that are discussed openly by managers and are accepted by members. They establish the standards for achievement in the organization. They are the essence of the organization's philosophy; they provide a sense of direction, guide daily behavior, serve as an informal control system, help set priorities, and plan strategies.

Heroes personify the organizational culture's values. They show that success is attainable, set a standard for performance, preserve what is special in the organization, motivate employees, serve as role models, and symbolize the organization to the outside world.

The cultural network is the primary informal means of communication within the organization that carries the corporate values and heroic mythology. Managers should use this network to understand what is going on and to get things done (Deal and Kennedy, 1982) (Box 11-1).

Artifacts, or articles made by human work, include a range of verbal and physical symbols such as stories, myths, verbal or visual forms of humor, rituals, ceremonies, analogies, and metaphors. Gestures are a nonverbal form of communication. Gossip is talk or rumors about others. Jargon is specialized vocabulary or idioms specific to a way of work. A joke is a funny anecdote. Slang is a specialized vocabulary of idioms outside the standard language. A signal is given by a gesture. Slogan is a catchword or motto. Stories may describe conflicts, heroes, or traditions. Legend is the story of a saint or some wonderful event. Myths are fictitious, traditional stories with a historical basis used to explain something. Saga is a long story of adventure or heroic deeds. Songs are poetry or verse that is sung. Verbal forms of

Box 11-1   CULTURAL FORMS

LANGUAGE	NARRATIVES
Gestures	Legends
Gossip	Myths
Humor	Sagas
Jargon	Stories
Jokes	
Metaphors	**PRACTICES**
Myths	
Proverbs	Ceremonies
Rituals	Rituals
Rumors	Taboos
Taboos	
Signals	**SYMBOLS**
Slang	
Slogans	Objects
Signs	Performances
Songs	Settings

humor could be jokes, whereas visual forms could be cartoons posted on bulletin boards.

Rituals are the day-to-day routines that show employees how they are to behave. Policies and procedures clarify routines. Inductions, promotions, planning retreats, and retirements are rituals that reinforce the values. Ceremonies are extravagant rituals that give visible evidence of the agency's values. Ceremonies keep the values, beliefs, and heroes visible.

Analogies speak to similarities between things that are otherwise unlike or that bear a partial resemblance. For example, the organization is like a battlefield. Metaphors are figures of speech in which one thing is likened to another and spoken of as if it were the other thing. Organizations can be spoken of as follows: (1) anthropology (a family, big daddy, the prodigal son), (2) mechanistic (an assembly line, a factory, a well-oiled machine), (3) television (sitcom, soap opera), (4) military (battles, battle zone, captain, enemies, troops), (5) sports (quarterback, stars, teams), and (6) zoo (chicken, sly fox) (Decker and Sullivan, 1992; Huber, 1996; Swansburg and Swansburg, 1999; Trice and Beyer, 1993; Wilkins, 1989).

Types of Cultures

William Schneider (1994) has identified four core cultures with a leadership and management focus. The *control culture* is authoritative, conservative, impersonal, tough-minded, realistic, systematic, task driven, objective, and prescriptive. The *collaborative culture* is adaptive, collegial, democratic, informal, participative, personal, relational, supportive, and trusting; the leader functions as a coach, integrator, team builder, and trust builder. The *competence culture* is challenging, efficient, emotionless, formal, impersonal, intense, objective, rational, and task driven; the leader is an assertive, visionary standard setter who recruits the most competent people and then stretches them. The *cultivation culture* is attentive, emotional, enabling, humanistic, nurturing, people driven, personal, promotive, and relaxed; the leader is a catalyst, cultivator, empowerer, inspirer, promoter, and steward.

Robert Cooke and Denise Rousseau (1987) have identified three culture types: (1) positive, (2) passive-defensive, and (3) aggressive-defensive. In a positive culture members are proactive and interactive to meet their satisfaction needs. That culture is based on humanism, affiliation norms, achievement, and self-actualization. In passive-defensive and aggressive-defensive cultures people protect their security and status in reactive, guarded ways. Passive-defensive culture is based on conventional, approval, dependent, and avoidance norms. Aggressive-defensive culture is based on power, oppositional, competitive, and perfectionistic norms. Leaders need to diffuse negativism in oppositional norms and act as role models for desirable behaviors, encouraging a cultural transition to more positive norms.

Integrated or Differentiated Frames of Reference

Organizations may have action, content, and symbolic consistency. *Action consistency* occurs when content themes are consistent with the formal and informal practices and the artifacts. *Content consistency* is congruence between content themes. *Symbolic consistency* happens when there is congruence between artifacts and informal and formal practices. Integration means that an organization has a single culture with a high level of consistency and consensus. Highly integrated cultures can be repressive and nonadaptive. Differentiation recognizes and allows for variation of cultures within the organization, such as subcultures (Sullivan and Decker, 1997).

Subcultures. Subcultures have the same elements that cultures have, including distinct patterns of shared ideologies and sets of cultural forms. They are collective, dynamic, emotionally charged, historically based, and inherently symbolic. The degree of distinctiveness of subcultures varies. Some resemble the dominant culture in which they are embedded, and others deviate greatly from it. The more unique the subculture, the more it encourages members to weaken their commitment to the dominant culture and violate significant aspects of it. Organizations are usually multicultural, having multiple subcultures within them. Frequency of interactions provides the basis of subcultures. Subcultures require long periods of close association to develop distinctive ideologies. It is shared experiences that stimulate that collective sense making. Shared personal characteristics such as age, education, ethnicity, occupational training, and social class also facilitate sense making because people do not need to displace their old beliefs and values very much when they find a common ground with each other. Cohesion is also important to subcultures and is facilitated by small groups; agreement of group goals; tasks requiring interdependence; similar characteristics of members, like interests and values; physical isolation from others; threats from the outside; and performance success, failure, or crisis. When groups are cohesive, the members are attracted to each other, spend time together, and consequently influence each other. Subcultures tend to form strong norms that govern the behavior of members.

Social cohesiveness is not the same as a subculture. When neighbors respond to a natural disaster, they have social cohesiveness for a while. But when the circumstances that brought them together end, so do the mutual influence and strong emotional bonds. Subcultures are more enduring than social cohesiveness. People's occupations are the most pervasive source of subcultures in an organization. An occupation consists of a set of tasks, and members of the occupation claim exclusive rights to perform and control those tasks. Members of the occupation identify themselves with other members of that occupation and come to share beliefs, norms, and values in a variety of ways. Language, myths, rituals, songs, and taboos help members vent their emotions and learn ways to frame their activities so they are not overwhelmed. Members then form favorable self-images and social identities from their work that then become part of their presentation of self. Members of occupations may live near one another, spend time together, encourage their children to enter the same profession, and link families

through marriage. The subculture then becomes prone to ethnocentrism.

Countercultures. Countercultures develop to oppose the dominant culture. Mergers, rebellious innovators, chronically discontented employees, and illegal or other deviant behaviors encourage the formation of countercultures (Trice and Beyer, 1993).

Leaders help shape the culture by identifying and projecting a vision, demonstrating a philosophy, modeling values, setting policies, creating systems, and supporting a reward system. Leaders must ensure congruity between strategic plans and decision-making processes. They need to identify the actual norms, establish desired norms, identify and close culture gaps, and sustain culture changes. Leaders help others understand and make sense of events and cope with change, instability, and the unexpected. Leaders need to help members of the organization adapt to the dynamic life cycle of the organization. Open and collaborative interaction between leaders and followers is important (Box 11-2).

MANAGEMENT OF CHANGE
Forces That Influence Change

There are internal and external forces that influence change. Internal forces originate from inside operations that may result from external changes and include changing priorities, need for increased productivity, need for cost containment, staffing pattern changes, shifts in philosophy, work process changes, and need for quality of work life. External forces include health care economics, technology, restructuring, diversity, and changing demographics (Douglas, 1996; Martin, 1995).

Leaders are visionary role models who focus on the future. Managers process the changes and understand the future directions (Box 11-3).

Strategies for Effecting Change

Whether working with individuals, groups, or systems, the nurse manager is sure to be involved with management of change. Several strategies for managing change have been identified.

TRENDS: PARADIGM SHIFTS EFFECTING CHANGE

From	To
Atomism	Holism
Fragmentation	Integration
Emphasis on separate parts	Emphasis on relationships
Determinate	Indeterminate
Control	Trust
Certainty/predictability	Uncertainty/ambiguity/rapid change
Reductive	Emergent
Isolated/controlled	Contextual/self-organizing
Parts defining the whole	Whole being greater than the sum of the parts
Top-down management	Bottom-up leadership
Hierarchy	Nonhierarchical networks
Reactive	Imaginative/experimental
Power from top	Power from interacting centers
Competition	Cooperation
Single viewpoint	Many viewpoints
Knowing	Discovering
Quality of work	Quality of life

Data from Zohar D: *Rewiring the corporate brain: using the new science to rethink how we structure and lead organizations*, San Francisco, 1997, Berrett-Koehler.

LEADERSHIP AND MANAGEMENT FOR CHANGE

Leader	Manager
Is visionary in identifying needed change	Assesses the driving and restraining forces
Is a role model	Identifies and implements strategies
Is sensitive to timing initiatives	Seeks subordinates' input
Is creative in identifying solutions	Supports and rewards individual efforts
Focuses on the future	Understands future directions

Data from Carr DK, Johansson HJ: *Best practices in reengineering: what works and what doesn't in the reengineering process*, New York, 1995, McGraw-Hill; Marquis BL, Huston CJ: *Leadership roles and management functions in nursing: theory and application*, ed 2, Philadelphia, 1996, Lippincott.

Empirical-rational strategies. Empirical-rational strategies are based on the assumption that people are rational and behave according to rational self-interest. It follows then that people should be willing to adopt a change if it is justified and if the people are shown how they can benefit from the change.

Nurse managers who use empirical-rational strategies are likely to want the appropriate persons for specific positions. Desirous of having people

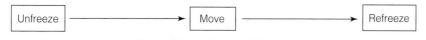

Figure 11-1 Process of change.

perform jobs for which they are well qualified, nurse managers give considerable attention to recruitment and selection of personnel. Staff development through independent study, in-service education, continuing education, and formal degree programs is encouraged. Systems analysis, operations research, and implementation of research findings are consistent with the empirical-rational philosophy, as is long-range futuristic planning.

Normative reeducative strategies. Normative reeducative strategies are based on the assumption that people act according to their commitment to sociocultural norms. The intelligence and rationality of people are not denied, but attitudes and values are also considered. The manager pays attention to changes in values, attitudes, skills, and relationships in addition to providing information.

Believing that the basic unit of the social organization is composed of individuals, the manager fosters the development of staff members through means such as personal counseling, training groups, small groups, and experiential learning because people need to participate in their own reeducation. Organizational development programs are fostered, and it is typical to collect data about the organization, give data feedback and analysis to appropriate people, plan ways to improve the system, and train managers and internal change agents. The relationships of internal change agents with other personnel can be a major tool in reeducating others.

Power-coercive strategies. Power-coercive strategies involve compliance of the less powerful to the leadership, plans, and directions of the more powerful. These strategies do not deny the intelligence and rationality of people or the importance of their values and attitudes, but rather they acknowledge the need to use sources of power to bring about change. Use of strikes, sit-ins, negotiations, conflict

confrontation, and administration decisions and rulings are power-coercive strategies (Bennis, Benne, and Chin, 1969).

Process of Change

Unfreezing, moving, and refreezing are the three phases of change (Figure 11-1). *Unfreezing* is the development through problem awareness of a need for change. Even if a problem has been identified, people must believe there can be an improvement before they are willing to change. Coercion and the induction of guilt and anxiety have been used for unfreezing. Removal of people from the source of their old attitudes to a new environment, punishment and humiliation for undesirable attitudes, and rewards for desirable attitudes effect change.

Stress may cause dissatisfaction with the status quo and become a motivating factor for change. Points of stress and strain should be assessed. Change may begin at a point of stress but ordinarily should not be started at the point of greatest stress. It is most appropriate for it to start with a policy-making body that considers both formal and informal structures. The effectiveness of the change may depend on the amount of involvement in fact finding and problem solving of all personnel.

Moving is working toward change by identifying the problem or the need for change, exploring the alternatives, defining goals and objectives, planning how to accomplish the goals, and implementing the plan for change.

Refreezing is the integration of the change into one's personality and the consequent stabilization of change. Frequently personnel return to old behaviors after change efforts cease. Related changes in neighboring systems, momentum to perpetuate the change, and structural alterations that support the procedural changes are stabilizing factors.

Types of Change

The variables of mutual goal setting, the power ratio between the change agent and the client system, and the deliberativeness of change are differentiating factors in the change process.

Coercive change. Nonmutual goal setting, imbalanced power ratio, and one-sided deliberativeness characterize coercive change.

Emulative change. In this case change is fostered through identification with and emulation of power figures.

Indoctrination. Indoctrination uses mutual goal setting, has an imbalanced power ratio, and is deliberative. Subordinates are instructed in the beliefs of the power sources.

Interactional change. Mutual goal setting, fairly equal power, but no deliberativeness characterize this. Parties may be unconsciously committed to changing one another.

Natural change. These changes include accidents and acts of God. They involve no goal setting or deliberativeness.

Socialization change. This has a direct relationship with interactional change. One conforms to the needs of a social group. When there is greater deliberativeness on the power side, change becomes indoctrination.

Technocratic change. Collecting and interpreting data bring about change. A technocrat merely reports the findings of the analysis to bring about change.

Planned change. Planned change involves mutual goal setting, an equal power ratio, and deliberativeness (Box 11-4).

Ronald Lippitt, Jeanne Watson, and Bruce Westley have identified seven phases of planned change. First, the client must feel a need for change. The manager, as the change agent, can stimulate an awareness of the need for change, help the client

Box 11-4 COMPARISON OF PLANNED CHANGE THEORIES

Lewin	Lippitt	Havelock	Rogers
1. Unfreezing	1. Diagnosing the problem	1. Building a relationship	1. Awareness
	2. Assessing motivation and capacity for change	2. Diagnosing the problem	2. Interest
	3. Assessing change agent's motivation and resources	3. Acquiring the relevant resources	3. Evaluation
2. Moving	4. Selecting progressive change objective	4. Choosing the solution	4. Trial
	5. Choosing the appropriate role for the change agent	5. Gaining acceptance	
3. Refreezing	6. Maintaining change	6. Stabilization and self-renewal	5. Adoption
	7. Terminating the helping relationship		

Data from Bennis, Benne, and Chin, 1969; Gillies, 1994; Havelock, 1973; Huber, 1996; Lippitt, Watson, and Westley, 1958; Rocchiccioli and Tilbury, 1998; Rogers, 1995; Swansburg, 1996; Swansburg and Swansburg, 1999; Tappen, 1995; Yoder-Wise, 1999.

become aware of the problems, and indicate that a more desirable state of affairs is possible. The change agent assesses the client's motivation and capacity for change and the change agent's motivation and resources. Thus unfreezing occurs.

Next, the helping relationship must be established, and the moving process begun. Managers, as change agents, must identify with clients' problems while remaining neutral so that they can remain objective. The change agent needs to be viewed as an understandable and approachable expert. The success or failure of most planned action will depend largely on the quality and workability of the relationship between the change agent and the client. The problem must be identified and clarified. Collecting and analyzing data can facilitate this process. Alternative possibilities for change should be examined. Goals and objectives are planned. The client's emotional and material resources are examined. Strategies for change are determined. The success of planned change is evaluated by the implementation of the plans. It is the active work of modification that completes the moving process.

The refreezing process occurs during the sixth phase—generalization and stabilization. All too often clients slip back to their old ways after change efforts cease. The spread of change to neighboring systems and to subparts of the same system aids the stabilization process. Change momentum, positive evaluation of the change, rewards for the change, and related procedural and structural changes increase the stabilization. The helping relationship ends, or a different type of continuing relationship is established. Dependency is the major factor determining when the relationship will end (Lippitt, Watson, and Westley, 1958).

Lippitt's seven phases, Ronald Havelock's six, and Everett Rogers' five can all be clustered in Kurt Lewin's three, as illustrated in Box 11-4. In addition, Margaret Wheatley (1992, 1996) discusses chaos theory. Organizations are self-organizing and self-renewing open systems that have chaotic, randomly appearing patterns. Wheatley points out that order emerges from chaos. She encourages leading in nonlinear ways, emphasizing the relationships of the parts in forming the whole. Vision, information, and relationships are particularly important. Edward Deevy (1995) speaks to the importance of resilience and hardiness to the survival of organizations. Daryl Conner (1993, 1998) has identified five personal characteristics of resilient behavior as follows: positive, focused, flexible, organized, and proactive. Peter Senge (1990) has addressed learning organizations that stress flexibility and responsiveness. He believes that what makes the difference between learning organizations and traditional organizations is mastery of the five disciplines of a learning organization: (1) systems thinking, (2) personal mastery, (3) mental models, (4) building shared vision, and (5) team learning. He presents strategies and tools for building a learning organization in *The Fifth Discipline Fieldbook* (Senge, Kleiner, Roberts et al., 1994).

Role of the Manager as Change Agent

As a change agent, the manager identifies the problem, assesses the client's motivations and capacities for change, determines alternatives, explores ramifications of those alternatives, assesses resources, determines appropriate helping roles, establishes and maintains a helping relationship, recognizes the phases of the change process and guides the client through them, and chooses and implements techniques for planned change (Grohar-Murray and Di-Croce, 1997; Lippitt, Watson, and Westley, 1958; Loveridge and Cummings, 1996; Swansburg, 1996; Tappen, 1995). Havelock (1973) indicates that change agents facilitate planned change by being a catalyst, solution giver, process helper, and resource linker. Harry Woodward, Steve Bucholz, and Karen Hess (1987) indicate change agents clarify, share, and engage commitment. They clarify by listening, focusing, and restating. They share by signaling the shift from listening to talking, explaining the purpose, overviewing the change, linking the change to the workers' concerns, and netting it out by specifying how their concerns will or will not be met. They engage for commitment by asking for understanding, asking for ideas, suggesting ideas, and agreeing on action steps.

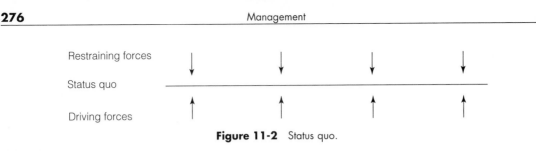

Figure 11-2 Status quo.

DRIVING AND RESTRAINING FORCES

Driving Forces		Restraining Forces	
Rank	**Factor**	**Rank**	**Factor**
1	Pressure from manager	4	Conformity
4	Please manager	4	Security
2	Improve self-image	2	Economic threat
2	Improve situation	3	Threat to prestige

Scale
1 = Little strength
2 = Moderate strength
3 = Important strength
4 = Major strength

Modified from Lippitt R, Watson J, Westley B: *The dynamics of planned change*, New York, 1958, Harcourt, Brace & World, p. 126.

Force-Field Analysis

Lewin's force-field analysis provides a framework for problem solving and planned change. Status quo is maintained when driving forces equal the restraining forces (Figure 11-2), and change will occur when the relative strength of opposing forces changes. Consequently, when planning change, the manager should identify the restraining and driving forces and assess their strengths.

Driving forces may include pressure from the manager, desire to please the manager, perception that the change will improve one's self-image, and belief that the change will improve the situation. Restraining forces include conformity to norms, morals, and ethics; desire for security; perception of economic threat or threat to one's prestige and homeostasis; and regulatory mechanisms for keeping the situation fairly constant.

Once the driving and restraining forces have been identified, the manager determines their relative strengths. Which are the major factors toward or resisting change? Which are important or moderately important? Which have little effect for or against change? These might be listed in columns under "driving" and "restraining" and ranked (Box 11-5).

To help visualize these forces, the manager can draw a diagram as shown in Figure 11-3, write in key words to identify the forces, and draw arrows toward the status quo line to represent the strength of the forces. The longer the line, the stronger the force.

Next, the manager plans strategies for reducing the restraining forces and strengthening the driving forces. Managers may do some experiential learning exercises to facilitate the change of group norms, explain each person's role in the change with emphasis on security, and provide some status symbols to reduce the threat to people's prestige. They should also help the workers identify how the

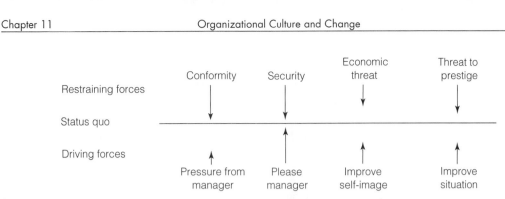

Figure 11-3 Strength of driving and restraining forces.

change will improve their situation. Steps should be taken to improve self-images. For instance, people may be taught new tasks to prepare themselves for the change, to reduce the threat to their prestige and their fear of making fools of themselves when doing something new, and to improve their self-images. If managers perceive that the workers want to please them, they may inform the workers that they desire the change and give positive reinforcement for it. Keeping the goals in mind, the manager should assess the results of implementing the strategies and revise plans as necessary.

Cultural Change in Organizations

In an adaptive culture members of an organization support each other's efforts to identify and solve problems. The members believe they can manage the problems; have confidence and enthusiasm; and are receptive to change. In a dysfunctional culture members continue behaviors that have worked in the past but are no longer effective. Culture rut occurs when members do not adapt to change and continue to function out of habit even when success is not forthcoming. Culture shock happens when the members realize that the organization is out of touch with its setting, mission, and assumptions.

Ralph Kilmann (1989, 1991) has identified five stages of organizational planned change: (1) initiate the integrated program for cultural change, (2) diagnose the problems, (3) schedule the tracks, (4) implement the tracks, and (5) evaluate the results (Box 11-6).

Box 11-6

FIVE STAGES OF ORGANIZATIONAL PLANNED CHANGE

Initiate the integrated program of cultural change.

Diagnose the problems.

Schedule the tracks.

Implement the tracks.

Evaluate the results.

Box 11-7

FIVE TRACKS FOR CULTURAL CHANGE

Culture

Management skills

Team building

Strategy structure

Reward system

The five tracks are as follows: (1) culture, (2) management skills, (3) team building, (4) strategy structure, and (5) reward system (Box 11-7). They require implementation in that order to be most successful. The culture track helps explain organizational differences in decision making and actions, much as personality explains differences in indi-

Task support norms

Task innovation norms

Social relationship norms

Personal freedom norms

Sensing problems

Defining problems

Deriving solutions

Implementing solutions

Evaluating outcomes

viduals. The culture track reveals the norms of the organization. It exposes the old culture and helps create a new culture. Without an adaptive culture it can be impossible to make improvements, so removing the cultural barriers has to be accomplished before proceeding to another track.

First, one needs to clarify the actual norms. For instance, one could ask members to list current dos and don'ts. The members can then list what they want the norms to be and identify the culture gaps. Culture gaps are often related to the following: (1) task support—norms related to helping others, information sharing, and concern for efficiency; (2) task innovation—norms related to performing new activities, trying different approaches, and being creative; (3) social relationship—norms about mixing business with pleasure and socializing with co-workers; and (4) personal freedom—norms for pleasing oneself, using self-expression, and exercising discretion (Box 11-8). Culture gaps are generally largest at lower levels in the organization.

Closing the culture gaps then becomes the issue. If the managers and associates decide that changes should occur, they can. Adaptive cultures have internal control. Control is a social reality but not necessarily an objective one. To establish desired norms, members can be asked to list norms they think would lead to organizational success. Then work groups need to develop a sanctioning system to monitor and enforce the new norms. Work groups should decide what will be done if a member violates a new norm or performs the desired behavior. The open sanctioning system is probably more equitable than the old unconscious sanctions.

Now it becomes important to sustain the cultural change. If the new culture is not supported by the remaining four tracks, it is likely that the culture will revert to the dysfunctional ways. The management skills and team-building tracks develop leadership to support the adaptive culture. The strategy-structure track will document the new systems, and the reward system track will support the new norms.

In the management skills track, managers are taught the five steps of problem management: (1) sensing problems, (2) defining problems, (3) deriving solutions, (4) implementing solutions, and (5) evaluating outcomes (Box 11-9). Next, managers examine their personality types. Because one's personality type determines how one will assimilate information and make decisions, managers should be aware of their style and the styles of associates so they can compensate for their natural inclinations and acknowledged limitations and develop strong work teams.

Managers also need to learn assumptional analysis: how to surface, classify by amount of certainty and importance, and synthesize assumptions. Outdated assumptions can lead to the wrong strategy-structure and reward systems. In a climate of trust and openness, associates should be able to examine previously unstated assumptions so they are not held back by faulty assumptions.

The team-building track activates the new culture and skills through the entire organization. Team building involves the following: (1) reuniting the work group, (2) identifying work-group prob-

Box 11-10　TEAM BUILDING

Reuniting the work groups

Identifying work-group problems

Identifying solutions and developing plans

Implementing the plans

Evaluating and monitoring the outcomes

Box 11-11　STRATEGY-STRUCTURE TRACK

Operationalizing strategy

Designing subunits

Implementing structure

Box 11-12　DEVELOPMENTAL STAGES OF AN ORGANIZATION

Birth—creation and survival as a viable system

Youth—stability, reputation, pride

Maturity—uniqueness, adaptability, contribution to society

lems, (3) identifying solutions and developing action plans, (4) implementing the plans, and (5) evaluating and monitoring the outcomes (Box 11-10). Interteam building is also included in this track. Everyone in the organization needs to learn how to cope with difficult people, understand her own personality style, and appreciate the styles of others.

In the strategy-structure track, strategy sets the direction and structure organizes the goals, tasks, people, and other resources to accomplish the plans. This involves operationalizing strategy, designing subunits, and implementing structure (Box 11-11). The reward-system track ensures that associates are rewarded for doing the right things for the right reasons.

ORGANIZATIONAL DEVELOPMENT

Organizations progress through developmental stages—birth, youth, and maturity (Box 11-12). The creation of a new organization and its survival as a viable system are primary concerns during the birth stage. Gaining stability and developing a reputation and pride are the focuses of the youth stage. The maturity stage involves achieving both uniqueness and adaptability and contributing to society.

As organizations are born and grow, they pass through increasingly complex stages of life. They must develop internally and generate new control processes to fit the amount of turbulence and complexity in the environment. At each stage the environment can become more unknown, unsettled, and difficult. A crisis develops in each stage. Changing its organizational and decision-making structures is needed to fit this new complexity. The new organization copes by developing job descriptions, programs, policies, and procedures. However, as the organization grows and becomes more complex, these policies do not cover the exceptions. As a result, the organization develops a set of hierarchical positions to make judgments about the exceptions to the existing job descriptions and policies. As the organization becomes larger and more complex, the managers in the hierarchy become overloaded. They do not have time to deal with all the exceptions and cannot make sense out of the situation.

Consequently, in the third stage accomplishing orderliness by developing broader goals is required. However, as the organization becomes increasingly complex, conflicts arise between factions, and the organization regresses to hierarchical referral again.

A decentralized system of departments reduces the interconnections between divisions and reduces the number of communications necessary to make decisions. But as the revolutionary cycle continues, conflict between decentralized departments develops.

In the last stage, a vertical information system is developed so that standardized accounting and statistical reporting systems from each department are consolidated at the top, and then resources are allocated among departments. Because all the complex information in turbulent systems cannot be reduced to numbers, human contacts made between department members become a major coping mechanism. Liaisons, teams, committees, task forces, and integrator roles are used.

BEHAVIORAL ASPECTS OF ORGANIZATIONAL CHANGE

Many people are unaware of the factors that initiate change or influence its direction. Even when known, some forces are beyond their control. Some factors that effect change in an agency stem from society, such as new knowledge and technology, new social requirements, changing client needs and demands, and increased competition. Even when known in advance and anticipated, they cannot be controlled by an agency.

The efficiency of an organizational structure is hard to measure, and the factors contributing to success or failure may be impossible to isolate. Organizational structure may not be the problem. A few ineffective people can disrupt an otherwise sound structure, and good people can make a bad structure work. High labor costs, inadequate equipment, ineffective advertising, changing client needs, and increased competition may contribute to inadequate profits.

Some symptoms reflect inefficiencies within the organization and indicate a need for change. If slow and erroneous decision making is a problem, one may question the qualifications of the person making decisions, the level at which responsibility is placed, and access to necessary information. Poor communications, a dearth of innovation, and failure in functional areas are other symptoms indicating a need for change. Diagnosis of the problem is extremely important for planned change. Minor adjustments rather than major reorganizations may correct some problems. However, even a small change in one part of an organization can cause a chain reaction throughout the agency. This domino effect creates problems with coordination and control and brings about a need for comprehensive planning.

Change disrupts equilibrium. Equilibrium can be maintained only when opposing forces are equal. Production may be maintained when the forces fostering production, such as pressure of the manager to produce, desire for favorable attention from the manager to foster one's own gain, and desire to earn more through the incentive plan, equal the forces limiting production, such as the informal group's standard against rate busting, resistance to training, and the feeling that the job and product are not important. However, when the forces in one direction or the other change in relation to each other, a new grouping forms and change is inevitable.

Changes involve endings, transitions, and beginnings. People grieve when they lose something, when they are threatened with the loss of something, and when they never had and never will have something (Jeffreys, 1995). With change, people go through the grieving process, which Elizabeth Kubler-Ross (1969) has identified as denial, anger, bargaining, depression, and then acceptance. Three stages of loss and mourning are (1) protest, (2) despair, and (3) reorganization. If people do not work through acceptance and reorganization, they may have disengagement (withdrawal), disidentification (sadness and worry), disorientation (confusion), or disenchantment (anger). Disengaged workers may quit and leave or quit and stay, or retire in place. They tend to not ask questions, not seek information, not discuss, and do only the basic requirements, and they may be hard to find. With disidentification, people have lost their self-identity and are vulnerable, like a lobster that has cast off its shell so it can grow. They may sulk, reminisce, dwell on the past, continue to do the old job, and resist new tasks. With disorientation, people have lost sight of where they fit in the organization. They do not know the priorities, do the wrong things, get very detail oriented, and get others to ask questions. The disenchanted people know that what is gone is gone and may become angry and negative. They may talk in a raised tone of voice or refuse to talk, show self-pity, walk out, sabotage, and do backstabbing. Disenchantment can lead to personal problems and destructive behavior (Belasco, 1990; Kanter, 1985, 1989; Loveridge and Cummings, 1996; Marquis and Huston, 1996, 1998; Woodward and Woodward, 1994).

Resistance to Change

Caution should be used when making organizational changes. Changes are disturbing to those affected, and resistance often develops. Giving the structure a chance to work may be better than changing it. Although changing the organizational structure may appear easy on paper, it is quite complicated in reality. It affects the attitudes and effectiveness of personnel whose prestige and status are threatened. Resistance to change is a common phenomenon whether it is initiated by positive stimuli, such as growth or promotion of an employee, or negative forces, such as poor management. Personnel develop vested interests, preferences, habits, and rigidities that attract them to the existing structure. People tend to consider the effects of the change on their personal lives, status, and future more than on the welfare of the agency. Change introduces the risk of error, fear of failure when trying something new, resistance to admission of weakness, fear of losing a current satisfaction, or a fatalistic expectation based on previous unsuccessful attempts to change. Change is most threatening in the presence of insecurity. Even logical, needed changes produce resistance (Maurer, 1996).

Causes of resistance to change include the following: threatened self-interest; embarrassment; insecurity; habits; complacency; inaccurate perceptions; perceived loss of power, rewards, or relationships; objective disagreement; psychological reactions; low tolerance for change; the change's going against the current trends; and the system's having been stable for a long time (Grohar-Murray and Di-Croce, 1997; Loveridge and Cummings, 1996; Morrison, 1993; Swansburg, 1996; Swansburg and Swansburg, 1999).

Robert Fritz (1996, 1999) explains that organizations either oscillate or advance. If they oscillate, success is neutralized. If they advance, success is possible. Successes breed further success, but with oscillation, success is short term. Because oscillation occurs over a long period of time and the organization is moving in the desired direction some of that time, oscillation can be hard to observe.

A conflict of interest causes oscillation between tension and resolution. For example, there is tension in a desire for change, which leads to the resolution in change effort. But that creates tension in a desire for continuity, which leads to change avoidance. That further leads to tension in a desire for change, which leads to change effort, which causes tension in a desire for continuity, which leads to change avoidance. Organizations often oscillate between centralized and decentralized decision making, expansion and limitation, growth and stability, investment and cost cutting, and long-term and short-term benefits (Figure 11-4).

Problem-solving approaches identify a problem and take action to solve the problem, which lessens the intensity of the problem, which leads to less action and then to reintensifying the problem. That is oscillation because as problems are solved, the motivation for change is reduced. Problem solving focuses on how to eliminate an unwanted situation instead of visioning the desired situation. Successful organizations often use a continuous quality improvement approach within structural tension. Personnel are clear about the desired outcomes and work on improving processes. Then success is measured against standards that reflect improvement toward the vision.

Organizations advance when there is structural tension. That requires structural understanding, leadership, and organizational learning. If the structure remains unchanged, behavior will revert to previous organizational behavior. A change in structure facilitates change in organizational behavior. The structural change is hierarchical because the organization's purpose gives direction to the strategies that are steps to move the organization from the current state to the desired vision. Progression creates a cycle that leads to results that are

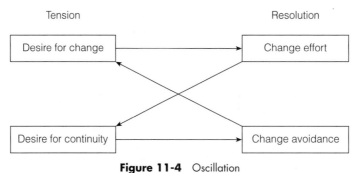

Figure 11-4 Oscillation
Modified from Fritz R: *Corporate tides: the inescapable laws of
organizational structure*, San Francisco, 1996, Berrett-Koehler.

evaluated. That leads to adjustments and refine-
ments, which lead to new actions or continuous
quality improvement and increased capacity over
time because it keeps renewing structural tension.
Organizations without vision cannot create structural tension and will oscillate instead of advance.
Values that dominate in an organization will displace competing lesser values, thus reducing oscillation. Leadership is a critical factor in clarifying the
vision. Leaders need to be clear about the vision
and the present reality to create the necessary structural tension. They make decisions about competing interests based on values. When leadership is
weak, workers support their own interests, which
leads to conflicts and oscillation. Leaders need to
create fair situations and reward people for their
merits and the accomplishments of the team. Organizations renew themselves by learning, which is
best motivated when it serves a desired outcome.
Training that is directly related to the organization's
vision and values is a powerful instrument for
change toward expanding capacity.

Gradual changes made in progressive phases
are usually less disturbing than radical, sweeping,
unpredicted changes. Changes in the structure resulting from sharply defined events that have
already been planned—such as changes in size,
scope, or objectives—are easier to execute than
shifts in personnel, which involve infinitely complex
human relations. Careful planning, appropriate
timing of communications, adequate feedback, and
employee confidence in management can reduce resistance to change.

Informing personnel of the reasons for change
can further reduce resistance, especially when the
advantages of the change are stressed. Personnel can
be involved by requests for their input, including
feelings, suggestions, and talents; their negative, as
well as positive, feelings should be respected. Communicating honestly about the changes, giving specific feedback, asking what assistance is needed to
help them cope, and recognizing their contributions to the implementation of the changes can further minimize resistance.

Types of Organizational Change

Organizational structure usually grows vertically,
then horizontally, and from a functional type to a
divisionalized type. Initially there is vertical growth,
but as the amount of work and its complexity increase, horizontal growth develops. Usually organizations develop from a functional type, which is
departmentalized by major functions, to one divisionalized by product or territory.

Planning for Change

Plans for change begin with an evaluation of the
existing organization. An organizational audit provides a detailed analysis of the organization, reveals
the extent to which goals are accomplished, and ex-
amines the use of personnel and the growth of individuals. One begins an organizational audit by
collecting and reviewing all available written material about the organization, including statement of

the mission or purpose, scope of the agency, goals and objectives, organizational chart, job descriptions, annual reports, performance appraisals, and qualifications needed and not needed by personnel in their present positions. The planner notes whether the reviewed materials are consistent, looks for gaps and overlapping of functioning, and determines if all activities contribute to the major goals of the agency.

Departmentalization, span of management, and balance and emphasis are analyzed. Authority relationships are studied. Leadership patterns, delegation, decentralization, use of committees, and provision of controls are considered. The agency may be compared with what is visualized as an ideal agency or with competitors to identify areas of need and to propose recommended changes. Personnel may be surveyed to identify areas needing improvement. The quantitative approach may be used where ratios are appropriate, such as figuring range of management. Then various organizational patterns are designed, and position breakdown using existing personnel is developed. Personnel who are needed but not presently available and people who are available but not qualified or needed are identified.

A job description and requirements are necessary for each position. Each person's qualifications can be compared with the job requirements. Notations are made of job requirements for which skills are not possessed. Those qualities that can be developed on the job within reasonable time limits should be separated from required skills that cannot be acquired. Unused abilities should be related to requirements of other jobs for which the individual may be better qualified.

Changes in personnel are normal, but they are accelerated during organizational changes. Unless managers are to become obsolete, they must change with the times. Some quickly increase their managerial knowledge and skills. Unfortunately, others are inflexible, overly conservative, and negative. Executive obsolescence is increasingly common with the rapid changes in our society. Managers who previously performed competently may be overwhelmed with increasingly complex duties, or they may have been promoted during an emergency

to a position for which they were inadequately prepared.

What can one do about an unqualified incumbent? In developing a strategy, one should consider the ramifications of the action on the individual and on the group. The strategy should depend on the particular circumstances. An incompetent staff associate may be counseled toward satisfactory performance. Weaknesses should be identified and means to overcome them defined. On-the-job training, in-service education, college courses, and independent study may be explored. A contract may be written between the employer and the incompetent subordinate, specifying what skills are to be developed to what level of achievement and in what time frame.

Incompetent executives may be transferred to positions for which they are more qualified. They may be moved from line to staff authority. The change is most attractive when the advisory staff position is at a higher organizational level than the present line position, carries prestige, and maintains the current salary. Executives may be told there is a problem in the new area that they are to solve. This method fosters high morale and loyalty. It removes incompetence from line authority when damage could be done but uses the executive's knowledge and skills to solve specific problems. This is an expensive method.

Termination is the most extreme way to handle incompetence. It is either direct or indirect. In the direct method employees are informed that their work does not meet the minimal criteria and they are expected to leave the agency. The indirect method may involve giving incompetent employees nothing to do, withholding information from them, leaving their names off memoranda, excluding them from conferences, and generally making them so miserable they will voluntarily resign.

New managers may be hired, particularly when new positions become available during reorganization. They often bring new ideas, objectivity, and enthusiasm to the job. Recruitment is important for development of an executive pool. The best managers do not need to hunt for jobs. The jobs hunt for them. The agency should let its need be known and seek good managers aggressively. Similar agencies may be a resource for managers with new ideas and different approaches. Graduates may be recruited from university programs. Recruiting through advertisements in professional journals and through employment agencies is useful for locating potential managers and well-qualified staff.

Promotions within the agency provide incentives and supply the executive pool. However, some personnel may not be interested in managerial work, and competent, satisfied employees may lack managerial potential.

After the revised organization is decided, developing operational procedures to expedite changes is required. These procedures define activities that are necessary for specific work and identify changes needed. The revised operational procedures should be inclusive, show all details, and ensure coordinated change. Work flow should be maintained and standards upheld. Special activities are likely to be needed during a transitional period. The revised operational procedures should be perceived as carefully thought-out, planned changes and not just as stopgap actions.

Strategies for Organizational Change

Visions of what the organization can become, instead of what it is or has been, allow for organizational change. To this end, managers need to create an open atmosphere where questions can be asked. Welcoming criticism instead of forbidding it helps personnel be adequately self-critical. Denying problems has serious consequences. A good recruitment plan is needed for hiring competent, highly motivated personnel. Career development programs should be provided. All employees need to feel that what they achieve is important to the agency and that needed change for the continuing vitality of the organization overrides their vested interests.

David Coleman and Raman Khanna (1995) have identified the issues in managing change as awareness, knowledge, trial, evaluation, and acceptance.

Michael McMaster (1996) has identified the phases of the transformation process as follows:

1. *Awakening.* There is an awareness that something is wanted or needed.
2. *Formulation.* The iterative process of dialogue facilitates movement from proposals to possibilities.
3. *Experimentation.* Isolated experiments and pilot projects test the propositions.
4. *Integration.* Isolated projects are added to other parts.
5. *Development.* Continuous improvements are implemented.
6. *Mastery.* Teaching and learning lead to understanding and excellence.

John Kotter (1996) outlines an eight-stage process for leading change as follows: (1) establishing a sense of urgency, (2) creating the guiding coalition, (3) developing a vision and strategy, (4) communicating the change vision, (5) empowering employees for broad-based action, (6) generating short-term wins, (7) consolidating gains and producing more change, and (8) anchoring new approaches in the culture. He discusses how not doing those things are reasons transformation efforts fail in James Champy and Nitin Nohria's book *Fast Forward: The Best Ideas on Managing Business Change* (1996).

David Carr and Henry Johansson (1995) outline 16 best practices in reengineering as follows:

1. Recognize and articulate an "extremely compelling" need to change. . . .
2. Start with and maintain executive-level support. . . .
3. Understand the organization's "readiness to change." . . .
4. Communicate effectively to create buy-in. Then communicate more. . . .
5. Create top-notch teams. . . .
6. Use a structured framework. . . .
7. Use consultants effectively. . . .
8. Link goals to corporate strategy. . . .
9. Listen to the "voice of the customer." . . .
10. Select the right processes for reengineering. . . .
11. Maintain focus: Don't try to reengineer too many processes. . . .
12. Maintain teams as the key vehicle for change. . . .

13. Quickly come to an as-is understanding of the processes to be reengineered. . . .
14. Choose and use the right metrics. . . .
15. Understand the risks and develop contingency plans. . . .
16. Have plans for continuous improvement. . . .

David Nadler (1998) has identified twelve steps in three categories to deal with power, anxiety, and control as follows:

A. Need to shape the political dynamics of change
    1. Build the support of key power groups
    2. Use leader behavior to generate support
    3. Use symbols and language deliberately
    4. Define points of stability
B. Need to motivate change
    5. Create dissatisfaction with the current state
    6. Build participation in planning and implementing change
    7. Reward behavior in support of change
    8. Provide people time and opportunity to disengage from the old
C. Need to manage the transition
    9. Develop and communicate a clear image of the future state
    10. Use multiple leverage points
    11. Develop transition management structures
    12. Collect and analyze feedback

Others speak to the importance of persuasive communications, participation, education, support, role modeling, new structural arrangements, extrinsic rewards, and moving slowly (Grohar-Murray and DiCroce, 1997; Morrison, 1993; Nadler, Shaw, Walton et al., 1995; Nevis, Lancourt, and Vassallo, 1996; Smith, 1996).

Timothy Galpin (1996) clarifies that resistance may be because people do not know, are not able, or are not willing. When they are not knowing, the leader should communicate the what, why, how, when, who, and where. When they are not able, the leader educates and trains in new skills and management techniques. When they are not willing, the leader sets goals, measures, provides coaching and feedback, rewards, and recognizes.

CHAPTER SUMMARY

Chapter 11 covered the following:
Culture of Individuals
  Values
  Attitudes
  Perceptions
  Cognitive Styles
  Attitudes Toward Change
  Interpersonal Needs
  Personality
  Roles
Myers-Briggs Type Indicator
Diversity
Management of Cultural Diversity
Organizational Culture
  Types of Cultures
    Integrated or Differentiated Frames of Reference
      Subcultures
      Countercultures
Management of Change
  Forces That Influence Change
  Strategies for Effecting Change
    Empirical-rational strategies
    Normative reeducative strategies
    Power-coercive strategies
  Process of Change
  Types of Change
    Coercive change
    Emulative change
    Indoctrination
    Interactional change
    Natural change
    Socialization change
    Technocratic change
    Planned change
  Role of the Manager as Change Agent
  Force-Field Analysis
  Cultural Change in Organizations
Organizational Development
Behavioral Aspects of Organizational Change
  Resistance to Change
  Types of Organizational Change
  Planning for Change
  Strategies for Organizational Change

REFERENCES

Barr L, Barr N: *The leadership equation: leadership, management, and the Myers-Briggs,* Austin, Tex, 1989, Eakin Press.

Belasco JA: *Teaching the elephant to dance: empowering change in your organization,* New York, 1990, Crown.

Bennis WG, Benne KD, Chin R: *The planning of change,* Fort Worth, 1969, Holt, Rinehart, & Winston.

Briggs-Myers I, Myers PB: *Gifts differing,* Palo Alto, Calif, 1980, Consulting Psychologists Press.

Carr DK, Johansson HJ: *Best practices in reengineering: what works and what doesn't in the reengineering process,* New York, 1995, McGraw-Hill.

Champy J, Nohria N: *Fast forward: the best ideas on managing business change,* Boston, 1996, Harvard Business Review.

Coleman D, Khanna R: *Groupware: technologies and applications,* Upper Saddle River, NJ, 1995, Prentice Hall.

Conner DR: *Managing at the speed of change,* New York, 1993, Villard.

Conner DR: *Leading at the edge of chaos: how to create the nimble organization,* New York, 1998, John Wiley & Sons.

Cooke R, Rousseau D: Behavioral norms and expectations: a quantitative approach to the assessment of organizational culture, *Group Organ Stud* 13:245-273, 1987.

Deal TE, Kennedy AA: *Corporate cultures: the rites and rituals of corporate life,* Reading, Mass, 1982, Addison-Wesley.

Deevy E: *Creating the resilient organization,* Englewood Cliffs, NJ, 1995, Prentice Hall.

Douglas LM: *The effective nurse leader and manager,* ed 5, St. Louis, 1996, Mosby.

Festinger L: *A theory of cognitive dissonance,* Stanford, Calif, 1957, Stanford University Press.

Fritz R: *Corporate tides: the inescapable laws of organizational structure,* San Francisco, 1996, Berrett-Koehler.

Fritz R: *The path of least resistance for managers: designing organizations to succeed,* San Francisco, 1999, Berrett-Koehler.

Galpin TJ: *The human side of change: a practical guide to organization redesign,* San Francisco, 1996, Jossey-Bass.

Gardenswartz L, Rowe A: *Diverse teams at work: capitalizing on the power of diversity,* Burr Ridge, Ill, 1995, Irwin Professional.

Gillies DA: *Nursing management: a systems approach,* ed 3, Philadelphia, 1994, WB Saunders.

Grohar-Murray ME, DiCroce HR: *Leadership and management in nursing,* Stamford, Conn, 1997, Appleton & Lange.

Havelock RG: *The change agent's guide to innovation in education,* Englewood Cliffs, NJ, 1973, Educational Technology Publications.

Huber D: *Leadership and nursing care management,* Philadelphia, 1996, WB Saunders.

Jeffreys JS: *Coping with workplace change: dealing with loss and grief,* Menlo Park, Calif, 1995, Crisp Publications.

Kanter RM: *The change masters,* New York, 1985, Simon & Schuster.

Kanter RM: *When giants learn to dance,* New York, 1989, Simon & Schuster.

Kilmann RH: *Managing beyond the quick fix: a completely integrated program for creating and maintaining organizational success,* San Francisco, 1989, Jossey-Bass.

Kilmann RH: *Managing beyond the quick fix,* San Francisco, Calif, 1991, Jossey-Bass.

Kotter JP: *Leading change,* Boston, 1996, Harvard Business School Press.

Kubler-Ross E: *On death and dying,* New York, 1969, Macmillan.

Lippitt R, Watson J, Westley B: *The dynamics of planned change,* New York, 1958, Harcourt, Brace & World.

Loden M, Rosener JB, Rosener J: *Workforce America! Managing employee diversity as a vital resource,* Burr Ridge, Ill, 1991, Irwin Professional.

Loveridge CE, Cummings SH: *Nursing management in the new paradigm,* Gaithersburg, Md, 1996, Aspen.

Marquis BL, Huston CJ: *Leadership roles and management functions in nursing: theory and application,* ed 2, Philadelphia, 1996, Lippincott.

Marquis BL, Huston CJ: *Management decision making for nurses: 124 case studies,* Philadelphia, 1998, Lippincott.

Martin J: *The great transition: using the seven disciplines of enterprise engineering to align people, technology, and strategy,* New York, 1995, American Management Association.

Maurer R: *Beyond the wall of resistance,* Austin, Tex, 1996, Bard Books.

McMaster MD: *The intelligence advantage: organizing for complexity,* Boston, 1996, Butterworth-Heinemann.

Morrison M: *Professional skills for leadership: foundations of a successful career,* St. Louis, 1993, Mosby.

Nadler DA, Nadler MB: *Champions of change: how CEOs and their companies are mastering the skills of radical change,* San Francisco, 1998, Jossey-Bass.

Nadler DA, Shaw RB, Walton AE et al.: *Discontinuous change: leading organizational transformation,* San Francisco, 1995, Jossey-Bass.

Nevis EC, Lancourt J, Vassallo HG: *Intentional revolutions: a seven-point strategy for transforming organizations,* San Francisco, 1996, Jossey-Bass.

Rocchiccioli JT, Tilbury MS: *Clinical leadership in nursing,* Philadelphia, 1998, WB Saunders.

Rogers EM: *Diffusion of innovations,* ed 4, New York, 1995, Free Press.

Schneider WE: *The reengineering alternative: a plan for making your current culture work,* Burr Ridge, Ill, 1994, IRWIN.

Senge PM: *The fifth discipline,* New York, 1990, Doubleday.

Senge PM, Kleiner A, Roberts C et al.: *The fifth discipline fieldbook,* New York, 1994, Currency Doubleday.

Smith DK: *Taking charge of change: 10 principles for managing people and performance,* Reading, Mass, 1996, Addison-Wesley.

Stewart EC, Bennett MJ: *American cultural patterns: a cross-cultural perspective,* Yarmouth, Me, 1991, Intercultural Press.

Sullivan EJ, Decker PJ: *Effective leadership and management in nursing,* Menlo Park, Calif, 1977, Addison Wesley Longman.

Swansburg RC: *Management and leadership for nurse managers,* ed 2, Boston, 1996, Jones & Bartlett.

Swansburg RC, Swansburg RJ: *Introductory management and leadership for nurses: an interactive text,* Boston, 1999, Jones & Bartlett.

Tappen RM: *Nursing leadership and management: concepts and practice,* ed 3, Philadelphia, 1995, FA Davis.

Trice HM, Beyer JM: *The cultures of work organizations,* Englewood Cliffs, NJ, 1993, Prentice Hall.

Wheatley MJ: *Leadership and the new science,* San Francisco, 1992, Berrett-Koehler.

Wheatley MJ, Kellner-Rogers M: *A simpler way,* San Francisco, 1996, Berrett-Koehler.

Whetten DA, Cameron KS: *Developing management skills,* ed 4, Reading, Mass, 1998, Addison-Wesley.

Wilkins AL: *Developing corporate character,* San Francisco, 1989, Jossey-Bass.

Woodward H, Bucholz S, Hess K: *Aftershock: helping people through corporate change,* New York, 1987, John Wiley & Sons.

Woodward H, Woodward MB: *Navigating through change,* Burr Ridge, Ill, 1994, Richard D Irwin.

Yoder-Wise PS: *Leading and managing in nursing,* ed 2, St. Louis, 1999, Mosby.

Zohar D: *Rewiring the corporate brain: using the new science to rethink how we structure and lead organizations,* San Francisco, 1997, Berrett-Koehler.

BIBLIOGRAPHY

Andrews MM: A model for cultural change, *Nurs Manage* 29:62-63, 66, Oct 1998.

Beyers M: Nurses responding to change, *Nurs Manage* 25:37-38, Nov 1994.

Bhola HS: The CLER model: thinking through change, *Nurs Manage* 25:59-63, May 1994.

Bruhn JG: Creating an organizational climate for multiculturalism, *Health Care Superv* 14(4):11-18, 1996.

Bruhn JG, Chesney AP: The organizational zoo: a fable, *Health Care Superv* 14(3):13-20, 1996.

Ciancio J: Organizational restructuring and the psychologic contract, *Nurs Manage* 29:81-82, Sept 1998.

Clark KH et al.: Turning the organization upside down: creating a culture for innovation and creativity, *Nurs Adm Q* 16(1):7-14, 1991.

Coccia C: Avoiding a "toxic" organization, *Nurs Manage* 29:32-33, May 1998.

Coeling HVE, Simms LM: Facilitating innovation at the unit level through cultural assessment, Part 2: adapting managerial ideas to the unit work group, *JONA* 13:13-20, May 1993.

DeLellis AJ: Creating a climate of mutual respect among employees: a workshop design, *Health Care Superv* 15(4):48-56, 1997.

Dienemann J: *Nursing administration: strategic perspectives and application,* Norwalk, Conn, 1990, Appleton & Lange.

Ellis JR, Hartley CL: *Managing and coordinating nursing care,* ed 2, Philadelphia, 1995, JB Lippincott.

Fetteroll EC, Hoffherr GD, Moran J: *Growing teams: a down-to-earth approach,* Methuen, Mass, 1993, GOAL/QPC.

Flarey DL: The social climate scale: a tool for organizational change and development, *JONA* 21:37-44, April 1991.

Fleeger ME: Assessing organizational culture: a planning strategy, *Nurs Manage* 24:39-41, Feb 1993.

Gelinas LS, Manthey M: The impact of organizational redesign on nurse executive leadership, *JONA* 27:35-42, Oct 1997.

Goodridge D, Hack B: Assessing the congruence of nursing models with organizational culture: a quality improvement perspective, *J Nurs Care Qual* 10:41-48, Jan 1996.

Hagerman ZJ, Tiffany CR: Evaluation of two planned change theories, *Nurs Manage* 25:57-60, April 1994.

Jeska S, Rounds R: Addressing the human side of change: career development and renewal, *Nurs Econ* 14:339-345, Nov-Dec 1996.

Johns J: Trust: key to acculturation in corporatized health care environments, *Nurs Adm Q* 20(2): 13-24, 1996.

Jones KR, DeBaca V, Yarbrough M: Organizational culture assessment before and after implementing patient-focused care, *Nurs Econ* 15:73-80, March-April 1997.

Knox S, Irving JA: Nurse manager perceptions of healthcare executive behaviors during organizational change, *JONA* 27:33-39, Nov 1997.

Kreitzer MJ, Wright D, Hamlin C et al.: Creating a healthy work environment in the midst of organizational change and transition, *JONA* 27:35-41, June 1997.

Luechauer D, Shulman GM: Using a metaphor exercise to explore the principles of organizational culture, *J Man Ed* 22:736-744, Dec 1998.

Lutjens LRJ, Tiffany CR: Evaluating planned change theories, *Nurs Manage* 25:54-57, March 1994.

Marino BL, Ganser CC: Sensitivity of patient report of care to organizational change, *JONA* 27: 32-36, April 1997.

McDermott K et al.: Work empowerment and organizational commitment, *Nurs Manage* 27:44-47, May 1996.

Murphy L, Gorham G: Organizational and operational redesign: if we should, then how? *Seminars Nurse Managers* 4:10-19, March 1996.

Murphy R, Pearlman F, Rea C et al.: Work redesign: a return to the basics, *Nurs Manage* 25:37-46, Feb 1994.

Nash MG, Everett LN: Cultural cohesion versus collision: a model for facilitating organizational mergers, *JONA* 26:11-17, July-Aug 1996.

Potter ML et al.: change . . . ouch! *Nurs Manage* 29:27-29, Nov 1998.

Rizzo JA, Gilman MP, Mersmann CA: Facilitating care delivery redesign using measures of unit culture and work characteristics, *JONA* 24:32-37, May 1994.

Schein EH: *Organizational culture and leadership,* San Francisco, 1989, Jossey-Bass.

Schoolfield M, Orduna A: Understanding staff nurse responses to change: utilization of a grief-change framework to facilitate innovation . . . introduction of patient-focused care, *Clinical Nurse Specialist* 8:57-62, Jan 1994.

Seago JA: Work group culture, stress, and hostility: correlations with organizational outcomes, *JONA* 26:39-47, June 1996.

Seago JA: Culture of troubled work groups, *JONA* 26:41-45, Sept 1996.

Seago JA: Five pitfalls of work redesign in acute care, *Nurs Manage* 28:49-50, Oct 1997.

Spiker BK: Making change stick, *Industry Week* 243:45, March 7, 1994.

Tiffany CR, Lutjens LRJ: *Planned change theories for nursing: review, analysis, and implications,* Thousand Oaks, 1998, Sage Publications.

Tillman HJ et al.: Environmental turbulence: staff nurse perspectives, *JONA* 27:15-22, Nov 1997.

Tye J: Never fear, never quit, *Nurs Manage* 28:38-40, July 1997.

CASE STUDY

Primary nursing with all nursing care given by RNs has been practiced for the past several years on the unit where you are the patient care coordinator. In an effort to cut costs, the hospital is going to hire technicians to work with RNs and implement a "partners in practice" model. What will you do as a patient care coordinator to help change the organizational culture?

CASE STUDY

You are going to start using critical pathways instead of nursing care plans on the unit. What are the driving and restraining forces related to this innovation? How would you go about implementing the five tracks for organizational planned change?

Critical Thinking Activities for this chapter begin on page 503.

CHAPTER 12

SELECTION AND DEVELOPMENT OF PERSONNEL

CHAPTER OBJECTIVES

- Describe why retention measures are at least as important as recruitment efforts.
- Identify three activities related to selection of personnel.
- Interpret affirmative action.
- Discuss at least four cultural phenomena and their influence on the interviewing process.
- Describe features of job descriptions.
- Describe advantages and disadvantages of career ladders.
- Describe the importance of orientation.
- List at least six ways to accomplish staff development.
- Describe career mapping as a part of career development.
- Diagram four stages of group, or team, process and the major activity in each stage.
- Compare groups and teams.

Chapter Overview

Chapter 12 outlines leadership and management for recruitment and development of personnel, screening of staff, equal opportunity and affirmative action, cultural diversity, Americans With Disabilities Act, job analysis, orientation, staff development, career planning, career mapping, group process, and team development.

MAJOR CONCEPTS AND DEFINITIONS	
Personnel	persons employed in an agency or department
Recruitment	the process of enlisting personnel for employment
Retention	capacity to retain employees once they are hired
Affirmative action	actions taken to remedy past discriminatory practices
Cultural diversity	communication, space, social organization, time, environmental control, and biological variations between cultures
Orientation	familiarization with and adaptation to an environment
Job analysis	the study of a position to determine what knowledge, skill, aptitude, and personal characteristics are needed to perform certain responsibilities
Job evaluation	process of measuring the remunerative worth of a job in relationship to other positions
Job design	specifies what the job requires, job methods, and the relationship between the organizational, social, and personal needs of the worker
Job rotation	a horizontal job enlargement technique
Job enrichment	vertical approach to job design that uses more abilities and skills of personnel
Job descriptions	specifications that are the requirements for the job
Career ladder	vertical clinical advancement
Staff development	education of the employees
Preceptor	teacher or instructor
Mentor	a wise and faithful counselor
Career mapping	strategic plan for one's career
Group process	how the group functions

SELECTION OF PERSONNEL

Leaders predict and plan for the future. They serve as role models, promote the image of the organization, identify and recruit well-qualified people, and assign the new personnel for success for them and the organization. Managers share responsibility for recruitment and retention of well-qualified people. They help establish criteria for selection of personnel and structure interviews to increase validity and reliability of recruitment. They apply their knowledge of legal requirements for hiring and make placement decisions based on employee strengths and the organization's needs (Box 12-1).

Box 12-1   RECRUITMENT LEADERSHIP AND MANAGEMENT

Leadership	Management
Predicts the future	Shares responsibility for recruitment and retention of staff
Plans for the future	Structures interview process
Role models for recruitment	Increases validity and reliability of recruitment
Uses interview process to promote image of the organization	Helps establish criteria for selection
Identifies and recruits well-qualified people	Applies knowledge of legal requirements for hiring
Assigns new personnel for success	Makes placement decisions based on employee strengths and organizational needs

Modified from Marquis BL, Huston CJ: *Leadership roles and management functions in nursing: theory and application*, Philadelphia, 1996, Lippincott.

Recruitment and Retention

The acquisition of qualified people in any agency is critical for the establishment, maintenance, and growth of the organization. Therefore active recruitment is important, and the attraction of qualified applicants is the first step in selection of personnel. Modes for active recruitment include employee recommendations and word of mouth; advertisements in local newspapers, nursing organization bulletins, and nursing journals; recruitment literature, such as flyers and newsletters; posters; career days; job fairs; contacts with schools' graduating classes; placement services; open houses; nursing conventions; and frequent, low-cost, credit-carrying continuing education courses for outsiders, as well as employees (Box 12-2).

Word of mouth can be very effective, but it can also lead to the hiring of friends and relatives of the current workforce; this practice may foster nepotism and violate equal opportunity employment requirements. The use of advertisements in professional journals, in newspapers, and on radio and television, employment agencies, and contacts with schools' graduating classes offers the prospective employer a broader field for selection and more opportunities to hire from minority groups. Hiring minority group members may require active recruitment to meet public policy.

Box 12-2   MODES FOR RECRUITMENT

Employee recommendations	Posters
Word of mouth	Career days
Advertisements	Job fairs
Flyers	Placement services
Newsletters	Open houses
Bulletins	Nursing conventions

Each institution should have someone who is responsible for recruitment. Recruiters should know nursing qualifications and the needs of the institution. They should be able to represent the institution with candor and enthusiasm. It is important that the recruiter relate well to people. Referrals from employees should be sought and in-house applicants encouraged; however, favoritism should not be shown. To aid in the selection of the best candidate for the job, an adequate budget should be provided for necessary advertisement, and these advertisements should depict an institution that cares about employees and patients. That image should also be reflected at open houses, during conventions, and at high school and college career days.

The content of advertising is more important than the form. The recruiter should determine the needs and desires of potential applicants and demonstrate how the institution will meet those needs. New graduates are likely to be interested in thorough orientation, in-service education, staff development, and intern programs. Some nurses will be interested in tuition reimbursement and release time to work on educational degrees. Single people will be more interested in health benefits than married people whose spouses have family coverage. Older nurses will be increasingly interested in retirement plans. Refresher courses, chartered buses for people who live in suburban areas, child care programs, part-time work, and flexible personnel policies may appeal to inactive nurses. The nurse recruiter needs to assess nurses' interests and show how the institution can address their concerns.

The recruiter should respond to inquiries immediately. Records of inquiries noting the origin (how the job applicant learned of the opening) and disposition (hired or not and length of tenure) should be compiled and evaluated. The most productive recruitment method should be maximized. Out-of-town or out-of-state applicants should be assisted with information about the community and housing.

The major sources of personnel are persons seeking their first jobs, dissatisfied employees, and the unemployed. These classifications are important, for the categories indicate types of information the nursing manager should obtain, and they influence the selection process. Recent graduates or nurses who have not practiced since graduation may have a limited idea of job opportunities. Their choice of a first job may be strongly influenced by their education, achievement level, geographical preference, salary, mate's occupation, and peer pressure. They are likely to take several jobs before settling down. This variety of jobs, along with growing family responsibilities and maturity, helps develop the nurse's capabilities.

The dissatisfied employees are often not actively seeking other employment but are likely to be receptive to news of openings and job offers. If nursing managers attribute the dissatisfaction to the misuse of the person's talents and abilities, they may explore how to employ that person more effectively within their own agency. Job dissatisfaction is not uncommon, for every job has disadvantages. Agencies that require special job skills should expect applications from nurses who are looking for a better job with fewer disadvantages.

Hiring an unemployed worker who has been released from a previous job because of an infraction or a quarrel with the previous employer demands careful assessment. The nursing manager may wish to hire nurses who were fired because they refused to falsify records or perform a task for which they were not adequately prepared. They would not want to hire a nurse who was terminated because of high absenteeism and irresponsibility, unless the nurse could adequately explain the situation and assure the nursing manager that the problem has been resolved. For instance, the prospective employee might have been caring for a dying child at that time or having a marital crisis that has since ended in divorce.

It is unlikely that nurse applicants have been laid off from previous jobs because of slack times. If so, the nursing manager should consider the chances of the nurses' returning to their old jobs when the slack has ended. Seniority and other vested interests may influence nurses' desires to return to their previous positions.

Because of the costs of recruiting, selecting, and training employees, the decreased quality of care while orienting new workers, and the emotional drain of turnover on continuing employees, serious attention should be given to retention efforts. Exit interviews, particularly anonymous questionnaires, can help identify the reasons people resign. Posttermination questions mailed to the homes of former employees a month or two after their resignation may obtain more accurate information than does the exit interview. After a period of time has elapsed, a person may be less emotional and more objective with some distance from the job and may feel more anonymous with less fear of retaliation. In addition, attitude surveys can be used with current employees to identify sources of dissatisfaction and concern. Focus groups can be used to identify and solve problems. Once stressors are identified, strategies to reduce them can be planned. It is important to meet personnel's psychosocial needs for advancement, responsibility, achievement, and recognition. Nurses want input into decision making and control over their own lives.

Screening of Potential Staff

Investment in well-qualified nurses can produce a high rate of return, and errors, whether they be failure to hire a promising nurse or hiring someone who fails to achieve the organization's expectations, can be expensive mistakes. In general there are three underlying philosophies in the screening process:

1. The manager should screen out applicants who do not fit the agency's image. Although this practice is common among some corporations, it is not a standard procedure for selecting health care personnel.
2. The manager should try to fit the job to a promising applicant. Examples include part-time positions, split-shift hours, and opportunities for handicapped people.
3. Usually the manager should try to fit the applicant to the job. This philosophy assumes that both the person and the position are unique.

The essential and desirable qualities for the applicant can be identified. Each of the search and screen committee members can list what she thinks are essential and desirable qualities for an applicant for a specific job; the committee members can then discuss the qualities and come to consensus (Worksheet 12-1—Systematic Selection Chart, p. 509). Next, a qualification assessment form (Worksheet 12-2, p. 509) can be developed listing the essential and desirable qualities with yes, ?, and no columns for if the applicant has the quality or not and with a column for comments.

Application forms and résumés. Once the applicants have been attracted, they should submit biographical data. The application form is a quick way to collect demographical information. Data in the personal history—educational background, work experience, and other pertinent information—can be used to do the following:

- Determine whether the applicant meets minimal hiring requirements such as minimal educational level or minimal job experience
- Furnish background data useful in planning the selection interview
- Obtain names of references who may be contacted for additional information about the applicant's work experience and general character
- Collect information for personnel administration, that is, Social Security number, number of dependents, and so forth

Letters of reference. Letters of recommendation may be requested from references listed on the application form, previous employers, or both. However, these letters may be inaccurate and misleading because the people writing may not have had sufficient exposure to the nurses to become familiar with their capabilities, or they may not have even known the nurse. Because of rapid turnover of nursing personnel, it is possible that few current staff members worked with the previous employee, and the current manager, who joined the agency after the applicant had resigned, may have to write the letter of reference based on an inadequate personnel file. The applicant may not know the current whereabouts of previous managers. To prevent these problems, employees could ask that a letter of reference be sent to a placement bureau at the time of termination, but this measure does not necessarily solve the problem. They have no assurance that the letter writers can express themselves well or are even willing to be accurate.

The preceding discussion indicates that letters of reference should be used cautiously. More emphasis should be placed on comments made by previous employers and co-workers, because they tend to give more critical evaluations than do subordinates and personal acquaintances. Most emphasis should be placed on characteristics consistently cited and on the general tone of the letters.

Interview. A preemployment interview to predict job success should be conducted with the most qualified applicants. Information obtained from the application form and letters of reference should be taken into consideration during the interview. The purposes of the interview are to obtain information, to give information, and to determine if the applicant meets the requirements for the position. The interviewer judges the applicant's dependability, willingness to assume responsibility for the job, willingness and ability to work with others, interest in the job, adaptability, consistency of goals with available opportunities, and conformance of manners and appearance to job requirements. The interviewer answers questions, explains policies and procedures, and helps acquaint the applicant with the position. Finally, the interviewer must predict whether the applicant's overall performance will be satisfactory. The value of the interview is determined by the interviewer's ability to evaluate applicants and to predict accurately their future success.

The interview has definite purposes and should avoid social chitchat, although a brief warm-up period may help put the interviewee at ease. One of the main purposes is to learn about the prospective employee. Therefore it behooves the interviewer to concentrate on listening, as well as to provide necessary information and answer questions from the applicant. Managers should avoid giving clues about what pleases or displeases them, should not be argumentative, and should try to avoid premature judgment. They should also beware of the halo effect: judgment based on appearances. Although individuals wear clothing that reflects their personality, they are likely to select clothes for the interview that project the image they wish to convey.

It is advisable to train managers in the art of interviewing. Training might include methods of establishing rapport with an interviewee, interviewing techniques, therapeutic communication, and predicting applicant job performance. It is helpful to construct an interview recording form designed for the needs of the agency or for a specific position. Use of the job description to define and specify job dimensions on the form increases interviewer reliability. A personal profile of what the person hired should be, including education, experience, abilities, aptitudes, and interests, is helpful. Standardization of the interview promotes nondiscriminatory hiring practices and is particularly important when more than one person does the interviewing.

The heading of the form contains the date, name of the applicant, position desired, and the interviewer's name. The body categorizes traits required for the position. This allows the interviewer to assess the applicant more systematically. One area might be work history. Does the applicants' work history indicate that they have the ability to learn and understand the requirements of the job for which they are applying? More specifically, is there any evidence of lack of ability? Have they had past experience in performing the same or similar tasks? Are they familiar with the equipment and procedures? Have they had special project or task force assignments? Have they had job progression? Education is another area to be evaluated. Have applicants had adequate formal education? Is there evidence of on-the-job training? Have they participated in continuing education or in self-initiated skill development by reading books and journals and watching related television specials? Are they active in professional organizations?

Certainly applicants' dependability demands assessment. Is it likely that they will have a good attendance record and maintain good work habits? Or is there evidence of poor work habits or work performance? What do past attendance and safety records indicate? Of equal concern is applicants' sense of responsibility. Will they seek assistance when needed and take initiative when appropriate to get the job done? Will they see jobs through to the end? Is there evidence of past independent thought and action, or do they tend to blame others for problems? Finally, are they capable of assuming leadership when required?

Are applicants cooperative and able to get along with others and work well as team members, or do they have a preference for working alone? Is there evidence of success or friction with managers, peers, and staff associates? Are they open to criticism, or do they react excessively? Are applicants involved in the community? Have they been open and candid during the interview? Job interest, poise, manners, appearance, and aspirations are other areas to investigate.

The interviewer greets the applicant, introduces herself to the applicant, and makes brief comments about the agency and the position available. The interviewer confirms the position for which the person is applying and explains the plan for the interview. Information on the application is discussed, and clarification is sought if necessary. The applicant qualifications are discussed preferably using the structured interview format. If the applicant appears qualified, the agency and position can be discussed in more detail, and subsequent hiring procedures can be explained before the interview is terminated.

During the interview the interviewer explains the purpose and plan of the interview. This helps create a positive climate. The interviewer learns the most by listening rather than talking and can encourage the job candidate to talk freely by asking open-ended questions. These are nondirective questions that help reveal feelings and attitudes. Examples of nondirective questions are as follows: What qualifies you for this job? What aspects of your last job appealed to you? How were your relations with your peers?

Closed-ended questions are directive and can often be answered yes or no. They solicit less information than open-ended questions but are appropriate for objective and factual information. The following are examples of closed-ended questions: Who was your last employer? How long did you work for that agency? Did you get along with your co-workers? Do you think you are qualified for this job?

The funnel technique incorporates both open-ended and closed-ended questions. When using the funnel technique, the interviewer starts with an open-ended question such as, What subjects did you like most in school? This gets objective information and sets a nonthreatening tone. The scope of the discussion is then funneled by asking a self-appraisal question such as, Why do you think you liked those courses in particular? This elicits subjective information. The interviewer closes the discussion of a particular subject by asking direct questions to clarify the self-appraisal. A direct question might be, What classes did you take for your nursing electives?

A grid of topics to explore and the funnel technique can help the interviewer sequence questions in a logical order and decide what kind of questions to ask. Initially it may be helpful to fill in the topics and potential questions. The questions may be modified during the interview (Table 12-1).

After obtaining information from the candidate, it is appropriate for the interviewer to share information about the job, policies, the agency, and how the interviewee will be informed of the decision. The applicant is given an opportunity to ask questions. The interviewer closes the interview by telling the applicant when and how she can expect to hear the decision. For example, the interviewer can say, "I will be interviewing a few more applicants this week. You can expect to hear from me by the first of next week." Or, "You should receive a letter regarding our decision within 2 weeks."

The facts collected during the interview are used as the basis for assumptions or inferences. They should be checked throughout the interview as new information is collected. It is possible to make both positive and negative assumptions from the same information. For example, if an applicant did not work for 3 months between jobs, the negative assumption could be that the person was escaping, undirected, or lazy. A positive inference could be that the applicant was clarifying goals and fulfilling personal objectives. Inferences are often more reflective of the person making them than of the applicant, thus making it particularly important to test interpretations.

Women, men, minority applicants, and persons with disabilities should be treated in the same professional manner. The same general questions and the same standards should be required for all applicants. One should follow a structured interview plan to help achieve fairness in interviewing and

Table 12-1 Topics and Questions to be Explored During an Employment Interview

Topic to Explore	Open-Ended Question	Self-Appraisal Question	Direct Question
Education	Why did you choose to go to that school?	What courses were most useful to you, and how were they useful?	What courses did you take as electives?
Prior employment	Where have you worked?	What did you like best about your last job? What did you like least about your last job?	How long did you work there? What was your title? On what service areas did you work?
Life experiences	What life experiences have you had that help qualify you for this job?	How will raising your own children help you in this job?	How long have you spoken Spanish? How frequently do you use sign language?
Professional	What are your professional goals?	How do you plan to accomplish your goals?	What do you plan to be doing 5 years from now?

should treat all applicants with fairness, equality, and consistency.

Interviewers can talk about applicants' qualifications, abilities, experiences, education, and interests; the duties and responsibilities of the job; where the job is located, travel, equipment, and facilities available; and the organization's missions, programs, and achievements. These are acceptable, but one may not ask about lineage, national origin, race, sex, age, marital status, number or age of children, former addresses, religious affiliations, or handicaps. While one may ask about academic and professional education, schools attended, and ability to read, write, and speak a foreign language, the interviewer may not ask about the racial or religious affiliation of the schools, the date of the schooling, or one's native language. One may ask about professional organizations but not all memberships. A photograph may not be required before employment. The name and address of a person to contact in case of an emergency may be solicited but not the name and address of a relative. Inquiries about relatives who work in the agency or name and address of parents if the applicant is a minor are acceptable. Inquiry into actual convictions that relate to job performance can be asked, not questions relating to arrests.

Discriminatory behavior is improper even when it is not intended, and appearance is as important as reality. Questions not related to the job have been used in a discriminatory way and should be avoided. Because improper significance might be given to questions regarding marriage plans or family matters, one should not inquire about marital status or nonmarital arrangements; what the significant other does or earns; how the significant other feels about the applicant's work life, travel arrangements, or possible relocation; medical history concerning pregnancy or any questions relating to pregnancy; or whether there are children, how many, and their ages. One should use either first or last names for all candidates and persons involved in the recruitment.

Applicants with disabilities should also be asked questions relevant to the job. Whether the individual needs any reasonable accommodations or assistance during the hiring or interviewing process and the individual's ability to perform essential job functions with or without reasonable accommodations may be discussed. One should avoid discussions of past or present serious illnesses or physical or mental conditions; the nature or severity of an apparent disability; problems an individual may have had because of a disability; or how the person became disabled.

Because people are presumed innocent until proven guilty, records of arrest without convictions are meaningless. One may inquire about an applicant's conviction record for jobs where that is relevant.

When discussing the location, one should mention the special features: lakes, parks, and urban areas; sports, cultural, and other recreational features; and renting and buying options.

One should avoid references to the applicant's personal happiness and not suggest that one is interested in hiring a woman, minority person, or person with a disability as a statistic to improve the Affirmative Action/Equal Opportunity profile. Applicants are being considered for a position based on qualifications.

Interviews do have limitations. Reliability and validity are questionable. The same interviewer has higher interrater reliability than different interviewers. Interrater reliability is lower in unstructured interviews than in structured interviews. Even if the interview has reliability, it may not be a valid predictor of job performance. Validity tends to increase with a team approach. Interviewers seem to be more influenced by unfavorable than by favorable information. Attitudes and biases of interviewers affect how applicants are rated. Fortunately, there are interventions to reduce subjectivity. Multiple interviews using a team approach with a structured interview format for each job classification reduce biases. Training people how to do interviews is helpful. Scenarios can be used to check problem-solving ability of applicants (Arthur, 1998; Champy, 1995; Gillies, 1994; Marquis and Huston, 1996; Sullivan and Decker, 1997).

Testing.   Personality and interest testing is sometimes done but does require a trained psychologist. Ability tests are rarely used when hiring nurses. However, in-basket exercises, problem analysis, mock selection interviews, oral presentations, and debates have been used to select management personnel. Testing is useful for selecting clerical help.

Tests can measure knowledge and skills possessed and estimate the rate at which the applicant can acquire the knowledge and skills required for the position. They measure clerical and mechanical aptitudes, general intelligence, and mental, perceptual, and psychomotor abilities.

EQUAL OPPORTUNITY AND AFFIRMATIVE ACTION

The employer is subject to a number of legal requirements that have been enacted to provide equal opportunity and affirmative action in the workplace. Requirements for providing equal opportunity are contained in Title VI and Title VII of the Civil Rights Act of 1964, Title IX of the Education Amendments of 1972, the Equal Pay Act of 1963, and the Age Discrimination in Employment Act of 1967. Affirmative action requirements are contained in Executive Order 11246, Section 503 of the Rehabilitation Act of 1973, and in Section 402 of the Vietnam Era Veterans Readjustment Assistance Act of 1974.

Title VI and Title VII of the Civil Rights Act of 1964, as amended by the Equal Employment Act of 1972, prohibit discrimination because of race, color, religion, sex, or national origin in any term, condition, or privilege of employment.

Title IX of the Education Amendments of 1972 prohibits discrimination on the basis of sex in any educational program or activity receiving federal financial assistance. The Equal Pay Act, as amended by the Education Amendments of 1972, requires the same pay for men and women doing substantially equal work, requiring substantially equal skill, effort, and responsibility under similar working conditions in the same establishment.

The Age Discrimination in Employment Act of 1967, as amended, prohibits age discrimination against individuals between 40 and 70 years of age.

Executive Order (EO) 11246 (as amended by EO 11375) prohibits all government contracting agencies from discriminating against any employee or applicant for employment and requires that contractors take affirmative action to ensure that applicants are employed and that employees are treated during employment without regard to their race, color, religion, sex, or national origin.

Sections 503 and 504 of the Rehabilitation Act of 1973 prohibit discrimination because of handicap in employment and in programs and activities receiving federal funds. Section 503, in addition, requires contractors to take affirmative action to employ and advance in employment qualified handicapped individuals.

Section 402 of the Vietnam Era Veterans Readjustment Assistance Act of 1974 requires contractors to take affirmative action to employ and advance in employment qualified disabled veterans and veterans of the Vietnam era.

Affirmative action in Executive Order 11246 requires the employer to make extra efforts to recruit, employ, and promote qualified members of formerly excluded groups. It is based on the premise that unless action is taken to overcome systematic exclusion and discrimination based on national origin, race, color, sex, or religion, employment practices will perpetuate the status quo indefinitely. In addition to the elimination of all existing discriminatory practices, affirmative action requires actions beyond neutral nondiscrimination.

A major portion of an affirmative action program must recognize and remove barriers and establish affirmative measures to remedy past discriminatory practices. Such measures include additional aid to prepare disadvantaged people for jobs. It is noteworthy that Supreme Court rulings state that such measures are not restricted to workers who have individually been victims of discrimination.

Development of an affirmative action program includes the addition of affirmative action intent to the agency's philosophy, development of affirmative action policies and procedures, appointment of a manager responsible for the program, inclusion of affirmative action responsibilities in appropriate job descriptions, and publication of the affirmative action commitment internally to all employees and externally to sources for recruitment, to minority and women's organizations, to organizations of handicapped individuals, to appropriate veterans'

service organizations, to community agencies, and to the community in general.

The affirmative action policy is disseminated internally by including it in the policy manual, annual reports, and other media, such as the agency newsletter. It can also be posted on bulletin boards. Nondiscrimination clauses are included in union agreements. Articles about the affirmative action program, its progress, and the activities of disadvantaged workers are published in agency publications. When employees are pictured in handbooks or advertising brochures, minority and nonminority men and women should be included.

Top administration should discuss the intent of the policy and individuals' responsibilities for its implementation with management personnel. Special meetings should be scheduled with all employees, and the policy discussed in orientation and management training classes.

A workforce analysis of job classifications by departments is the first step toward identifying where minorities, women, and men are currently employed and discovering areas of concentration and underuse. The availability of minorities, women, and handicapped persons having requisite skills is considered when determining whether there is underuse: How many minorities, women, and handicapped persons are in the geographical area from which the institution recruits? What percentage of the total workforce in the area is minorities, women, and handicapped persons? How many are unemployed? How many can be recruited from the local community or the nation? Are there training programs available to prepare minorities, women, and handicapped people with skills the agency can use? Can the agency prepare minorities, women, and handicapped personnel? An agency may be able to prepare nurse's aides or assistants but would need to rely on other institutions to prepare licensed practical, or vocational, nurses (LPNs or LVNs) and registered nurses (RNs). Are there disadvantaged people already employed by the agency who are transferable or promotable? Programs to correct underuse must be developed when there are fewer minorities, women, and handicapped persons in a job classification than would be expected by their availability.

Once management has completed its use and availability analysis, it establishes goals and timetables to improve use. To correct identifiable deficiencies, management needs goals that are measurable and attainable. Goals for minorities and women are presented separately. Those goals and the timetables for completion, along with supportive data and analysis, are major parts of the written affirmative action program.

Programs to achieve these goals must be developed and implemented next. This phase begins with a review of the employment process to identify barriers. Recruitment procedures and the selection process—including job requirements, job descriptions, application forms, testing, and interviewing—are examined. The upward mobility system, including training, assignments, job progressions, seniority, transfers, promotions, and disciplinary action policies, is reviewed. Wage and salary structure, benefits, conditions of employment, and union contracts are also studied. Appropriate changes are made, and an internal audit and reporting system to monitor and evaluate the affirmative action program is implemented. Records of referrals, placements, transfers, promotions, and terminations should be maintained for 3 years. Formal reports regarding attainment of goals and timetables are prepared on a regular basis. The manager of the affirmative action program reviews the reports with other managers, advises top administration of the program's effectiveness, and submits recommendations for improvement of unsatisfactory performance.

Compliance status is not judged solely by whether goals have been met by the time set for achieving them. A review of the program's content and the efforts made toward realization of the goals are factors that are considered in determining its effectiveness.

It is important to keep in mind that goals are not inflexible quotas that must be met but are targets that are reasonably attainable through good faith efforts. Goals therefore should be realistic, measurable, and achievable by the time established.

When interviewing applicants for positions, one should remember that some employment inquiries are acceptable, whereas others are not. The purpose of the question determines its propriety. Appropriate inquiries have a direct relationship to the applicant's capacity to do the job. Inappropriate questions may receive answers that will limit the person's opportunities because of ancestry, race, color, age, religion, sex, marital or parental status, or handicap. Some information needed for payroll or personnel purposes—such as age, proof of citizenship, and number of dependents—can be obtained after the person has been hired. Questions about the applicant's religious preferences, sex, marital status, credit rating, number and ages of dependents, or marital and family plans are not appropriate. Questions that would identify the person as being over 40 or general questions about disabilities are not acceptable. Applicants may be asked to prove they are over 18 years of age and able to perform job-related functions. One can ask for an address and length of residence in a city or state but not for rental or ownership information. Questions about ability to read, write, or speak a language are acceptable, but questions about one's primary language or the way one acquired the ability to use a language are unacceptable. One's legal right to remain in the United States can be questioned, but questions about naturalization of parents or spouse are unacceptable. The applicant may be asked to list membership in clubs, organizations, societies, and associations, excluding those that would indicate the national origin, race, color, or religion of the membership. Requests for all memberships are not appropriate. General questions about military service are inappropriate.

When interviewing minority candidates, one should not pretend interest in, or knowledge of, an ethnic culture or use ethnic vernacular or a foreign language one does not speak well. It is inappropriate to talk about one's minority friends or to expect the candidate to know all other minority members. Lack of eye contact should not be judged negatively, since some cultures interpret direct eye contact as disrespectful. The interviewer should be aware that body language and voice tone give messages that provoke confidence or mistrust and suggest support or indifference.

The manager should be aware that some minority applicants may not have well-defined aspirations and career goals because their opportunities may have been limited and they may feel they have little control over their careers. Minority applicants often have frequently changed jobs in search of better pay. Therefore steady work and work progression histories may be of little use in evaluating minority applicants who have had limited opportunities.

CULTURAL DIVERSITY

People bring with them assumptions, attitudes, and behaviors related to their cultural heritage. The recognition of and respect for cultural differences help foster positive relationships. Leaders and managers need to have an awareness of how their own cultural background affects their performance.

Individuals within a cultural group vary widely, but the majority of individuals within a cultural group generally agree on common norms and traits. Communication is an important aspect of one's culture. It includes spoken and nonverbal expressions. Misunderstandings can result from silence, words used, tone of voice, pitch, and body movements. What a person says and does can be interpreted in a variety of ways. Unless the person's cultural heritage is understood, an interpretation could be wrong. Someone speaking loudly with animation might be misinterpreted as being aggressive, pushy, or rude. Someone speaking in a soft, low voice may be viewed as passive, afraid, or shy.

Context of speech refers to use of emotion in communications. Mexican Americans, Irish, and Italian Americans often use emotions, whereas Black Americans, German Americans, and the Jewish rarely do. Kinesics is the use of gestures, stances, and eye movements when communicating. Alaskan Eskimos blink to indicate agreement. Irish and Italian Americans use gestures, stances, and eye movements to emphasize points. Persons in certain socioeconomic groups in India are to avoid eye contact with persons in lower or higher socioeconomic groups and persons of the opposite sex.

Dialect and language styles often differ between cultural groups. Some cultures convey feelings and emotions through touch. Others find touch intrusive or consider it to have sexual connotations.

There are four zones of interpersonal space: (1) intimate, (2) personal, (3) social consultative, and (4) public. Each zone has distinctive distance and intimacy techniques for verbal and nonverbal communication. The intimate zone is 0 to 18 inches, is reserved for close personal relationships, and is considered taboo in some cultures.

The personal space, 18 inches to 4 feet, is where touching family and friends and some counseling interactions are permitted. The social consultative zone, 4 to 12 feet, is for casual social interactions. The public zone, beyond 12 feet, is beyond the sphere of personal involvement, and verbal communication is usually formal. The preferred space between people in the United States is 2 to 3 feet. In general, Asians do not mind closer spaces, whereas Black Americans do not want their personal space invaded.

People tend to be past, present, or future oriented. People who value the past maintain tradition and are not likely to set goals for the future. People who focus on the present tend to be unappreciative of the past and do not plan for the future. People with future orientations plan and organize for the future.

People in the United States tend to be individualistic and desire to control their own lives. Chinese, Mexican, Vietnamese, and Puerto Rican Americans tend to consider the family as the most important social organization. Some cultural groups, such as the Italians and Appalachians, extend their family beyond blood lines.

Environmental control relates to the ability to control nature and direct the environment. Some groups believe they can control nature; others feel controlled by it. Still others, such as many Native American nations, believe humanity should attempt to live in harmony with nature.

There are also biological variations between cultures. Features, skin color, body size, and enzyme differences are related to cultural heritage. Understanding cultural variables can help leaders and managers recruit, retain, direct, and evaluate personnel. Understanding cultural variables can help one understand oneself better, as well (Giger and Davidhizar, 1990).

AMERICANS WITH DISABILITIES ACT

Three categories of individuals with disabilities are protected by the Americans with Disabilities Act (ADA): (1) individuals who have a physical or mental impairment that substantially limits one or more major life activities; (2) individuals who have a record or history of a physical or mental impairment that substantially limits one or more major life activities; and (3) individuals who are regarded as having such an impairment whether they have the impairment or not. Disability in a major life activity includes caring for one's self, walking, breathing, hearing, seeing, speaking, and learning.

Physical impairments include but are not limited to orthopedic, visual, speech, and hearing impairments; cerebral palsy, epilepsy, muscular dystrophy, multiple sclerosis, cancer, diabetes, tuberculosis, and HIV-positive status; drug addiction; and alcoholism.

Mental impairments include but are not limited to mental retardation, organic brain syndrome, emotional or mental illness, and specific learning disabilities.

Other conditions covered by the ADA include homosexuality or bisexuality; transvestism, transsexualism, pedophilia, exhibitionism, voyeurism, gender identity disorders, compulsive gambling, kleptomania, and psychoactive substance use disorders. ADA excludes current drug users from coverage when an adverse action is taken against an individual based on such use.

Temporary conditions may be considered a disability depending on the duration and the extent to which one or more major life activities are limited. Qualified individuals with a disability must meet the essential eligibility requirements of the agency, with or without (1) reasonable modification to the agency's rules, policies, or practices; (2) removal of architectural, communication, or transportation barriers; or (3) provisions of auxiliary aids or services.

People who pose a direct threat to the health or safety of others are not qualified for protection under the ADA. Determination may not be based on generalizations or stereotypes but must be based on an individualized assessment that relies on current medical evidence or the best available objective evidence to assess (1) the nature, duration, and severity of the risk; (2) the probability that the potential injury will actually occur; and (3) whether reasonable modification of policies, practices, or procedures will mitigate or eliminate the risk. Modifications that fundamentally alter the nature of the program, service, or activities are not required.

An agency should have procedures by which people who identify potential difficulties with meeting essential performance standards can receive appropriate assistance and guidance. When a person believes that she cannot meet one or more of the standards without accommodations or modifications, the agency must determine on an individual basis whether or not the necessary accommodations or modifications can be made. Reasonable accommodations are defined by the ADA to include (1) making existing facilities readily accessible to and usable by individuals with disabilities and (2) job restructuring, part-time or modified work schedules, acquisition or modification of equipment or devices, appropriate adjustment or modification of examinations, training materials, or policies, the provision of qualified readers or interpreters, and other similar accommodations for individuals with disabilities. Each agency should rely on its legal resources to make informed decisions.

JOB REDESIGN
Job Analysis

Job analysis affects employee recruitment, hiring, orientation and training programs, performance appraisal, placement, transfers, and promotions; it consequently influences nursing care. It can determine equitable rates of pay and grade nursing positions within the total agency personnel system. By reviewing national, state, regional, and local wage surveys and using wage scales and performance appraisal, nursing personnel can be compensated satisfactorily for performance. It is the nurse administrator's responsibility to inform the analyst of the scope of authority in nursing positions so that they might be upgraded. This is especially pressing in the nursing profession, because nursing positions have long been rated lower than those of other professionals with comparable education, experience, and responsibility.

Job analysis is the study of a position to determine what knowledge, skill, aptitude, and personal characteristics are needed to perform certain responsibilities successfully. Analysis does not include any attempt to change the task. Rather, one starts by locating or developing a job description and position requirements. Questionnaires, interviews, observation, and logs furnish information about the job title and summary, duties performed, type of supervision given and received, equipment used, working conditions, and relationship to other positions. Job analysis determines minimum requirements (type and level of knowledge, skill, aptitude, and personal characteristics) and consequently sets standards for such factors as education, experience, intelligence, personality, and physical strength (Caroselli, 1992).

Job Evaluation

Job evaluation is a process of measuring the remunerative worth of a job in relation to other positions, both internal and external to the organization. On the assumption that workers will be more satisfied if they perceive pay rates as consistent, the objective of evaluation is to compare jobs and establish a consistent pay base, providing employees in responsible positions with more pay than those with less demanding jobs. A point system, ranking of jobs, job grading, and job-to-job comparison are used. Consideration is given to education, mental and manual skills, responsibility for resources (personnel, materials, and finances), mental and physical effort, and working conditions, such as exposure to dangerous or disagreeable elements.

With the point system the nurse manager assigns numerical values to specific qualifications. An example appears in Box 12-3.

Once point values have been assigned to various job factors, they can be added to determine a grade. The grades for various jobs can be ranked, and job-to-job comparisons can provide a basis for determining pay.

Job evaluation is a systematic rather than a scientific process, and its high reliability does not ensure validity. The management values used to choose and weigh factors may not be consistent with the values of other personnel, or the selected values may be different between work groups. Although relative pay rates can be determined by job evaluation, the absolute levels are often negotiated by the individual or unions.

The number of grievances related to pay rates commonly increases after the introduction of job evaluation because personnel now have an objective basis for a grievance. Before job evaluation, employees had little concrete justification on which to file grievances. They complained that they were not getting paid enough; management insisted that they were. With job evaluation, employees have criteria on which to base grievances.

The transition period is especially troublesome. Problems related to adjusting the worker's present pay to the new pay structure may interfere with traditional lines of promotion. Adjusting a worker's pay upward to the new rate is acceptable to employees, but some may then file grievances for back pay. Back pay, however, could undermine the agency's budget. Therefore management may decide that back pay is retroactive only to a specified date. The case of an employee who has previously been overcompensated creates a more difficult situation. To prevent dissatisfaction, personnel can be assured that no one's pay will be reduced as a result of the new pay schedule. However, it is possible to deny any pay increase to the individual who was overcompensated until others' salaries have been raised and all have been realigned to the new pay schedule. That, of course, can be demoralizing to the overpaid individual, but the previous situation is demoralizing to other employees. More acceptable options may be to promote the individual to a job commensurate with the pay or give the overpaid employee additional responsibilities in the present

Box 12-3 JOB EVALUATION

Qualifications	Points
Education	
Less than a high school diploma	10
High school diploma	20
High school diploma plus a special training course	30
Associate degree or three years in work study program and passage of accrediting examinations	40
Baccalaureate degree and passage of accrediting examinations	50
Master's degree in area of specialty needed for the position	60
Doctorate in area of specialty appropriate for the position	70
Mental skills	
Work is simple and repetitive and is performed according to instructions	10
Work involves a variety of duties that are performed according to procedures but require alertness to identify needed changes	20
Work involves a variety of complicated duties and some independent actions in adapting procedures to specific situations	30
Work involves planning, organization, implementing, and evaluating actions related to patient care	40
Work involves development of policies and procedures, organization of functions, development of staffing patterns, and budget preparations	50
Manual skills	
Work involves the normal manual skills, such as lifting, pushing, folding, writing, filing	10
Work involves about-normal manual skills, such as accurate measurements, administration of medications and treatments, manipulation of instruments, typing, bookkeeping	40
Work involves considerable manual skill, such as administering complex treatments and manipulation of complex equipment	50
Responsibility for resources	
Personnel	
Supervises no one	10
Supervises fewer than 10 people	20
Directs up to 25 people	30
Directs up to 50 people	40
Directs up to 100 people	50
Directs more than 100 people	60
Finances	
No responsibility for budget	10
Responsible for budget up to $10,000	20
Responsible for budget up to $25,000	30
Responsible for budget up to $100,000	40
Responsible for budget over $100,000	50

Continued

JOB EVALUATION—cont'd

Qualifications	Points
Effort	
Mental	
Requires little thinking or judgment	10
Requires some alertness while performing repetitious tasks according to directions	20
Requires mental effort for problem solving	30
Requires considerable mental effort for decision making and problem solving	40
Requires continuous mental effort for dealing with the most difficult situations	50
Physical	
Light work requiring little physical effort, usually seated	10
Light physical effort, use of light materials, frequently seated	20
Sustained physical effort, seldom seated, continuous activity	30
Considerable physical effort, continuous activity, lifting	40
Working conditions	
Good working conditions—light, ventilation, freedom from disagreeable elements such as dirt, heat, wetness, odors, noise	10
Average working conditions with occasional exposure to disagreeable elements and danger	20
Fair working conditions with frequent exposure to disagreeable elements and danger	30
Poor working conditions with continuous exposure to disagreeable elements and danger	40

position to make the current job commensurate with the salary. After the individual vacates the position, the salary for the job can be realigned at a lower salary level according to the pay schedule.

Job Design

Job design specifies the job content (what the job requires), job methods (how to do it), and the relationship between the organizational, social, and personal needs of the worker. It involves observation, recording, and analysis of current jobs to make work more efficient and to provide incentives for the workers, thereby reducing costs and improving job satisfaction.

Job Simplification

Another technique, job simplification, removes the more difficult parts of the job so that the worker can do more of what remains. For example, a nurse

can be hired to start all IVs. The treatment nurse, team leader, and primary nurse, then, do not have to start any IVs but can give other medications and treatments to more patients. Work simplification, however, tends to lead to further boredom.

Personnel may also be assigned more tasks. For instance, staff nurses can teach aides to do additional treatments. This may relieve some monotony, but many workers are already very busy, and the new tasks may prove to be no more meaningful than the others.

Job Rotation

Job rotation is another horizontal job-enlargement technique. Nurses may rotate shifts and assignments between different units and different patients on the units, but this practice complicates continuity of care and often leads to additional frustration. Community health nurses may be rotated through clinic assignments. For instance, a nurse may work well-baby clinics one month; family planning the next; and immunization, tuberculosis, or venereal disease clinics at other times. Again, this can disrupt continuity of care.

Job Enrichment

Job enrichment is a vertical approach to job design that uses a fuller range of abilities and skills of the personnel. When planning job enrichment, one should consider skill variety—the number of different talents and skills needed to do a job; task identity—the degree to which one can do a job from beginning to end with a visible outcome; task significance—the degree to which the job has an impact on others; autonomy—the degree of independence and discretion one has to plan and implement the job; and feedback—the degree to which one receives clear feedback about the effectiveness of one's performance. These core job dimensions contribute to the psychological states that affect the work outcomes. Skill variety, task identity, and task significance contribute to the experience of meaningfulness of work. One may experience responsibility for outcomes through autonomy and knowledge of the results through feedback. That should contribute to motivation, high-quality work performance, and satisfaction, which in turn contribute to lower absenteeism and turnover.

For example, community health nurses may have "their own" assortment of clinics in addition to their family case load. Continuity is preserved because nurses are always at that clinic. They need to develop their expertise, knowledge, and skill in all of the clinical areas. Previously hospital units have switched from functional or team nursing to primary nursing so nurses could give total patient care and so nurses could assume additional responsibility and accountability.

Job enrichment is intended to increase motivation and productivity while reducing absenteeism and turnover. It can, however, increase anxiety, conflict, and feelings of exploitation. Skill levels of personnel limit the amount of job enrichment possible, because some workers lack managerial skills and may not be able or willing to plan and control

their jobs. Supervisors may not be willing to trust workers, and personnel may feel they are being exploited.

Job Descriptions

Job descriptions are derived from job analysis and are affected by job evaluation and design. They generally contain specifications that are the requirements for the job, major duties and responsibilities, and the organizational relationships of a given position. The title of the job indicates the major responsibilities and sets that job apart from others. The job description is a summary of primary duties in a complete but not detailed fashion. Job relationships and professional affiliations may be cited. Education, experience, and worker traits such as aptitude, interests, and temperament may be included. The physical demands and working conditions of the job may be mentioned. Job descriptions should be up to date, accurate, and realistic in terms of the resources available. Standard forms for all jobs within a category facilitate comparison.

Job descriptions should arrange duties in a logical order, state them separately and concisely, and use verbs to describe the action. They should be specific rather than vague and should avoid generalizations by using quantitative words whenever possible. To indicate frequency, one can note daily, periodically, or occasionally when the percentage of total time spent on a specific activity cannot be determined.

Job descriptions are useful for recruitment, placement, and transfer decisions. They can also be used to guide and evaluate personnel. Job descriptions help prevent conflict, frustration, and overlapping of duties. Box 12-4 provides a sample job description.

Career Ladders

Marie Zimmer designed a clinical ladder to create a work environment that would nurture and challenge professional growth and recognize clinical excellence to meet the professional's needs for growth

**Box
12-4**   **SAMPLE JOB DESCRIPTION**

SAMPLE JOB DESCRIPTION

Nursing Service Director
Description of Work

General statement of duties: Performs administrative work in planning, coordinating, and directing the nursing service.

    Supervision received: Works under general direction of the hospital administrator.

    Supervision exercised: Supervises assigned personnel as a significant part of the duties.

Examples of Duties

(Any one position may not include all of the duties listed, nor do the listed examples include all tasks that may be found in positions of this class.)

    Directs and administers the nursing service, including inpatient and ambulatory care; develops and implements policies and patient care standards for all nursing service areas.

    Participates in the planning and development of hospital policies and practices; works closely with administrative and medical personnel in coordinating nursing service functions with those of all other hospital departments and services.

    Develops and implements staffing and ratio patterns to meet patient care and medical service needs; directs the broad planning of in-service training and orientation programs for nursing staff; directs research activities for continuing education and coordinates the clinical experience of nursing students.

    Develops nursing service philosophies and goals in accordance with hospital policies; encourages and provides channels for staff participation in achieving these goals; interprets nursing service objectives to administrative and medical staff.

    Serves on various hospital and community committees for the coordination of nursing services with other patient care and educational services; participates in professional organizational activities and represents the hospital in working with various service agencies and volunteer groups.

    Directs the preparation of budget for nursing service staffing, equipment, and supplies; develops systems and standards for patient care records and reports.

    Directs the recruitment, selection, transfer, and promotion of nursing personnel and the maintenance of personnel records.

    Performs related work as required.

Qualifications for Appointment

Knowledge, skills, and abilities: Extensive knowledge of professional nursing theory and practice. Extensive knowledge of modern principles and practices of hospital operation and nursing administration. Ability to plan, organize, and direct large-scale and comprehensive nursing activities. Ability to supervise, train, and motivate employees. Ability to communicate effectively orally and in writing. Ability to establish and maintain effective working relationships with administrative and medical personnel, employees, the public, and other agencies.

    Education: Graduation from a four-year college with attainment of a master's degree in nursing and major course work in nursing administration or education.

    Experience: Five years' professional nursing experience including three years in an administrative capacity.

    Necessary special requirement: Possession of a license or permit to practice as a registered nurse as issued by the State Board of Nursing, permit to be used only until such time as a decision on licensure is made.

Clinical Specialist I
Description of Work

General statement of duties: Performs advanced professional nursing work in a recognized medical specialty field.

> *Supervision received:* Works under the general supervision of an administrative superior.
> *Supervision exercised:* Supervises personnel as assigned, or full supervision incidental to the other duties.

Examples of Duties

(Any one position may not include all of the duties listed, nor do the listed examples include all tasks that may be found in positions of this class.)

> Performs advanced professional nursing work in specialized medical fields such as mental health, respiratory care, and other recognized medical specialties in accordance with standard nursing procedures and medical direction.

> Interviews patient to obtain general background information and problem identification; evaluates patient's behavior and assesses immediate and long-range needs; schedules and conducts individual and group psychotherapy sessions.

> Participates as a member of a professional medical, psychiatric, or social public health team in evaluating, developing, and implementing health care plans.

> Makes rounds with physician to review condition of patients; develops nursing care plans; participates in the care of the critically ill.

> Participates in the orientation and in-service training of professional nursing personnel in teaching new, advanced, or complicated methods and procedures; interprets nursing services to patients and hospital personnel.

> Performs related work as required.

Qualifications for Appointment

Knowledge, skills, and abilities: Thorough knowledge of professional nursing theory and practice. Thorough knowledge of modern nursing care principles and practices in a recognized medical specialty. Ability to motivate and train employees. Ability to communicate effectively orally and in writing. Ability to establish and maintain effective working relationships with patients, employees, the public, and other agencies.

> *Education:* Attainment of a master's degree in nursing.
> *Experience:* Two years' experience in an appropriate nursing clinical specialty.
> *Necessary special requirement:* Possession of a license or permit as a registered nurse by the State Board of Nursing, permit to be used only until such time as a decision on licensure is made.

Graduate Nurse I
Description of Work

General statement of duties: Performs professional general duty nursing work.

> *Supervision received:* Works under direct supervision of a higher-level nurse.
> *Supervision exercised:* Supervises personnel as assigned, or full supervision incidental to the other duties.

Continued

Examples of Duties

(Any one position may not include all of the duties listed, nor do the listed examples include all tasks that may be found in positions of this class.)

Performs professional nursing care in accordance with standard nursing procedures and medical direction.

Evaluates patient care needs; initiates nursing care plans; coordinates patient services.

Takes temperature, pulse, respiration, and blood pressure; administers prescribed medication and reports symptoms, reactions, and condition of patients; assists physicians with examinations, treatments, and diagnostic tests; prepares and applies dressings, compresses, and bandages; instructs patients in health measures and self-care; instructs nonprofessional nursing personnel and hospital attendants.

Performs related work as required.

Qualifications for Appointment

Knowledge, skills, and abilities: Working knowledge of professional nursing theory and practice. Ability to communicate effectively orally and in writing. Ability to establish and maintain effective working relationships with patients, employees, the public, and other agencies.

Education: Graduation from a school of nursing.

Experience: None.

Necessary special requirement: Possession of a license or permit to practice as a registered nurse as issued by the State Board of Nursing, permit to be used only until such time as a decision on licensure is made.

Modified from Job Descriptions, Denver General Hospital, Denver.

and recognition and the institution's requirement for a stable, experienced nursing staff. It was a ladder for clinical advancement with rungs for vertical advancement, which provided recognition for nurses who chose to stay at the bedside. Career ladders proliferated during the 1970s and early 1980s.

Ladders were designed in various sizes and shapes. Most initially had three to five rungs for vertical clinical advancement. Now ladders may have one to five tracks and are more likely to be called career ladders. Career programs may vary from a simple two-level clinical ladder to multitrack and multileveled systems that include provisions for evaluation.

Practice Alternatives for Career Expansion (PACE) is a six-level, four-track career mobility program that includes clinical, research, education, and administration tracks. Special aspects include a residency program, a PACE consultation team, a performance appraisal system, and a career consultant. The residency program is a course developed to groom nurses for advancement to higher levels. Advancement to level four is mandatory on any track. It has structured didactic classes and individually designed practical experiences. The PACE consultation team is composed of a nursing director, patient care coordinator, and several staff nurses who respond to a unit's invitation for consultation about the PACE program. The PACE program stimulated the development of new job descriptions and performance appraisal systems. Job descriptions are behaviorally defined for each level of each track and serve as the performance evaluation tool. The career consultant is available to discuss career opportunities within the institution, aspects of the career development program, educational opportunities, and general issues of concern about upward mobility (Vestal, 1995).

Advantages of career ladders include potential to increase positive self-image, increase motivation, improve personal and professional satisfaction, provide opportunity for professional growth, provide a system of rewards for accomplishments, encourage development of peer review, improve recruitment and retention, and improve cost-effectiveness through lower attrition rate and retention of experienced nurses.

Potential problems with career ladders include the difficulty of designing them and their potential negative psychological effect. A newly hired experienced nurse may enter the career ladder at the same level as an inexperienced, newly graduated nurse; there may be fewer monetary rewards between clinical levels than administrative levels. Competency is difficult to define, and nurses on tracks may be evaluated by administrators instead of peers (McKay, 1986).

ORIENTATION

Induction is the first 2 or 3 days of orientation. It can be done by personnel department employees for all new employees. It includes a history of the organization, the vision, purpose, structure, working hours, holiday time, vacation, sick time, paydays, performance standards and evaluation, labor contracts, grievance procedures, parking facilities, eating facilities, health services, and education opportunities. That is more information than new employees can remember. It is advisable to have the information in a handbook and to reference the handbook during the induction. Both the new employees and experienced nurses in new positions need orientation. The manager introduces the nurse to the new job, agency policies, facilities, and co-workers. Orientation is important, and the manager who does not take the time to assist a new employee is making a serious mistake. Communicating regulations and exactly what is expected of the nurse diminishes uncertainty, relieves anxiety, and prevents unnecessary misunderstandings. One's security usually increases when someone is considerate enough to help one adjust to a new situation. The manner in which nurses are treated during

their first day at a new job may be critical to their future job satisfaction and performance.

Because of information overload, induction and further orientation should be conducted over time. A checklist for orientation that indicates the content, time frame, and who is responsible to teach it can be helpful (Box 12-5).

It is appropriate to use an orientation schedule (Box 12-6).

Orientation to the institution typically includes a tour of the facilities; a description of the organizational structure; a discussion of different departmental functions; a presentation of the philosophy, goals, and standards; an interpretation of administrative policies and procedures; and possibly an explanation of hospital relationships with the community. Next, the nurse will need an orientation to the nursing service, including interdepartmental relationships, departmental organization, administrative controls, philosophy, goals, policies, procedures, and job descriptions.

After the general orientation, new nurses may be assigned to an experienced nurse for orientation to their specific job. New nurses will need a tour of the unit so that they know the location of supplies, equipment, and policy and procedure books. Information about how the unit is run, specific methods of practice, and communication systems is important. Introductions to other personnel can help the new person feel welcome.

Frequent visits to see that the nurse is comfortable and that the orientation is progressing satisfactorily are helpful. Documentation of the orientation process is useful. The documentation may be a simple checklist that itemizes information such as the organizational structure, specific policies, fire and disaster plans, tour of the facilities, and procedures, with space for a signature. It can be retained in the personnel file.

Nurse internship programs are common to assist newly graduated nurses in making the adjustment from the student role to a staff nurse position. The instructor and head nurse usually work together to identify teaching-learning needs, plan rotation schedules, and evaluate the intern's performance. Classes are held on a regular basis for

> ## Box 12-5 SAMPLE ORIENTATION CHECKLIST

Activity	Time Frame	Who is Responsible
History of organization	Day 1	Personnel Department
Vision, purpose of organization	Day 1	Personnel Department
Structure of organization	Day 1	Personnel Department
Payroll information	Day 1	Personnel Department
Tour of facilities	Day 1	Staff Development Department
Introduction to unit heads and purpose of departments	Day 1	Staff Development Department
Employee and organizational responsibilities, rules of conduct	Day 1	Personnel Department
Fire and safety video	Day 1	Staff Development Department
Personnel policies	Day 2	Personnel Department
Tour of unit	Day 2	Preceptor
Introductions to unit personnel	Day 2	Preceptor
Work schedules, staffing, scheduling policies	Day 2	Preceptor
CPR recertification	Day 2	Staff Development Department
Workload assignments	Day 3	Preceptor
Introductions to charting	Day 3	Preceptor
Reporting of accidents	Day 3	Preceptor
Use of services such as nutrition, OT, PT, pharmacy, x-ray, clinical lab	Day 3	Preceptor
Job description	Day 3	Preceptor
Standards of performance	Day 3	Preceptor
Staff development	Day 3	Preceptor
Employee appraisal system	Day 3	Preceptor
Promotion and transfer policies	Day 3	Preceptor
Work with preceptor while assuming more responsibility	Week 2	Preceptor

orientation, role adjustment, problem solving, and information about pathophysiology. There is a concentration on the mastery of technical skills. Some programs also present leadership instruction. Nurse internship programs help new graduates build self-confidence, lower frustration levels, increase nursing care planning, improve patient care, improve job satisfaction, and reduce turnover.

In-service education helps keep employees' skills and knowledge up to date. It usually involves how to use new equipment, new patient care procedures, and new services. The Joint Commission on Accreditation of Healthcare Organizations (JCAHO) requires that nursing in-service be offered on a continuing basis and that employee attendance be documented.

Near the end of the probationary period, it is advisable to have a systematic evaluation. The nurse should know what characteristics will be evaluated. Two independent judgments, such as those of the manager and a head nurse, may be secured and used to check reliability of the evaluation. The results of the evaluation are indicative of the success of the selection process.

Orientation alone does not socialize people to the organization. Socialization is the sharing of attitudes and values through role modeling, myths, and legends. It is less structured than orientation.

Box 12-6   **SAMPLE ORIENTATION SCHEDULE**

DAY 1

8:00-10:00 AM	Welcome by Personnel Department
	Employee Handbook distributed; overview of organizational history, vision, purpose, structure, payroll information
10:00-10:15 AM	Bread, coffee, and fruit provided
10:15-11:30 AM	Tour of facilities by Staff Development Department
11:30 AM-12:00 PM	Introduction of unit heads and purpose of units by Staff Development Department
12:00-1:00 PM	Lunch with unit heads
1:00-2:15 PM	Employee and organizational responsibilities, rules of conduct by Personnel Department
2:15-2:30 PM	Break, refreshments provided
2:30-4:00 PM	Fire and safety video by Staff Development Department

DAY 2

8:00-10:00 AM	Personnel policies by Personnel Department
10:00-10:30 AM	Report to unit, have break with preceptor
10:30 AM-12:00 PM	Tour unit with preceptor
	Introduction to unit personnel
	Work schedules, staffing, scheduling policies
12:00-1:00 PM	Lunch with unit personnel
1:00-4:00 PM	CPR recertification by Staff Development Department

DAY 3

Work all day with preceptor on unit and shift
Workload assignment
Introduction to charting
Reporting of accidents
Use of services such as nutrition, physical therapy, occupational therapy, pharmacy, x-ray, clinical laboratory services

DAY 4

Work all day with preceptor on unit and shift
Job description
Standards of performance

DAY 5

Work all day with preceptor on unit and shift
Staff development
Employee appraisal system
Promotion and transfer policies

WEEK 2

Work with preceptor on unit and shift, gradually assuming more responsibilities to full workload day 5 of week 2

All employees need socialization. Instilling clarity of the value system throughout the organization is the socialization process for team spirit found in excellent organizations. It is correlated with reduced dissatisfaction, absenteeism, and attrition (Gillies, 1994; Marquis and Houston, 1996, 1998; Sullivan and Decker, 1997).

STAFF DEVELOPMENT

Staff development goes beyond orientation. It is a continuing liberal education of the whole person to develop her potential fully. It deals with aesthetic senses, as well as technical and professional education, and may include orientation, preceptorships, mentorships, skill checklists, internships, in-service education, courses, conferences, seminars, journal or book clubs, programmed learning, and independent study and refresher courses.

Nurse managers play an important role in the support of staff development and have a responsibility to review the goals for the staff development program and to provide a budget for those activities. They participate in needs identification and analyze how education effects change in nursing services. In addition, they must be careful to differentiate staff development needs from administrative needs. If staff nurses know how to do a procedure properly but do not do it because the necessary supplies and equipment are not available to them, the need is administrative rather than educational. Nursing managers are legally liable for the quality of nursing services. Their ability to document staff development provides strong supportive evidence for them. Conversely, the reception of staff development will be largely related to the reward system developed. Positive reinforcement through recognition, such as oral praise on the unit or acknowledgment of accomplishments in a newsletter, is useful. Staff development can also be related to retention, pay raises, advancement to other positions, or termination.

Preceptorship

Preceptorships may be used to help recruit, retain, orient, and develop staff. They may be used before students graduate to orient them to the agency and to recruit them for hire. If students have worked at an agency before graduation and are familiar with it, they can make sounder decisions about where to work, are not as likely to be unprepared for the work situation, and, consequently, are likely to be retained longer. The preceptorship also gives agency personnel an opportunity to evaluate students and determine if they are suitable candidates for employment.

During the preceptorship faculty facilitate, monitor, and evaluate student learning. Faculty direct students to resources, offer suggestions regarding patient care problems, and lead discussions at conferences. The faculty member is responsible for student learning and encourages students to apply class content.

The preceptor is responsible for the quality of patient care and facilitates the student's learning. Preceptors are liaisons between students and the agency. They help students learn skills and learn how to organize their work. They provide real-life experiences for students before graduation to help reduce the difficulties of transition from school to work.

The professional nurturance of a preceptorship can be likened to the "good old boy" network or godfathers who look after godsons. It allows students to use and increase their knowledge and skills so they can assume increasing responsibilities. They gain experience with a variety of patients and different levels of staff. They have opportunities to discuss and adjust to professional-bureaucratic conflicts. Preceptorships are a potential recruitment tool for the agency and can increase the job satisfaction of nurses. Preceptors may even learn from the students and are likely to find the preceptor role challenging and stimulating.

There are also disadvantages to preceptorships. They add to staff nurse responsibilities and require time. Sometimes busy nurses have little time to spend with students. It becomes difficult for faculty to evaluate students because they have little direct observation of the students' work. The use of preceptors requires considerable planning and coordination. Role descriptions should clarify who chooses learning experiences for the student, who supervises the student, and who evaluates the student. Practical evaluation tools of the student, preceptor, and faculty should be developed and used. Educational and service administrative support is needed.

The faculty member serves as a preceptor of preceptors. A workshop to prepare preceptors is desirable. It is appropriate to discuss and clarify role descriptions, skill inventory lists for students, and guidelines for preceptor evaluation of students. Information about teaching methods, counseling, and evaluation is useful. Finding a time and place for the workshop and getting release time for the preceptors may create problems. Awarding continuing education credits for the workshop and preceptor experience may be considered as a way to reward preceptors.

The preceptor model can also be used by the staff development department and nurses after a graduate has been hired. The staff development faculty may present formal content in orientation and development programs that are reinforced by preceptors on the units.

Mentorship

Preceptors are role models who may become mentors. Mentors give their time, energy, and material support to teach, guide, assist, counsel, and inspire a younger nurse. It is a nurturing relationship that cannot be forced. Close, trusted counselors, usually in their forties or fifties, acquaint younger nurses, usually in their twenties or thirties, with the values, customs, and resources of the profession. The mentor is a confidant who personalizes role modeling and serves as a sounding board for decisions. The mentor is a resource person who supports the development of the younger person through influence and promotion.

There are phases to the mentoring process (Box 12-7). At first, during the invitational stage, mentors must be willing to use their time and energy to nurture someone who is goal directed, willing to learn, and respectfully trusting of the mentor. The younger professionals have a career goal, a vision of what they want to become; the mentors are people who have reached that goal and are willing to share the secrets of their success. Then there is a period of questioning, when the younger person has self-doubt and fears of being unable to meet the goals. The mentor helps clarify those goals through self-discrimination. Next, mentors share information about power and politics, tell how they became successful, and serve as a sounding board. The transitional phase is the final phase, when mentors help students personalize learning and become aware of their own strengths and uniqueness. Younger nurses are then prepared to be mentors and to tell others how they became what they are.

Mentorship should provide an opportunity to share information, review work, provide feedback, explore issues, plan strategies, and solve problems. It helps socialize novices into professional norms, values, and standards. Career advancement and success are promoted, thus increasing self-confidence, self-esteem, and greater personal satisfaction.

Box 12-7	**PHASES OF THE MENTORING PROCESS**

Invitational:	Mentor uses time and energy to nurture a younger professional who is goal directed, willing to learn, and respectfully trusting of the mentor.
Questioning:	Mentee experiences self-doubt and questioning of goals.
	Mentor helps clarify goals and provides guidance.
Transitional:	Mentor helps student personalize learning and become aware of own strengths and uniqueness.
	Mentee is now prepared to be a mentor.

CAREER PLANNING
Choosing a Field of Nursing

There are many opportunities in nursing. From the 1930s until the 1990s about 70% of nursing was done in hospitals. Hospital nurses can do medical, surgical, obstetrical, pediatric, and psychiatric nursing or nursing in subspecialties such as intensive cardiac care. Community health nursing, home care, hospice care, industrial nursing, school nursing, working in a physician office or clinic, rehabilitation nursing, long-term care, and health promotion are other opportunities. The federal government offers additional options, such as a career in the Army, Navy, or Air Force, and working for the nursing service of the Veterans' Administration or the Indian Health Services. Teaching, consulting, conducting research, serving as a staff member of a professional organization, and being an independent nurse practitioner are possibilities.

To set short-term and long-range goals, one considers the importance of salary, fringe benefits, retirement plans, work hours, and opportunities for advancement. Desirable climate and geographical location are also considerations. Short-term goals help position one for long-range goals. It is advisable to get some clinical experience before applying for teaching or consultation positions. Trends should be taken into consideration for long-term goals. The population is growing older and acquiring chronic diseases; health care reform is focusing on access to high-quality, economical care; care is moving from the hospital to the community; ambulatory care and home care are increasing; and health promotion is being encouraged.

Locating Job Openings

After deciding what type of nursing one wants to do and the geographical area where one wants to practice, one needs to locate job openings. Professional journals advertise positions, and college placement services and employment agencies maintain job listings. Recruiters are often at professional meetings. One can ask friends, acquaintances, and relatives if they know of openings. Employers can be contacted directly.

Résumé

A résumé is a summary of information about one's education, employment, and professional and personal history. It is typically a prerequisite for an interview, because the employer uses the résumé to determine who will be interviewed. Consequently, the résumé should be carefully developed and updated periodically.

Résumés should be printed on high-quality 8½ inch-by-11 inch typing paper with a laser printer; they should never be handwritten. The contents should be well arranged, with major and minor headings to facilitate reading. The content should be concise yet complete, but not crowded. Résumés should contain the following information:

Identification. Full name, address, and telephone number should appear at the beginning of the résumé.

Job objective. Including or excluding a job objective is controversial. Some say it limits one's scope of employment, whereas others argue that the personnel manager should know what position the nurse is seeking. Separate résumés for each job, customizing the job objective, and accenting the characteristics that qualify the nurse for a particular job are appropriate.

Education. In reverse chronological order, one should list the names and locations of schools attended, dates of attendance, and diploma or degrees conferred. Continuing education, such as workshops, in-service education, and home study courses, indicates an interest in self-improvement and is appropriate to list. If the grade point average is high, it is appropriate to cite it.

Work experience. Previous employment should be listed in reverse chronological order by identifying the name and location of each agency, dates of employment, position title, and responsibilities. New graduates can list their student clinical experiences. It is appropriate to give a reason for leaving the position.

Military service.   If the applicant has served in the armed forces, a summary of the military record should be included. Branch of service, years in the service, rank achieved, awards and distinctions, special assignments, skills, and knowledge acquired are some of the items appropriate to include.

Affiliations.   Memberships, offices, committee activities in professional organizations, learned societies, and civic and social groups may be listed. Religious and political affiliations should be used with discretion.

Honors and awards.   Scholarships, honors, and awards may be cited by stating the honor, the organization that conferred it, the location, and the date.

References.   If references are available, it should be stated that they will be provided upon request. One should always check the willingness of people who might serve as references. One may also compile a letters of reference file by asking teachers, supervisors, or peers to write letters of reference "to whom it may concern" at the time of termination. This is an opportune moment to make such a request because the nurse's performance is vivid in the reviewer's mind. It may prevent the reviewer from having to write more than one letter when copies are acceptable, and the applicant does not have to be concerned about locating the person later. Compiling one's own letter file allows one to send the most informative and appropriate letters of reference. One keeps the original letters and sends the appropriate photocopies with the résumé. Multiple copies with the original signature can be made to save time.

Cover letter.   The résumé should be accompanied by a cover letter stating the applicant's interest in working for the specific agency, the special qualifications and interests the applicant brings, the applicant's availability, and how the applicant can be reached.

Interview.   An interview allows the employer to determine if the applicant meets the requirements for the position being sought, and it allows the applicant to obtain information about the agency. First impressions are important. The interviewer will quickly assess the applicant's manners and appearance. The applicant may be questioned about dependability, responsibility, and ability to work with others. The compatibility of the applicant's goals with available opportunities may be explored.

Job procurement.   A nurse is likely to apply for more than one job at a time. Once a position has been accepted, the other agencies should be informed of the decision in a friendly and professional way because the nurse may apply to that agency again in the future.

CAREER MAPPING

Career mapping is a strategic plan for one's career. It provides direction for formal education, experience, continuing education, professional associations, and networking. Nurses need to assess their own values and define success for themselves. Job security, sense of accomplishment, and opportunities for professional advancement are often considered important. Other issues to consider are work hours, salary, fringe benefits, retirement plans, organizational and geographical climate, and location.

Nurses also need to assess their skills. What do they do well, do poorly, want to do, not want to do, or have the potential to develop?

Once one has (1) assessed interests and skills, one should (2) determine goals, (3) develop a map, and (4) pursue strategies to maintain the map. It is appropriate to make a list of interests and skills and to set 1-, 5-, and 10-year plans. The time frame can be illustrated in a career map with a 10-year time frame across the top of the paper. Then one can write in years of specific experience under "Dates" and types of education under "Experiences." One might focus on continuing education classes for a time or work on an advanced degree during certain periods.

Ongoing maintenance of the map will reflect advancement efforts: writing, personal presentations, networking, and professional development.

The curriculum vitae (CV) and the résumé are used interchangeably to present oneself in writing. The CV is a listing of educational, professional, and scholarly accomplishments most commonly used in academic settings. The résumé is a concise history of education and experiences in a few pages. The vitae should have an attractive format and contain such information as professional goal, education, work experience, professional memberships, continuing education, research, publications, and presentations. If there have been no accomplishments in a category to date it is best to omit that category from the vitae. Résumés are updated periodically, especially when one is applying for a job. It is helpful to keep information files listing continuing education, organizational memberships, offices, committees, research, publications, and presentations so that accurate information is available for updating the résumé. A cover letter should accompany a résumé to introduce the sender and explain the purpose for sending the résumé: interest in a position.

One must present oneself in person for an interview. One-on-one interviews are common. The applicant is typically asked, What are your goals? What are your strengths and weaknesses? Why do you want to work here? What do you have to offer this agency? In serial interviews the applicant sees one person after another. Looking attractive, having a positive attitude, remaining consistent, and treating each interviewer as if that person alone will make the decision are appropriate. Serial interviews are increasingly common as one applies for jobs higher in the hierarchy. The interviewers are interested in the interrelationship with their specific area of responsibility. One's communication skills are tested during group interviews, when the applicant is interviewed by several people at once. Stress interviews are sometimes used to test an applicant's reactions to stress. They may leave a very negative feeling about the job; the applicant should try to remember such a test is not a personal attack. After the initial screening the most serious candidates may be asked back for an interview.

It is helpful to network with colleagues inside and outside the organization. Identify individuals who have influence over your career, who can serve as mentors, who can give you career guidance, and who can serve as references. Join professional organizations where you can meet colleagues with similar interests. Volunteer for committee work. Attend conventions and meetings. Have business cards made and swap them with colleagues. Keep in touch with your colleagues, ask for what you need, give feedback, and follow up with contacts.

Careers typically progress through stages of exploration, early career trial and establishment, middle career growth and maintenance, and later career plateau and decline. The exploration stage involves identifying the right career and getting the appropriate education. Early career involves getting the first job, adjusting to a daily work routine, choosing a specialty, transfers and promotions, and broadening one's perspective of the organization and profession. During the middle career people establish their professional identity, choose between alternative career paths, and take on more responsibility. In the later career people develop others, shape the future of the organization, plan for retirement, deal with a reduced workload and less power, and may help develop their replacement.

Exploration typically occurs during ages 15 to 22, early career during ages 22 to 38, middle career 38 to 55, and later career 55 to 70. However, some women raise a family before they start the exploration stage, and many interrupt their career to raise a family. It is more common for women than men to have discontinuous careers because of family responsibilities. People may change careers during their lifetime too (Steers and Black, 1994).

One progresses in professional development by systematically reviewing professional journals, collecting and filing articles and materials topically, developing a professional library, achieving professional certification, chairing a committee to develop leadership skills, presenting an in-service, and fostering a support group.

GROUP PROCESS

Group process is critical for group development. How the group functions, communicates, and sets and achieves objectives are all related to group dynamics. Both task-oriented behavior and maintenance-oriented behavior are necessary for adequate group development.

People who assume group task roles coordinate and facilitate the group's efforts to identify the problem, explore alternative options, identify the ramifications of the options, choose the most viable option, and implement and evaluate the plan. There are numerous group task roles, and any member of the group may fulfill a number of these roles in successive participation (Box 12-8).

Initiator-contributors propose new ideas or different ways of approaching a problem. Their task is to identify the problem, clarify the objectives, offer solutions, suggest agenda items, and set time limits. The *information seeker* searches for factual information about the problem, whereas the *opinion seeker* clarifies values pertinent to the problem and its solutions. Unlike the information seeker, the *information giver* identifies facts, shares experiences, and makes generalizations. *Opinion givers* state their beliefs and what they think the group should value. Their focus is on values rather than on facts. The *elaborator* develops suggestions, illustrates points, and predicts outcomes. Relationships are clarified by the *coordinator*. The *orienter* summarizes the discussion, activities, and points of departure to pro-

vide perspective on the group's progress toward its goal. Evaluation of the problem, content, and process is done by the *critic*, who may measure the group's achievement against a set of standards. The *energizer* stimulates the group to increase the quantity and quality of their work. The *procedural technician* facilitates group action by arranging the room for the meeting, distributing the materials, working the audiovisual equipment, and generally functioning as the "go-for"—the person who goes for what is needed. An account of the discussion, suggestions, and decisions is kept by the *recorder*.

The roles of group building and group maintenance focus on how people treat each other while accomplishing a task. The *gatekeeper* regulates communication and takes actions to ensure everyone an opportunity to be heard. *Encouragers* radiate warmth and approval. They offer commendation and praise and indicate acceptance and understanding of others' ideas and values. *Harmonizers* create and maintain group cohesion, relieving tension through their sense of humor and helping others reconcile their disagreements. *Compromisers* promote group process by yielding status, admitting mistakes, modifying their ideas for the sake of group cohesiveness, maintaining self-control for group harmony, or by generally making compromises to

---

Box 12-8   GROUP PROCESS ROLES

GROUP TASK ROLES	GROUP MAINTENANCE ROLES	DYSFUNCTIONAL ROLES
Initiator-contributor	Gatekeeper	Aggressor
Information seeker	Encourager	Dominator
Opinion seeker	Harmonizer	Recognition seeker
Information giver	Compromiser	Special-interest pleader
Opinion giver	Follower	Blocker
Elaborator	Group observer	Self-confessor
Coordinator	Standard setter	Help seeker
Orienter		Playboy
Critic		
Energizer		
Procedural technician		
Recorder		

keep the group action oriented. The *follower,* acting as a passive audience, goes along with the group. The *group observer* keeps records of the group process and gives interpretations for evaluation of the proceedings. The quality of the group process is compared with standards by the *standard setters.*

Some members of the group may try to satisfy their individual needs irrespective of the group tasks or maintenance roles. For example, *aggressors* meet their needs at the expense of others by disapproving of others and deflating their status. The *dominator* asserts authority or superiority through flattery, interrupting others, and by giving directions authoritatively. *Recognition seekers* call attention to themselves by boasting and acting in unusual ways. The *special-interest pleader* speaks for an interest group and addresses issues that best meet that need. The *blocker* is negative, resistant, and disagreeable without apparent reason and brings issues back to the floor after the group has rejected them. The *self-confessor* uses the group to express personal feelings, whereas the *help seeker* expresses depreciation, insecurity, and personal confusion that elicit sympathetic responses. The *playboy* has a lack of involvement in the group process and appears nonchalant. A high incidence of individual roles in a group requires self-diagnosis to suggest what group-training efforts are needed. Having a trained observer record who is fulfilling what roles during a meeting can be revealing. On a form similar to the one shown in Worksheet 12-6 on p. 513, an observer records each time a participant plays a certain role (Tuckman, 1965).

TEAM DEVELOPMENT

Groups go through stages of development (Box 12-9). They typically form, organize, solve problems, implement solutions, and disband. During the forming stage, individuals are likely to feel anxious, fearful, doubtful, and self-protective. The leader concentrates on putting the members at ease, explaining the purpose, developing a workable climate, and exerting leadership. Tension tends to be high, suspiciousness, hostility, and resistance are common, and disagreement emerges with the

Box 12-9	STAGES OF GROUP DEVELOPMENT

Form

Storm

Norm

Perform

Adjourn

Data from Caroselli M: *Quality driven designs: 36 activities to reinforce TQM concepts,* San Diego, 1992, Pfeiffer; Parker GM: *Team players and teamwork: the new competitive business strategy,* San Francisco, 1990, Jossey-Bass; Tuckman BW: Developmental sequence in small groups, *Psych Bull* 63(6):384-399, 1965; Zenger JH et al.: *Leading teams: mastering the new role,* New York, 1994, Irwin.

power struggles that occur during the organizing, or storming, phase. The leader needs to clarify goals, policies and procedures, code of conduct, and communication patterns to help the members progress. Loyalty, trust, confidence, dignity, pride, and group cohesiveness develop during problem solving. The leader seeks to approve recommendations by consensus through a systematic and logical approach. The group has structure and purpose, roles are clarified, and interpersonal relationships are stabilized during the performing stage. The leader should help the group focus on issues, behaviors, or problems, not on a person. The leader should encourage group members to help build self-confidence and self-esteem of others, maintain constructive relationships, and take initiative to make things better. The leader should lead by example. Members may have positive or negative feelings about disbanding. The leader should express appreciation and give positive reinforcement.

According to James Lundy (1992) TEAMS means Together Each Achieves More Success. Dilenschneider has said, "In our age, independence and the ability to get things done are often mutually exclusive" (Lucas, 1998). David Coleman and Raman Khanna (1995) have described individualism like sprinters who are uncoordinated individuals work-

Box 12-10   DIFFERENCES BETWEEN GROUPS AND TEAMS

Group	Team
Sharing of information	Collective performance goals
Members not necessarily accepting common objectives	Objectives understood and accepted by members
Tending to have majority and minority opinions	Decisions by consensus with members heard and valued
Destructive criticism	Dialogue with resolution
Hidden personal feelings	Free expression accompanied by listening
Little discussion about how the group is functioning	Self-examination about team functioning
Individuals protecting their role and niche	Understood roles
Individual accountability	Individual and mutual accountability
Varied and random skills	Complementary skills
Neutral and sometimes negative energy	Synergy
Leadership that is appointed or elected	Shared leadership

Modified from Mears P, Voehl F: *Team building: a structured learning approach*, Delray Beach, Fla, St. Lucie Press; Robbins SP: *Organization behavior: concepts, controversies, applications*, ed 7, Englewood Cliffs, NJ, 1996, Prentice Hall.

ing toward a goal. The coordination level of group work is like a relay where there is coordinated but independent effort. Group dynamics level is like a rowing crew that puts a concerted effort toward a goal. Just as there are differences between individuals and groups, there are differences between groups and teams (Box 12-10).

The team is empowered to do what is required. The team members need to know the purpose of the team, the goals, and the targets for accomplishment. Goal setting and planning strategies to meet the goals are important. There should be plans to measure accomplishments (Box 12-11).

The leader should recruit and hire talented people. The inventory of talent on the team should be known. Team members should know each other's strengths and weaknesses. Team members need to continually develop their knowledge and skills. While the organizations should use selection procedures and provide training and education opportunities, individual team members have responsibility for updating their own knowledge and skills too. Team members should know their roles and develop themselves to fulfill those roles. Listening,

problem solving, conflict management, communication skills, assertiveness, and basic teamwork are important skills to learn.

Teams need policies and procedures for a disciplined but not overly rigid way to get things done. It is also helpful for team members to be familiar with their own and each other's personalities. Knowledge of the Myers-Briggs Type Indicator can help team members plan strategies for resolving conflict between them. Validating different values and motives, building respect for diverse points of view, and integrating a range of perspectives into decision making by ensuring that all team members participate are important. Symbols such as shirts, jackets, or hats can be used to emphasize team identity.

Team members should show respect for and appreciation of each other. It is also important for the organization to have an evaluation and reward system for reinforcing desirable behaviors. Team members need to understand that they will not bad-mouth each other. They also need to develop diplomatic ties with key players outside their own team (Carr, 1996; Harrington-Mackin, 1996; Har-

Box 12-11 KEY COMPONENTS OF EFFECTIVE TEAMS

Clear sense of direction

Talented members

Clear and enticing responsibilities

Efficient operating procedures

Constructive interpersonal relationships

Active reinforcement system

Constructive external relationships

Data from Huszczo GE: *Tools for team excellence: getting your team into high gear and keeping it there,* Palo Alto, Calif, 1996, Davies-Black.

Box 12-12 CHARACTERISTICS OF CULTURES THAT SUPPORT TEAMS

Value employees' interpersonal requirements
Promote cooperative rather than competitive relationships
Encourage individual accountability and responsibility
Recognize individual contributions
Have positive visions of the future
Have short- and long-term goals
Have quality standards
Believe in their products and services
Are people oriented
Support the community

From Hicks RF, Bone D: *Self-managing teams,* Menlo Park, Calif, 1990, Crisp Publications.

vey and Drolet, 1994; Huszczo, 1996; Lewis, 1993; Parker, 1990; Porter-O'Grady, 1998; Robbins, 1996; Zenger et al., 1994).

Organizational cultures that are people oriented, goal directed, and quality driven are conducive to team development (Box 12-12). The role of the manager in the development of self-managing teams is as follows:

- Show a willingness to help establish teams.

- Set goals and expectations.

- Monitor performance.

- Give the team feedback to help it self-correct as it proceeds.

- Build relationships.

- Train and educate team members.

- Acquire needed resources such as education, consultation, supplies, and equipment.

- Allow processing time.

- Protect the team from the political obstacles and roadblocks that may occur when people in the hierarchy feel threatened because they believe they are losing decision-making power.

Box 12-13 lists the benefits of self-managed teams.

The manager can help ensure the team's success through its infancy by selecting members who work well together, are mature problem solvers, have positive attitudes, are future oriented, are willing to take risks, and are interested in working on a self-managing team. The leader should meet privately with an ineffective team player and confront the person about the undesirable behavior. The leader should listen to understand the other person's point of view, reestablish team norms, and negotiate an agreement on a new behavior. Positive reinforcement should be given for desirable changes. If the person's behavior remains ineffective, reassignment for a better fit or dismissal are options.

Building a successful experience is also important. Documenting and communicating success make it easier to take the next steps. Verbal feedback to the organization about the successes of the team is very powerful. The manager should make sure that the commitment, time, and resources are available for success. She should encourage the team to go slowly enough to do it right and consequently move faster in the long run. Employees should then

Box 12-13	BENEFITS OF SELF-MANAGED TEAMS

Increased productivity
Commitment to the organization
Commitment to the job
Common commitment to goals and values
Increased effort toward stated goals
Shared ownership and responsibility for tasks
Proactive approach to problems
Faster response to change
Increased employee development
Flexible work practices
Motivation through peer pressure rather than
  management mandates
Less need for management interventions
Increased employee satisfaction
Better work climate
Synergy

Modified from Harrington-Mackin D: *The team building tool kit,*
New York, 1994, American Management Association; Hicks RF,
Bone D: *Self-managing teams,* Menlo Park, Calif, 1990, Crisp
Publications.

start feeling autonomy, responsibility, accomplishment, and belongingness that contribute to job satisfaction and synergy (Hicks and Bone, 1990).

The leader can educate team members so they know what to do; enable them so they know how to do it, and empower them by authorizing them to do it (Harrington-Mackin, 1996; McCoy, 1996; Parker, 1990).

It is appropriate to do a needs assessment to plan for staff development. First, identify the desired knowledge and skills. Then identify the present level of knowledge and skill and determine the discrepancy. Next, identify the resources available to meet the needs, plan and implement appropriate learning strategies, and evaluate the results. How did the learners react to the learning process? Was there behavior change indicating learning occurred? Was there an impact on the organization? Was the staff development cost-effective? Benefits of staff development could be improved job performance, less cost for rework and

fixing errors, lowered supervision costs, enhanced service reputation, increased job security, increased job enrichment, enhanced cross training, higher morale, lower attrition, less expense for recruitment, more use of technology, faster implementation of strategic directions, and a more competitive strategic advantage. Benjamin Franklin said, "An investment in knowledge pays the best interest" (Bowsher, 1998; Davenport and Prusak, 1998, p. ix; Marquis and Houston, 1998).

Diversity should be considered when planning learning activities. Learners have diverse learning styles, so it is advisable to use a variety of teaching methods. Cultural variables should also be considered. People raised in a traditional hierarchical system may regard the teacher as an unquestionable authority and may be reticent to speak in class. Nonnative speakers of English may feel insecure to speak in group discussions or activities. Requesting their views may help them speak out. Leaders and managers should not underestimate the power of talk. A story is a good way to convey meaningful knowledge. Organizations should probably shift their focus from documents to discussions. We structure our reality with language. Consequently, Sue Hammond (1998) recommends appreciative inquiry, which appreciates and values the best of what is; envisions what might be; dialogues about what should be; and then innovates what will be. What we focus on becomes our reality. The use of successful history, tradition, and facts distinguishes appreciative inquiry from other visions based on dreams and wishes. People feel more comfortable taking what they know into the future. Dialogue is a powerful tool. It differs from debate, which uses power and knowing answers to prove and win a point. Dialogue uses questions to find out through respectful sharing and listening. Dialoging together can help build bonds and personal relationships (Davenport and Prusak, 1998; Marquis and Houston, 1998; McMaster, 1996; Odenwald, 1996; Zohar, 1997).

Pedagogy (teaching children) differs from andragogy (teaching adults). To teach children, it is appropriate to create an authoritative climate where the teacher makes the decisions, sets the goals, lectures, evaluates, and encourages competition. A more relaxed and informal climate is used for adults, where the teacher and the students make decisions, set goals, process activities, evaluate together, and encourage collaboration (Marquis and Huston, 1998).

There are several principles of learning and transfer of knowledge. People need to be able to attach what they are learning to what they already know. They need underlying knowledge and skills. They also need confidence to believe they can learn and to be willing to try new skills. They are more motivated to learn if they believe the learning will lead to desirable outcomes. Immediate and specific feedback improves performance. Self-monitoring and feedback become important as people increase their competency. Content can be taught in a concentrated or distributed way. Complex material that is learned over time is usually retained longer than material taught in a concentrated way. Storage of knowledge and skills in long-term memory is necessary to transfer it. Identical elements or training in a context similar to the real work environment facilitates transfer, as does stimulus variability, which incorporates a variety of situations one would encounter on the job into the training. General principles also enhance transfer of knowledge by having learners apply principles to a variety of situations they might encounter in the workplace. Relapse prevention then facilitates long-term maintenance of learned behaviors. People can identify high-risk situations and plan coping strategies to deal with them and can use "what if" scenarios to practice new knowledge and skills.

There are numerous teaching methods and tools available, including but not limited to lecture, discussion, role-playing, case studies, simulations, games, small group activities, movies, audiotapes, videotapes, overheads, models, graphic materials, still pictures, drawings, graphs, posters, cartoons, and handouts. Technology has made Web pages, Internet, e-mail, listservs, chat rooms, telephone calls, telephone bridges, conference calls, voice mail, fax, audio conferencing, video conferencing, virtual instrumentation, interactive video, and multimedia possible. Videotelephone (a form of videoconferencing or desktop conferencing), videoconferenc-

ing, video/image mailboxes, image/fax transmission, and desk-to-desk conferencing, or integrated voice/data communications, are increasing (Billings and Halstead, 1998; Lloyd, 1994).

CHAPTER SUMMARY

Chapter 12 covered the following:
Selection of Personnel
    Recruitment and Retention
    Screening of Potential Staff
        Application forms and résumés
        Letters of reference
        Interview
        Testing
Equal Opportunity and Affirmative Action
Cultural Diversity
Americans with Disabilities Act
Job Redesign
    Job Analysis
    Job Evaluation
    Job Design
    Job Simplification
    Job Rotation
    Job Enrichment
    Job Descriptions
    Career Ladders
Orientation
Staff Development
    Preceptorship
    Mentorship
Career Planning
    Choosing a Field of Nursing
    Locating Job Openings
    Résumé
        Identification
        Job objective
        Education
        Work experience
        Military service
        Affiliations
        Honors and awards
        References
        Cover letter
        Interview
        Job procurement

Career Mapping
Group Process
Team Development

REFERENCES

Arthur D: *Recruiting, interviewing, selecting & orienting new employees,* ed 3, New York, 1998, AMACOM.

Billings DM, Halstead JA: *Teaching in nursing: a guide for faculty,* Philadelphia, 1998, WB Saunders.

Bowsher JE: *Revolutionizing workforce performance: a systems approach to mastery,* San Francisco, 1998, Jossey-Bass Pfeiffer.

Caroselli M: *Quality driven designs: 36 activities to reinforce TQM concepts,* San Diego, 1992, Pfeiffer.

Carr C: *Choice, change & organizational change: practical insights from evolution for business leaders & thinkers,* New York, 1996, American Management Association.

Champy J: *Reengineering management: the mandate for new leadership,* New York, 1995, Harper Business.

Coleman D, Khanna R: *Groupware: technologies and applications,* Upper Saddle River, NJ, 1995, Prentice Hall.

Davenport TH, Prusak L: *Working knowledge: how organizations manage to know,* Boston, 1998, Harvard Business School Press.

Giger JN, Davidhizar R: Transcultural nursing assessment: a method for advancing nursing practice, *Int Nurs Rev* 37:199-202, 1990.

Gillies DA: *Nursing management: a systems approach,* Philadelphia, 1994, WB Saunders.

Hammond SA: *The thin book of appreciative inquiry,* ed 2, Plano, Tex, 1998, Thin Book.

Harrington-Mackin D: *The team building tool kit,* New York, 1994, American Management Association.

Harrington-Mackin D: *Keeping the team going: a tool kit to renew & refuel your workplace teams,* New York, 1996, American Management Association.

Harvey TR, Drolet B: *Building teams building people: expanding the fifth resource,* Lancaster, Pa, 1994, Technomic.

Hicks RF, Bone D: *Self-managing teams,* Menlo Park, Calif, 1990, Crisp Publications.

Huszczo GE: *Tools for team excellence: getting your team into high gear and keeping it there,* Palo Alto, Calif, 1996, Davies-Black.

Job Descriptions, Denver General Hospital, Denver.

Lewis JP: *How to build and manage a winning project team,* New York, 1993, American Management Association.

Lloyd P: *Groupware in the 21st century: computer supported cooperative working toward the millennium,* Westport, Conn, 1994, Praeger.

Lucas JR: *Balance of power,* New York, 1998, American Management Association.

Lundy JL: *Teams: together each achieves more success: how to develop peak performance teams for world-class results,* Chicago, 1992, Dartnell.

Marquis BL, Huston CJ: *Leadership roles and management functions in nursing: theory and application,* Philadelphia, 1996, Lippincott.

Marquis BL, Huston CJ: *Management decision making for nurses: 124 case studies,* Philadelphia, 1998, Lippincott.

McCoy TJ: *Creating an open book organization . . . where employees think & act like business partners,* New York, 1996, American Management Association.

McKay DI: Career ladders in nursing: an overview, *Am J Nurs* 12:272-278, Sept-Oct 1986.

McMaster MD: *The intelligence advantage: organizing for complexity,* Boston, 1996, Butterworth/Heinmann.

Mears P, Voehl F: *Team building: a structured learning approach,* Delray Beach, Fla, St. Lucie Press.

Odenwald SB: *Global solutions for teams: moving from collision to collaboration,* Chicago, 1996, Irwin.

Parker GM: *Team players and teamwork: the new competitive business strategy,* San Francisco, 1990, Jossey-Bass.

Porter-O'Grady T: *The health care teambook,* St. Louis, 1998, Mosby.

Robbins SP: *Organization behavior: concepts, controversies, applications,* ed 7, Englewood Cliffs, NJ, 1996, Prentice Hall.

Steers RM, Black JS: *Organization behavior,* ed 5, New York, 1994, HarperCollins College.

Sullivan EJ, Decker PJ: *Effective leadership and management in nursing,* Menlo Park, Calif, 1997, Addison Wesley Longman.

Tuckman BW: Developmental sequence in small groups, *Psych Bull* 63(6):384-399, 1965.

Vestal KW: *Nursing management: concepts and issues,* ed 2, Philadelphia, 1995, JB Lippincott.

Zenger JH et al.: *Leading teams: mastering the new role,* New York, 1994, Irwin.

Zimmer M: Rationale for a ladder for clinical advancement in nursing practice, *JONA* 2(6):18-24, Nov-Dec 1972.

Zohar D: *Dewiring the corporate brain: using the new science to rethink how we structure and lead organizations,* San Francisco, 1997, Berrett-Koehler.

BIBLIOGRAPHY

Allen SR, Thrasher T, Wesolowski C et al.: Peer interviewing: sharing the selection process, *Nurs Manage* 29:46+, May 1998.

Anderson JK: Orientation with style: matching teaching/learning style, *J Nurses Staff Develop* 192-197, July-Aug 1998.

Barter M, McLaughlin FE, Thomas SA: Use of unlicensed assistive personnel by hospitals, *Nurs Eco* 12:82-87, March-April 1994.

Blount K, Nahigian E: How to build teams in the midst of change, *Nurs Manage* 29:27-29, Aug 1998.

Britton BP, Raper JT, Walden CM: From development to evaluation: making a competency plan work, *J Nurs Staff Develop* 11:210-214, July-Aug 1995.

Cardona SM, Bernreuter M: Graduate nurse overhires: a cost analysis, *JONA* 26:10-15, March 1996.

DeSilets LD: Assessing registered nurses' reasons for participating in continuing education, *J Contin Ed Nurs* 26:202-208, Sept-Oct 1995.

Hayes PM: Team building: bringing RNs and NAs together, *Nurs Manage* 25:52-54, May 1994.

Hetherington LT: Becoming involved: the nurse leader's role in encouraging teamwork, *Nurs Adm Q* 23(1):29-40, 1998.

Howell SB: It's a match! *Nurs Manage* 30:25-29, Feb 1999.

Madison J: The value of mentoring in nursing leadership: a descriptive study, *Nurs Forum* 29:16-23, Oct-Dec 1994.

Mahaffey T, Kaplan T, Triolo PK: A nursing fellowship: building leadership skills, *Nurs Manage* 28:30-32, March 1998.

Mueller A, Ladewig P, Falco J: The use of group process in developing articulation models, *Nurs Ed* 18:29-32, Jan-Feb 1993.

Muus K et al.: Retaining registered nurses in rural community hospitals, *JONA* 23:38-43, March 1993.

Neubauer J: Thriving in chaos: personal and career development, *Nurs Adm Q* 19(4):71-82, 1995.

Noyes BJ: Hiring to build a better team, *Semin Nurs Man* 3:11-15, March 1995.

Nuccio SA, Lingen D, Burke LJ et al.: The clinical practice development model: the transition process, *JONA* 26:29-37, Dec 1996.

Pedersen A, Easton LS: Teamwork: bringing order out of chaos, *Nurs Manage* 26:34-35, June 1995.

Shaffer SC: Automation: it can help solve staff scheduling—maybe, *Nurs Homes* 43:44+, Jan-Feb 1994.

Stevenson B, Doorley J, Moddeman G, Benson-Landau M: The preceptor experience: a qualitative study of perceptions of nurse preceptors regarding the preceptor role, *J Staff Develop* 11:160-165, May-June 1995.

Strzalka A, Havens DS: Nursing care quality: comparison of unit-hired, hospital float pool, and agency nurses, *J Nurs Care Qual* 10(4):59-65, 1996.

Sullivan PD et al.: Management development: preparing nurse managers for the future: Part 1, program model, *JONA* 24:32-38, June 1994.

Swart JC, Wendt AC, Slonaker WM: Employment discrimination experiences of registered nurses, *JONA* 26:37-43, July-Aug 1996.

Waddell DL: Why do nurses participate in continuing education? A meta-analysis, *J Contin Ed Nurs* 24:52-55, March-April 1993.

Wells RB, Mueller JF: Revisioning the recruitment of talented professionals, *JONA* 26:21-30, Jan 1996.

Wheaton M: Cross-training: meeting staffing needs in the ICU, *Nurs Manage* 27(11):32B, 1996.

Worthy CH: Clinical ladders: can we afford them? *Nurs Manage* 27:33-34, Sept 1996.

Zabkar FK: We hired our boss, *RN* XXIV:19-22, April 1997.

CASE STUDY

You are responsible for hiring staff for your unit. You have one staff nurse position available. You have four applicants. They have all graduated from the same school of nursing with the same level of education, and they have all had similar clinical experiences. Three are white, and one is black. What criteria will you use to make your decision? What is the affirmative action policy at your institution? What is the diversity mix on your unit? What is the cultural background of the clients you serve? What will your decision be and why?

CASE STUDY

A new graduate is starting on your unit next week. Using Worksheet 12-4, make a list of what the employee needs to be oriented to and identify who should tell the employee about what. Would you assign the new graduate to a preceptor, and if so what part would the preceptor play in the orientation? What is your role as patient care coordinator? What might the in-service department of the hospital do? Identify some of the new graduate's learning needs and identify means for facilitating the nurse's lifelong learning needs.

Critical Thinking Activities for this chapter begin on page 508.

CHAPTER 13

STAFFING AND SCHEDULING

CHAPTER OBJECTIVES

- Identify at least five patient care delivery modes or assignment systems.
- Compare and contrast at least three patient care delivery modes or assignment systems.
- Discuss the relationship between case management and managed care if any.
- List at least six policy issues related to staffing schedules.
- Describe the pros and cons of centralized and decentralized scheduling.
- Identify at least three different staffing patterns and discuss the pros and cons of each.
- Describe how to calculate the number of full-time staff needed for vacation, holiday, and absentee coverage per year.

Chapter Overview

Chapter 13 presents assignment systems for staffing, staffing schedules, variable staffing, variables affecting staffing, reductions in force, the evolution to health promotion in the community, and managed care.

MAJOR CONCEPTS AND DEFINITIONS	
Case method	assigning each patient to a nurse for total patient care
Functional nursing	hierarchical division of labor
Team nursing	RNs supervising auxiliary nursing staff
Modular nursing	district nursing
Primary nursing	RNs giving total patient care to a few patients
Managed care	comprehensive health care system services through established networks of hospitals, physicians, and other health care providers to give population-wide access to economical, high-quality care
Case management	management and coordination of the care a patient receives in all settings throughout an episode of illness
Collaborative practice	cooperative interdisciplinary practice
Differential practice	distinction between professional and technical nursing
Partners in practice	interdisciplinary team
Staffing schedules	work schedules for personnel
Centralized scheduling	scheduling done in one location
Decentralized scheduling	scheduling done in local areas
Self-scheduling	staff coordinating their own work schedules
Rotating work shifts	alternating work hours between days, evenings, and nights
Permanent shifts	personnel working the same hours repeatedly
Block scheduling	using the same schedule repeatedly
Variable staffing	determining the number and mix of staff based on patient needs
Patient classification systems	calculating staffing needs based on patient acuity
Staffing formulas	calculations used to determine staffing needs

ASSIGNMENT SYSTEMS FOR STAFFING

Changes in assignment systems are a response to changing needs. In the 1920s the case method and private duty nursing were popular. By 1950 functional nursing was predominant in response to the shortage of nurses. During that decade team nursing was introduced to maximize use of the knowledge and skills of professional nurses and to supervise auxiliary workers. The late 1960s and 1970s witnessed a shift back to care of the patient by a professional nurse through primary nursing. Case management became popular during the 1980s, and managed competition emerged as an economic strategy guiding health care reform during the 1990s. It stimulated partners in practice, which is an interdisciplinary team. Each system has advantages and disadvantages (Box 13-1).

Case Method

In the case method each patient is assigned to a nurse for total patient care while that nurse is on duty. The patient has a different nurse each shift and no guarantee of having the same nurses the next day. The patient care coordinator, with no obligation to assign nurses to the same patient, supervises and evaluates all of the care given on the unit. Popular during the 1920s along with private duty nursing, the case method emphasized following physicians' orders (Tappen, 1995).

Functional Nursing

In the 1950s, when few registered and only some practical nurses were available, nurses' aides gave much patient care. In functional nursing hierarchical structure predominates. The medication nurse, treatment nurse, and bedside nurse are all products of this system. The functional method implements classic scientific management, which emphasizes efficiency, division of labor, and rigid controls. It is an efficient system that is the least costly and requires few RNs. Procedural descriptions are used to describe the standard of care, and psychological needs typically are slighted. Care tends to be fragmented and depersonalized. RNs keep busy with managerial and nonnursing duties, and nurse's aides deliver the majority of patient care.

Although efficient, the functional assignment method does not encourage patient and staff satisfaction. Regimentation of tasks may bore nurses because they no longer have the satisfaction of seeing the effects of their total patient care. On the other hand, the functional system may work satisfactorily during critical staffing shortages. Routinized patient care for patients with similar needs may meet those

needs more consistently than other systems, and some staff members may be satisfied by doing repetitious jobs well (Gillies, 1994; Huber, 1996; Marrelli, 1993; Tappen, 1995).

Team Nursing

After World War II RNs were still scarce, although the number of auxiliary personnel had increased. Team nursing was introduced during the 1950s to improve nursing services in hospitals and nursing homes by using the knowledge and skills of professional nurses and to supervise the increasing numbers of auxiliary nursing staff. The result was an improvement in patient and staff satisfaction. Team nursing is based on a philosophy that supports the achievement of goals through group action. Each team member is encouraged to make suggestions and share ideas. When team members see their suggestions implemented, their job satisfaction increases, and they are motivated to give even better care.

The team is led by a professional or technical nurse who plans, interprets, coordinates, supervises, and evaluates the nursing care. Team leaders assign team members to patients by matching patient needs with staff's knowledge and skills. They also do the work other members of the team are not qualified to perform. They set goals and priorities for patient care; centralize information through the use of a Kardex; direct the planning of care by directing care conferences and developing care plans; fix responsibility for the work; provide for coverage during absences, such as breaks, meals, and conferences; and coordinate and evaluate team activities. The team members report to the team leader, who reports to the patient care coordinator. This is a form of decentralization that frees the patient care coordinator to manage the unit.

One of the main features of team nursing is the nursing care conference. Its primary purpose is the development and revision of nursing care plans by providing an opportunity to identify and solve problems. Precision in the identification of problems is increased through information sharing. The belief that the total group has more information

Box 13-1   PROS AND CONS OF VARIOUS ASSIGNMENT SYSTEMS

Assignment System	Pros	Cons
Case method	Total patient care	Different nurse, different shifts, different days
Functional nursing	Efficiency	Nurses do managerial work Nurses' aides do patient care
Team nursing	Team effort Frees patient care coordinator to manage the unit Nursing care conferences help problem solve and develop staff Nursing care plan	Time needed to coordinate delegated work
Modular nursing	Useful where there are few RNs RNs plan care	Paraprofessionals do technical aspects of care
Primary nursing	RNs give total patient care Primary nurse has 24 hour-a-day responsibility Associate nurse works with patient while the primary nurse is off duty Accountability in place Continuity of care is facilitated Reduces number of errors from relay of orders Fewer patient complaints Shorter hospitalization	Confines nurse's talents to a limited number of patients Associate nurse may change care plan without discussing with primary nurse
Managed care	Unit-based Can be used with any nursing care delivery system Standard critical paths	Questionable continuity of care
Case management	Focuses on entire episode of illness Emphasizes achievement of outcomes Incorporates managed care Care is coordinated by a case manager Second-generation primary nursing Critical paths Variation analysis Intershift reports Health care team meetings Quality assurance Interdisciplinary approach	Effort to coordinate

about a topic than any one person enhances the staff's appreciation of group work. A resulting consensus increases the commitment to the decisions made. Identification of the problem and determination of goals early in the conference necessarily precede planning intervention. During the conference, one care plan can be developed or the care plans for a caseload can be updated.

Team conferences also provide the opportunity to identify and work through staff educational needs. Nurses can review standards of care by comparing the actual patient's condition with the textbook example. They can review procedures and learn specialized nursing care and the operation of infrequently used equipment. By studying critical incidents, they may prevent problems from recurring and identify the contributing components of excellent care. Team conferences also provide an opportunity to discuss and resolve interpersonal problems and the chance to prevent future ones. Consequently, team spirit is fostered.

The team leader is responsible for planning and conducting the team conference, which should be limited in time and scope. Meeting for 15 to 30 minutes at the same time each day helps the conference become a part of the daily routine. A time that least interferes with other activities and a place away from the hub of activity are preferable. The team leader must arrange for coverage of the unit during the conference, because relief from patient care responsibilities is essential to prevent interruptions. Staff should be informed of the time, place, and purpose of the conference, so that they can plan their other work around the conference and be well prepared on arrival. Interest can be stimulated by allowing the staff to decide which patient they wish to discuss at the next conference and by having one of the team members record patient problems and solutions during the conference.

Preparation of the meeting area is also a responsibility of the team leader. Temperature, ventilation, lighting, and chair arrangements should be controlled. Refreshments may be appropriate. The team leader introduces the topic and starts the meeting on time to motivate latecomers to be more prompt. A brief review of the patient's condition is appropriate. The team leader monitors the group process, records problems and solutions on the nursing care plan or delegates that task, does appropriate teaching, and summarizes the major points. The nursing care plan is then available to the staff. The team leader serves as a role model by referring to the care plan while receiving and giving reports, making out assignments, and administering nursing care.

The nursing care plan is another main feature of team nursing. A care plan identifying present and potential problems and long- and short-term objectives should be developed for each patient. The care plan should be realistic to prevent morale problems that result from setting unattainable objectives. Care plans should be individualized, reflecting the interrelatedness of psychosocial and physiological needs and involving patient and family participation. Problems, mutually acceptable goals, objectives, actions, and responses are identified. The care is evaluated according to how well the objectives are met.

Team nursing contributes to the satisfaction of patient and staff needs. Each patient is treated as a unique individual. Staff can identify their contributions and the correlation between their work and patient outcomes. The closer interaction of staff contributes to *esprit de corps.*

Because each staff member does many tasks for a limited number of patients instead of a single task for a large number of patients, there is an increased likelihood of errors and a need to spend more time monitoring for them. It also takes time to coordinate delegated work. Although team leaders probably have the least contact with the patients, they are responsible for assessment, planning, and communicating with the physician. Continuity of care is not a given, because patients are not assigned to the same staff all of the time and large assignments make individualized patient care difficult. Changing team membership makes it difficult for the team leader to know team members well enough to match their talents with patient needs. Team nursing is similar to functional nursing when the team leader administers medications and treatments other team members are not qualified to give. Team conferences are often omitted because they are difficult to fit into busy days, and care plans (if done) usually note functional duties relative to the physician's orders. Care plans rarely depict the patient as a total person and consequently are not comprehensive. Medication precautions, fluid intake requirements, dietary and environmental adaptations, protective measures, psychological support, teaching, rehabilitation, and referrals are seldom mentioned. In reality the key features of team nursing—nursing care conferences and nursing care plans—often receive inadequate attention, resulting in routinized care (Gillies, 1994; Huber, 1996; Marrelli, 1993; Tappen, 1995).

Modular, or District, Nursing

Modular, or district, nursing is a modification of team and primary nursing. It uses smaller teams for patients who are grouped geographically. It is sometimes used when there are not enough RNs to practice primary nursing. Each RN, assisted by paraprofessionals, delivers as much care as possible to a group of patients. The RN plans the care, delivers as much of it as possible, and directs the paraprofessionals for the more technical aspects of care. The RN's role is closer to that of a coordinator and information processor than that of a charge nurse.

Modular nursing decreases the sense of isolation and unrealistic expectations often associated with primary nursing. When nurses are consistently assigned to the same module, continuity and quality of care can increase. More time may be spent in direct care. Closer monitoring is possible. Morale can improve when staff know they are making a difference. It is less costly than primary nursing but more costly and less efficient than team nursing.

Some physical changes may be necessary to implement modular, or district, nursing. For example, a medication cart may be placed in the hall instead of using a medication room. Kardexes may be kept on the medication cart. Charts may be moved to the patient's room. Patient Kardexes and staff identification badges may be color coded (Huber, 1996; Marrelli, 1993).

Primary Nursing

During the late 1960s and early 1970s, primary nursing was instituted in some hospitals by professional nurses who were unhappy with fragmented care and lack of direct patient contact. Based on the philosophy that patients, instead of tasks, should be the focus of professional nurses, primary nursing features an RN who gives total patient care to four

to six patients. The RN remains responsible for the care of those patients 24 hours a day throughout the patient's hospitalization. The associate nurse cares for the patient by using the care plan developed by the primary nurse while the primary nurse is off duty. The associate nurse is expected to contact the primary nurse regarding changes in the care plan. The number of patients assigned to one nurse varies according to length of hospitalization, complexity of care, number of medical and paramedical personnel involved with the patient's care, availability of support systems, and the shift worked. Day-shift nurses are assigned the greatest number of patients; evening nurses have some; and night nurses are primarily auxiliary nurses because of their reduced contact with patients and families.

The primary nurse does the admission interview and develops the nursing care plan, including teaching and discharge planning, which is shared with the associate nurse. Primary nurses have autonomy and authority for the care of their patients. Consequently, accountability is placed and continuity of care is facilitated. Primary nursing decreases the number of people in the chain of command and reduces the number of errors that can result from a relay of orders. Other advantages include mobile use of auxiliary workers and increased satisfaction by both nurse and patient. Nurses can identify patient outcomes as a result of their work. Patients have the security of knowing the nurse is available and has to cope with fewer people than in other assignment systems. Research suggests that patients have fewer complications and a shorter hospitalization when cared for by a primary nurse.

Unfortunately, primary nursing confines a nurse's talents to a limited number of patients. Other patients cannot benefit, and if a patient has a nurse who is not capable, the patient may be worse off than if cared for by numerous people, some of whom might meet the patient's needs. Another problem occurs when the associate nurse changes the care plan without discussing the reasons with the primary nurse. Thus it is critical that the primary nurse communicate verbal and written plans to the associate nurse. The success of primary nursing seems to depend on the quality of the nursing staff and administrative support (Gillies, 1994; Huber, 1996; Marrelli, 1993; Tappen, 1995).

Case Management

Case management has its roots in psychiatry and social work that focused on chronic long-term outpatient care in the 1920s. It was used by community health nursing in the 1930s, and it was adapted to acute-care settings and outpatient services during the mid-1980s. It focuses on an entire episode of illness, including all settings in which the client receives care. A case manager coordinates services for the patient and family. Options for alternative health care, living arrangements, and community and social services are considered. Arrangements with nonpreferred providers may be negotiated to reduce claim costs. Case management can cross departmental and disciplinary boundaries.

There are a variety of models for case management. The nurse may give care and coordinate it or just coordinate it. The nurse may work across agencies such as an ambulatory clinic, acute care, and long-term care facilities or may make site visits to the home or health care agencies. Case management emphasizes achievement of outcomes in designated time frames with limited resources. Case management is sometimes called second-generation primary nursing.

Case management involves critical paths, variation analysis, intershift reports, case consultation, health care team meetings, and quality assurance. Critical paths visualize outcomes within a time frame. Variation analysis notes positive or negative changes from the critical path, the cause, and the corrective action taken. This information is reported in intershift reports. Case consultation may be indicated when the client's condition differs from the critical path as noted in the intershift report. Case consultation is conducted about once a week for a few minutes immediately after intershift report to deal with variations. It can also be conducted informally whenever a staff member identifies a variation and consults others. The problem solvers focus on the variation and the desired outcomes, brainstorm ideas to achieve desired outcomes, and use open communication to evaluate a plan. A summary can be used to close the session.

Health care team meetings provide an interdisciplinary approach to problem solving. The case manager needs to identify no more than three priority goals and decide what team members should be present after considering the patient, family, physician, social service, various therapists, and others involved. The case manager should set the time and place for the meeting, make the arrangements, and post the date, time, place, and people to attend in the Kardex. The case manager calls the meeting to order, states the goals, initiates discussion, documents the plans, and sets time limits for follow-through. The variance between what is expected and what happens is assessed for quality assurance. Collaboration is important (Bower, 1992; Cesta, 1998; Cohen and Cesta, 1997; Easterling et al., 1995; Gillies, 1994; Marrelli, 1993; Mullahy, 1998 a,b; Murer et al., 1997; Powell, 1996; Siefker, Garrett, and Genderen, 1997; Tappen, 1995).

Collaborative Practice

Collaborative practice can include interdisciplinary teams, nurse-physician interaction in joint practice, or nurse-physician collaboration in caregiving. Collaboration is cooperative and assertive. The interaction between nurses and physicians or other health care team members in collaborative practice should enable the knowledge and skills of the professions to influence the quality of patient care provided synergistically. It is important to the managed care models that proliferated during the 1990s (Del Togno-Armanasco, 1993; Etheredge, 1989).

The ANA and the American Medical Association established the National Joint Practice Committee (NJPC) in 1972 with funding from the W.K. Kellogg Foundation. The report supported collaborative practice and suggested that increased collaboration results in improved quality of care and patient and nurse satisfaction, and a decreased need for physician supervision of nurses. Primary nursing, nurse decision making, integrated patient record, a joint practice committee, and a joint record review were found to enhance nurse-physician collaboration.

During the 1990s there was a rapid move of health care from the hospital to the community. With the rapidly aging population, accompanying increase in chronic diseases, interdisciplinary teams, and advancing technology, a computer and network based community infrastructure became increasingly important. A prototype of an information system in community nursing was developed in Delphi programming environment, and an international classification of nursing practice was published. A common classification system became increasingly important for communication. The first nurse-initiated classification system began in 1973 and is known as NANDA, North American Nursing Diagnosis Association. Nurses have worked at refining that over the decades, and a research team at the University of Iowa formed the Nursing Diagnosis and Extension Classification to refine, extend, validate, and classify nursing diagnoses in collaboration with NANDA to produce a comprehensive and validated taxonomy of nursing diagnoses (University of Iowa College of Nursing Web site a, accessed July 15, 1999). Researchers have been leading the classification work through the Center for Nursing Classification at the University of Iowa College of Nursing. NIC, Nursing Interventions Classification, interventions have been linked with NANDA nursing diagnoses and the Omaha System problems and are being linked with NOC, Nursing Outcomes Classification. NOC has been recognized by the ANA Congress of Nursing Practice Steering Committee on Databases to Support Clinical Nursing Practice as useful for clinical nursing practice and has been included in the National Library of Medicine for inclusion in the Unified Medical Language System (UMLS) Metathesaurus (University of Iowa College of Nursing Web site b, accessed July 15, 1999; University of Iowa College of Nursing Web site c, accessed July 15, 1999). The Omaha classification system was developed by staff and supervisors of the Visiting Nurses Association of Omaha. The three parts—(1) problem classification, (2) intervention scheme, and (3) problem rating scale for outcomes—were developed for com-

munity health nursing (Pesut and Herman, 1999). The 1999 ANA House of Delegates passed a recommendation to "advocate the timely implementation of ANA recognized standardized nursing languages (SNLs) including the Nursing Management Minimum Data Set (NMMDS) to establish comparability nursing data across clinical settings populations, geography and time" (ANA House of Delegates materials).

During the 1990s primary care became a focus of health care. Nurse practitioner programs had a marked increase in enrollment as advanced practice nurses played a key role in primary care. Medical education made some shift from specialties to general medicine. HMOs, PPOs, and integrated health care systems increased.

Managed Care

During the 1980s managed care referred to unit-based acute care. During the 1990s the focus shifted from acute care to promotion of health and disease management of chronic and terminal care. Managed care involves financing care and risk management of acute, chronic, and terminal diseases as HMOs, PPOs, and integrated care systems proliferated. Managed care is shaped by fluid market forces and changes quickly and frequently. No single definition of managed care has endured for long, and continuous change is probable. There are several differences between traditional insurance programs and managed care. Traditional insurance allowed patients to see any health care professional with unlimited access to specialty providers and coverage for acute illness or injury only. Managed care uses a network of credentialed care professionals, covers primary and preventive care, and restricts access to specialty providers. Traditional insurance assumed all financial risk and used multiple providers to deliver care without knowledge of the total patient plan of care. Retrospective audits were done on claims data only. Managed care transfers risk to the providers, has the patient care provider manage and coordinate the patient's care, and does prospective review of the costs, use, and quality of treatment (Hicks, Stallmeyer, and Coleman, 1993; Knight,

1998; Kongstvedt, 1997; Kongstvedt and Plocher, 1998; Steinberg, 1997).

Differentiated Practice

Differentiated practice generally refers to the difference between professional and technical nursing. Complexity of decision making, timeline of care, and structure of the setting are its main distinctive features. The Midwest Alliance in Nursing organization facilitated clarification of differentiated practice. Professional nurses have received a baccalaureate or graduate degree. They give direct care to patients with complex interactions of nursing diagnoses and relate to their families from preadmission to postdischarge in a variety of more or less structured settings. Until the 1990s the technical nurse received a diploma or an associate degree and gave nursing care to patients with common conditions and to their families in structured settings. With the movement of health care into the community and an attempt to lower health care costs, technical nurses, LPNs, and unlicensed personnel are used in the community and less structured situations too.

The original Integrated Competencies of Nurses (ICON) model addressed entry into practice roles by developing a differentiated practice model. The baccalaureate degree–prepared nurses assessed, planned, and evaluated. The associate degree–prepared nurses implemented care. One professional and two or three associate nurses cared for 10 to 15 patients during the day. ICON II responded to the shortage of nurses by "grandfathering" all RNs into the professional role. LPNs then filled the technical role.

Mathey's Primary Practice Partners model responds to the nursing shortage by recommending former military corpsmen, emergency medical technicians (EMTs), and registered certified technicians (RCTs) with special technical training to be nurse extenders. These and other job categories may expand differentiated practice models.

The partners in practice models of the 1990s cross-trained cleaning personnel, who had less downtime than previous nurses' aides, to be nursing assistants. Use of unlicensed personnel increased during the 1990s.

LEVEL OF STAFF

The level of staff available greatly influences the assignment system used. When there are a few RNs and a few practical nurses, many aides are quickly oriented and used. This is an expensive and relatively dangerous mix, because aides do not have the educational background to do most of what is required or to recognize what should be reported. After the aides have done all they can, there is still much work to be done. Consequently, there is considerable downtime. This staffing mix lends itself best to functional nursing.

Team nursing is appropriate when there are some RNs, even more practical nurses, and fewer aides. The RNs plan and direct the care, pass medications, and do the more complicated treatments. Although this provides better physical care, the staff is still not adequately educated to understand the pathophysiological basis of symptoms, to plan nursing intervention, and to detect changes in the status of the patient at an early stage so they may promptly report pertinent information to the physician. There is also a dearth of patient education and response to psychosocial needs.

Modular nursing is appropriate when more RNs are available, and primary nursing works best with a staff of only RNs. Research regarding exclusively RN staffs indicates an increase in staff, patient, and physician satisfaction. There is an increase in professional orientation, personal liking of colleagues, and cooperation with others. Collegial relationships are more common, and there is more mobility on units because nurses can cover for each other. There is greater competence in skills, creative interventions, personalized care, and continuity of care.

All-RN staffing is economical. It has been found to save money through decreased turnover, sick leave, unpaid absences, float hours, and overtime. RNs can give better care in fewer hours. Patients have fewer complications, shorter hospitalizations, and lower readmission rates. Hospitals also generate more revenue when patients have shorter stays with a concentration of treatments. Unfortunately, frequent shortages of nurses make all-RN staffs unlikely.

Pure applications of case method, functional method, team nursing, modular nursing, and primary nursing are possible, but they seldom exist in pristine form. Rather, it is common to find elements from more than one assignment system combined and used at the same time. Case management is used across settings. During the 1980s managed care was considered unit based. During the 1990s disease management and case management became a part of managed care through community-focused, collaborative arrangements and structures such as HMOs.

STAFFING SCHEDULES

Staffing policies largely influence staffing schedules. To determine staffing policies, one must consider the following questions (Marquis and Huston, 1996, 1998; Swansburg, 1993; Swansburg and Swansburg, 1999):

- What is the best organization for staffing—centralized or decentralized to clinical areas or nursing units?

- Who is responsible for the original scheduling or daily adjustments?

- Where are nursing hours posted and an accurate copy kept?

- For what period will schedules be prepared—1, 2, 4, or 6 weeks?

- How far in advance will personnel know their work schedule?

- Will there be an adjustment in staffing based on the identification of patient needs?

- Will there be shift rotation?

- If there is shift rotation, how often—daily, weekly, monthly?

- How much time should elapse between rotated shifts?

- What day starts a calendar week—Sunday or Monday?

- Will there be 2 days off each week or an average of 2 days a week?

- How often are weekends off guaranteed?

- What days does a weekend comprise—Friday, Saturday, Sunday?

- Will days off be split or consecutive?

- What are the maximum and minimum work spans?

- How many holidays and vacation days are allowed?

- How far in advance of scheduling should employees request time off?

- How will holiday time off be determined?

- Will part-time help be used?

- If so, what is the most economical ratio between full- and part-time personnel?

- Will part-time help be allowed to specify when they can and cannot work?

- Will part-time help be required to work weekends? If so, how often?

- Will "float" personnel be used?

- What are the low-census procedures?

- Is there a policy for trading days off?

- What is the emergency request policy?

Centralized Scheduling

Two major advantages of centralized scheduling are fairness to employees through consistent, objective, and impartial application of policies and opportunities for cost containment through better use of resources. Centralized scheduling also relieves nurse managers from time-consuming duties, freeing them for other activities. Centralized scheduling is not without its critics, however. Lack of individualized treatment of employees is a chief complaint, and centralized scheduling has brought to the surface previously unrecognized organizational and managerial problems.

Organizational and managerial problems can be reduced when (1) the philosophy and goals of the agency are identified; (2) the goals, objectives, and organizational structure are defined; (3) scheduling policies are stated; (4) standards of nursing care practices are set; (5) acuity of care as it relates to staffing needs is determined; (6) patient needs, personnel policies such as vacation and personal leave, and staff development are taken into account in personnel schedules; and (7) quality of care is measured.

Resistance to centralized scheduling may be reduced when head nurses prepare and control their own budgets, understand and approve the scheduling policies, and have open communication with the scheduler. Line and staff accountability should be carefully defined to prevent confusion over responsibility and authority when staff personnel make decisions where line managers are accountable. Line authority is accountable for decisions, and staff provides support to help line make decisions.

The staff functions of the scheduler include scheduling employees according to staffing policies, implementing procedures for position control and reallocation of staff, maintaining records for line managers, gathering information and preparing reports to help line authority prepare personnel budgets, and maintaining communications with other appropriate departments, such as personnel and payroll.

Line responsibilities of managers include developing a master staffing pattern; establishing procedures for adjustment of staff; clarifying requirements for each job description and staff position; hiring, developing, promoting, disciplining, and fir-

ing employees when appropriate; and defining and controlling the personnel budget.

Computers can be used for centralized scheduling. Before implementing a computer system, an analysis of policies and procedures is done and baseline data collected. Agency policies regarding the nature of the schedule—straight, alternating, or rotating shifts; frequency of alternating or rotating shifts; work stretch; weekends-off sequence; and use of part-time help—are constants in the information processing system. Variables such as census, acute conditions of patients, special requests, special assignments, vacations, and holidays can be fed into the computer.

Advantages of centralized computer scheduling include cost-effectiveness through the reduction of clerical staff and better use of professional nurses by decreasing the time spent in non–patient-care activities; unbiased, consistent scheduling; equitable application of agency policies; an easy-to-read work schedule developed in advance so employees know what their schedules are and can plan their personal lives accordingly; and availability of data for monitoring the effect of staff size and composition, quality of care, and cost. However, staff may not trust the machine and nurse managers may feel a loss of control and may resist the use of technology (Decker and Sullivan, 1992; Saba and McCormick, 1996) (Box 13-2).

Decentralized Staffing

When managers are given authority and assume responsibility, they can staff their own units through decentralized staffing. Personnel feel that they get more personalized attention with decentralized staffing. Staffing is easier and less complicated when done for a small area instead of for the whole agency. Each manager learns the responsibility and challenges of staffing. With a philosophy of sharing and mutual trust, managers can work together to solve chronic staffing problems. Because of their knowledge and experience, managers can form a support system and offer each other informed advice. Nurse managers and charge nurses are freed

Box 13-2	PROS AND CONS OF CENTRALIZED AND DECENTRALIZED STAFFING

	Pros	Cons
Centralized	Fairness	Lack of individualized treatment
	Cost containment	
Decentralized	Managers have authority	Unfair treatment
	Staff get personalized attention	Schedule used to punish and reward
	Staffing is easier	Time-consuming for managers
	Staffing is less complicated	Less efficient use of resources
		Cost containment is more difficult

from staffing responsibilities and have more time for other tasks.

Unfortunately, some staff members may receive individualized treatment at the expense of others, and work schedules can be used as a punishment-reward system. Staffing, which is very time-consuming, takes managers away from other duties or forces them to do the scheduling while off duty. Decentralized staffing may use resources less efficiently and consequently make cost containment more difficult.

Self-Scheduling

Self-scheduling is a system that is coordinated by staff nurses (Box 13-3). It is a process by which nurses and other staff collectively develop and implement work schedules, taking policies and variables affecting staffing into consideration. A process might allow about 2 weeks for staff to indicate the days, shifts, weekends, holidays, and vacation days that they want. Then about 2 weeks are needed for negotiations to finalize a schedule that accommodates both the staff's and the unit's needs. Staff may negotiate before and after work and during break and lunchtime. They may also write notes to each other and wait for responses.

Self-scheduling can help create a climate where professional nursing can be practiced. It saves the manager considerable scheduling time and changes the role of the manager from supervisor to coach. It

increases the amount of time the staff spends on scheduling and helps develop a more accountable and professional staff. It also increases staff members' ability to negotiate with each other.

Self-scheduling has been associated with increased perception of autonomy, increased job satisfaction, increased cooperative atmosphere, improved team spirit, improved morale, decreased absenteeism, reduced turnover, and shortened scheduling time. It has also been effective in recruitment and retention. Staff do need negotiation and conflict negotiation skills (Decker and Sullivan, 1992; Swansburg, 1996; Swansburg and Swansburg, 1999; Tappen, 1995; Yoder-Wise, 1999).

Alternating or Rotating Work Shifts

Although straight shifts are used by some institutions or for some personnel within institutions, rotating work shifts are common for staff nurses. The frequency of alternating between days and evenings, or days and nights, or rotating through all three shifts varies among institutions. Some nurses may work all three shifts within 7 days.

Alternating and rotating work shifts create stress for staff nurses. Environmental cues, such as sunrise and sunset, fluctuate in a predictable cycle. Instruments that designate hours, minutes, and seconds correspond to the natural daily cycle and allow knowledge of one's location in that cycle. Social and work routines synchronize with the internal circa-

Box 13-3   ADVANTAGES AND DISADVANTAGES OF VARIOUS SCHEDULING METHODS

Scheduling Method	Pros	Cons
Self-scheduling	Coordinated by staff nurses Saves manager scheduling time Helps develop accountability Increased perception of autonomy Increased job satisfaction Improved team spirit Improved morale Decreased absenteeism Reduced turnover Effective for recruitment and reten- tion	Increases amount of time staff spends on scheduling
Rotating work shifts	Can rotate teams	Rotate among shifts Increases stress Affects health Affects quality of work Disrupts development of work groups High turnover
Permanent shifts	Can participate in social activities Job satisfaction Commitment to the organization Fewer health problems Less tardiness Less absenteeism Less turnover	Most people want day shift New graduates predominately staff evenings and nights Difficulty evaluating evening and night staff Nurses may not appreciate the work- load or problems of other shifts
Block, or cyclical, scheduling	Same schedule repeatedly Nurses not so exhausted Sick time reduced Personnel know schedule in advance Personnel can schedule social events Decreased time spent on scheduling Staff treated fairly Helps establish stable work groups Decreases floating Promotes team spirit Promotes continuity of care	Rigidity
Variable staffing	Use census to determine number and mix of staff Little need to call in unscheduled staff	

dian rhythms as the body rhythms are timed to co-incide with the usual activities. Thus when environmental conditions are changed by altering work hours, sleep time, hour for rising, mealtimes, and social and recreational activities, the body must make accommodations for the environmental changes. Body rhythms need time to adjust to the discrepancy between the person's activity cycle and the new demands of the environment. The ability of the body functions to adjust varies considerably among individuals. It may take 2 to 3 days to 2 weeks for a person to adjust to a different sleep-wake cycle.

Alternating and rotating work shifts affect the health of nurses and the quality of their work. The rapid shift of work schedules causes stress. Nurses complain of restlessness and nervousness while trying to sleep, wakefulness or sleepiness at inappropriate times, anorexia, digestive disturbance, disruption in bowel habits, fatigue, slower reaction time, lower job performance, and error proneness. There are changes in the patterning of temperature, blood pressure, and urine excretory cycles, and a possible lowered resistance to disease. Resultant increase in medication errors, equipment failures, and errors in problem solving are probable.

To guarantee that nurses work their share of weekends, holidays, and unpopular evening and night hours, alternating and rotating assignments currently focus on the time patterns of an individual nurse rather than on well-integrated work groups. The rotation of personnel on an individual basis is disruptive to the development of work groups.

The Federal Aviation Agency's (FAA) rotation of teams of airport personnel may be used as a model by nursing services. The FAA rotates entire teams consisting of four or five controllers plus trainees and a leader, chosen because of their qualifications, amount of experience, and anticipated compatibility. Their schedules are planned a year in advance so that team members can plan their personal lives with confidence. Emergencies and vacations are handled within the team. Absenteeism affects the workload of the peers with whom one must continue to work; therefore team identifica-

tion reduces absenteeism because of team pressure. Controllers have a low turnover rate.

In hospitals, rotation of teams instead of individuals could contribute to team development. If a group of personnel work together consistently, they can help each other through the dependence of the orientation phase of group development and the conflict experienced during the organizational phase, when the role negotiations of who will be responsible for what occur. The staff has a chance to become an interdependent, cohesive group with good communication and effective problem-solving abilities. Unfortunately, there is usually a high turnover of nursing personnel, which complicates team development. Perhaps more attention to team development would reduce turnover.

Permanent Shifts

Permanent shifts relieve nurses from stress and health-related problems associated with alternating and rotating shifts. They also provide social, educational, and psychological advantages. When nurses are able to choose the shift that best suits their personal life, they can participate in social activities (such as hobbies, sports, and community, professional, or church organizations) even when they require regular attendance. They may be able to continue their education by planning courses around their work schedule. Child care arrangements can be stable. Nurses may develop a sense of belonging to a shift and feel and work better because the shift suits them. In studies conducted with Montreal nurses, those working permanent shifts had higher averages on psychological scales such as mental health, job satisfaction, social involvement, and commitment to the organization. They had fewer health problems and less tardiness, absenteeism, and turnover.

Although the day shift is not always the preferred shift, it is likely to be. Consequently, assignment to preferred shift may have to be done on a seniority-priority basis. This usually results in a predominance of new graduates staffing the evening and night shifts. Managers may have difficulty evaluating the evening and night shift personnel unless they make some observations during those shifts; therefore it may be easier for evening and night supervisors to evaluate permanent staff on those shifts. One disadvantage of permanent shifts is that nurses may not develop an appreciation for the workload or problems of other shifts.

Block, or Cyclical, Scheduling

Block, or cyclical, scheduling uses the same schedule repeatedly. With a 6-day forward rotation, personnel are scheduled to work 6 successive days followed by at least 2 days off. The schedule repeats itself every 6 weeks.

Personnel can be scheduled with every other weekend off and 1 day during the week so that there are no more than 4 consecutive days of work. Several blocks are possible. Because nurses are not exhausted by working too many consecutive days, sick leave can be reduced. By having one team member at a time on vacation and by rotating holidays among the workers, vacations and holidays can be scheduled to avoid changes in the block. However, some nurses fear that 1 day off at a time is not adequate to feel rested. But nurses who currently do not work more than 4 consecutive days report that 1 day is adequate to refresh themselves.

There are several advantages to established rotations. Personnel know their schedules in advance and consequently can plan their personal lives. Absences because of social events decrease because staff can plan their social activities around their work schedules. There is a decrease in preoccupation with staffing, time for scheduling, time for maintenance of schedule, and conflict over preferred days off. Staff are treated more fairly by equitable distribution of popular and unpopular days on duty. The scheduling of appropriate number and category mix of personnel is simplified. Once the appropriate mix is determined, it is repeated. This helps establish stable work groups and decreases floating, thus promoting team spirit and continuity of care. The initial schedule is time-consuming, and a decrease in flexibility of staffing may be perceived as a disadvantage, especially by people who need flexibility (Decker and Sullivan,

1992; Swansburg, 1993; Swansburg, 1996; Swansburg and Swansburg, 1999).

Variable Staffing

Variable staffing is a method that uses patient needs to determine the number and mix of staff. Time measures are done for direct and indirect patient care. A patient classification system is developed, and tables are designed to determine the number of nursing hours required, depending on the number of patients in each category. This provides the information to determine staff needs by skill levels. Nursing pools, floats, and part-time help can be used to supplement the regular staff to accomplish the variable staffing. With a study of previous staffing needs, redistribution of peak routine work, and slight overstaffing in some areas to create float personnel for last-moment needs, there may be little need to call in unscheduled staff (Box 13-4).

Eight-Hour Shift, Five-Day Workweek

The 5-day, 40-hour workweek became popular during the late 1940s. It was a radical change from the 10-hour day, 5-day workweek that contained split shifts and few holidays. It has been a predominant pattern since then. The shifts are usually 7 AM to 3:30 PM, 3 PM to 11:30 PM, and 11 PM to 7:30 AM, allowing for a half-hour lunch break and a half-hour overlap time between shifts to provide for continuity of care (Grohar-Murray and DiCroce, 1997; Marrelli, 1993).

Ten-Hour Day, Four-Day Workweek

The Intensive Coronary Care Unit at Saint Elizabeth Community Health Center in Lincoln, Nebraska, implemented the 10-hour day, 4-day workweek with an every-other-weekend-off staffing pattern. The shifts were 7 AM to 5:30 PM, 1 PM to 11:30 PM, and 9 PM to 7:30 AM. A cyclical schedule allowed at least 14 hours off between shifts and a 4-day weekend every 6 weeks for those who rotated. The workweek began on Sunday, and the weekend was Saturday

Box 13-4	PROS AND CONS OF VARIABLE STAFFING

	Pros	Cons
8 hours	Traditional	
10 hours	Time to complete work	Longer workday
	Long weekends	Fatigue
	Extra days off	Overlap
	Decreased overtime	Difficult to find substitute
	Cover peak workloads	
	Decreases costs	
12 hours	Lower staffing requirements	Overtime
	Lowers cost per patient day	Exhaustion increases at end of work-week
	Increased knowledge of patients	week
	Get new admissions settled	Tension increases at end of workweek
	Not so rushed	Increases in minor accidents
	Better continuity of care	Increases medication errors
	Team development is possible	Home and social life suffers the week
	Less daily reporting	worked
	Less time to do staffing	
	Reduced travel time	
	Less personal expenses for gas, meals, babysitting	
Baylor plan/weekend option	Fewer people need to work weekends	Illness increased
	Weekends off more frequently	Absences increased
	Work fewer hours for greater pay	
	Staffing improved	
	Morale improved	

and Sunday for all shifts. The main problem was fatigue, but it was not found to be as serious a problem as anticipated. The long weekends and extra days off were attractions (Bauer, 1971). In addition, there is time to finish work, peak workloads can be covered, and there is decreased overtime and decreased costs. Ten-hour days, however, are considered long workdays to some, and there is overlap (Grohar-Murray and DiCroce, 1997; Marrelli, 1993; Swansburg, 1993, 1996).

Ten-Hour Day Plus Five- or Six-Hour Shift

Roger Williams General Hospital in Providence, Rhode Island, implemented two 10-hour shifts and one 5-hour shift. The shifts were 7 AM to 5 PM, 5 PM to 10 PM, and 9 PM to 7 AM. A 2-week cyclical schedule posted 2 days on, 2 days off, 3 on, 2 off, 2 on, and 3 off with two teams working complementary schedules. The younger nurses seemed to have a more positive attitude toward the 10-hour shift and cited the social opportunities as a major benefit. However, the 10-hour system did contribute to greater fatigue, poorer communication between physicians and nurses, and discontinuity of patient care (Colt and Corley, 1974).

Nursing service at Sacred Heart Hospital in Eau Claire, Wisconsin, was able to capitalize on a pool of inactive RNs by developing a 6-hour evening shift and a 10-hour day shift. Shifts were

7 AM to 5 PM, 5 PM to 11 PM, and 11 PM to 7 AM. Problems encountered were overtime, which may have been partially due to adjustment, and absences of ill nurses from 10-hour shifts—a difficult deficit to fill, and one that burdened other staff members and lowered morale (Minor, 1971).

Ten-Hour Shift, Seven-Day Workweek

Evergreen General Hospital in Kirkland, Washington, implemented a 7-70 plan that included a 10-hour shift 7 days a week, followed by 7 consecutive days off. Two teams alternated weeks from Tuesday through Monday. There was no rotation of shifts. Each team contained permanent day, evening, and night shifts. The shifts were 6:45 AM to 5:15 PM, 12:45 PM to 11:15 PM, and 9:15 PM to 7:45 AM. Initially there was no extra pay for holiday or vacation time, because that was compensated for in the pay for 80 hours when only 70 hours were worked. Later, vacation time was instituted, dependent on length of employment and ranging from 70 hours annually for 1 to 3 years of employment to 140 hours per year for 11 or more years of employment.

Advantages of the 10-hour day, 7-day workweek include increased continuity of care, more consistency of care between weekdays and weekends, improved communications, better understanding of the patients' needs resulting from longer time with patients, more consistent patient teaching, more flexibility for meeting patient needs instead of hospital regimens, and improved job satisfaction because of advanced knowledge of work schedule and prolonged rest periods that facilitated a more normal home life and more control over one's personal affairs. Sick leave and resignations decreased. However, nurses were tired at the end of the 7-day workweek (Hutchins and Cleveland, 1978).

Twelve-Hour Shift, Seven-Day Workweek

The 12-hour shift, starting at 7 or 7:30 AM and ending at 7 or 7:30 PM, was adopted by some institutions. The better use of nursing personnel lowers staffing requirements; this consequently lowers the cost per patient day. Nurses find they get to know their patients better because they have more time to study charts and can visit patients more frequently. They have more time to get new admissions settled before the change of shift and feel that they can give better patient care because they are not so rushed. They find that there are fewer communication gaps and better continuity of care. Consequently, there are improved nurse-patient relations, job satisfaction, and morale.

Working relations are improved. Personnel work with the same group of people, so team development is possible. There is less friction and no 3-to-11 shift to blame for problems. Less daily reporting results in less confusion about physicians' orders and changes in procedures and routines. Less time is required for staffing, thus freeing supervisors and head nurses for other duties.

Total time off is increased with an increased usefulness of time. Travel time is reduced. There is less personal expense for babysitting, gas, and meals. Nurses find they have more time to relax and enjoy their days off and are able to return to work refreshed. Flexibility for personal schedules improves staff morale.

Overtime pay has been of some concern. The 1966 Amendments to the Fair Labor Standards Act permit agencies to calculate overtime pay on a 14-consecutive-day work period. Consequently, overtime pay is required only for more than 80 hours in a 2-week period.

Some nurses complain that the extra time they have for learning and research becomes boring. Mental exhaustion and tension increase by the end of the workweek. Increases in minor accidents and medication errors have been reported. Others, however, have reported no such increases as a result of the cumulative fatigue. Nurses also complain that their home and social lives suffer the week they work.

The wide variety of staffing practices suggests there is no right or wrong staffing schedule. Rather, there is much variability to consider when designing the best staffing schedule for a given situation (Grohar-Murray and DiCroce, 1997; Marrelli, 1993; Swansburg, 1993, 1996).

Baylor Plan—Weekend Alternative

Baylor University Medical Center in Dallas, Texas, started a 2-day alternative plan. Nurses have the option to work two 12-hour days on the weekends and be paid for 36 hours for day shifts, or 40 hours for night shifts, or to work five 8-hour shifts Monday through Friday. This plan required a larger nursing staff, filled weekend positions, and reduced turnover. Some hospitals have implemented the Baylor plan, indicating that the extra pay on weekends compensated for vacations, holidays, and sick time.

Some hospitals have nurses work 12-hour shifts when they work weekends. This way fewer people have to work weekends and, consequently, staff can have weekends off more frequently. While illness and absences increased, recruitment and staffing improved (Grohar-Murray and DiCroce, 1997; Marrelli, 1993; Swansburg, 1993, 1996).

VARIABLES AFFECTING STAFFING

Although institutional and nursing service philosophy and objectives guide staffing, various patient, staff, and environmental factors also affect staffing patterns. The types of patients, their expectations, fluctuations in admissions, length of stay, and complexity of care complicate staffing (Box 13-5). Personnel policies, educational and experiential levels of staff, job descriptions, the mix of work titles or leveling, hour and rotation policies, absenteeism, and the competitive market also affect staffing. Environmental factors, such as the floor plan of the unit and hospital, number of patient beds, availability of supplies and equipment, the organizational structure, and support services from other departments and agencies, are also considered when planning staffing patterns.

Budget submission is done periodically by submitting a summarization of the revenue and

---

Box 13-5   VARIABLES THAT AFFECT STAFFING

Workload budgets indicate the amount of work produced by a unit in terms of units of service, which are used to calculate expense budgets.

Activity reports measure statistics about current activity centering on the number of units of service given compared with the capacity.

Average daily census is the average number of patients cared for per day for a period of time.

Average length of stay is the average number of days that patients stay in the agency.

Adjusted units of service allows budgeting based on expected workload units of service adjusted for the expected mix of patients.

Care hours calculation determines the average required care hours per patient per 24 hours for each classification level and the sum or the total hours of care needed for all patients.

Personnel expense budget is the budget for all personnel assigned to a unit.

Fixed staff are employees who do not vary with the patient volume.

Variable staff are responsive to the projected number of care hours needed.

Establishing positions should involve the manager's discretion for use of full-time and part-time personnel to total the number of full-time equivalents needed to meet the care needs.

Labor costs are determined by calculating the dollar basis of the straight-time salary, differentials, overtime, raises, and fringe benefits for each employee used by the unit.

Expense budget (other than personnel) is a combination of the direct unit expenses plus the indirect overhead expenses.

Revenue budget is the unit's income.

Modified from Finkler SA, Kovner CT: *Financial management for nurse managers and executives*, Philadelphia, 1993, WB Saunders, pp. 315-347.

expense sections of the budget for review. A narrative justification is used to negotiate changes in the budget.

Managers are responsible for implementation of the budget to meet the staffing needs of the unit, including weekends, holidays, vacations, and sick leave coverage through busy and slow periods.

Staffing Studies

Three major types of staffing studies are used to predict the number, level, and mix of personnel required for staffing. Nursing care needed may be predicted from patient classification systems by assigning patients to categories according to diagnosis, acuity of care, or amount of self-sufficiency. Number, level, and mix of staff needed can be determined by noting the number of patients in each category. Then a cost-effective nursing personnel budget based on the needs of patients and the qualifications of nursing personnel can be determined. Patient classification systems can be combined with nursing care plans, and costs to individual patients can be determined. Systems that charge patients for the care they receive can be designed.

Time standards can be determined for nursing procedures by listing and analyzing the procedures required by each patient. The time required for each patient and the sum for all patients on a unit can then be calculated. Formulas deduced from statistical analysis of work sampling data can be used to predict the number of nursing care hours needed. However, staffing is a function of fiscal factors, market availability, creativity, and innovation.

Patient Classification Systems

Patient classification systems were introduced when managers realized that nurse staffing needs were more dependent upon the patient's dependency on care than on the medical diagnosis. The three basic styles of patient classification systems are (1) descriptive, (2) checklist, and (3) time of relative value unit standard. In the descriptive style, the nurse classifies the patient in the category that most

closely describes the care received. The tool used is a narrative on a concise acuity table. Category 1 may be self-care and category 4 complete care, including feeding, frequent skin care, complete bath, complete bed rest, and frequent positioning. The patient does not have to receive all of the care in a category to be classified in that category. The nurse chooses the category that best describes the patient. The major problem with this style is interrater reliability, caused by the subjectivity of the interpretation of the patient's degree of care. The descriptive style is a quick-check guide, but the poor interrater reliability leads to a wide range of requested nurse-to-patient ratios. Many administrators have moved away from this subjective style of patient classification.

The checklist-style acuity table divides descriptions of care routines into activity categories, such as eating and bathing. Activity levels are described in each category. Levels in the eating category might be self-care, help setting up, feed, and frequent feedings. Each activity is assigned an activity level point score, such as 1 for routine or self-care and 4 for comprehensive care. The nurse checks the activity level for each patient in each category and totals the points for each patient to determine the level of care. This is usually done at each shift or daily. It, too, is a subjective system.

Time standard or relative value unit (RVU) systems assign a value unit (usually a measure of time) to various activities of patient care. Those activities are usually clustered according to categories, such as diet, bathing, and mobility. There is considerable variation in the complexity of these systems (Ellis and Hartley, 1995; Gillies, 1994; Lewis and Carini, 1984; Swansburg, 1993, 1996; Swansburg and Swansburg, 1999).

Time Standards

When figuring time standards for nursing care, one should consider both direct and indirect care. Direct care involves the patient and includes feeding, bathing, treating, and giving medications. Indirect care involves all activities that are not direct care, such as preparation of and cleaning up after medications and treatments, clinical work, reporting, communications, and coffee and lunch breaks.

Once the number and kind of care activities required by each patient are identified and the length of time it takes to do the activities calculated, one can add up the time required by all patients on a unit and divide by the number of productive work hours on a shift to determine the number of personnel needed. The mix of nursing personnel can be predicted by categorizing the care needed by the qualifications needed to give it, adding the time in each category, dividing by productive hours on a shift, and obtaining the number of specific types of personnel required to meet the patients' needs. Once this is accomplished, patients can be charged by the level of care required.

Public health nurses deal with health needs of aggregate groups in the community, whereas visiting nurses provide care to clients in their own homes. There are also health care clinics and nurse practitioner clinics in the community. For visiting nurse services and home health agencies, staffing is determined by the number of clients who need to be seen in a day. A standard amount of time is often allocated per visit. A standard of 45 minutes per visit for four to six clients depending on the amount of driving has been used, but the acuity of clients treated at home has increased. Thus an acuity system is merited and RVUs can be used (Loveridge and Cummings, 1996).

Staffing Formulas

When determining the number of staff to hire, one must consider hours for which coverage is required, vacations, holidays, absenteeism, and staff development time. If nurses work 5 days a week and coverage is needed for 7 days, it takes 1.4 nurses to have one nurse on duty 7 days and 2.8 nurses to have two nurses on duty for 7 days. This is calculated by multiplying the number needed on duty by days of the week for which coverage is required and dividing by the number of days each employee works per week to determine the number of personnel needed for coverage. Table 13-1 provides some examples.

This figure does not allow for vacations, holidays, absenteeism, or staff development time.

To calculate vacation coverage, multiply the number of vacation days per year by the number of people at that skill level. Dividing the total number of vacation days per skill level by the total days worked per year per person determines the number of people needed for vacation coverage. For example:

$$\begin{array}{c}\text{Number of} \\ \text{vacation days} \\ \text{per year}\end{array} \times \begin{array}{c}\text{Number of} \\ \text{full-time people} \\ \text{at that skill level}\end{array} = \begin{array}{c}\text{Total vacation} \\ \text{days by} \\ \text{skill level}\end{array}$$

$$\begin{array}{c}\text{Total} \\ \text{vacation} \\ \text{days by} \\ \text{skill level}\end{array} \div \begin{array}{c}\text{Total days} \\ \text{worked per} \\ \text{person per year}\end{array} = \begin{array}{c}\text{Number of} \\ \text{full-time people} \\ \text{needed for} \\ \text{vacation} \\ \text{relief coverage}\end{array}$$

To determine holiday coverage, multiply total number of personnel required (7-day coverage per skill level) by the number of holidays to determine the number of holiday days to be staffed. Then di-

Table 13-1   Staffing Formulas

Number Needed		Days of Week		Number of Days Each Workweek		Number of People Required
1	×	7	÷	5	=	1.4
2	×	7	÷	5	=	2.8
3	×	7	÷	5	=	4.2
4	×	7	÷	5	=	5.6
5	×	7	÷	5	=	7.0

Table 13-2 Staffing Formulas

Number Needed on Duty	Number Needed to Cover Days Off	15.6 Extra Days + 6%	18.2 Extra Days + 7%	20.8 Extra Days + 8%	23.4 Extra Days + 9%
1	1.4	1.46	1.47	1.48	1.49
2	2.8	2.92	2.94	2.96	2.98
3	4.2	4.38	4.41	4.44	4.47
4	5.6	5.84	5.88	5.92	5.96
5	7.0	7.30	7.35	7.40	7.45

Data from Decker PJ, Sullivan EJ: *Nursing administration: a micro/macro approach for effective nurse executives,* Norwalk, Conn, 1992, Appleton & Lange; Marquis BL, Huston CJ: *Management decision making for nurses: 124 case studies,* Philadelphia, 1998, Lippincott; Yoder-Wise PS: *Leading and managing in nursing,* ed 2, St. Louis, 1999, Mosby.

vide the total holiday relief days by the total days worked per year per person to obtain the number of personnel required per skill level for holiday coverage per year.

$$\text{Number of personnel} \times \text{Number of holidays} = \text{Number of holidays needing coverage}$$

$$\text{Number of holiday relief days} \div \text{Number of days worked per year per person} = \text{Number of personnel required for holiday coverage per year}$$

The percentage of absenteeism is used to calculate absentee relief coverage.

$$\text{Weeks/year} \times \text{Days worked/week} \times \% = \text{Absentee days/person/year of absenteeism}$$

$$\text{Personnel requirements (7 days/week)} \times \text{Absenteeism days/person/year} = \text{Absentee coverage for staffing}$$

$$\text{Absentee coverage required} \div \text{Total days worked/person/year} = \text{Full-time personnel required for absentee coverage per year}$$

Personnel required for staff development relief per year can also be calculated.

$$\text{Number of hours required or recommended for staff development per year per person} \times \text{Number of staff} = \text{Number of hours per year for staff development needing relief coverage}$$

$$\text{Number of staff development hours needing coverage} \div \text{Hours worked/day} \div \text{Total days worked/person}$$

$$= \text{Full-time personnel required for staff development coverage}$$

A staffing slide rule can be developed to save time when computing the number of budgeted positions needed to meet staffing standards by preparing a table that identifies the number of persons needed on duty, number of persons needed to cover days off, and number of persons needed to cover additional days off for vacation, holiday, sick, and personal leaves. Table 13-2 provides examples.

Staffing to Meet Fluctuating Needs

Full-time staff. Full-time staff may be hired to meet the average staffing needs of an institution. The most common adjustment for an increased workload is to transfer staff from a less busy area to the overloaded area. This is economical for the agency but disrupts the unity of work groups, causes the transferred nurse to feel insecure, and contributes to job dissatisfaction and turnover. Some units require specialized knowledge and skill that not every nurse has. Cross-training is helpful.

In the companion floor system, two units relieve each other. Staff nurses are oriented to the second unit and know that if they are transferred, it will be to the companion unit. Thus staff aggravation is minimized, flexibility is possible, and quality of care is maintained.

At best, a complementary, or float, staff is composed of full-time staff nurses who are oriented to many areas and like the challenge of different types of patients and settings. Unfortunately, most nurses prefer stability. Consequently, the float staff is likely to be part-time staff or new personnel waiting for a permanent assignment.

Having full-time staff work double shifts and overtime is another option. The nurse is already oriented to the area, and continuity of care is facilitated. There are also disadvantages, however. Institutional costs increase. The nurses may become tired, errors are likely to increase with fatigue, and overtime may interfere with the nurses' personal lives (Decker and Sullivan, 1992; Swansburg, 1993; Swansburg and Swansburg, 1999).

Part-time staff. Flexible working hours can be an incentive for inactive nurses to start part-time employment and can thus reduce staffing shortages. Most nurses are women who have to combine their nursing role with many others, such as wife, mother, and homemaker. A part-time job can broaden the woman's horizons beyond her home, increase her income, give her ego satisfaction, and help her maintain her nursing skills. It is not uncommon for nurses to want to work part-time while continuing their education. Part-time nurses tend to work more than their share of unpopular hours, and some prefer evening and night duty exclusively. When part-time nurses' other responsibilities decrease, they are likely candidates for full-time work. It is sometimes possible for two people to share a job.

There are, of course, disadvantages to the use of part-time nurses. Educational and administrative expenses are higher proportionately for part-time than for full-time help. For example, it is likely to cost as much to orient a part-time nurse as a full-time nurse, thus costing more per hours worked. Maintaining continuity of care is complicated, because two or more part-time people may fill budgeted full-time positions. There are also disadvantages for the employee. The part-time nurse may not receive benefits such as paid sick or vacation days and is not likely to be considered for promotion. Sometimes benefits are prorated for part-time workers.

Temporary help is another option. Some institutions hire temporary help for the summer to give relief for vacations. The University of Virginia Hospital in Charlottesville has used temporary bed and bath teams to reduce weekend staffing shortages (Rinker, Norris, and Jordan, 1975). Rochester Methodist Hospital in Rochester, Minnesota, has used a "premium day" approach to reduce the weekend staffing shortage. Staff nurses get an extra day off (a premium day) if they work one additional weekend within a 4-week schedule (Fisher and Thomas, 1974). Some nurses may be willing to work on an on-call basis the year around.

External temporary help agencies are available in some areas. The use of such agencies can greatly reduce the amount of time middle management must spend on staffing. The supervisor merely calls the external agency and requests so many nurses, and the agency makes the necessary contacts. The agency has a registry of available nurses who are allowed to have highly flexible, self-determined schedules. This allows some nurses to work who could not otherwise and consequently helps those nurses maintain their skills. It is then more likely for those nurses to return to nursing practice on a full-time basis than if they had remained inactive. Their availability may boost morale, and they may introduce new ideas and stimulate creativity among the regular staff.

Unfortunately, there are also disadvantages to temporary help agencies. The matching of the nurses' credentials and qualifications with assignments and orientation to assignments are severe problems. Although some temporary help agencies do keep orientation information and procedure manuals for their client institutions on file, their use may still be optional. It is likely to take considerable time for the regular staff to orient the temporary help, errors are likely to increase, and continuity of care is jeopardized. The temporary nurses get preferred schedules, leaving the regular staff with more of the less-attractive hours. Consequently, morale may be lowered.

A central placement service run by the state board of nursing or the state nurses' association could be useful for matching nurses' qualifications and interests with vacancies and anticipated vacancies throughout the state.

There are many variables to be considered when planning staffing schedules. The more accurately those variables are assessed, the better one is able to contain costs while providing high-quality care (Douglas, 1996; Grohar-Murray and DiCroce, 1997; Koch and Fairly, 1993).

Managers have several relatively undesirable options for handling a called-in absence or otherwise uncovered shift. They can consider the following (Marrelli, 1993):

1. Using a float, per diem, or agency nurse
2. Asking a nurse to work for the sick person and canceling a shift for that person later in the week
3. Asking a part-time person to work an extra shift
4. Substituting one type of classification for another, such as an LPN for an RN
5. Asking one staff member to stay a few hours overtime and another to come in a few hours early

6. Doing without a substitute
7. Covering the shift themselves

Reductions in Force

Declining inpatient activity and changing patient care patterns have caused some institutions to rightsize or downsize. Proactive rightsizing measures may eliminate or minimize the need for downsizing. Rightsizing is a comprehensive and systematic process that studies ineffective, costly programs and generates ideas for replacing them with revenue-generating programs. Units that should be investigated include those where the occupancy rate is below 60%, where caregiver worked hours per patient have increased by several percentage points in a year, where fixed staffing levels have increased by a small percentage of the full-time equivalents, where productivity goals are not met, where costs exceed revenues, and where the units have been out of service (Bruce and Patterson, 1985).

Finding new work for present departments can delay the need for downsizing. Examples are contracting out continuing education and laundry services and attracting work through expanded or new services such as geriatrics. Slow times can be used for in-servicing personnel to increase competence, for cross-training personnel to work in more than one area, for carrying out special projects, and for updating policies and procedures. Reducing overtime, encouraging use of holidays, vacation time, and leaves of absence without pay, reducing temporary help, and deferring hiring can decrease the budgetary deficit (Borg and Jensen, 1985).

Use of attrition, temporary early retirement, and conversion of full-time to part-time positions may be considered before termination. When it becomes necessary to implement layoffs, there are many issues to consider: Will they be based on seniority, job skills, job classification, or a combination of those factors? It is beneficial to involve managers from the patient care coordinator position up in deciding the criteria for layoffs. If seniority is used, is there a bumping policy? Bumping through transfers, demotions, and layoffs makes layoffs much more complicated and time-consuming and

involves about five times more people than origi-
nally targeted. People who know their positions are
in jeopardy may experience more stress than those
who have actually been bumped. Nurses may be angry and frustrated that they are transferred outside
their specialty area. They may not be suited to their
new position and may file grievances that are time-
consuming and costly to both staff and management. Many nurses would rather be laid off and be
eligible for unemployment compensation than
work where they do not feel qualified. Orientation
and training for the new positions also cost time
and money. Nurses may be too angry to orient
people who will replace them. Those who are stay-
ing may worry about being responsible for inexperienced nurses placed on their units. Those who re-
train may leave the institution as soon as they find
another position in their area of interest. Many
qualified people may leave voluntarily but will discuss their unhappy experiences in the community.

There are also communication issues. Many
people prefer to be informed about the layoff by
personal communication rather than in writing. It
is common to have a public meeting with immediate written follow-up. Many want information
about why cuts are needed, the extent of the cuts,
and the potential effects. They may want to be informed as soon as possible so they can make necessary arrangements.

Attention must be given to morale building
through increased communication and input into
decision making. A central communication office
may be helpful by allowing personnel to call or stop
in for clarification or information. A meeting may be
scheduled to explain rules, present facts, and answer
questions in an attempt to reduce anxiety. Discussion of the organization's bumping policy and procedures is particularly appropriate. Recall policy
should also be discussed so that retained and laid-off
personnel know their rights and responsibilities
concerning future vacancies. Support groups can be
formed to allow for venting anger and sharing feelings. Stress management workshops are appropriate.

A placement committee may be formed to
match affected personnel to openings, or a review
process implemented to respond to objections. Job

skill evaluation and job counseling may be offered
to affected personnel. Clear-cut procedures for
matching personnel skills and openings are essential. Training opportunities to prepare people for
new jobs should be provided, and prospective employees should be informed of the organization's
layoff policies before they are hired (Meehan and
Price, 1988). Public relations efforts for community
image will require attention.

Productivity.   Productivity is the product or work
produced through a specific amount of resources,
measured as outputs divided by inputs. For example, productivity can be measured as required
staff hours divided by provided staff hours multiplied by 100. Improvements in productivity involve
more work or product produced for less overall
cost. Productivity can be increased by decreasing
the staff hours provided while holding the required
staff hours constant or increasing them. It is often
measured through the patient classification system:
average daily census, number of patient days per
month, number of patients treated, and number of
procedures performed are productivity measures.

Many actions can be taken to increase outputs
while maintaining or reducing inputs. Recognizing
the need to do better, involving staff, seeking staff
ideas and recommendations, creating challenges,
management interest in staff achievements and
concerns, and praise and reward for good performance can help. Evaluating the problems, resources,
and realities in the organization; using work flow
analysis and work simplification procedures; and
improving use of time by helping personnel keep
and analyze time diaries, and decreasing waiting
time can make a difference. There are many ways to
improve productivity: set a climate for productivity
by asking personnel what would help them be more
productive and implementing their ideas. Set targets for increasing outputs. Have personnel set personal objectives and measure performance against
them. Seek new approaches to old problems and
improve products and services. Staff development,
attention to process, ethics, and aesthetics enhance
productivity through attention to doing the right
things the right way (Swansburg, 1996).

CHAPTER SUMMARY

Chapter 13 covered the following:
Assignment Systems for Staffing
    Case Method
    Functional Nursing
    Team Nursing
    Modular, or District, Nursing
    Primary Nursing
    Case Management
    Collaborative Practice
    Managed Care
    Differentiated Practice
Level of Staff
Staffing Schedules
    Centralized Scheduling
    Decentralized Staffing
    Self-Scheduling
    Alternating or Rotating Work Shifts
    Permanent Shifts
    Block, or Cyclical, Scheduling
    Variable Staffing
    Eight-Hour Shift, Five-Day Workweek
    Ten-Hour Day, Four-Day Workweek
    Ten-Hour Day Plus Five- or Six-Hour Shift
    Ten-Hour Shift, Seven-Day Workweek
    Twelve-Hour Shift, Seven-Day Workweek
    Baylor Plan—Weekend Alternative
Variables Affecting Staffing
    Staffing Studies
    Patient Classification Systems
    Time Standards
    Staffing Formulas
    Staffing to Meet Fluctuating Needs
        Full-time staff
        Part-time staff
    Reductions in Force
        Productivity

REFERENCES

ANA House of Delegates materials, 1999.

Bauer J: Clinical staffing with a 10-hour day, 4-day work-week, *JONA* 1:12-14, Nov-Dec 1971.

Borg JH, Jensen DL: Managing layoffs: a comprehensive approach, *Nurs Manage* 16:31-37, Aug 1985.

Bower KA: *Case management by nurses,* Washington, DC, 1992, American Nurses Association.

Bruce A, Patterson D: Resizing hospital nursing organizations, an alternative to downsizing, *Nurs Manage* 18:33-35, Aug 1985.

Cesta TG, Tahan HA, Fink LF: *The case manager's survival guide: winning strategies for clinical practice,* St. Louis, 1998, Mosby.

Cohen EL, Cesta TG: *Nursing case management: from concept to evaluation,* ed 2, St. Louis, 1997, Mosby.

Colt AM, Corley TF: What nurses think of the 10-hour shift, *Hospitals* 48:134-142, Feb 1974.

Decker PJ, Sullivan EJ: *Nursing administration: a micro/macro approach for effective nurse executives,* Norwalk, Conn, 1992, Appleton & Lange.

Del Togno-Armanasco V, Hopkin LA, Harter S: *Collaborative nursing case management: a handbook for development and implementation,* New York, 1993, Springer.

Douglas LM: *The effective nurse leader and manager,* ed 5, St. Louis, 1996, Mosby.

Easterling A et al.: *The case manager's guide: acquiring the skills for success,* Chicago, 1995, American Hospital Publishing.

Ellis JR, Hartley CL: *Managing and coordinating nursing care,* ed 2, Philadelphia, 1995, Lippincott.

Etheredge MLS, editor: *Collaborative care: nursing case management,* Chicago, 1989, American Hospital Publishing.

Finkler SA, Kovner CT: *Financial management for nurse managers and executives,* Philadelphia, 1993, WB Saunders, pp. 315-347.

Fisher DW, Thomas E: A "premium day" approach to weekend nurse staffing, *JONA* 4:59-60, Sept-Oct 1974.

Gillies DA: *Nursing management: a systems approach,* ed 3, Philadelphia, 1994, WB Saunders.

Grohar-Murray ME, DiCroce HR: *Leadership and management in nursing,* Stamford, Conn, 1997, Appleton & Lange.

Hicks LL, Stallmeyer JM, Coleman JR: *Role of the nurse in managed care,* Washington, DC, 1993, American Nurses Association.

Huber D: *Leadership and nursing care management,* Philadelphia, 1996, WB Saunders. Hutchins C, Cleveland R: For staff nurses and patients—the 7-70 plan, *Am J Nurs* 78:230-233, Feb 1978.

Knight W: *Managed care: what it is and how it works,* Gaithersburg, Md, 1998, Aspen.

Koch MW, Fairly TM: *Integrated quality management: the key to improving nursing care quality,* St. Louis, 1993, Mosby.

Kongstvedt PR: *Essentials of managed health care,* ed 2, Gaithersburg, Md, 1997, Aspen.

Kongstvedt PR, Plocher DW: *Best practices in medical management,* Gaithersburg, Md, 1998, Aspen.

Lewis EN, Carini PV: *Nurse staffing and patient classification: strategies for success,* Rockville, Md, 1984, Aspen.

Loveridge CE, Cummings SH: *Nursing management in the new paradigm,* Gaithersburg, Md, 1996, Aspen.

Marquis BL, Huston CJ: *Leadership roles and management functions in nursing: theory and application,* ed 2, Philadelphia, 1996, Lippincott.

Marquis BL, Huston CJ: *Management decision making for nurses: 124 case studies,* Philadelphia, 1998, Lippincott.

Marrelli TM: *The nurse manager's survival guide: practical answers to everyday problems,* St. Louis, 1993, Mosby.

Meehan M, Price C: Managing layoffs with minimum loss of productivity, *Nurs Adm Q* 13:26-32, Fall 1988.

Minor MA: Ten- and 6-hour nursing shifts solve staffing problem, *Hosp Prog* 52:62-66, July 1971.

Mullahy CM: *The case manager's handbook,* Gaithersburg, Md, 1998a, Aspen.

Mullahy CM: *Essential reading and case management,* Gaithersburg, Md, 1998b, Aspen.

Murer CG et al.: *The case management sourcebook,* Blacklick, Ohio, 1997, Richard Irwin.

Pesut DJ, Herman J: *Clinical reasoning: the art & science of critical & creative thinking,* Albany, NY, 1999, Delmar.

Powell SK: *Nursing case management: a practical guide to success in managed care,* Philadelphia, 1996, Lippincott-Raven.

Rinker KL, Norris CL, Jordan MF: "Bed and bath teams": one solution to the weekend staffing shortage, *JONA* 4:34-35, May 1975.

Saba VK, McCormick KA: *Essentials of computers for nurses,* ed 2, New York, 1996, McGraw-Hill.

Seifker JM, Garrett MB, Genderen AV: *Fundamentals of case management: guidelines for practicing case managers,* St. Louis, 1997, Mosby.

Steinberg AJ: *The insider's guide to HMOs: how to navigate the managed-care system and get the health care you deserve,* New York, 1997, Plume.

Swansburg RC: *Introductory management and leadership for clinical nurses: a text-workbook,* Boston, 1993, Jones & Bartlett.

Swansburg RC: *Management and leadership for nurse managers,* ed 2, Boston, 1996, Jones & Bartlett.

Swansburg RC, Swansburg RJ: *Introductory management and leadership for nurses: an interactive text,* Boston, 1999, Jones & Bartlett.

Tappen RM: *Nursing leadership and management: concepts and practice,* ed 3, Philadelphia, 1995, FA Davis.

University of Iowa College of Nursing: *Nursing diagnosis and extension classification* (http://www.nursing.uiowa.edu/ndec/index.htm), accessed July 15, 1999 a.

University of Iowa College of Nursing: *Nursing interventions classification* (http://www.nursing.uiowa.edu/nic/overview.htm), accessed July 15, 1999 b.

University of Iowa College of Nursing: *Nursing outcomes classification* (http://www.nursing.uiowa.edu/noc/index.htm), accessed July 15, 1999 c.

Yoder-Wise PS: *Leading and managing in nursing,* ed 2, St. Louis, 1999, Mosby.

BIBLIOGRAPHY

Abts D, Hofer M, Leafgreen PK: Redefining care delivery: a modular system, *Nurs Manage* 25:40-46, Feb 1994.

American Nurses Association: *Principles for nurse staffing,* Washington, DC, 1999, American Nurses Publishing.

Arthur T: Determining nurse staffing levels: a critical review of the literature, *J Adv Nurs* 19:558-565, 1994.

Baldwin L, McGinnis C: A computer-generated shift report, *Nurs Manage* 25:61-64, Sept 1994.

Barratt CC, Schultz MK: Staffing the operating room: time and space factors, *JONA* 27:27-31, Dec 1997.

Buerhaus PI: Economics of managed competition and consequences to nursing part 1, *Nurs Econ* 12:10-17, Jan-Feb 1994.

Buerhaus PI: What is the harm in imposing mandatory hospital nurse staffing regulations? *Nurs Econ* 15:66-72, March-April 1997.

Davidhizar R, Dowd SB, Brownson K: An equitable nursing assignment structure, *Nurs Manage* 29:33-35, April 1998.

DeGroot HZ: Patient classification systems and staffing: part 2, practice and process, *JONA* 24:17-23, Oct 1994.

Douglas DA, Mayewski J: Census variation staffing, *Nurs Manage* 27:32-36, Feb 1996.

Fielo SB, Crowe RL: A nursing center in Brooklyn, *Nurs Health Care* 13:488-493, Nov 1992.

Grimaldi PL: Manage authorizations to manage care, *Nurs Manage* (suppl) 27:110-112, Oct 1996.

Hall LM: Staff mix models: complementary or substitution roles for nurses, *Nurs Adm Q* 21(2):31-39, 1997.

Hayes PM: Team building: bringing RNs and NAs together, *Nurs Manage* 25:52-54, May 1994.

Hoffart N, Willdermood S: Self-scheduling in five med/surg units, *Nurs Manage* 28:42-45, April 1997.

Hollabauch S, Kendrick S: Staffing: the five-level pyramid, *Nurs Manage* 29:34-36, Feb 1998.

Huber DG, Blegen MA, McCloskey JC: Use of nursing assistants: staff nurse opinions, *Nurs Manage* 25:64-68, May 1994.

Ingersoll GL: Licensed practical nurses in critical care areas: intensive care unit nurses' perceptions about the role, *Heart Lung* 24:83-88, Jan-Feb 1995.

Kielyka CA, Robertson S, Bebner KG: A flexible staffing model for patient service associates, *JONA* 27:48-54, Jan 1997.

Kirkby MP: Moving to computerized scheduling: a smooth transition, *Nurs Manage* 28:42-44, Aug 1997.

Kirkby MP, Dost P, Holdwick CC et al.: Improving staffing with a resource management plan, *JONA* 28:25-29, Nov 1998.

Moniz DM: Too few staff, too much risk, *Montvale* 61:63-65, Dec 1998.

Morrow KL: Using staffing and scheduling information to support change, *Nurs Manage* 25:78-80, May 1994.

Reid N, Robinson G, Todd C: The 12-hour shift: the views of nurse educators and students, *J Adv Nurs* 19:938-946, 1994.

Schmidt L, Nelson D: A seasonal staffing model, *JONA* 26:52-55, April 1996.

Snyder J, Nethersole-Chong D: Is cross-training medical/surgical RNs to ISU the answer? *Nurs Manage* 30:58-60, Feb 1999.

Strickland B, Neely S: Using a standard staffing index to allocate nursing staff, *JONA* 25:13-21, March 1995.

Strzalka A, Havens DS: Nursing care quality: comparison of unit-hired, hospital float pool, and agency nurses, *J Nurs Care Qual* 10(4):59-65, 1996.

Uzark K, LeRoy S, Callow L et al.: The pediatric nurse practitioner as case manager in the delivery of services to children with heart disease, *J Pediatr Health Care* 8:74-78, March-April 1994.

Warren IB, Rozell BR: Supplemental staffing: nurse manager views of costs, benefits, and quality of care, *JONA* 25:51-57, June 1995.

CASE STUDY

You are responsible for the budget on your unit. You have a registered nurse vacancy, which you may fill with one registered nurse or two unlicensed personnel. What will you do and why?

CASE STUDY

Using the case study in the Appendix, determine an assignment system to be used on one of the units at Lake View Hospital. Determine how the scheduling will be done and how shifts and workweeks will be defined (8-, 10-, 12-hour days on a permanent or rotating basis). Determine the number and level of staff needed. Discuss the rationale for and advantages and disadvantages of your decisions with your classmates.

Critical Thinking Activities for this chapter begin on page 514.

CHAPTER 14

EVALUATION AND DISCIPLINE OF PERSONNEL

CHAPTER OBJECTIVES

- List at least five purposes of personnel evaluation.
- List at least six common errors in performance evaluation.
- Describe five methods of personnel evaluation.
- Discuss 360 degree evaluation.
- Explain various ways to arrange a room for performance evaluations.
- List at least five principles of disciplinary action.
- Identify at least three components of a disciplinary action program.
- Compare discipline without punishment with progressive discipline.
- Explain behavior modification.
- List at least three types of problem employees.
- Identify at least three types of employee counseling.
- Explain outplacement counseling.

Chapter Overview

Chapter 15 differentiates methods of performance management, appraisal interviews and reports, legal implications, principles of disciplinary action, penalties, components of a disciplinary action program, modification of employee behavior, problem employees, employee counseling, and outplacement counseling.

MAJOR CONCEPTS AND DEFINITIONS	
Evaluation	valuation, appraisal, determination of worth
Peer review	group evaluation of a group member
Appraisal interview	verbal evaluation
Appraisal report	written evaluation
Discipline	to train, control, punish
Penalties	punishment; negative consequences
Behavior modification	changes in behavior
Reinforcement	actions that strengthen a behavior or increase its probability
Shaping	reinforcing successive attempts at achieving the desired behavior
Extinction	annihilation, destruction
Substance abuse	misuse of drugs
Angry	furious, raging, tumultuous
Withdrawn	retreated, isolated
Productivity	results
Absenteeism	absence from work
Due process	procedural requirements to ensure fairness
Termination	end of something
Directive counseling	counselor telling one what to do
Nondirective counseling	client deciding what to do
Outplacement counseling	helping dismissed personnel find another job

Leaders encourage peer review, promote motivation and growth through it, reduce the anxiety related to it, and develop trust by being honest and fair. Leaders facilitate two-way communication, facilitate growth through coaching, and support employees attempting to correct performance deficiencies. Managers use a formalized system, document standards, gather fair and objective data, determine educational and training needs, follow up on performance deficiencies, maintain documentation of the appraisal process, and give frequent informal feedback (Box 14-1).

Box 14-1

LEADERSHIP AND MANAGEMENT FOR PERFORMANCE MANAGEMENT

Leader	Manager
Encourages peer review process	Uses a formalized system for performance appraisal
Promotes motivation and growth through the appraisal process	Uses documented standards as bases for performance appraisal
Reduces anxiety inherent in the appraisal process	Gathers fair and objective data for performance appraisals
Develops trust by being honest and fair	Determines education and training needs from appraisal process
Facilitates two-way communication through appraisal interviews	Follows up on performance deficiencies
Encourages growth through coaching	Maintains documentation of the appraisal process
Supports employees attempting to correct performance deficiencies	Provides frequent informal feedback

Modified from Marquis BL, Huston CJ: *Leadership roles and management functions in nursing: theory and application*, ed 2, Philadelphia, 1996, Lippincott.

PURPOSES

Performance appraisal is a periodic formal evaluation of how well personnel have performed their duties during a specific period. Purposes of the evaluation are as follows: (1) to determine job competence, (2) to enhance staff development and motivate personnel toward higher achievement, (3) to discover the employee's aspirations and to recognize accomplishments, (4) to improve communications between managers and staff associates and to reach an understanding about the objectives of the job and agency, (5) to improve performance by examining and encouraging better relationships between nurses, (6) to aid the manager's coaching and counseling, (7) to determine training and developmental needs of nurses, (8) to make inventories of talent within the organization and reassess assignments, (9) to select qualified nurses for advancement and salary increases, and (10) to identify unsatisfactory employees (Swansburg, 1996; Tappen, 1995).

COMMON ERRORS IN EVALUATION

Criteria involving judgments are used for performance evaluation. Because human judgment is sub-ject to the influences of prejudice, bias, and other subjective and extraneous factors, the attempt to get objective, accurate evaluations is extremely difficult. A number of errors may affect performance ratings. The manager should be aware of the most common ones and try to minimize them.

The halo error is the result of allowing one trait to influence the evaluation of other traits or of rating all traits on the basis of a general impression. A logical error is rating a nurse high on one characteristic because the nurse possesses another characteristic that is logically related. Sometimes employees are given a good rating in the recent past because they did good work in the distant past, or outstanding performance on a recent job may offset a mediocre performance during the rest of the evaluation period. A manager is likely to rate personnel who are compatible with the manager higher than they deserve and may not see certain types of defects that are like the manager's. The person who does not complain is likely to have higher ratings than the person who does.

The horns error is the opposite of the halo effect. The evaluator is hypercritical. Managers who are perfectionists may rate personnel lower than they should. Managers may compare how they used to do the job with how it is done now and are more likely to rate people doing jobs with which they are familiar lower than those with whose jobs they are not familiar. Good workers on weak teams are more likely to get lower ratings than if they were working on a better team. Persons who are not well known may be judged by the company they keep. A recent mistake may offset a year's good work. If the worker is contrary, managers may vent their irritation by lowering the rating. The nonconformist or person with a personality trait that is not appreciated is likely to be rated lower than that person's work merits.

The contrast error is produced by the tendency of managers to rate the nurse opposite from the way they perceive themselves. A small range of scores may be a result of the central tendency error. When the rating on a preceding characteristic influences the rating on the following trait, a proximity error exists. Because raters tend to have their own built-in set of standards or frame of reference on which to make evaluations, it becomes a major problem comparing different raters' scores. Some managers may be easy and lenient, whereas others may be severe in their judgments.

The manager can take precautions to minimize judgment errors. For instance, a forced-distribution technique may be used to overcome the leniency and central tendency errors. A critical incident checklist can reduce the halo effect and logical rating errors. Ranking systems, paired comparisons, and force-choice techniques may be used (Decker and Sullivan, 1992; Gillies, 1994; Huber, 1996; Marquis and Huston, 1996; Yoder-Wise, 1999).

METHODS OF PERFORMANCE MANAGEMENT
Anecdotal Notes

Anecdotal records are objective descriptions of behavior recorded on plain paper or a form. The notations should include who was observed, by whom, when, and where. The notation comprises a description of the setting or background and the incident, and interpretation and recommendations may be included. Value-laden words such as good and bad should be avoided.

Characteristic behavior cannot be determined without several incidents depicting similar behavior. The director or patient care coordinator may use time sampling to accumulate observations. The time that is set aside specifically for observations may be divided by the number of staff to be observed. The manager then concentrates on the scheduled staff member for a short period. It is advisable to make several brief observations over a time span to allow for temporary variables and to identify patterns of behavior.

An advantage of anecdotal recordings is that the description is not coerced into a rigid structure. However, this latitude becomes a problem when the interpreter tries to develop relationships between notations that may have little or no relationship to each other. Although anecdotal records provide a systematic means for recording observations, they do not guarantee that observations will be made systematically or that specific, relevant behaviors will be observed. It also takes considerable time to record the observations (Yoder-Wise, 1999).

Checklists

With a checklist the manager can categorically assess the presence or absence of desired characteristics or behaviors. Checklists are most useful for tangible variables, such as inventory of supplies, but they can be used for evaluation of nursing skills as well. It is advisable to list only the behaviors essential to successful performance, and it is advantageous to determine the behavior to be observed in advance. The same criteria can then be used in each situation. Unfortunately, this does not guarantee that the observed behavior is a persistent one or that a representative situation is being observed. Nor is the checklist practical for evaluating interpersonal relations (Dienemann, 1990; Douglas, 1996; Ellis and Hartley, 1995; Gillies, 1994; Marquis and Huston, 1996).

Rating Scales

The rating scale does more than just note the absence or presence of desirable behavior. It locates

Nurse	Observation of working hours				
	Lowest (1)	Below average (2)	Average (3)	Above average (4)	Highest (5)
Betty Green	X				
Sara Smith		X			
Pam Peterson			X		
Sue Jones				X	
Anita Anderson					X

Figure 14-1 Nurse-to-nurse comparison scale.

Box 14-2 RATING SCALE

Rate the staff member on the items below. Responses have the following values:

1 = Never

2 = Sometimes

3 = About half the time

4 = Usually

5 = Always

A. Observation of working hours   1 2 3 4 5

B. Ability to get along with others   1 2 3 4 5

the behavior at a point on a continuum and notes quantitative and qualitative abilities. The numerical rating scale usually includes numbers against which a list of behaviors is evaluated:

Observation of working hours 1 2 3 4 5

Ability to get along with others 1 2 3 4 5

This is not a very reliable tool because of the inconsistent value attributed to the number. That fault can be partially overcome by adding a few quantitative terms, as shown in Box 14-2.

The tool can be made even more reliable by developing a standard scale by using comparative examples to establish a set of standards. The difficulty is finding appropriate comparative standards. A nurse-to-nurse comparison scale might be developed (Figure 14-1).

As long as the managers can agree on the qualifications of a few nurses known to all of them, a comparison scale that gives a common reference for rating the rest of the staff nurses can be developed.

The graphic rating scale is different from the numerical rating scale in that words rather than numbers are used (Figure 14-2).

Graphic rating scales usually list extremely broad and general personal characteristics that are to be rated from poor to excellent or from low to high. Raters are given little if any guidance about what work behavior qualifies a person for a particular rating and must consequently use their own judgment about how to classify the behaviors.

The descriptive graphic rating scale is similar to the graphic rating scale except that it presents a more elaborate description of the behavior being rated (Figure 14-3).

BARS is an acronym for behaviorally anchored rating scales, sometimes known as BES, behavioral expectation scales. They are similar to graphic rating scales in that a person is rated on a series of dimensions or qualities. However, BARS differs from graphic rating scales in the ways that the criteria are identified and the alternative responses along the rating scale are anchored or described. BARS evalu-

Unsatisfactory / Below average / Average / Above average / Outstanding

Observation of working hours

Figure 14-2 Graphic rating scale.

ates behavior relevant to specific demands of the job and provides examples of specific job behaviors corresponding to good, average, and poor performances. This reduces the amount of personal judgment needed by the rater.

The major disadvantage of BARS is the time and expense required to involve large numbers of employees in determining the dimensions of effective performance and behavioral examples of various levels of performance of each variable. Separate BARS are needed for each job. It is primarily applicable to physically observable behaviors rather than to conceptual skills. However, it should reduce rating errors and provide more reliable, valid, meaningful, and complete data. Employees give more acceptance and commitment to this appraisal system because of their involvement in designing it. They have full knowledge of the requirements of the job, and they evidence less defensiveness and conflict because people are evaluated on the basis of specific behaviors rather than personalities. This system

thereby identifies performance deficiencies and needs for development.

BOS is an acronym for behavioral observation scales. This system capitalizes on some of the strengths of BARS while avoiding some of the disadvantages. BOS also uses critical incidents of worker behavior. The evaluator lists a number of critical incidents for each performance dimension and rates the extent to which the behavior has been observed on a five-point scale ranging from almost never to almost always. It too is relatively reliable, well accepted and understood, and provides useful feedback, but it is relatively time-consuming and expensive to develop.

Instead of a descriptive choice, a frequency-rating scale provides a quantitative choice. The manager may rank the employee's behavior on any given criterion as among the bottom 10% of staff, next 20%, middle 40%, next 20%, or top 10% of staff (Figures 14-3 and 14-4).

To maintain perspective, the manager may list staff names down the side of a paper and the behavior to be rated across the top. Rating one behavior at a time, the manager checks for variation in evaluations because one expects variation in performance. Forced distribution should be used cautiously. It is based on a normal bell-shaped curve with a few people ranked high, a few ranked low, and the majority ranked in the middle. However, this assumes that the group is representative of the

Observation of working hours

Figure 14-3 Descriptive graphic rating scale.

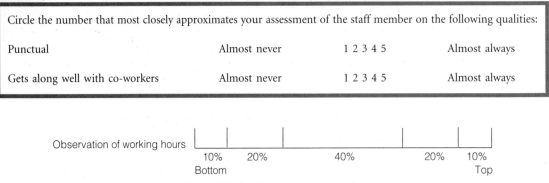

Figure 14-4 Percentage rating scale.

total population, and this is not true for a group of nurses (Dienemann, 1990; Douglas, 1996; Ellis and Hartley, 1995; Gillies, 1994; Marquis and Huston, 1996; Yoder-Wise, 1999).

Ranking

Ranking forces managers to rank staff in descending order from highest to lowest even if they do not think there is a difference. Ranking implicitly requires the manager to compare each nurse with others, but that comparison is not systematically built into the method. Paired comparison forces the supervisor to compare each nurse with each other nurse. As shown in Box 14-4, if managers are ranking four nurses, they must deal with six possible pairs; this number can be calculated as follows:

$$N(N - 1)/2 = 4(3)/2 = 12/2 = 6$$

Then each pair is presented to the manager, who must determine which of the two she thinks is better. Choices should be marked (Figure 14-5).

Tally marks can be placed in a matrix to help visualize the ranking (Figure 14-6).

The major disadvantages of paired comparisons are that they do not lend themselves to large numbers of staff and demand considerable time

of the manager (Douglas, 1996; Marquis and Huston, 1998).

Management by Objectives

Management by objectives (MBO) is a tool for effective planning and appraisal. It emphasizes the achievement of objectives instead of personality characteristics. It focuses attention on individual achievement, motivates individuals to accomplishment, and measures performance in terms of results. MBO is a managerial method whereby the manager and staff nurse identify major areas in which the nurse will work, set standards for performance, and measure results against those standards. It determines the results that the nurse is to achieve in a given time frame.

To develop management by objectives, nurses should first review the mission and group objectives. They can determine the mission and objectives by analyzing what they do or what they think they should do. They describe their job and clarify its purpose. This helps identify major job responsibilities.

Next, they list their major job responsibilities. Results expected, rather than activities, should be listed. This can be accomplished by asking themselves why the activity is being done or why it is important. For example:

- What is the task? To help team members organize their work for the day.

- Why? To improve use of their time.

Box 14-4   **EXAMPLE OF RANKING USING PAIRED COMPARISON**

Nurses	Possible Pairs	
Anita Anderson	AA with SJ	SJ with PP
Sue Jones	AA with PP	SJ with SS
Pam Peterson	AA with SS	PP with SS
Sara Smith		

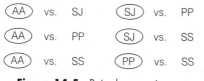

Figure 14-5 Paired comparisons.

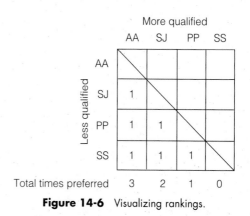

Figure 14-6 Visualizing rankings.

- Why? To be as productive as possible.

- Why? To give good, cost-effective nursing care by completing the work identified on nursing care plans efficiently.

Major job responsibilities of a nurse manager are related to productivity, quality of care, morale, turnover, staff development, self-development, and affirmative action.

Once the major job responsibilities are identified, expected levels of accomplishment are determined. Criteria for expected levels of accomplishment should be results oriented, established before the fact, time bound, realistic and attainable, measurable and verifiable, written, and agreed on by both the manager and the staff associate. Common errors to avoid when developing objectives are writing too many objectives or too complex objectives; having too high or too low of standards; using too long or too short a time period; and having imbalanced emphasis, objectives that are not measurable, or objectives for which the cost of measurement is too high.

After staff associates have reviewed the mission and group objectives and determined their major job responsibilities and the expected levels of accomplishment, they should meet with the manager to establish priorities and to develop plans for the accomplishment of the objectives. The manager will determine whether the objectives are compatible with the overall goals of the organization. The manager and staff associate should hold periodic reviews to check the progress and make adjustments. An annual review should be held to compare the actual results with the expected levels of accomplishment and to set the objectives for the next period.

The underlying philosophy is a belief that people perform best and develop most in an environment of participative management, high performance standards that build on individual strengths, prompt feedback that accentuates the positive, and appropriate rewards. Staff are encouraged to "do their thing" while maintaining individual accountability. The manager is a listener and clarifier who readjusts responsibilities on the basis of individual differences.

Higher frequencies of appraisal are associated with a more favorable attitude toward MBO, higher goal success, improvement of manager–staff associate relationships, clarity of goals, an opinion that the manager was helpful and supportive, the attitude that staff associates had influence in matters affecting them, and esteem for and satisfaction with the manager. More praise and less criticism of the objectives by the manager are associated with higher goal success. It is advisable to use an incentive system that rewards effective planning, as well as goal achievement, when using MBO.

Advantages of MBO for the staff nurse are that the standard of evaluation is based on the characteristics of a specific person and job; nurses have input and some control over their future; nurses know the standard by which they will be judged; nurses have knowledge of the manager's goals, priorities, and deadlines; staff nurses have a greater understanding of where they stand with the manager in relation to relative progress; there is a better basis for evaluation than personality traits; MBO emphasizes the future, which can be changed, instead of the past; and it stimulates higher individual performance and morale.

Advantages for the manager include a reservoir of personnel data and performance information for updating personnel files, an indication of personnel development needs within the agency, a basis for promotion and compensation, a relationship with the staff that makes the manager a coach rather than a judge, and better managerial planning and use of the employee.

MBO directs work activities toward organizational goals, facilitates planning, provides standards for control, provides objective appraisal criteria, reduces role conflict and ambiguity, and uses and motivates human resources.

MBO is limited because it is not an easy system to implement and requires hard work for maintenance; the process must be taught and reinforced for managers to become and remain proficient in applying the principles of the system; the MBO system assumes that staff nurses and managers will define suitable standards that will serve the agency; it presumes that managers understand their limitations; managers are responsible for assessing actual results rather than activities that seem to indicate results; some managers are unable to manage by objectives; some staff nurses may not want to be involved in setting goals; managers and staffs may give lip service to MBO, although managers really set the goals; staff nurses may set their goals according to what they know their managers expect; MBO stresses results but does not supply the methods for achieving them; nurses can become frustrated if they believe that increasingly higher goals will be expected of them; overlapping objectives are difficult to evaluate; MBO lends itself to quantitative assessment but may neglect qualitative factors; and MBO does not provide comparative data for promotions and salary increases (Ellis and Hartley, 1995; Gillies, 1994; Marquis and Huston, 1996; Marquis and Huston, 1998; Marrelli, 1993; Odiorne, 1965, 1969; Tappen, 1995; Yoder-Wise, 1999).

Self-Appraisal

Self-appraisal promotes dignity and self-respect. It is a less structured approach used in participative organizations that promotes employee acceptance of plans for improvement and uses the manager as a coach instead of a judge. Personnel are the best source of information about their work. Self-appraisal ensures that the person is prepared for the discussion and it increases the perception of fairness. Personnel may be fearful of punishment; rate themselves low to avoid disagreement with the boss; or evaluate themselves high to influence the supervisor. Sometimes employees undervalue their achievements or feel uncomfortable giving themselves high ratings. If used alone, self-appraisal could provide an inaccurate picture. If the self-appraisal is not consistent with other available data, the manager should confront the differences (Grote, 1996; Marquis and Huston, 1996; Rocchiccioli and Tilbury, 1998; Swansburg, 1996; Swansburg and Swansburg, 1999).

Peer Review

Peer review is a process whereby a group of practicing RNs evaluate the quality of another RN's pro-

fessional performance. It provides a feedback mechanism for sharing ideas, comparing the consistency of the nurse's performance with standards, recognizing outstanding performance, and identifying areas in which further development is required. This process can increase personal and professional growth and job satisfaction because of the recognition from peers.

Once it has been decided that an institution will use peer review, appraisal tools must be developed. A review of the evaluation tools currently used and the literature on evaluation tools is in order. Various standards may also be reviewed. The tool developed may address technical competence and human relationship, communication, organizational, leadership, and other skills. The process must also be determined, and then staff must be oriented to the system.

The staff should be oriented to the components of the peer review before it is implemented and thereafter during orientation. It is appropriate to give them copies of the peer review process and forms used for peer review. Opportunities to learn how to fill out the forms, how the peer review committee uses the materials, and what questions are to be expected during the peer review interview should be provided.

The peer evaluation process typically includes a review of an employee's self-evaluation form (including short- and long-term goals), reference letters, committee work, special projects, additional education, and contributions to nursing; a performance evaluation by the nurse's immediate manager; a review of past performance; care plans and charting done by the nurse; assessment; observation of the nurse; interviews with clients; a summary of the findings; a presentation of the findings; and recommendations to the nurse. It is appropriate to allow the candidate some agency time to prepare a review folder. A leader is assigned to the nurse to help clarify policy and procedures and to check the documents for completeness.

Who will evaluate whom must be determined. A committee may be appointed, elected, or randomly selected, but it should represent a number of job titles and a wide variety of specialty areas. The members should be familiar with committee responsibilities. The committee's recommendations should be made by consensus, with dissenting opinions recorded.

Once the candidate has been evaluated, there should be a peer review interview for feedback. All feedback must be well documented in the review materials. Hearsay reports are not permitted. The review committee chairperson or designee is responsible for arranging the interview and helping the candidate feel welcome and comfortable. The interview may provide recognition of outstanding performance, identification of areas in which further development is required, recommendations regarding learning needs, and possibly a recommendation for classification.

Peer review can be threatening and time-consuming. There is a risk of rating candidates too high or too low. Friends may inflate evaluations. Peers may omit suggestions for improvement for people with whom they work. Managers may feel threatened. However, nurses will be held accountable and responsible for their nursing performance when they are measured against realistic and attainable standards (Marquis and Huston, 1996, 1998; Rocchiccioli and Tilbury, 1998; Swansburg, 1996; Swansburg and Swansburg, 1999; Tappen, 1995).

Customer or Subordinate Evaluation

Student evaluation of teachers is common in education. Patients can evaluate their care. Staff can evaluate their managers and leaders (Rocchiccioli and Tilbury, 1998).

360 Degree Feedback

360 degree feedback is a multisource system of assessment including self-appraisal and subordinate, peer, and administrative feedback. It creates credible feedback, reduces supervisor bias, supports a team environment, supports career development, moves from a seniority to a performance system, and allows rewarding high performers. Unfortunately, friendships or competition may bias the process; some people may collude; some respondents are more critical than others; and some teams are harder than others. Computers with safeguard for confidentiality can be used for on-line assessment (Edwards and Ewen, 1996; Grote, 1996).

Appraisal Interview

There are several kinds of appraisal interviews. They include tell and sell, tell and listen, problem solving, and goal setting. When using the tell-and-sell technique, the manager does most of the talking while the staff associate listens. The manager reports the results of the evaluation to the employee and tries to persuade the staff associate to improve. This assumes that managers are qualified to evaluate staff associates and that staff associates will want to correct their weaknesses. In this role of judge, the interviewer risks losing the loyalty of the employee and inhibiting independent judgment. Face-saving problems are created. Employees usually suppress defensive behavior and attempt to cover their hostility to protect themselves. The tell-and-sell method uses positive and negative extrinsic motivation and is most likely to be successful when the employee respects the interviewer. It tends to perpetuate existing values and practices. The tell-and-sell method works best with young or new employees or individuals who are new to an assignment. These employees may want advice and assurance from an authority figure. Under these conditions managers are most likely to be respected because of their position, knowledge, and experience. Unfortunately, the tell-and-sell method fosters either dependent and docile or rebellious behavior. After a tell-and-sell style evaluation, the employee often feels like looking for another job.

When using the tell-and-listen method, the manager speaks for about half the time and lets the staff associate speak for the remainder. The interviewer outlines the strong and weak points of the staff associate's job performance and then listens to the interviewee's response. Although still in the role of judge, the interviewer listens to disagreement and allows defensive behavior without attempting to refute any responses. This tends to remove defensive behavior. The employee expresses defensive-

Interviewer

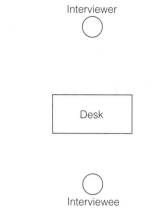

Desk

Interviewee

Figure 14-7 Tell-and-sell arrangement.

ness and feels accepted while the interviewer listens, reflects, and summarizes. Thus resistance to change is reduced, and the staff associate develops a more favorable attitude toward the manager. Although this method fosters upward communication and allows the interviewer to learn and change views, the need for change may not be developed in the employee. Tell and listen works best when there is a good relationship between the interviewer and interviewee. Interviewers can learn about staff associates' needs and aspirations, but the latter may not know where they stand. There are no plans for personnel development.

With the problem-solving method, the interviewer assumes the role of helper to stimulate growth and development in the interviewee. It assumes that change can occur without correcting faults and that discussing problems can lead to improvements because the discussion develops new ideas and mutual interests. The staff associate does most of the talking while the interviewer listens, reflects ideas and feelings, asks exploratory questions, and summarizes. Intrinsic motivation is stimulated through increased freedom, increased responsibility, and problem-solving behavior; thus change is facilitated. Both the manager and staff associate learn from each other. Staff associates may view their job in relation to others more accurately, and managers gain insights into staff associates' working conditions. Unfortunately, the employee may

lack ideas, and change may be other than what the interviewer had planned. Although this method is excellent for problem solving and personnel development, it does not warn staff associates or let them know where they stand, evaluate them for lateral transfers or promotional purposes, provide a rating or furnish an evaluation record, or supply top administration with an inventory of talent.

Goal setting is future oriented. It focuses attention on the employee's achievement and consequently stimulates accomplishment. The philosophy behind MBO is teamwork. Top administration sets the organization's objectives, and employees set individual objectives. This method integrates institutional and personal achievement goals. It clarifies objectives and, because it focuses on results and not methods, encourages the person closest to a job to decide how to do it. MBO involves participative management. An autocratic leader is likely to dictate goals to a staff associate. Although that is not consistent with a participative management philosophy, it is better for staff associates to know what is expected of them than not to know.

Which appraisal interview style is used largely depends on the purpose of the evaluation, the manager's philosophy of management, and the institutional guidelines. The manager can create an atmosphere during the interview that is consistent with the appraisal interview style. To create an authoritative image for the tell-and-sell method, managers should have the interview in their office and sit behind a desk, preferably looking down on the staff associate (Figure 14-7).

To create an atmosphere of equality for the tell-and-listen, problem-solving, or goal-setting style, the interviewer and employee may sit at a corner table looking at each other (Figure 14-8).

Sitting at a table helps create a working situation for problem solving and goal setting. Sitting either side by side or at the corner of the table helps create a sense of equality and a working relationship (Figure 14-9).

Nonverbal communication is important and should be consistent with verbal communication. Active listening can be expressed through eye contact, a responsive posture, and facial expressions and lets the interviewee know that the interviewer is trying to understand the employee's attitudes and feelings. Pauses give the employee time to think and respond. The interviewer may restate what the employee said. Although this helps the interviewee know the interviewer is listening, it does not guarantee that the meaning of the message was understood. Paraphrasing states the message in fewer and simpler words. If the interviewee says, "I don't understand! One minute she tells me to do it this way, and the next minute she tells me to do it that way," the interviewer may paraphrase, "She confuses you." One should ask for clarification if the intent is not clear or say, for example, "Do you mean . . . ?" Reflection of feelings, such as "You sound proud of that," helps show understanding. Summarizing what has been said at the end of the interview is particularly important.

The manager's assessment of the staff nurse's performance should be continuous rather than annual. This maximizes feedback for learning. The manager and staff nurse should have an appointment to do the appraisal interview when both are unhurried and should meet where they have privacy. Adequate time should be allowed and interruptions prevented. The purpose of the interview should be clear; both should enter it ready to compare notes, knowing that the counseling notes will not become part of the personnel file. Emphasis should be on the growth of the nurse and on accomplishments related to specific targets. Actual, observed behavior rather than broad personality traits should be discussed during the exchange of ideas between the manager and the staff nurse. The staff nurse should be encouraged to take the initiative in setting goals for improving performance, with the manager supporting, guiding, and validating the nurse's plans.

If managers find it necessary to make unfavorable comments, they should insert them between favorable comments. It is important that the managers not create an atmosphere in which they appear to be sitting in judgment. When the manager enumerates improvement needs, the staff nurse's self-esteem is threatened, and the nurse may become defensive. The greater the threat to the self-image, the poorer the attitude toward evaluations will be, and less improvement in job performance results. If the staff nurse becomes defensive or aggressive, the manager should accept comments without a fight. Keeping quiet and not exposing alibis can help the staff nurse save face.

Before the interview is terminated, ways in which the manager can help the staff nurse accomplish goals should be explored. Staff nurses will probably approach their work with more enthusiasm and confidence if they believe they have the respect and support of the manager (Maier, 1976).

Appraisal Reports

The appraisal report is to be written jointly by the manager and staff nurse. It should be reliable, valid, and accurate, showing progress made by the nurse

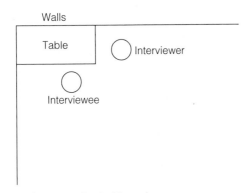

Figure 14-8   Problem-solving arrangement.

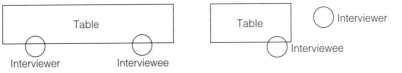

Figure 14-9   Goal-setting arrangement.

and giving illustrations to substantiate value judgments. If both have kept notes that they have periodically assessed, and if the staff nurse believes the manager's intent is to help rather than to blame, the nurse will feel more free to be honest in an evaluation of strengths and weaknesses. If staff nurses have not been functioning satisfactorily, they will already be aware of it. If their performance has not improved adequately since previous interviews, they should be informed that the weakness will be included in the report. Any improvements are to be noted, and staff nurses should know exactly where they stand. It may be necessary to tell them they have to make certain improvements within a definite time period or they will be fired.

Permanent, cumulative evaluation records can be used to assess how the nurse can best be used in the agency. They can be used as a basis for pay increases and promotions or terminations. These records are frequently used as a source of information for letters of reference to be sent to other agencies.

Legal Implications for Performance Appraisals

The Equal Pay Act of 1963, which prohibits paying personnel of one sex at a different rate from personnel of the other sex for the same work; the Civil Rights Act of 1964, which prohibits discrimination on the basis of race, color, religion, sex, or national origin; and the Age Discrimination in Employment Act of 1967, which prohibits discrimination against persons 40 to 70 years of age all require that employers document the quality of employee performance before making decisions about selection, training, transfer, retention, and promotion (Gillies, 1994).

The most legally defensible content of performance appraisals should be based on job analysis, should be objective and verifiable, and should be specific and job related rather than global. Individual traits such as attitudes should not be evaluated. Legally defensible procedures should be a formal, standardized system and uniform for all personnel in a job category. Performance standards,

performance results, appeal process, and antidiscrimination laws should all be communicated to personnel. Raters should have written instructions for how to do an unbiased appraisal. Using more than one rater is desirable, and raters should observe the worker firsthand. Documentation requirements should be consistent for all personnel within a job category, documentation of critical incidents for extreme ratings should be required, and a thorough written record of evidence should be collected about evaluations, counseling about performance deficits, and help to take corrective actions before termination decisions are made (Decker and Sullivan, 1992).

DISCIPLINE OF PERSONNEL
Need for Discipline

Lack of knowledge about policies and procedures is a major cause of the need for disciplinary action. Management should provide orientation from the first day of employment. Nurses cannot be expected to follow rules that are unknown to them, vague, or loosely enforced. Consequently, each new employee should be given an employee's handbook. The handbook itemizes the rules and procedures of the agency and specifies the type of discipline that will be imposed for infractions. New employees should be encouraged to read the handbook and ask questions about it.

During orientation the manager should explain in detail the most frequently violated rules and discuss their significance and rationale. It is recommended that the manager conduct regularly scheduled meetings with staff to discuss changes or to review policies. Rules and regulations also may be posted in a consistent and conspicuous manner.

Most employees are not disciplinary problems, but a minority requires more than positive stimuli. These few cases are potentially explosive. About half of the grievance cases appealed to an arbitrator by labor unions involve disciplinary action. In about half of those cases, management either reversed or modified its decision when the individual's appeal was upheld. Consequently, it is of utmost importance that disciplinary action be undertaken in a judicious manner. The disciplinary action program and grievance procedure must be uniform for all personnel of a specific grade or classification. A standard disciplinary action program with procedures outlined and forms provided should be available to managers.

Principles of Disciplinary Action

Have a positive attitude.   The manager's attitude is very important in preventing or correcting undesirable behavior. If personnel are treated as suspect, they are more likely to provide the trouble that the manager anticipates. People tend to do what is expected of them; therefore it is the manager's duty to maintain a positive attitude by expecting the best from the staff.

Investigate carefully.   The ramifications of disciplinary action are so serious that managers must proceed with caution. They should collect the facts, check allegations, talk to witnesses, and ask accused employees for their side of the story. Managers should accept the employee's account until and unless the allegations are proven. The manager may wish to consult other managers or the director. If the situation is serious enough to require action before a full investigation can be conducted, it is better to suspend the employee subject to reinstatement after investigation than to take more drastic action.

Be prompt.   Managers should not be so expeditious that they neglect to be thorough in ascertaining the facts. If a staff nurse is disciplined unfairly or unnecessarily, the effects on the entire staff may be severe. However, if the discipline is delayed, the relationship between the punishment and the offense may become less clear. Because of the distastefulness of disciplinary action, the manager may tend to postpone the punishment as long as possible. The longer the delay, the more the staff forget their actions, the more likely they are to feel that the discipline is not deserved, and the fewer are the positive educational effects for the future.

Protect privacy.   Disciplinary action affects the ego of the staff nurse. Thus it is better to discuss the situation in private. By helping the nurse save face, there is less possibility of future resentment and a greater chance for future cooperation. However, a public reprimand may be necessary for the nurse who does not take private criticism seriously.

Focus on the act.   When disciplining a staff nurse, the manager should emphasize that it was the act that was unacceptable, not the employee. If the employee is not acceptable, the person should be fired.

Enforce rules consistently.   Offending employees should be treated equally or consistently for similar transgressions. Equal treatment is based on rules with specific penalties for various acts and the number of offenses. Consistency reduces the possibility of favoritism, promotes predictability, and fosters acceptance of penalties.

Be flexible.   Consistent implementation is complicated by the fact that individuals and circumstances are never the same. A penalty should be determined only after the entire record of the employee is reviewed. The manager should consider length of service, past accomplishments or problems, level of skill, and expendability to the organization. The intent of the staff nurse, the extenuating circumstances, and whether this situation constitutes a test case and will set precedent for the future should also be taken into consideration. If managers enforce identical penalties for seemingly similar offenses, they may be excessively severe with one person and lenient with the other.

Advise the employee.   The employees must be informed that their conduct is not acceptable. Personnel files containing anecdotal notes can be a useful management tool, but they are of little value in upholding disciplinary action if the staff nurse is not informed of the contents promptly.

Take corrective, constructive action.   The manager should be sure that the staff nurse understands that the behavior was contrary to the organization's requirements and should explain why such regulations are necessary. The staff nurse should be counseled as to what behavior is required and how to prevent future disciplinary action.

Follow up.   The manager should quietly investigate to determine whether the staff nurse's behavior has changed. If the staff nurse continues to invite disciplinary action, the manager should reevaluate the situation to try to determine the reason for the nurse's attitude. The manager must try to come to terms with the offender and the reasons for the transgression.

Penalties

Oral reprimand.   For minor violations that have occurred for the first time, managers may opt to give an oral warning in private. They might tactfully correct the deviation by telling the staff nurse the proper way to deal with the situation or by rebuking the nurse. An oral reprimand is of limited value beyond alerting the nurse in a relatively friendly way to a need for correction. Because nothing is in writing and the reprimand is given in private, it is difficult to prove that a warning was given. Over time the manager may become unsure and inexact about what was said to whom and under what conditions. When an oral warning is given, the manager is advised to make an anecdotal note of the time, place, occasion, and the gist of the reprimand. Oral comments may be easily forgotten, but too formal handling of initial minor offenses can be counterproductive.

Written reprimand.   If the offense is more serious or repeated, the reprimand may be written. It is suggested that the manager and staff associate develop a written plan for improvement that defines what the staff associate will do to make the performance acceptable and what the manager will do to change the environmental situation if appropriate. A time limit should be set. Additional penalties may be defined in case the employee's behavior does not adequately improve during the allowed time period. The written notice should include the name of the worker, the name of the manager, the nature of the problem, the plan for correction, and the consequences of future repetition. It is recommended that the worker sign the report to indicate that she has read it, received a copy of it, or both. A copy should be given to the employee and one retained for the personnel file. If the employee believes that signing such a document would be considered an admission of guilt and hence refuses to sign, the manager may ask another managerial person to sign as witness to the fact that the document was discussed with the worker and that a copy was given to the worker. It is appropriate for higher management and the personnel department to review this report. At the end of the designated time, the manager and worker should have another conference to determine if the terms of the agreement have been met. It is hoped that the nurse can be complimented for having made progress and that no further action is deemed necessary. However, if no change or inadequate change has occurred, the continuing nature of the problem should be identified and documented. Additional penalties will probably be necessary.

Other penalties.   Fines may be charged for offenses such as tardiness. Loss of privileges might include transfer to a less desirable shift and loss of preference of assignment.

Layoff, demotion, and discharge are the most serious penalties and require approval beyond the manager. Layoff may be appropriate in situations where it is best to remove the nurse while an investigation is conducted. The staff nurse may be reinstated with no loss of pay if cleared through the investigation or may be suspended if found guilty of a serious offense. Demotion is a questionable solution. It creates hard feelings, which may be contagious, and more than likely places offenders in a position for which they are overqualified. Termination becomes necessary as a last resort.

Components of a Disciplinary Action Program

Codes of conduct.   Employees must be informed of the nature and meaning of codes of conduct.

Agency handbooks, policy manuals, and orientation programs may be used. The staff nurse must understand that the rules are reasonable and directly related to efficient, effective operation of the agency.

Authorized penalties. During disciplinary action the personnel record should indicate that a fair investigation was made of charges before the assessment of guilt and determination of penalties. The agency's disciplinary action program should indicate that the current action is being administered without bias and is directly related to the offense.

Records of offenses and corrective measures. Records are of utmost importance when disciplinary action is appealed. The personnel record should clearly indicate the offense, management's efforts to correct the problem, and resulting penalties.

Right of appeal. Formal provision for the right of employee appeal is a part of each disciplinary action program. Appeal beyond the manager ensures equitable treatment and encourages more employee acceptance of the disciplinary process. At the same time, fair managers need not fear a review of their actions by others.

Discipline Without Punishment

Progressive discipline starts with an oral reprimand, then a written reprimand, then suspension without pay, and if no corrective action is taken, the last step is termination. Discipline without punishment gives disciplinary suspension with pay to demonstrate that management is sincere in the desire to see the worker change and stay. It starts with complete documentation to recognize and reinforce desirable performance, to confront the few who do not meet the standards, and to support workers to correct problems while maintaining self-esteem. The system is designed to influence the worker to accept responsibility, to change behavior, and to return to an acceptable standard of performance. Without punishment there is an oral reminder, a written reminder, and a decision-making leave. This allows solving problems and enhancing relationships. It focuses on personal responsibility and decision making. Initially the manager lets the employee know what is expected and the employee's responsibility to do what is expected. A memo is used to document the interaction. By making the correction, the employee can "wipe the slate clean" and have information about the incident removed from the record. Otherwise, the employee gets one day with pay to take responsibility for her behavior and do what is best for her and the organization. That helps reduce the anger associated with the final step. If necessarily, people are discharged from the organization fairly, humanely, and permanently. The decisions to perform well or poorly and to follow the rules or not are the employee's. Requiring them to take responsibility for their own behavior is more effective than punishing. Punishment can produce compliance but not commitment. Seeking agreement about why a problem must be solved and the logical consequences to the employee if it is not helps get commitment (Douglas, 1996; Ellis and Hartley, 1995; Grote, 1995).

MODIFICATION OF EMPLOYEE BEHAVIOR

Can an employee's behavior be changed by changing the manager's behavior? Is behavior that recurs in the presence of the manager being reinforced by the manager? Is it possible that doing nothing is doing something? In all three instances the answer is yes. Behavior leads to consequences, and the consequences that follow the behavior affect the probability of recurrence of that behavior. Because behavior is a function of the consequence, it is important for nurse managers to identify the contingency relationship.

Consequences may be favorable, punitive, absent, or insufficient. Positive consequences increase the probability of recurrence of the behavior that preceded them. Absence of consequences decreases the probability, and insufficient consequences have little effect. Punishing consequences have varied and unpredictable effects. Punishment is not the opposite of a favorable consequence. No consequence is.

Reinforcement

Positive reinforcement increases the probability of a recurrence of desired behavior. It is more effective the sooner it follows the desired behavior, and it should be clearly connected to the behavior that the manager wishes to increase. Positive reinforcement may be as subtle as a smile or a nod of the head when someone speaks. Whatever is being said when the manager smiles or nods is reinforced and will recur with increasing frequency. Recognition is a powerful reinforcer. "Mr. Jones must feel so much better now since you have completed his morning care" and "You collected a lot of valuable information during your interview with Mrs. Smith" are examples. "I'm glad to see you here today" reinforces attendance, whereas "I see you were absent again yesterday" gives attention to the absence.

The nurse manager can even stimulate new behavior by verbal acknowledgment of the desired response. Words are used to describe the behavior the nurse manager wants to encourage. A comment such as "I really appreciate nurses' attending in-services" is likely to increase attendance at in-services. A number of stimuli—such as feedback, attention, praise, avoidance of punishment, merit pay increases, special assignments, assistance with tuition, or tickets to a ball game or play—can be used to reinforce behavior. However, nurse managers must consider that any stimulus can be reinforcing or aversive depending on the person and the situation, so they should carefully select stimuli that are reinforcers for the individual in a given situation. For example, tickets to a ball game may be reinforcing to some and aversive to others. Recognition is one of the easiest, cheapest, and most universally effective reinforcers.

Shaping

Shaping is a behavior-modification technique used when the response does not meet the criteria. By systematically reinforcing successive approximations, the nurse manager can shape the responses into the desired behavior and get the nurse to do something new. The manager provides favorable consequences after any attempt at the desired behavior, then withholds consequences until improvement is made. When working with the staff nurse who is chronically absent or late, the manager may acknowledge that the nurse is at work: "I see you were only 30 minutes late today." Later, "I see you were only 15 minutes late today." Still later, "I noticed you were only 5 minutes late today." The manager may initially praise a new employee for attempting a new task and then note improvements in skill as they occur. Once the level of desired performance has been reached, it can be maintained by providing favorable consequences intermittently. Too many positive consequences cause satiation, and they lose their effect on the behavior. Performance that has been intermittently reinforced is most resistant to extinction.

Extinction

Withholding reinforcers will decrease the probability of the occurrence of the behavior and contribute to its extinction. Therefore if the manager does not mention or otherwise reward undesirable behavior, the lack of action should contribute to extinction. Conversely, any reinforcer that is presented frequently but not paired with another reinforcer will lose its effectiveness. Promises of "raises" or "hiring more help and getting some relief" become meaningless if not paired with a pay increase or recruitment and selection of personnel. Managers who praise everyone for everything all of the time will find that their words lose their effectiveness as reinforcers. When the consequences are not worth the effort, the behavior will decrease also.

Punishment

The manager can decrease the probability of a response by pairing the behavior with an aversive stimulus. People who are late to work will not be paid for the time they are absent. There will be no overtime pay for people who did not complete their work on time. Employees who do not meet work standards will be fired. Firing a few workers who were not meeting standards can have an immediate impact on the remaining personnel, who initially work harder to avoid being fired. However, if management does nothing to reinforce the more productive work behavior, avoidance behavior is likely to occur. Employees may cover up for each other, steal from the agency what they rationalize is theirs, or resign. By using aversive stimuli to control behavior, management pairs itself with those stimuli and becomes viewed as aversive.

Once managers have started an aversive stimulus, they should not stop it until the behavior has been corrected or the cessation may act as a positive reinforcer. Absences, tardiness, excuse making, rationalizing, placing blame elsewhere, and other avoidance behaviors will increase if they successfully reduce the aversive stimuli. If the manager gruffly asks a nurse why some work has not been done (aversive stimulus), and the manager backs off when the staff nurse replies that she thought someone else was doing it, blaming others is reinforced. Although punishment causes behavior to occur less frequently, it does not teach new behaviors and is likely to increase avoidance behaviors. Most motivation problems are caused by punishment, absence of consequences, or insufficient consequences (Berni and Fordyce, 1973).

Behavior Modification for the Employee With a Performance Problem

Besides being aware of the subtle ways that one's behavior may reinforce, shape, or reduce behavior of others, the nurse manager may apply behavior modification to personnel with performance problems. First, one must identify the performance problem and analyze the antecedent, behavior, and consequence. What happened before the behavior occurred? Each time nurse A was late to work, she had worked the evening shift the night before. Each time nurse B yelled at her staff, an emergency treatment was being performed. Head nurse C was condescending to her staff after a physician had scolded her. What happened after the behavior occurred? Someone had already done part of nurse A's work by the time she got to the ward. Staff nurses responded quickly when nurse B yelled at them during an emergency procedure. Nurse C's staff avoided her.

Once the performance problem has been identified, the baseline frequency is determined. The baseline measure is the frequency before any attempts to change it. If nurses are interested in modifying their own behavior, they may collect the baseline data themselves. The behavior must be precisely defined, observable, and consequently countable. Written records should be kept, preferably on a portable recording system that is present when the behavior occurs, so the nurse can record it immediately. A tailor-made tally sheet is useful because one can see data in relation to time. If the behavior occurs daily, it should be recorded for 1 week. If there are large variations in the behavior from one day to the next, observations should be recorded for 2

	M	T	W	Th	F	Sat	Sun
7:00	I I I	I I	I I	I I I	I I		
8:00			I				
9:00	I I			I	I		
10:00		I		I			
11:00			I		I		
12:00				I	I		
1:00		I	I		I		
2:00	I I	I	I I	I I	I		
3:00	I I I	I I	I I I	I I	I I I		

Figure 14-10 Tally sheet.

weeks. A time-sampling technique can be used by busy managers by randomly selecting short periods to observe and tally behaviors. This is effective only for high-frequency behavior. The manager must consider if the period of data collection was representative of the normal situation and use a stable baseline rate as a cue to start the intervention (Figure 14-10).

If one transfers the information from the tally sheet to a graph that depicts frequency over time, it is easy to visualize the effect of the intervention strategy. One can put a wavy vertical line on the graph to depict the point where intervention was started (Figure 14-11).

After identifying the relevant variables, the supervisor and nurse select appropriate reinforcement, extinction, punishment, or any combination of intervention strategies to decrease the frequency of the undesirable behavior. If the desired performance is punished, the punishment should be removed. Instead of making fast workers finish everyone else's work, they can be allowed time to do what they choose, such as read in the library or meditate in the chapel, receive a bonus day at a specified frequency, or be given a merit pay increase specifically for doing more than their share of the work. If undesirable behavior is rewarded, the reward should be removed. Instead of having slow employees' work completed by others, the manager should inform the workers that they are responsible for so much work by themselves, must have that

work completed before going home, and will receive no overtime pay for completion of the normal workload.

If desired behavior has not been rewarded, the manager should arrange a consequence. This may be as simple as orally acknowledging a nurse's accomplishment occasionally. Nurses' accomplishments can be acknowledged in the agency's newsletter. Awards can be created to recognize desirable behavior.

If obstacles are identified, they should be removed. Nurses can be referred to professional counseling to help them work through situational crises that are interfering with their work performance. The manager can try to get the resources nurses need to do their job. Nurses should also have the necessary education to do what is expected of them. They may need formal education, on-the-job training, practice sessions, or simply feedback. The staff associate is the best source of information for what can serve as a positive reinforcer because what may be desirable for the manager may be aversive to the staff associate.

Once the intervention strategy has been planned, it should be implemented and the response frequency recorded. The strategy should be evaluated for effectiveness. If it is not working, it should be analyzed and revised. Once the desired behavior is obtained, it should be maintained through intermittent reinforcement (Berni and Fordyce, 1973).

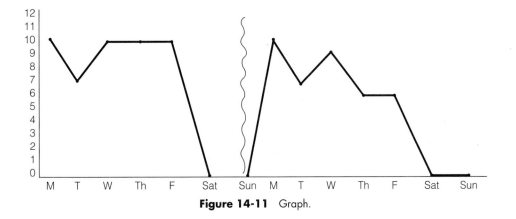

Figure 14-11 Graph.

PROBLEM EMPLOYEES

Substance abusers, angry or withdrawn workers, personnel with excessive absenteeism, and the terminating employee provide challenges to nurse managers. In each case the manager must be alert to symptoms of problems, help the employee solve the problem, and evaluate the results.

Substance Abusers

Substance abuse is not uncommon among nurses. It affects all socioeconomic classes, cultures, and races. Only 5% or less of all alcoholics are skid-row bums. Among alcoholic nurses studied, most had been in the top third of their class, held advanced degrees, held responsible and demanding jobs, and had an excellent work history.

Nurses with alcohol or other drug addictions often exhibit psychosocial problems (Box 14-5). Personality changes may be noted as the nurse be-

comes more irritable, withdrawn, and moody. Because of a decreased interest in outside activities, isolation increases. Related social changes include eating alone and avoiding social gatherings.

Changes in personal appearance become apparent. Changes in dress, an unkempt appearance, flushed complexion, red eyes, swollen face, and hand tremors are common. Mental status changes include forgetfulness, confusion, and decreased alertness.

General behavior changes too. Inappropriate responses and irritability occur more frequently. Excuses for behavior become more elaborate. Intolerance and suspicion of others and nervousness increase. Avoidance of others is noted. Work efficiency drops, there is a decline in the quality and quantity of work, and the work pace becomes uneven. Some assigned tasks are forgotten. Arriving late and leaving early and extended lunch hours and break times become patterns of behavior. Accidents increase. It is important for staff to know the importance of their reporting chemical abuse, because it is often not the manager who identifies the problem, especially as the manager covers more than one unit (Hutchinson, 1987).

When a nurse reports to work in a state of acute intoxication, the manager notes the signs objectively and asks a second person to validate the observations. The odor of alcohol, slurred speech, unsteady gait, and errors in judgment are symptoms of intoxication. The intoxicated nurse is removed from the situation, confronted briefly and firmly about the behavior, and sent home to rest and recuperate. Then the incident is recorded. The manager describes the observation, states the action taken, indicates future plans, and has the employee sign and date the memo after returning to work. Refusal to sign and date the memo should be noted by the manager and a witness.

Sally Hutchinson (1986) has described three stages in the self-annihilation trajectory that nurses experience as they become addicted: the experience, the commitment, and the compulsion. The experience is the nurse's introduction to alcohol or drugs and involves the three phases of initiating, connecting, and experimenting. Initiating is the first expe-

---

| **Box 14-5** | **SIGNS AND SYMPTOMS OF POSSIBLE SUBSTANCE ABUSE** |

SIGNS	
Psychosocial problems	Confusion
Irritability	Decreased alertness
Moodiness	General behavior
Tendency to isolate self	changes
Social changes	Inappropriate responses
Eating alone	Elaborate excuses
Avoiding social gatherings	for behavior
Changes in personal appearance	Intolerance of others
Changes in dress	Suspiciousness
Unkempt appearance	Nervousness
Flushed complexion	
Red eyes	**SYMPTOMS**
Swollen face	
Hand tremors	Odor of alcohol
Mental status changes	Slurred speech
Forgetfulness	Unsteady gait
	Errors in judgment

rience with drugs and is often experienced as a patient. The use of alcohol or drugs is associated with the relief of pain in the connecting phase. During the experimenting phase the person uses a variety of drugs to find the one of choice.

The commitment stage has three phases, too: dialogue with self, disengaging, and routinizing. Commitment is the decision to use alcohol or drugs in one's lifestyle. It requires finding a source. After finding the chemical of choice, the person dialogues with self to justify the use of the chemical to alleviate psychological or physical pain. Denying, bargaining, and justifying are common dialogues. After the self-diagnosis, a disengaging process occurs. People disengage from their conscience and their usual behavior. They disengage from their family, friends, and colleagues, and the values of nursing and society. They transform themselves into alcohol or drug users. They start using chemicals routinely to relieve their distress. Alcoholism is easier than drug addiction. The alcoholic nurse is more likely to miss work because of hangovers, whereas the drug-addicted nurse is likely to work overtime to have additional access to drugs. Many conning strategies are used to obtain chemicals.

The third stage, compulsion, has two phases—craving and surrendering. It is when the physical addiction becomes dominant. Some people stay in the experience stage for up to a year, but once they become committed, the compulsion stage follows.

Chronic performance problems are more common than acute intoxication. Each time performance problems are observed, they should be documented, including date, time, who was observed by whom, and a description of the incident and circumstances. At a prearranged conference, the nurse is confronted with the observations and how they affect job performance and patient care. The nurse is allowed to give an explanation. Alternatives are explored, and a course of action is planned. When substance abuse is identified as the problem, the offender is encouraged to take voluntary action. The manager refers the nurse to a local treatment facility and meets with the nurse periodically to monitor progress. The manager is not to serve the role of therapist.

Hutchinson (1987) has identified four phases of recovery: premotivation, breakthrough, early recovery, and extended recovery. During the premotivation phase the person may decide to stop using drugs to please someone. The person may hope to use chemicals only occasionally and employ a strong denial system. Denial decreases and the person admits to an addiction problem during the breakthrough phase. The person begins to cope with loss of the chemical, rediscovers values, and gains an image of self as a drug-free person during early recovery. The extended recovery begins after about 6 months in early recovery. People acknowledge their feelings about themselves and their relationships. They gain respect for themselves and their skills. They acquire control of their lives. This is the stage when the nurse can return to work and be productive.

Instead of disciplining and firing personnel whose job performance is impaired, more and more health care organizations are trying to help them regain their health and productivity through employee assistance programs (EAPs). At first EAPs focused on alcohol and drug abuse, but the services have broadened to include financial, legal, and marital problems; gambling; work addiction; and eating disorders. EAPs have increased productivity, reduced absenteeism, and lowered insurance costs. Assessment, diagnosis, and early intervention benefit the employee and the organization.

Many state nurses associations have started peer assistance programs. Ideally the association intervenes early in the addiction process before legal action is necessary. Often reports of impairment are made through a confidential telephone call or as a referral to the chairperson of the peer assistance program. The chairperson verifies that an impairment exists and may coach the nurse manager about documentation, verification, and intervention. A regional representative or local intervener contacts the person in question and makes an appointment.

The local intervener typically outlines the purpose of the visit with the impaired person, presents information about chemical abuse, and identifies behavior and circumstances in which the impairment has been evident. The fact that the disease is progressive is stressed. Various treatment options are presented. Issues such as hospitalization, insurance coverage, use of sick time and accrued vacation time, and family responsibilities are discussed. If the person denies impairment or refuses treatment, the impaired nurse may be reported to the state board of nursing by the employer.

When an impaired nurse participates in a peer assistance program, an advocate is assigned. The advocate maintains contact with the impaired nurse during treatment and until a solid recovery is established. A contract made by the peer review program advocate and the impaired nurse typically identifies employment restrictions, random urine screens, attendance at Alcoholics Anonymous or Narcotics Anonymous meetings, attendance at nurses' support groups, and contacts with the advocate.

When alcoholics or drug abusers refuse counseling or fail to follow the plan of care, they are told treatment is mandatory for continued employment. If they still refuse mandatory participation in the treatment, they are terminated in accordance with the hospital's policies.

Angry or Withdrawn Employees

Nurse managers often deal with angry or withdrawn employees. Anger and withdrawal are the fight and flight responses to anxiety. The angry nurse is more likely to be considered a troublemaker. The withdrawn person may be viewed as nice. However, both need help.

Anxiety occurs from the frustration of unmet expectations or loss of self-respect. The anxiety is transformed into feelings or actions and relief is felt. Angry, hostile, and destructive behavior is a primary response to frustration. It is intended to gain mastery over the situation. The angry employee may become hostile and use critical, sarcastic, and obscene language with others. Consequently, interpersonal relationships suffer, and productive work may be impaired. Anger can also be displaced to patients and others.

Withdrawn persons do not invest emotional energy in others. Fear of self-disclosure or having others become attached to them is frightening. Withdrawal is a protective mechanism to avoid hurt. Withdrawn persons sit through meetings without becoming involved. They are not assertive and do not protect their rights. They may be delegated more than their fair share of the work because they are so cooperative and polite. This leads to more feelings of use, abuse, and helplessness.

Nurse managers need to recognize aggressive and passive behaviors among employees, teach and display assertive behavior, and encourage problem solving. They should help personnel understand themselves and their job responsibilities, develop trust, and promote group harmony. Employees should be encouraged to express themselves without fear of reprisals. Managers should be sincere, firm, and fair. Job expectations should be clear and personnel rewarded liberally and disciplined justly.

Decreased Productivity

Decreased productivity is a side effect of personnel problems. Managers should make sure that desired performance is not being punished or undesirable behavior rewarded. Expectations are clarified. Employees are taught how to do what they are expected to do. If boredom is a problem, job rotation and special projects are considered.

Absenteeism

Absenteeism is also a side effect of personnel problems. Ineffective management, poor working relationships, boredom, lack of control over decisions affecting one's life, and overwork are contributing factors. Some workers are immature and lack the self-discipline to get themselves to work. Others stay away to avoid an unpleasant or boring job. Some are poorly motivated, do as little as possible to prevent being fired, and do not see their job as a means toward an end. The hypochondriac uses absenteeism to get attention and sympathy from others. Abusive absenteeism may be used to get even with a manager. Some personnel are exhausted from overwork, have lost their enthusiasm for the job, or are burned out.

Managers should make sure that there are attendance policies, that the policies do not reward nonattendance, and that they are enforced consistently. Attendance records should be maintained, and grievance procedures should be established.

Documented attendance policies greatly influence absence rates. Traditional sick leave policies have rewarded employees for absenteeism and have encouraged them to be dishonest to collect sick pay or be punished by losing it. Employees who receive sick pay are absent considerably more than those who do not. Some agencies have required a physician's excuse before an employee can receive sick pay to decrease the dishonest use of sick time. Because most people are sick only 1 or 2 days at a time, some hospitals do not compensate for the first 2 days of any sickness. The third and successive days are compensated. Other agencies have gone to paid time off. Each employee receives a certain amount of paid time off inclusive of holiday, vacation, and sick leave with few restrictions as to its use. It is typically collected at a rate calculated by length of continuous service. It simplifies record keeping but provides incentive to use the days whether sick or not.

Absenteeism data should be collected and analyzed to determine trends and patterns of individuals and personnel in general. Recording the date of absence, the reason and whether excused or unexcused, day of the week, preceding or following a day off, the employee's job classification, shift, tenure, age, sex, marital status, or any other information thought to be useful provides information to detect trends and pinpoint problems. Absenteeism often occurs more frequently in certain job classifications or departments, on specific days or shifts, or among a group working under a specific manager. Problems need to be identified so managers can develop control measures. Baseline data are also useful to determine the success of the control program.

A progressive discipline policy that imposes increasingly severe penalties is appropriate. Such a policy allows employees to know in advance the consequences of their behavior. Progressive discipline often starts with an oral reprimand that is documented and progresses through a written warning, pay deduction, suspension without pay, and dismissal.

Terminating Employees

Working with a terminating employee (whether voluntary or involuntary) is also challenging for the nurse manager. The manager must help the employee deal with the related feelings. A sense of loss and grief is common. A period of shock or denial that is then followed by disorganization, anger, guilt, and loneliness is normal. This is followed by a deorientation period and a reestablishment phase.

The manager can help terminating employees by providing an opportunity to talk about their feelings. Airing feelings about leaving, self-image, not working anymore or filling another position, and other interests that may be pursued helps relieve the anxiety. Helping the employee plan for the future is also useful.

It is not uncommon for terminating employees to detach themselves from the job and do little for some time before the termination. The manager can assign tasks that are considered important that can either be finished or transferred to someone else at the time of the employee's termination.

Rituals such as best wishes cards and going away parties serve to acknowledge the termination and provide a rite of separation that facilitates the termination process.

EMPLOYEE COUNSELING

Counseling helps improve employees' mental health, thus enhancing understanding, self-control, self-confidence, and consequently their ability to work effectively. Counseling accomplishes several activities on a directive to nondirective scale. It provides an opportunity to give advice, offer reassurance, improve communication, release emotional tension, clarify thinking, and reorient.

When giving advice, a counselor tells the employee what the counselor thinks the employee should do. Unfortunately, it is almost impossible to understand another person's complicated problems, and consequently the advice may not be sound. Advice may foster feelings of inferiority and dependence on the counselor.

Reassurance provides courage to face a problem and confidence that one is handling the situation appropriately. False reassurance is dangerous. It may prevent the employee from getting the professional help needed. It offers little comfort when the counselee knows that the counselor cannot predict the outcome. Even if there is some comfort obtained, it tends to dissipate when the person faces the problem again.

Counseling improves both upward and downward communication. It allows employees to express their feelings to management. Although individual names must be kept confidential, feelings can be grouped into categories and interpreted to higher management. The counseling session allows the counselor to explain company policies and activities to the employee, thus achieving downward communication.

Catharsis, or the release of emotional tension, often occurs when people have the opportunity to talk about their frustrations. They become more relaxed, and their speech becomes more coherent and rational as they explain their problems to a sympathetic listener. Then, as emotional blocks to clear thinking are eliminated, thinking becomes more rational. People may realize that their emotions are not appropriate for the situation. This may help people recognize and accept their limitations and bring about a reorientation or change in values and goals. The manager should refer an employee to professional help when reorientation is needed.

Directive counseling occurs when the counselor listens to the employee's problems, decides how to solve the problems, and tells the employee what to do. The counselor predominantly gives advice. This type of counseling does give some emotional release, can be reassuring, and fosters communication. Thinking may be clarified in a limited way. Reorientation seldom occurs.

Nondirective counseling is client centered. The counselor listens and encourages employees to explain their problems, identify alternatives, explore the ramifications of each option, and determine the most appropriate solution. Emotional release occurs more frequently in nondirective than in directive counseling. Clear thinking and reorientation are fostered. Reassurance may be used, but advice should be limited. This approach can be very beneficial, but managers must be cautious not to neglect their normal directive leadership responsibilities.

Nondirective counseling is more time-consuming and costly than directive counseling. To be effective, the employee must have the intelligence to identify problems and assess solutions and the emotional stability to deal with them. The nondirective counselor must be cautious not to allow emotionally dependent employees to avoid their work responsibilities.

Cooperative counseling is a compromise between directive and nondirective counseling. It is the cooperative effort by the counselor and employee through an exchange of ideas to help solve the problem. The cooperative counselor starts by listening, as would a nondirective counselor. As the interview progresses, however, the cooperative counselor offers information and insight and is likely to discuss the problems with a broad knowledge of the organization's point of view. This may help change the employee's perspective. Cooperative counseling combines the advantages of both directive and nondirective counseling and avoids most of the disadvantages.

Because of employees' rights to privacy, it is appropriate for the manager to refer an employee to professional help when personal problems are interfering with job performance or when a person needs reorientation. Managers are to be coaches, not counselors (Davis, 1981).

OUTPLACEMENT COUNSELING

Although not many RNs are fired, during economic recessions there is an increasing incidence in reduction in workforces. Outplacement counseling can be used to minimize the emotional and professional scarring that results from being dismissed from one's position.

Poor job performance, tardiness, absenteeism, substance abuse, inappropriate behavior, and staff reduction are the most common reasons for discharging nurses. A termination of this nature is usually a progressive process. However, for some offenses nurses can be terminated immediately. These are likely to include abuse of patients and visitors, insubordination, intoxication, possession of drugs, theft, gambling, disorderly conduct, willful destruction of property, sleeping on duty, or falsification of records.

The termination procedures used must be consistent with the agency policies. Termination usually involves several steps, beginning with an oral warning. If the employee does not change the offending behavior in response to the oral warning, written warnings with corrective interviews are used. There should be well-documented, sufficient grounds for termination. The nurse manager can use anecdotal notes to record both strong and weak attributes of the worker. They should contain factual information about who was observed by whom, where, and the background of the incident. There should be a sufficient number of observations to establish a pattern of behavior.

Written warnings used with corrective interviews should state the expected level of performance and the consequence if that standard is not met. Suspension is typically used before termination. The counseling note should be signed by both the nurse manager and the worker. If the worker refuses to sign, a witness can validate that the worker has read the counseling notes and refuses to sign them.

Poor job performance should be analyzed. Have employees been taught how to do what is expected of them? If not, they should be taught. Do they practice the skill often enough to keep their talents refined? If not, practice sessions could be made available. Specific, descriptive feedback should be given. Demonstrations and return demonstrations are appropriate. The feedback should be as close to the act as possible. Positive reinforcement for what was done well is as important as identifying weaknesses and making plans to overcome them. Follow-up by noting changes is also important.

A problem-solving approach can be used for tardiness and absenteeism. Why is the person late or absent so often? If a person has difficulty getting children to a babysitter and to work by 7 AM, could that person's hours be changed to 8:00 AM to 4:30 PM? This will allow the employee to fulfill her parental responsibilities, and it will also help provide a smooth transition at the change of shift. If the person is a night owl who has difficulty getting up in the morning, could that person be assigned the evening shift? Is the person working two jobs to make ends meet? Are financial assistance and counseling available? Are family problems interfering with attendance? Is the person hungover when reporting to duty? The social services that are available for patients should also be used for staff, for example, self-help groups such as Alcoholics Anonymous, single parents, and shelters for women. Social services, the chaplain, or family counseling is also useful.

Repeated failure to meet performance standards, lack of compliance with company policies, and staff reductions are just causes for termination. Each should be a progressive process. The employee should know what level of performance is expected to prevent termination and the risk of termination.

Support services are needed by people who are terminated. The agency should have termination policies regarding severance pay, terminal vacation, accrued holidays and sick time, and insurance. The person may need information about unemployment. This is an opportune time for a counselor in personnel to help terminating employees reassess their location and vocation. Where do they want to live? What type of climate do they like? What type of work interests them and provides the most satisfaction? What do their educational background and skills prepare them to do? What can they do to prepare themselves better to reach their goals? How important are salary, fringe benefits, retirement plans, work hours, and opportunities for advancement?

Once terminating employees decide what they want to do and where, they may need assistance to locate job openings. Professional journals, employment agencies, and college placement services are sources of information. Recruiters are often present at professional meetings. Friends, relatives, and acquaintances may help locate positions, and employers can be contacted directly.

Terminating employees are likely to need help preparing résumés, writing marketing letters, and interviewing. They do not need to state the reason that they left the last job on this marketing letter, résumé, or job application. However, they should be prepared to address the issue during an interview. They should be honest about the reason for termination, speak about the treatment they have had, if any, and focus on the knowledge and skills they have learned on the last job that they can transfer to the new one. They should not be critical of the last employer.

The sooner one accepts the fact that one has been fired, the sooner one can put the pieces back together and move on. The boss should be very clear about the reason. The termination should not come as a surprise. With the progressive process the employee should know the consequences of not meeting the performance standards. Any reduction in workforce should be done with fair warning and target dates. Employees should be informed of the grievance policy and procedure when reflecting if they have been fairly treated. The outplacement counseling can help the person know what questions to ask about pay and benefits, how to tell the family, how to solicit help from friends and acquaintances, and how to budget to protect securities until another job can be obtained. Career counseling and job placement counseling are useful.

Being fired initiates stress and can be quite devastating. Outplacement counseling can help reduce the related personal and professional scarring that inevitably results from being dismissed.

CHAPTER SUMMARY

Chapter 14 covered the following:
Purposes
Common Errors in Evaluation
Methods of Performance Management
    Anecdotal Notes
    Checklists
    Rating Scales

    Ranking
    Management by Objectives
    Self-Appraisal
    Peer Review
    Customer or Subordinate Evaluation
    360 Degree Feedback
    Appraisal Interview
    Appraisal Reports
    Legal Implications for Performance Appraisals
Discipline of Personnel
    Need for Discipline
    Principles of Disciplinary Action
        Have a positive attitude
        Investigate carefully
        Be prompt
        Protect privacy
        Focus on the act
        Enforce rules consistently
        Be flexible
        Advise the employee
        Take corrective, constructive action
        Follow up
    Penalties
        Oral reprimand
        Written reprimand
        Other penalties
    Components of a Disciplinary Action Program
        Codes of conduct
        Authorized penalties
        Records of offenses and corrective
            measures
        Right of appeal
    Discipline Without Punishment
Modification of Employee Behavior
    Reinforcement
    Shaping
    Extinction
    Punishment
    Behavior Modification for the Employee With a
        Performance Problem
Problem Employees
    Substance Abusers
    Angry or Withdrawn Employees
    Decreased Productivity
    Absenteeism
    Terminating Employees

Employee Counseling
Outplacement Counseling

REFERENCES

Berni R, Fordyce WE: *Behavior modification and the nursing process,* St. Louis, 1973, Mosby.

Davis K: *Human behavior at work: organizational behavior,* New York, 1981, McGraw-Hill.

Decker PJ, Sullivan EJ: *Nursing administration: a micro/macro approach for effective nurse executives,* Norwalk, Conn, 1992, Appleton & Lange.

Dienemann J: *Nursing administration: strategic perspectives and application,* Norwalk, Conn, 1990, Appleton & Lange.

Douglas LM: *The effective nurse leader and manager,* ed 5, St. Louis, 1996, Mosby.

Edwards MR, Ewen AJ: *360 feedback: the powerful new model for employee assessment & performance improvement,* New York, 1996, American Management Association.

Ellis JR, Hartley CL: *Managing and coordinating nursing care,* ed 2, Philadelphia, 1995, Lippincott.

Gillies DA: *Nursing management: a systems approach,* ed 3, Philadelphia, 1994, WB Saunders.

Grote D: *Discipline without punishment,* New York, 1995, American Management Association.

Grote D: *The complete guide to performance appraisal,* New York, 1996, American Management Association.

Huber D: *Leadership and nursing care management,* Philadelphia, 1996, WB Saunders.

Hutchinson S: Chemically dependent nurses: the trajectory toward self-annihilation, *Nurs Res* 35:196-200, July-Aug 1986.

Hutchinson S: Chemically dependent nurses: implications for nurse executives, *JONA* 17:23-29, Sept 1987.

Hutchinson S: Toward self integration: the recovery process of chemically dependent nurses, *Nurs Res* 36:339-343, Nov-Dec 1987.

Maier NRF: *The appraisal interview: three basic approaches,* La Jolla, Calif, 1976, University Associates.

Marquis BL, Huston CJ: *Leadership roles and management functions in nursing: theory and application,* ed 2, Philadelphia, 1996, Lippincott.

Marquis BL, Huston CJ: *Management decision making for nurses: 124 case studies,* Philadelphia, 1998, Lippincott.

Marrelli TM: *The nurse manager's survival guide: practical answers to everyday problems,* St. Louis, 1993, Mosby.

Odiorne GS: *Management by objectives: a system of managerial leadership,* Belmont, Calif, 1965, Pitman Publishing.

Odiorne GS: *Management decisions by objectives,* Englewood Cliffs, NJ, 1969, Prentice-Hall.

Rocchiccioli JT, Tilbury MS: *Clinical leadership in nursing,* Philadelphia, 1998, WB Saunders.

Swansburg RC: *Introductory management and leadership for clinical nurses: a text-workbook,* Boston, 1993, Jones & Bartlett.

Swansburg RC: *Management and leadership for nurse managers,* ed 2, Boston, 1996, Jones & Bartlett.

Swansburg RC, Swansburg RJ: *Introductory management and leadership for nurses: an interactive text,* Boston, 1999, Jones & Bartlett.

Tappen RM: *Nursing leadership and management: concepts and practice,* ed 3, Philadelphia, 1995, FA Davis.

Yoder-Wise PS: *Leading and managing in nursing,* ed 2, St. Louis, 1999, Mosby.

BIBLIOGRAPHY

Anderson JL: Treatment considerations for the addicted nurse, *Behav Health Man* 14:22, Sept 1994.

Ashton JT, Bay J: Investigating narcotic diversion, *Nurs Manage* 25:35, May 1994.

Curtin LL: Ethics, discipline and discharge, *Nurs Manage* 27:51, March 1996.

Davidhizar R, Giger JN, Poole V: Taking the dread out of annual performance evaluations, *Health Care Superv* 19(4):33-37, 1995.

Ellis P: Addressing chemical dependency: a need for consistent measures, *Nurs Manage* 26(8):56-58.

Falcone P: *101 sample write-ups for documenting employee performance problems: a guide to progressive discipline & termination,* New York, 1999, AMACOM.

Fiesta J: Labor law update—part 1, *Nurs Manage* 28:27-28, Jan 1997.

Fiesta J: Labor law update—part 5, *Nurs Manage* 28:16, Oct 1997.

Forte PS, Forstrom SJ: Work complexity assessment: decision support data to address cost and culture issues, *JONA* 28:46-53, Jan 1998.

Hughs TL: Chief nurse executives' responses to chemically dependent nurses, *Nurs Manage* 26:37-40, March 1995.

Keyes MAK: Recognition and reward: a unit-based program, *Nurs Manage* 25:52-54, Feb 1994.

McAllister M, Osborne Y: Peer review: a strategy to enhance cooperative student learning, *Nurs Ed* 22(1):40-44, Jan-Feb 1997.

McConnell CR: "We missed you": the absence that fails to make the heart grow fonder, *Health Care Superv* 14(2):78-84, 1995.

Neal JE: *Effective phrases for performance appraisals: a guide to successful evaluations,* Perrysburg, Ohio, 1997, Neal Publications.

Nelson B: Dealing with inappropriate behavior on a multidisciplinary level: a policy is formed, *JONA* 25:58-61, June 1995.

Peery BL, Rimler GW: Chemical dependency among nurses: are policies adequate? *Nurs Manage* 26:52-56, May 1995.

Queen VA: Performance evaluation: building blocks for credentialing and career advancement, *Nurs Manage* 26:52-57, Sept 1995.

Raper JL, Myaya SN: Employee discipline: a changing paradigm, *Health Care Superv* 12(2):67-77, 1993.

Recker D, Bless C, Wellens H: A decision-making process in shared governance, *Nurs Manage* 27:48A-48D, May 1996.

Seago JA: Culture of troubled work groups, *JONA* 26:41-46, Sept 1996.

Shaffer F, Kobs A: Measuring competencies of temporary staff, *Nurs Manage* 28:41-45, May 1997.

Smither JW: *Performance appraisal: state of the art in practice,* San Francisco, 1998, Jossey-Bass.

Taunton RL et al.: Predictors of absenteeism among hospital staff nurses, *Nurs Econ* 13:217-227, Aug 1995.

Tranbarger RE: A nurse executive's nightmare: the rogue nurse, *Nurs Manage* 28:33-36, Feb 1997.

Weinstein M et al.: Build consensus and develop collaborative practice guidelines, *Nurs Manage* 29:48-52, Sept 1998.

CASE STUDY

You do appraisal interviews with appraisal report follow-ups once a year with the personnel who work with you. You want to create an atmosphere of equality for planning and problem solving. What will you do to create that atmosphere?

CASE STUDY

A staff member has violated a policy. What principles of disciplinary action will you observe as you give the staff member an oral reprimand? How will you proceed if the violation is repeated?

CASE STUDY

One of the nurses with whom you work has developed an unkempt appearance, frequently has red eyes, has increased irritability, and has been late to work several times in the past few weeks. Today you smell alcohol on the nurse's breath when the nurse reports to work. How are you going to handle the situation as the manager for the unit?

Critical Thinking Activities for this chapter begin on page 518.

CHAPTER 15

CHAPTER OBJECTIVES

- Compare and contrast the roles of leaders and managers regarding quality improvement.
- Discuss trends in the history of continuous quality improvement.
- Identify three quality management heroes and their contributions to the field.
- Identify and describe at least five tools that can be used to facilitate continuous quality improvement.
- Outline a process for continuous quality improvement.
- Itemize activities that could be on a calendar of events for program evaluation.
- Identify and discuss at least six internal and six external sources of invalidity.
- Identify and discuss at least six research designs. In the discussion identify which sources of invalidity the design controls for and which could still be a problem.
- List the five steps in the risk management process.
- Identify at least three sources for identifying potential risks.
- Describe the importance of customer satisfaction in relation to risk management.
- Describe the research process as applied to quality improvement.
- Discuss the relationship between torts, negligence, and malpractice.

CONTINUOUS QUALITY IMPROVEMENT, RISK MANAGEMENT, AND PROGRAM EVALUATION

Chapter Overview

Chapter 15 outlines history, tools, and processes for continuous quality improvement (CQI), program evaluation, regulatory influences, changing regulations, and risk management.

MAJOR CONCEPTS AND DEFINITIONS	
Continuous quality improvement	preventive problem solving that results in exemplary service
Risk management	development and implementation of strategies to prevent patient injury, minimize financial loss, and preserve agency assets
Customer satisfaction	risk management of public relations is striving for customer satisfaction
Evaluation	valuation
Validity	measurement of what is to be measured
Internal invalidity	extraneous variables that confound the effects of the experimental variable
External invalidity	factors that reduce the findings' generalizability
Statistics	facts or data of a numerical kind that are assembled, classified, and tabulated so as to present significant information about a given subject
Torts	legal wrongs
Negligence	unintentional tort where harm results by not behaving in a reasonable and prudent manner
Malpractice	negligent acts of people with professional education
Legally liable	legally responsible
Plaintiff	complaining party
Defendant	answering party

Leaders envision high-quality care, encourage others to be involved in quality improvement, encourage setting high standards, are proactive, facilitate interdisciplinary quality, and consequently build a culture of quality. Managers organize quality-driven services; select standards, measures of those standards, and tools to measure them with others; facilitate collecting and analyzing data; determine discrepancies between care provided and standards; and facilitate ongoing quality improvement (Box 15-1).

HISTORY OF CONTINUOUS QUALITY IMPROVEMENT

In the late 1950s planning, organizing, and evaluating health care services became a public concern. In 1952 the Joint Commission on Accreditation of Hospitals—now the Joint Commission on Accreditation of Healthcare Organizations (JCAHO)—was formed. The American Nurses Association (ANA) and the National League for Nursing (NLN) both published manuals in 1959 to help establish standards for health care.

During the 1960s the ANA started a division of

QUALITY IMPROVEMENT LEADERSHIP AND MANAGEMENT

Leader	Manager
Envisions high-quality care	Organizes quality-driven services
Encourages others to be involved in quality improvement	Selects standards and measures of those standards with others
Encourages setting high standards	Selects tools with others
Is proactive versus reactive	Facilitates collecting and analyzing data
Facilitates interdisciplinary quality improvement	Determines discrepancies between care provided and standards
Builds a culture of quality	Facilitates ongoing quality improvement

Modified from Huber D: *Leadership and nursing care management,* Philadelphia, 1996, WB Saunders; Marquis BL, Huston CJ: *Leadership roles and management functions in nursing: theory and application,* ed 2, Philadelphia, 1996, Lippincott.

nursing practice to develop standards for nursing practice, which became the basis for quality assurance programs. The ANA also developed a process to evaluate the quality of patient care.

In October 1972 the Ninety-second Congress passed Public Health Law 92-603, an amendment to the Social Security Act that mandated the establishment of Professional Standards Review Organizations (PSROs) to review the quality and cost of care received by clients of Medicare, Medicaid, and Maternal Child Health programs. Health care facilities were to develop quality control programs by 1976 or the government would do it for them. Consequently, quality assurance has received considerable attention. The ANA developed guidelines for standards of nursing practice under the PSRO system; the American Hospital Association and the JCAHO developed a retrospective review of care. Individuals and agencies developed criteria and processes for the measurement of quality of care.

JCAHO required audits of care, delivered in its initial quality assurance standards, and increased the number of multidisciplinary audits required in 1975. Nursing then became a major contributor for evaluation of documentation. More recently, JCAHO has had nursing examine a nursing care problem quarterly, document assessment of the problem, develop and implement the plan for cor-

rection, and evaluate the effectiveness of the implemented actions.

Instruments for measuring nursing care were developed during the 1970s, but limited data were generated or published in quality assurance studies. The quality assurance program recommended by the Joint Commission on Accreditation of Hospitals was a retrospective review of patient care through a closed-chart audit that focused on patient-care outcomes.

Cost containment became a major issue in the 1980s. The federal Prospective Payment System (PPS), which uses a series of DRGs to determine a hospital's reimbursement for care provided to Medicare patients, was introduced. Outpatient services that were often uncovered for reimbursement in the 1970s became the preferred alternatives to health care in the 1980s. Outpatient services, long-term care, and home care were less expensive ways to deliver some care. The power in health care shifted from the provider to the consumer, primarily the third-party payers and insurers (Huber, 1996; Koch and Fairly, 1993; Loveridge and Cummings, 1996; Vestal, 1995).

Total quality management as the right thing to do the first time, on time, all the time was introduced in health care during the 1980s for improvement and customer satisfaction. Factories in Europe during the Industrial Revolution used measurement and standardization. Industry in the United States adopted quality management and product inspection after the turn of the century. During World War II industry in the United States produced large quantities of military products with declining quality. The boom in industry continued after World War II. The Japanese started focusing on quality through total workforce training and participation in quality improvement efforts. They called upon quality experts from the United States to train Japanese personnel. W. Edwards Deming, Joseph Juran, Philip Crosby, Avedis Donabedian, and Donald Berwick were important in the quality improvement movement. Deming (1982), with his 14-point management philosophy, was primarily responsible for training engineers in the United States to improve quality of military goods during World War II and was a key figure in training the Japanese. Juran (1981, 1989) and his trilogy of interrelated processes of quality planning, quality control, and quality improvement were also used to train Japanese. Crosby (1979) has 14 steps that emphasize training all employees, using teams, setting goals, and recognizing employees for their involvement. He is known for his zero defects concept. Donabedian and Berwick applied quality management principles to health care. Donabedian (1986) is known for his structure, process, and outcome criteria for quality assessment. Berwick (1989) stressed the importance of improving process toward quality improvement.

Quality became the issue in the 1990s. The objective became to provide quality health care in the most appropriate health care setting at the most economical cost. Customers started wanting involvement in decision making and wanted information about quality and costs. This brought intense competition between health care providers, and quality improvement became the key to survival and success.

QUALITY MANAGEMENT HEROES

Deming is the genius who revitalized Japanese industry with his focus on total quality management and CQI. The Deming chain reaction is as follows: (1) improve quality, (2) decrease costs with fewer mistakes, less rework, fewer delays, and better use of time and materials, (3) improve productivity, (4) capture the market with better quality at lower prices, (5) stay in business, and (6) provide jobs. Box 15-2 outlines the 14 key points of the Deming management method (Aguayo, 1990; Hunt, 1993; Mears, 1994; Walton, 1986, 1990).

Juran is an advocate for total quality management (TQM). His quality trilogy is composed of three activities: quality planning, control, and improvement (Hunt, 1993; Juran, 1988, 1989, 1992; Juran, Goyna, and Bingham, 1979) (Box 15-3).

Crosby defines quality as conformance to requirements. He believes that the system for creating quality is prevention of errors instead of appraisal. He has identified 14 steps to quality improvement, some of which are parallel (Crosby, 1979, 1984, 1992; Hunt, 1993) (Box 15-4).

Quality improvement differs from quality assurance (Table 15-1). The process of quality improvement includes the following steps:

- Identify the customers and their expectations and the outputs using brainstorming, focus groups, and interviews.

- Describe the current process using flowcharts and focus groups.

- Measure and analyze the discrepancy between desired expectations and reality using check sheets, logs, time charts, trend charts, histograms, and surveys.

- Focus on an improvement opportunity using decision matrix, Pareto charts, and voting.

- Identify root causes of inefficiencies through brainstorming, affinity charts, cause-and-effect diagrams, tree diagrams, relationship diagrams, force field analysis, and focus groups.

- Generate and select solutions to the problem by brainstorming and using decision matrices and tree diagrams.

- Map out a trial run through brainstorming, force field analysis, action planning, tree diagrams, and flowcharting.

| Box 15-2 | **FOURTEEN POINTS OF THE DEMING MANAGEMENT METHOD** |

1. Create constancy of purpose for improvement of products and services. Deming suggests that the purpose is to stay in business and provide jobs through maintenance, research, innovation, and constant improvement.

2. Adopt the new philosophy. Mistakes and negativism should be unacceptable.

3. Cease dependence on mass inspection. Deming maintains that quality arises from improvement in the process rather than from inspection and that workers should participate in improvement in the process. When quality is addressed at the inspection phase, workers are paid to make the mistake and then paid to correct it, which is very expensive.

4. End the practice of awarding business on the price tag alone. Buyers should get the best quality in a long-term relationship with a single supplier for any specific item rather than purchasing the lowest-priced and often poor-quality items from the cheapest vendor.

5. Constantly improve the system of production and service. Management must always look for ways to reduce waste and improve quality.

6. Institute training. Workers cannot be expected to do their jobs well if no one tells them how to do so.

7. Institute leadership. Deming believes that people who do not do well are just misplaced. It is the leader's responsibility to identify workers who need individual attention, find an appropriate place for them in the organization, and help them do a better job.

8. Drive out fear. Many workers are afraid to ask questions or point out problems for fear of being blamed for the problem. They may continue to do something wrong or not at all. For the best quality and productivity, people need to feel secure.

9. Break down barriers between staff areas. Often departments compete with each other or have goals that conflict. It is better to have teamwork to solve problems.

10. Eliminate slogans, exhortations, and targets for the workforce. It is better for workers to develop their own slogans.

11. Eliminate numerical quotas because they deal with numbers, not quality. They often contribute to inefficiency and high cost because workers meet quotas at any cost to keep their jobs.

12. Remove barriers to pride of workmanship. People are eager to do a good job. Barriers such as faulty equipment, defective materials, and misguided managers should be removed.

13. Institute a vigorous program of education and retraining. Both managers and staff need to be educated about new methods and teamwork.

14. Take action to accomplish the transformation. Managers and staff need a plan of action to carry out the quality mission. A critical mass of people must understand the 14 points about continuous quality improvement.

Modified from Walton M: *The Deming management method*, New York, 1986, Putnam; Walton M: *Deming management at work*, New York, 1990, Putnam's Sons.

Box 15-3 — JURAN'S QUALITY TRILOGY

QUALITY PLANNING

1. Determine who the customers are.

2. Determine the needs of the customers.

3. Develop product features that respond to the customers' needs.

4. Develop the processes that produce those product features.

5. Transfer the resulting plans to the operating forces.

QUALITY CONTROL

1. Evaluate actual quality performance.

2. Compare actual performance with quality goals.

3. Act on the difference.

QUALITY IMPROVEMENT

1. Establish the infrastructure needed to secure annual quality improvement.

2. Identify the specific needs for improvement, which become the improvement projects.

3. Establish a project team with responsibilities for bringing the project to successful closure.

4. Provide the resources and training needed by teams to diagnose the problems, develop a remedy, and establish controls to maintain the gains.

Modified from Juran JM: *Juran on leadership for quality: an executive handbook*, New York, 1989, Free Press.

Box 15-4 — CROSBY'S 14 STEPS TO QUALITY IMPROVEMENT

1. Commitment from management

2. Use of quality improvement teams composed of people with process knowledge and commitment to actions

3. Quality measurement to identify areas that need improvement and change

4. Measuring the cost of quality and nonquality

5. Quality awareness by all personnel

6. Corrective actions through opportunities for improvement

7. Zero defects planning—do it right the first time

8. Employee education for quality improvement

9. Zero defect day as demonstration of commitment to quality

10. Goal setting toward zero defects

11. Error-causal removal by removing barriers

12. Recognition for meeting goals

13. Quality councils to assist people in quality improvement

14. Do it all over again

Modified from Crosby PB: *Quality is free: the art of making quality certain*, New York, 1979, McGraw-Hill; Crosby PB: *Quality without tears: the art of hassle-free management*, New York, 1984, Penguin Group; Crosby PB: *Let's talk quality*, New York, 1989, McGraw-Hill.

- Implement the trial run using check sheets, logs, and histograms.

- Evaluate the results using check sheets, logs, surveys, focus groups, histograms, and trend charts.

- Draw conclusions using Pareto diagrams, focus groups, and force field analysis.

- Standardize the change using force field analysis, brainstorming, action planning, tree diagrams, and flowcharting.

- Monitor holding the gains through check sheets, trend charts, surveys, histograms, and control charts.

Table 15-1 Comparison of Quality Assurance and Quality Improvement

Quality Assurance	Quality Improvement
Detection oriented	Prevention oriented
Reactive	Proactive
Narrow focus	Cross-functional
Getting by	Raising standards
Tradition and safety	Experimentation and risk
Busyness	Productivity
Leadership not vested	Leadership leading
Leader as director	Leader as empowerer
Employee as expendable	Employee as customer
Responsibility of few	Responsibility of all
Problem solving by authority	Problem solving by all
We-they thinking	Organizational perspective
Cynicism	New optimism

CONTINUOUS QUALITY IMPROVEMENT

Deming introduced the *plan-do-check-act cycle* (PDCA) (Walton, 1990). FOCUS-PDCA is an acronym for the following (Walton, 1990, p. 107):

Find a process to improve.
Organize a team that knows the process.
Clarify current knowledge of the process.
Understand causes of process variation.
Select the process improvement.
Plan the improvement and continue data collection.
Do the improvement, data collection and analysis.
Check the results and lessons learned from the team effort.
Act to hold the gain and to continue to improve the process.

The basic assumptions for the PDCA cycle are that (1) decisions should be based on facts instead of on hunches and intuition, (2) people who perform the work know it best, (3) teams can have more success than individuals working alone, (4) teams need to be trained in problem solving processes, and (5) it helps to display information graphically (Sandras, 1989; Walton, 1990).

PDCA cycle methods include the following (Cofer and Greeley, 1998; Martin, 1995; Ritter and Brassard, 1998; Swansburg, 1996):

Plan	Plan the change.
	Identify opportunities.
	Develop vision statement.
	Collect data to define problems and opportunities.
	Use CQI tools to organize data and thinking.
	Decide on improvement initiatives.
Do	Implement the planned change.
	Implement initiatives.
	Test with a trial run.
	Identify costs, people, and materials.
	Educate staff and management about changes in process.
Check	Observe the effect of the change.
	Monitor progress of initiatives.
	Meet with staff to discuss changes.
	Delegate staff to monitor results.
	Compare new data with original data, using CQI tools.
	Use CQI tools to monitor results.
Act	Adjust as necessary.
	Incorporate changes into department policies.
	Inform and educate all involved.
	Distribute new policies to key individuals.
	Look for new opportunities.

The planning phase involves identifying customers, their needs, areas not meeting those needs, and improvement proposals. Deming identified the following seven helpful charts: cause-and-effect chart, flow chart, Pareto chart, histogram, run (trend) chart, scatter diagram, and control chart. Other tools that can be used to display information graphically include checklists, pie charts, time charts, decision matrices, affinity charts, tree diagrams, relationship diagrams, force field analysis, and bar graphs. Processes that can be used to vision

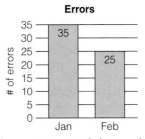

Figure 15-1 Simple bar graph.

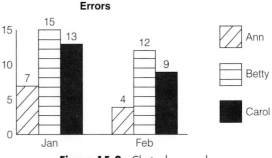

Figure 15-2 Cluster bar graph.

and make decisions include benchmarking, observations, interviews, questionnaires, record audits, nominal group technique, brainstorming, quality circles, focus groups, action planning, and voting.

Tools and Processes for Continuous Quality Improvement

A *bar graph* is a series of bars representing successive changes in the value of a variable or different data sets. A simple bar graph can measure one set of data that does not need to be subcategorized (Figure 15-1). The cluster bar graph can divide simple bar graph totals into subtotals (Figure 15-2). The histogram and Pareto chart are bar graphs (Cofer and Greeley, 1998).

Benchmarking is a process of identifying best practices and comparing them with the agency's practices to improve performance. It is learning and borrowing from others. The process is as follows: (1) identify the benchmark team, (2) identify what to benchmark, (3) gather information through search of the literature, (4) survey benchmark partners through written or telephone surveys or site visits, (5) compare benchmark data with organization's current practices and outcomes, (6) borrow ideas from the best and adapt them to important processes within the organization, and (7) monitor the results (Gift and Mosel, 1994; Hunt, 1993; Karlof and Ostblom, 1993; Nicholas, 1998; Stowell, 1997; Swansburg and Swansburg, 1999).

Brainstorming is a process of creating a free flow of ideas without fear of criticism and then thinking about the good in the wild ideas generated

(Cofer and Greeley, 1998; King and Schlicksupp, 1998; Ritter and Brassard, 1998). (See Chapter 3.)

A *cause-and-effect diagram* or *fishbone diagram* is used to identify the root causes of a problem or outcome. Identify a problem and then use brainstorming to identify root causes. Start with the outcome and then identify causal categories, such as facilities or equipment, materials or supplies, methods, and people, and items within those categories that cause the problem. Ask "why" four or five times. Identify first-, second-, and third-level causes until the causes become narrow enough to address. This can be outlined to look like a fish skeleton or can be done as hierarchical outlining on the computer (Brassard and Ritter, 1994; Cofer and Greeley, 1998; McCloskey and Collett, 1993; Oddo, 1995; Rocchiccioli and Tilbury, 1998; Yoder-Wise, 1999) (Figure 15-3).

Check sheets are grids that can be used to collect and classify raw data. They are good tools for monitoring key performance indicators. That raw data can be used to generate histograms, Pareto charts, run charts, and other tools that display information graphically (Band, 1994; Cofer and Greeley, 1998; McCloskey and Collett, 1993; Oddo, 1995; Sandras, 1989; Thomas, Gallace, and Martin, 1992; Wheatley, 1997) (Table 15-2).

A *decision matrix* is a grid that helps prioritize options. First, there is brainstorming to identify options. Those options are then evaluated, and unfeasible options are eliminated, leaving viable alternatives. The viable options are then listed down the left side of the grid. Criteria for evaluating each option are identified at the top of columns. How well

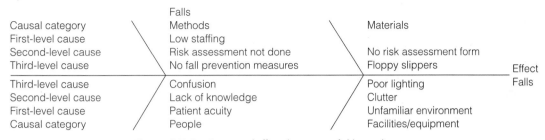

Figure 15-3   Cause-and-effect diagram or fishbone diagram.

Table 15-2   Check Sheet

Staff/day	Sunday	Monday	Tuesday	Wednesday	Thursday	Friday	Saturday	Weekly total/person
Ann		///	//	/	/		/	8
Betty	/	//	//	//	//			9
Carol		//	///	///	////	///		15
Daily total	1	7	7	6	7	3	1	32

Table 15-3   Decision Matrix

	Criteria						
	Ease of Implementation 2	Cost 3	Timeliness 2	Value Added 3	Quality Impact 3	Weighted Score	Rank
Surveys	3╱6	3╱9	3╱6	2╱6	3╱9	36	1
Interviews	1╱2	1╱3	1╱2	3╱9	2╱6	22	2
Observations	1╱2	1╱3	1╱2	2╱6	2╱6	19	3

the item meets the criterion can be rated as follows: 1 = poorly, 2 = adequately, and 3 = well. The criterion can be weighted as follows: 1 = unimportant, 2 = important, and 3 = very important. Then a weighted score can be calculated by multiplying the score by the criterion weight. The score can be recorded to the left of the diagonal dividing the score box, with the weighted score to the right of the diagonal (Band, 1994; Cofer and Greely, 1998; Sandras, 1989) (Table 15-3).

A *histogram* is a bar graph that can be used to compare patterns of occurrence over time. It displays the frequency with which comparable events occur and illustrates the variations in the occurrences. It can be used to identify trends and analyze variations. The measurement should occur at least 25 times during the period studied to get useful data. Raw data is gathered possibly using a checklist to plot the histogram. The range of the data is calculated by subtracting the smallest from the largest data point. The square root of the total number of data points collected will determine how many bars to use in the histogram. Divide the overall range by the number of bars to determine the inter-

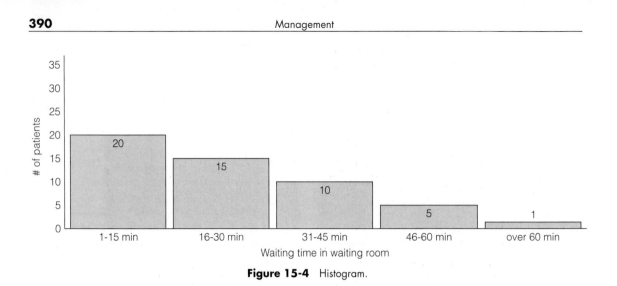

Figure 15-4 Histogram.

val for each bar. Use the check sheet to group the raw data by intervals. The number of data points per interval determines the height of the bar for that interval. A histogram that peaks in the middle with a narrow base indicates little performance variance. A histogram that peaks in the middle with a wide base indicates much performance variance. Histograms that peak to the right or left are skewed histograms and probably indicate that something unexpected happened during the process. Histograms with two peaks are bimodal and probably contain incompatible data sets that should be separated. Recalculate abnormal histograms before considering defective processes (Band, 1994; Cofer and Greely, 1998; McCloskey and Collett, 1993; Oddo, 1995) (Figure 15-4).

A *flow process chart* helps analyze how a task is being performed (Figure 15-5). Flow process chart symbols include ○ for operation, → for transportation, □ for inspection, **D** for delay, and △ for storage. An operation is the actual performance of the work, such as giving an injection. Transportation represents physical movement—the relocation of a person or thing from one place to another, such as movement of the syringe from the medication room to the patient's bedside. Inspection is to determine whether the necessary work has been properly performed. Nurses make sure that they are giving the right medication to the right patient and using the right mode at the right time. A delay is an

unplanned interruption in the flow of the process. Storage is an anticipated interruption in the process or at the end of it. When making a flow process chart, one must decide whether to follow the flow of material or the activities of the worker, because they may not be the same.

As a result of methods improvement, one should eliminate activities or combine steps when possible and change the sequence of activities as necessary to improve the performance of various steps. The proposed method is then analyzed using flowcharting. The potential impact on people is considered. Trial runs are conducted, and debugging is done (Band, 1994; Cofer and Greeley, 1998; Harbour, 1994; Jackson and Twaddle, 1997; McCloskey and Collett, 1993; Oddo, 1995; Rocchiccioli and Tilbury, 1998).

A *Gantt chart* is a grid with a time frame across the top that could be in minutes, hours, days, weeks, months, years, or decades depending on the time frame of the process. Tasks to be accomplished are listed down the left side of the grid. An *x* is put in the cell when a certain task is to be done. A line is drawn through cells when the task takes a period of time. This tool is used for managing production activities to complete a project (Swansburg and Swansburg, 1999). (See Chapter 3.)

Nominal group technique is a process for developing team goals and priorities. Individuals list ideas on a paper during silent generation of ideas.

Procedure: Injection

Distance traveled ___ Present ☐ Proposed ☐

Person ☐

Material ☐

	Present		Proposed		Savings	
	No	Hr	No	Hr	No	Hr
Operation	8					
Transportation	2					
Inspection	2					
Delay	0					
Storage	1					

Steps in procedure	○ → ☐ D △	Distance (ft)	Time (hr)	Remarks
Read medication order	○ → ☐ D △			
Collect vial and syringe	○ → ☐ D △			
Open vial	○ → ☐ D △			
Open disposable syringe	○ → ☐ D △			
Draw up solution	○ → ☐ D △			
Recheck medication order	○ → ☐ D △			
Put vial in medication drawer	○ → ☐ D △			
Take shot to patient	○ → ☐ D △			
Check patient identification	○ → ☐ D △			
Administer shot	○ → ☐ D △			
Return to medicine room	○ → ☐ D △			
Dispose of syringe	○ → ☐ D △			
Chart medication	○ → ☐ D △			
Store chart	○ → ☐ D △			

Key:

○   Operation

→   Transportation

☐   Inspection

D   Delay

△   Storage

Figure 15-5 Flow process chart.

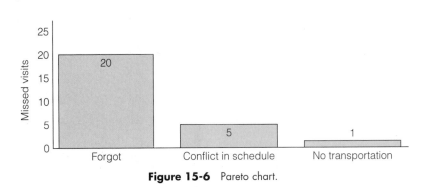

Figure 15-6 Pareto chart.

Each participant may give one idea at a time during a round-robin session. The ideas are written onto a chalkboard or paper. Ideas are expressed around and around the circle until all ideas have been expressed. Then there is a discussion for clarification before the preliminary vote. Participants may rank the first five to seven items, with the highest number being the highest weighting. Then the votes are weighted by multiplying the number of votes per priority for each item. If more than nine items surface as priorities, there can be further discussion and a second vote weighting the top items. Once items have been identified, brainstorming can be used to address the issues (Cofer and Greeley, 1998; Oddo, 1995). (See Chapter 3.)

A *Pareto chart* is a bar graph that displays categories of data in descending order of frequency or significance from the left to right. It is named after Pareto, an economist who noticed that 80% of the wealth in Italy in the nineteenth century was controlled by 20% of the population. The Pareto principle is that most effects come from a few causes (Figure 15-6). Once the major cause of a problem is identified, it can be problem solved, leading to considerable impact (Band, 1994; Brassard and Ritter, 1994; Cofer and Greeley, 1998; Martin, 1995; McCloskey and Collett, 1993; Oddo, 1995; Sandras, 1989; Swansburg, 1996; Yoder-Wise, 1999).

Pie charts compare relative size of different data sets in a circle instead of as bars on graphs. Data are collected and assigned percentages of the whole (Figure 15-7). A circle is drawn and divided into proportional pieces equal to the percentage of each

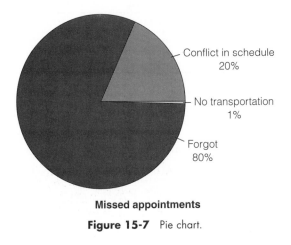

Missed appointments

Figure 15-7 Pie chart.

indicator subtotal. Different segments can be shaded differently (Cofer and Greeley, 1998).

Program evaluation and review technique (PERT) is a system model for planning that identifies key activities in a project and sequencing of those activities in a flow diagram with duration of each phase of the program assigned (Swansburg and Swansburg, 1999). (See Chapter 3.)

Radar charts are circular displays of before-and-after data to demonstrate progress made or lost. Decide what indicators to measure. Draw a circle and divide it into equal segments numbering the number of indicators. Establish the rating scale. Rate each indicator using the rating scale and post the finding on the segment line for that indicator. Draw a line connecting the posted ratings. Repeat the process later, use a different type line to connect

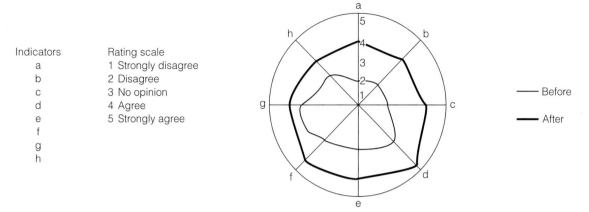

Indicators
a
b
c
d
e
f
g
h

Rating scale
1 Strongly disagree
2 Disagree
3 No opinion
4 Agree
5 Strongly agree

—— Before

—— After

Figure 15-8 Radar chart.

the second posted ratings, and compare the old and new ratings (Cofer and Greeley, 1998; Oddo, 1995) (Figure 15-8).

A *run chart* is a line graph that displays the variations in data over time. It allows a quick assessment of patterns and trends. It is good for monitoring time-related trends and shifts in processes (Cofer and Greeley, 1998; McCloskey and Collett, 1993; Oddo, 1995; Yoder-Wise, 1999) (Figure 15-9).

Scatter diagrams help determine relationships between two variables. They reflect correlations but do not explain causation. Identify two variables to compare. Collect the data and note the highest and lowest values for each variable. Draw axes for each variable ranging from the lowest to the highest value for each variable. Plot each data point where the two measurements intersect and analyze the pattern. If the points are clustered together from the lower left to the upper right, there is a positive correlation. If the points are clustered together from the upper left to the lower right, there is a negative correlation. If the points are scattered randomly, there is no correlation between the variables (Band, 1994; Cofer and Greeley, 1998; McCloskey and Collett, 1993; Oddo, 1994; Sandras, 1989) (Figure 15-10).

Several authors of the 1990s have outlined processes for risk management and change for quality

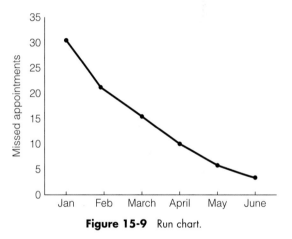

Figure 15-9 Run chart.

improvement. Otto Lerbinger (1997) outlines lessons learned from crises as follows (pp. 343-350):

Assess personal and organizational vulnerability. . . .
Look for ways to reduce vulnerability. . . .
Exercise constant vigilance and establish monitoring systems. . . .
Communicate with and relate to a wide range of stakeholders. . . .
Speed up and broaden the decision-making process. . . .
Apply a variable time perspective . . . examine immediate, short-term, and long-term impacts. . . .

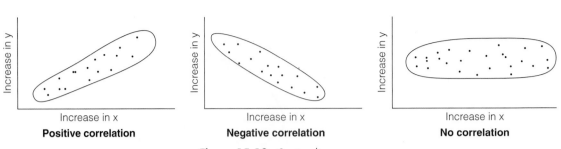

Figure 15-10 Scatter diagrams.

Recognize the importance of the corporate culture and its supporting structures.

Steve Albrecht (1996) wrote about how to protect an organization in crisis and how to stop a crisis before it begins. He outlined a five-step approach as follows (pp. 114-117):

Step One: Initiate a risk assessment survey. . . .
Step Two: Assign roles and discuss duties. . . .
Step Three: Respond to the risk assessment report. . . .
Step Four: Write crisis response plans. . . .
Step Five: Create an incident review subcommittee. . . .

David Ulrich (1997) identified four steps for building the capacity for change as follows (pp. 158-166):

Step One: Identify key success factors for building capacity for change. . . .

- Leading change: Having a sponsor of change who owns and leads the change initiative.
- Creating a shared need: Ensuring that individuals know why they should change and that the need for change is greater than the resistance to change.
- Shaping a vision: Articulating the desired outcome from the change.
- Mobilizing commitment: Identifying, involving, and pledging the key stakeholders who must be involved to accomplish the change.
- Changing systems and structures: Using human resources (HR) and management tools (staffing, development, appraisal, rewards, organization design, communication, systems, and so on) to

ensure that the change is build into the organization's infrastructure.
- Monitoring progress: Defining benchmarks, milestones, and experiments with which to measure and demonstrate progress.
- Making change last: Ensuring that change happens through implementation plans, follow-through, and ongoing commitments. . . .

Step Two: Profile the extent to which these key success factors are being managed. . . .
Step Three: Identify the improvement activities for each success factor. . . .
Step Four: See the seven factors as an iterative process, not an event. . . .

Michael Hammer (1996, p. 104) said, "Superior process performance is achieved by having a superior process design, the right people to perform it, and the right environment for them to work in." Jim Fuller (1997) outlined the five steps in the process of project definition as follows (pp. 8-13):

Step One: Identify the project. . . .

- Define why something must be done. . . .
- Define what would be done and the intended outcomes. . . .
- Create a preliminary cost-benefit analysis. . . .
- Analyze the risk. . . .
- Define the project's relationship to other performance improvement projects. . . .
- Evaluate future opportunities. . . .
- Assess organizational readiness. . . .

Step Two: Create a written definition document. . . .
Step Three: Create a project objective statement. . . .
Step Four: Validate the definition. . . .
Step Five: Create a project priority matrix. . . .

Jack Hagan (1994) says, "Developing a quality plan requires a framework from which to start. The following basic model can be applied to any plan."

Phase One—A Philosophy for Quality. This phase includes the establishment of:

a. A vision.
b. A clear policy.
c. Primary quality objectives.
d. Guidelines for meeting those objectives.

Once these are established, a company quality philosophy exists.

Phase Two—Tactics. This phase provides the ways and means for putting the philosophy into operation through:

a. Specific programs and projects.
b. The creation of an ongoing review process to help the business to understand its progress and make necessary adjustments when appropriate.

This basic model can be specifically adapted to a quality plan using the following eight-step process (pp. 60-62).

1. Obtain management commitment through sponsorship. . . .
2. Form the team. . . .
3. Develop a vision. . . .
4. Develop a policy statement. . . .
5. Develop objectives and guidelines. . . .
6. Review current programs and projects. . . .
7. Develop and implement a formal review process. . . .
8. Implement the plan. . . .

Hagan (1994) recommends the following guidelines (p. 63):

Plan it right—keep it short and simple.
Make it fun—be innovative.
Implement it—involve everyone.
Monitor it—show results.
Make it last—stress continuous improvement.
Make it rewarding—recognize excellence.
Sustain its success—focus on customer enthusiasm.

Rolf Smith (1997, p. 3) has identified seven levels of change as follows:

Level One: Effectiveness—doing the right things

- Set priorities.
- Focus.
- Do what is important first.
- Become more effective.

Level Two: Efficiency—doing the right things right

- Follow procedures.
- Understand standards.
- Clean up your mess.
- Become more efficient.

Level Three: Improving—doing things better

- Think about what you are doing.
- Find ways to improve things.
- Listen to suggestions.
- Help, coach, and mentor others.

Level Four: Cutting—doing away with things

- Stop doing what does not count.
- Simplify.
- Ask "why?"
- Refocus continuously.

Level Five: Adapting—doing things other people are doing

- Notice and observe more.
- Read about best practices.
- Think before you think.
- Copy!

Level Six: Different—doing things no one else is doing

- Think about thinking.
- Ask "Why not?"
- Combine new technologies.
- Focus on different, not similar.

Level Seven: Impossible—doing things that cannot be done

- Question assumptions.
- Defocus: Get a little crazy.
- Break the rules!
- What is impossible today, but . . . ?
- Wouldn't it be amazing if . . . ?
- Where will it take real magic?

George Land and Beth Jarman (1992, p. 69) said, ". . . growth no longer occurs through the limited extension of likeness or similarities but in sharing, exchanging differences, creating what has never before existed, and fulfilling the unrealized and unknown potential of the system."

PROGRAM EVALUATION

Program evaluation is an essential part of effective administration. It is the evaluation of a set of activities designed to determine the value of the program or of the program elements. Evaluative research is the use of scientific research methods to make an evaluation. Program evaluation may be formative or summative. Formative evaluations provide information about the program during the developmental stages. Summative evaluations provide information for judging a developed program. Evaluation may be descriptive or comparative.

Programs are evaluated for any number of reasons. Federal, state, or local agencies may require program evaluation. Program evaluation can be used to improve programs systematically or to determine the state of the programs. It can be used to evaluate the effect of new technologies on programs and help determine if parts responsible for success in one program can be used in other parts of the system.

Once the program to be evaluated and the purpose for its evaluation have been decided, someone should be made accountable for the evaluation. Credibility is the major argument in favor of an external evaluator. A person who is part of the program may have difficulty in being objective about the program's strengths and weaknesses because of pride, loyalty, or job security. On the other hand, an internal evaluator may be as objective as an external one and has knowledge about the program, its history, and circumstances; such knowledge facilitates the evaluation.

Calendar of Events

One of the first things the evaluator should do is develop a calendar of events that depicts the tasks to be done, the schedule, and organization of the project. A calendar of events for program evaluation itemizes activities to be done down the left margin and projected dates across the top. The projected date for each activity is estimated. This is a valuable tool for planning and judging the progress of the program evaluation (Box 15-5).

Committee Selection and Functions

Each agency needs multidisciplinary committees to establish criteria and a process for continuous quality improvement and to evaluate care, make recommendations, and do follow-up work. A chairperson with enthusiasm and attention to detail helps ensure a successful program. Members also need to be interested in quality assurance and knowledgeable about channels of communication, hospital resources, patient population, and nursing needs. Representation of nurses, physicians, pharmacists, therapists, nutritionists, and housekeepers from various units helps produce a wide variety of ideas. Preset meeting times allow for staffing to accommodate attendance, and large committee membership supplies personnel to do the work.

Conceptual Framework

Structure, process, and outcome or any combination of these is the common approach to evaluation. The structure approach focuses on the delivery system by which nursing care is implemented. Committee members evaluate policies, procedures, job descriptions, orientation schedules, in-service schedules, and charting. The process approach measures what the nurse does while delivering patient care. Both nurse and patient may be interviewed to collect evidence of professional judgment and functions. The outcome approach measures the results of the care administered to the patient and evaluates whether the goals were reached by considering clinical manifestations, patient knowledge, and the client's self-care. Outcomes became the focus of accreditation standards during the 1990s.

Audits may be concurrent or retrospective. Concurrent audits evaluate care as it is being ad-

Box 15-5	CALENDAR OF EVENTS

	Jan.-Feb.	March-April	May-June	July-Aug.	Sept.-Oct.	Nov.-Dec.
Inform personnel of purpose of the evaluation and who is responsible	X					
Define goals	X					
Determine criteria	X					
Develop instrument		X				
Train data collectors		X				
Pilot test			X			
Collect data			X			
Analyze data				X		
Report findings				X		
Correct deficiencies					X	
Reassess (follow up)						X

ministered and may include observation of staff; inspection of patient; open-chart auditing; staff and patient interviews; and group conferences including participation from the client, family, and staff. Retrospective audits judge care after it has been delivered through the study of patient charts or care plans after the patient has been discharged, postcare questionnaires, patient interviews, or all of these.

Review of the Literature

A review of the literature locates instruments, criteria, and standards that have been developed and allows committee members to benefit from others' accomplishments and mistakes.

Program Evaluation Model

The formulation of program goals is essential for program evaluation. The goals should be clear, specific, and measurable. The evaluator will need to develop indicators to measure the extent to which the goals are achieved. These program-outcome indicators are the dependent variables of the study. The standards set by accrediting agencies such as ANA, NLN, and the Joint Commission on Accreditation of Healthcare Organizations

can be used to determine goals and criteria (American Nurses Association, 1996 a, b).

Methods of data collection should be decided next. There are numerous sources for the collection of data, including questionnaires, interviews, observations, ratings, government statistics, instructional records, policy and procedure manuals, financial records, documents such as minutes of meetings or transcripts of trials, and tests.

Instrument Development

An operational definition of quality of care gives direction to instrument development. Instruments may be general and appropriate for all patients or structures or applicable only to a specific process or to a homogeneous group in which differences in scores are due to variations in the concept being evaluated rather than to other factors. Medical diagnosis, symptom, acuity, age, and health care settings often are used to determine homogeneity. A taxonomy of nursing diagnoses is being developed. Identification of homogeneous patient groups for the development and application of instruments necessitates the development of numerous tools.

Once the patient group or specific process has been identified, selection of goals, criteria, and items is the priority. The goal is a statement of the end that one strives to attain. Criteria are the standards or scales against which judgments are made. Criteria describe what is implied in the goal in concise, measurable statements of desired structure, process, or outcome. They are written for a specific condition and are understandable, clinically sound, and achievable.

Brainstorming is a common approach for identifying items. Actual problems—those that patients generally experience—and potential problems—those with a high risk of occurring—are identified, and the structure, process, or outcome to resolve or prevent them is determined. The generation of as many ideas as possible without immediate evaluation is recommended initially. Later, items can be eliminated, checked for comprehensiveness, put into a uniform format, precisely defined, and quantified. A pilot study to collect data with the instrument can clarify which items should be retained, discarded, or rewritten.

Scales and measurements must be developed. A checklist to determine whether a characteristic is present; ratings to give each item a measure of worth such as good, average, or poor; and ranking by comparison, such as more or less than the standard, are common measurements. Scales are either nominal, ordinal, interval, or ratio. The simplest type is the nominal. Its categories are collectively exhaustive, and each is mutually exclusive, meaning that there is a category for all the observations and that each observation can fit only one category. Sex, marital status, and the presence or absence of a condition are examples. Ordinal scales classify observations into a specific order of more or less, such as good, average, or poor. Interval scales are ordered with equal measurement between each class, but the unit of measurement is determined arbitrarily. Examples are the thermometer and sphygmomanometer. Ratio scales contain the properties of the other scales plus an absolute-zero point. Multiplication and division are possible because each number has a relationship to any other number. Currency systems are examples.

Sources of Internal and External Invalidity

Establishment of validity and reliability is important. Validity is the measurement of what is supposed to be measured and is difficult to establish. Face validity is an analysis of the instrument's appearance as valid. Someone simply looks at an instrument and decides if it has face validity. It is the easiest assessment of validity but is a questionable criterion because of its high degree of subjectivity. Content validity is a judgment that the content of the instrument is appropriate and closely related to what is to be measured. It is best determined by a jury of experts. Construct validity is particularly important when phenomena or concepts that are not directly observable, such as intellectual skills, human characteristics, and personal adjustment, are involved. The construct is a hypothetical definition that clearly defines observable phenomena. Construct validity is theory oriented. An instrument contains predictive validity to the extent that it predicts future behavior. It can be determined by checking the prediction after a period of time. Concurrent validity reveals the behavior that is being demonstrated presently and is particularly important for concurrent audits.

When designing research, the evaluator gives careful consideration to sources of internal and external invalidity. Extraneous variables can confound the effects of the experimental variable and are therefore sources of *internal invalidity*. Factors that reduce the generalizability are sources of *external invalidity*.

There are several sources of *internal invalidity*. *History* is a problem when an event extraneous to the purpose of the study occurs between the pretest and posttest and confounds the effect of the experimental variable. It is a hidden treatment or a change-producing event that occurred in addition to the treatment. The problem of history is a more plausible explanation of the change the longer the time lapse between pretests and posttests. It can be controlled with experimental isolation, which can almost never be used when human subjects are involved. For example, a group-training technique to reduce racial prejudice against African Americans has been developed. A group of prejudiced individuals is convened, pretested, trained, and posttested. If an African American political leader is assassinated during that time, one would suspect that history confounded the experimental effect. The reduced prejudice can probably be attributed to sympathy for the assassinated African American politician rather than to the therapy.

Maturation is another internal invalidity problem. It is a systematic change over time in a person's biological or psychological condition, including growing older or becoming tired or hungry. Prescribed plan activities to promote walking for 12- to 15-month-olds or bladder control for 2- to 3-year-olds would be questionable because children normally learn those skills during those times.

Testing is a practice effect or the effect on the scores of the posttest of taking the pretest. The practice effect is larger for the same test than for an alternative form of the test. A form of test wiseness, the practice effect lasts about 3 months. People taking an achievement, intelligence, or personality test for a second time within a 3-month period will usually do better than people taking it for the first time, although it is unlikely that they have become brighter or better adjusted.

Instrumentation becomes a problem when there are changes in the measuring instrument over time. Changes in tests, judges, measuring devices, or calibrations cause instrumentation problems. Results from one test cannot usually be compared with results of a different test. Instrument decay or the fatiguing of spring scales causes invalidity problems. Observations produce instrumentation problems. There are intrahuman differences of the observer through fatiguing, the process of learning, the process of increased skill with practice, and learning to establish rapport. There are differences in observations by the same person at different times. One may be more lenient at one time than at another. One becomes more skillful with experience. There are also interhuman differences, such as knowledge and skill. Researchers observing disruptive behavior in psychiatric patients before and af-

ter a treatment may become more aware of disruptive behavior by the second observation and record more behaviors, or they may record fewer minor disruptions the second time because of the high level of disruptive behavior they had observed. In either case, the treatment effect is difficult to determine.

Statistical regression becomes a problem when groups have been selected because of their extreme scores. The phenomenon of regression toward the mean is the inevitable tendency of persons whose scores are extreme (far above or below the norm) on the first test to be less extreme on the second test. Patients chosen for a therapy group because of their high anxiety would show less anxiety on a second test regardless of the treatment.

Selection is a problem when the experimental group differs from the control group. For example, a selection problem may exist when one is trying to compare a control ward with an experimental ward because patients were assigned as a function of systematic characteristics, such as presenting symptoms or histories. Randomization is a control for selection. This problem often occurs when the subjects are already formed into groups for reasons other than the study.

Experimental mortality is a differential loss of subjects from comparison groups. It includes lost cases, cases on which only partial data are available, and cases who refuse to participate. The experimental group may appear stronger or more intelligent only because the weak and stupid dropped out of it. Heavy smokers and drinkers are likely to be the first to drop out of therapy groups to reduce smoking and drinking, leaving the clients who appear most successful with the therapy.

Researchers must also be aware of *external invalidity* problems that complicate the generalizability of the findings. Subjects who are available to the experimenter may not represent the population, and consequently the results of the research are not generalizable. Random *sampling* solves this problem. The independent variable needs to be operationally defined so that replication of the research is possible. Multiple-treatment interference, Hawthorne effect, novelty effect, and experimenter effect are considered. When two or more treatments are given consecutively to the same subjects, it is difficult, if not impossible, to know the cause of the results, and *multiple-treatment interference* occurs. When one knows one is a subject, one may change one's behavior, not because of the treatment, but because one knows one is being observed. This is the *Hawthorne effect.* The subject may react either positively or negatively because of the newness of the treatment, thus producing the *novelty effect.* The *experimenter effect* occurs when the subject is influenced by the experimenter. Such subtle behavior as smiling and nodding one's head during an interview may unintentionally influence the subject.

Pretest sensitization is the same as the testing internal validity problem except as it relates to generalizability of the results, which makes it an external validity problem. Identification of the dependent variables and selection of instruments to measure those variables are necessary for external validity. One must also consider if the effect will be lasting or if one is likely to get different results at different times. In the situation where the African American political leader was assassinated, thereby reducing prejudice against African Americans among those in group therapy, we had a history internal validity problem. Now we have an *interaction-of-treatment-with-time* external validity problem. The racial prejudice may have been temporarily reduced as a result of the assassination but will probably not be maintained for long. Treatments to reduce smoking may appear most successful right after a cancer scare but not as successful later. One must have internal validity to obtain external validity, which is the ability to generalize the research results. With program evaluation there may be little intent to generalize the results.

Reliability is repeatability and is easier to determine than validity. Scores obtained by different raters' observations of the same event at the same time or by the same rater at different times can be compared. The *test-retest method* involves administration of the same test again after a period of time with the hope that the results will be consistent. The fact that people may remember items from the first

administration or that people change over time is a problem. This method is appropriate for stable characteristics but is problematic for unstable traits. The *split-half method* compares halves of the test to determine internal consistency. Reliability is suggested when the results of both halves are similar. To use the split-half method, both halves need to contain enough items to be reliable. *Statistical methods* to check reliability include the Kuder-Richardson test for internal consistency and the Spearman-Brown formula for a coefficient for the total test.

Research Designs

Next, the evaluator should design the evaluation. Will the evaluation be one shot only or a continuous process? Will a program be assessed, or will programs be compared? Will an experimental or a quasiexperimental design be used? The pretest-posttest control group, posttest-only control group, Solomon four group design, and factoral design are experimental designs.

Experimental designs. In the *pretest-posttest control group,* experimental subjects are randomly divided into two comparison groups as follows:

$$R \ O \ X \ O$$

$$R \ O \qquad O$$

where:

R = Randomly assigned individuals
O = Observation
X = Experimental treatment

The control and experimental groups are randomly assigned. The two groups are considered equivalent during initial observation. During final observation, the difference between groups should be the result of a variable being applied to one group but not to the other. The pretest-posttest control group true experimental design controls for history, maturation, testing, instrumentation, regression, selection, and mortality. One should consider the Hawthorne and novelty effects because the interaction of the testing and the experiment are not controlled.

In the *posttest-only control group,* experimental subjects are randomly divided into two groups to be compared as follows:

R X O

R   O

The control and experimental groups are randomly assigned. A pretest is not administered. A treatment is applied to one group only. Because of the random selection, it is assumed that the groups are equivalent before the treatment is administered to one group and that the difference noted on the posttest is due to the treatment. This design controls for history, maturation, testing, instrumentation, regression, selection, mortality, and the interaction of the testing and the experiment. It is superior to the pretest-posttest control design unless there is a question about the randomness. This design is appropriate when a pretest is awkward and is convenient for maintaining anonymity. The Solomon four group design is a better design but may not be worth more than double the effort.

The *Solomon four group design* uses four randomly selected groups. It combines the pretest-posttest control group and the posttest-only control group designs as follows:

R O X O

R O   O

R   X O

R   O

It is considered the most desirable of the experimental designs because it allows the investigator to examine the effects of the treatment in four independent comparisons. The Solomon four group design controls for history, maturation, testing, instrumentation, regression, selection, mortality, and the interaction of testing and the experiment. However, it may not be worth the effort.

Factoral design allows for observation of some subjects at all levels of all experimental variables and can be used when the situation is under the complete control of the experimenter, which is rarely the situation.

Quasiexperimental designs. The evaluator usually cannot control the time and subjects to whom experimental variables are applied. However, the evaluator may be able to select the time and persons on whom observations will be made and can consequently gain some control through the use of quasiexperimental designs.

A *time series* involves a series of measurements over a period of time with an experimental variable introduced at some point in the sequence as follows:

O O O O X O O O O

Maturation is controlled because it is not likely to cause the difference between each of the observations. Testing, regression, and selection are controlled. History is the most probable problem, and the longer the time over which the observations are made, the more probable the problem. Instrumentation is also a potential problem. It is important not to change the instruments or their calibration. It is best if this design is repeated by several researchers in separate situations.

When the *equivalent-time-samples design* is used, the time available for making the observations is divided into equal time periods as follows:

XO XO XO XO XO

The times to make observations are randomly selected. This design controls for history, maturation, testing, instrumentation, regression, selection, and mortality. The multiple-treatment effect is a problem, and generalization of the findings is limited to similar populations.

In the *nonequivalent control group,* the broken

line (- - - -) means the groups are not equivalent samples:

$$O\ X\ O$$
$$\text{- - - - -}$$
$$O\ \ \ \ O$$

For this design a control and an experimental group are both given a pretest and posttest. However, the groups are not randomly selected and do not have sampling equivalence. It is better than a one-group pretest-posttest design because it controls for history, maturation, testing, and instrumentation. Regression, mortality, and interaction between selection and maturation need to be considered as potential problems.

The *counterbalanced designs* are sometimes called Latin square, switchover designs, crossover designs, and rotation experiments. The following is an example:

$$X_1O\quad X_2O\quad X_3O\quad X_4O$$

$$X_2O\quad X_4O\quad X_1O\quad X_3O$$

$$X_3O\quad X_1O\quad X_4O\quad X_2O$$

$$X_4O\quad X_3O\quad X_2O\quad X_1O$$

Four experimental treatments are applied in a random manner in turn to four individuals or groups. Counterbalanced designs control for history, maturation, testing, instrumentation, regression, selection, and mortality. Multiple treatment interference is a problem. Strength can be obtained through replication.

For *separate-sample pretest-posttest design,* a pretest is given on one group and a posttest on another as follows:

$$R\ O\ (X)$$

$$R\quad X\ O$$

This simulated before-and-after design is weak, but it is better than a single-group pretest-posttest design because it controls for testing, regression, and selection. History, maturation, and mortality are not controlled, and the instrumentation needs to be questioned.

For the *separate-sample pretest-posttest control group,* two groups are pretested, one receives the experiment, and the two are posttested. This excellent design controls for history, maturation, testing, instrumentation, regression, selection, and mortality. Because it is an expensive design, it has probably never been used.

$$R\ O\ (X)$$

$$R\quad X\ O$$

$$R\ O$$

$$R\ O$$

For the *multiple time-series design,* a series of measurements is taken over a period of time on two separate groups with an experimental variable introduced at some point in the sequence of one of the groups as follows:

$$O\ O\ O\ X\ O\ O\ O$$
$$\text{- - - - - - - - - - - - -}$$
$$O\ O\ O\quad O\ O\ O$$

This excellent design can be used to compare one agency with a similar one. Controlling for history, maturation, testing, instrumentation, regression, selection, and mortality, it is the best of the more feasible designs. Power is increased through repeated measures.

The *recurrent institutional cycle design* is a patched-up design that starts with an inadequate design and adds features to control for sources of invalidity. It becomes an accumulation of precautionary checks that approaches experimentation.

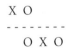

$$X\ O$$
$$\text{- - - - - - - -}$$
$$O\ X\ O$$

In *regression-discontinuity analysis design,* the solid line (—) means the groups are not equivalent. They differ by known amounts along a variable. The treatment is applied to individuals or groups that exceed a certain level of a variable rather than randomly. This design controls for history, maturation, testing, regression, and selection. Instrumentation and mortality would need to be questioned.

$$
\begin{array}{c}
X\ O \\
\text{——} \\
X\ O \\
\text{——} \\
X\ O \\
\text{——} \\
O \\
\text{——} \\
O \\
\text{——} \\
O
\end{array}
$$

Methods of Data Collection

Observation, interviews, questionnaires, and content analysis of charts and care plans are the most common methods for data collection. When *observation* is used, the quality assurance committee determines what to observe, develops observational procedures, and trains observers. Observations should be planned and recorded systematically and subjected to controls. Observation is suitable for concurrent audits. Behavior is observed and recorded as it occurs, and the process can be noted. Because observation does not demand participation of the observed, it is relatively independent of the subject's willingness to cooperate and therefore makes subjects readily available. Observation is a comparatively inexpensive method that lends itself to simple data-gathering instruments and recording equipment. Although it can be stopped at any time, it is limited to the length of the occurrence. The timing of an event may be difficult to predict, and consequently the observer may waste time waiting for something to happen. The presence of an observer also may influence the subject's behavior. Observations may

be difficult to record, are subject to observer bias, and may vary between observers. Consequently, observers need training. Specifications of observer tasks; detailed instructions; sharp, measurable categories; immediate, detailed recording; observation averaging; and the use of recording equipment such as cameras and tape recorders help overcome observer bias and variability.

Interviews of both clients and staff may be used to evaluate care. Interviews may be (1) nondirective—subjects talk about whatever they desire; (2) focused—the subject speaks to a list of topics; (3) nonstandardized—the interviewer makes up the questions; (4) semistandardized—the interviewer asks a specific number of questions and probes; or (5) standardized—the interviewer conducts each interview in exactly the same manner using the same wording without probing. The interviewer can minimize misunderstanding by probing, clarifying, pursuing topics in depth, and observing nonverbal communication. Subjects do not need to be literate. Interviewing provides more flexibility and a greater response rate than questionnaires. However, it is an expensive method because it requires so much time. The subject may be nervous or may attempt to please the interviewer, and the recording of answers is problematic.

Questionnaires are less time-consuming and consequently less expensive than interviews. They are particularly useful when subjects are dispersed over a large geographical area. Less skill is needed to administer a questionnaire than to conduct an interview. Questionnaires put less pressure on the subject for immediate response, standardize instructions and questions, and offer anonymity. The participants, however, must be literate. Unfortunately, often only a small percentage of questionnaires are returned, and the effect of nonrespondents is difficult to evaluate. Items may be omitted or misunderstood. A forced choice may not be an actual choice, and probing is not possible.

When preparing a questionnaire, the subjects' frame of reference and information level and the social acceptability of the item should be considered. Language should be gauged to the level of the subjects. Lengthy or leading questions and double negatives are to be avoided, and each question should contain only a single idea. Questions are arranged from general to specific. A pretest is helpful for identifying problems with the instrument. A high proportion of omissions, "other," "don't know," or all-or-none responses suggests poor questions. Added qualifications and comments and variation in answers when questions are reordered also suggest problems.

The percentage of returns of the questionnaires is influenced by a personal cover letter requesting cooperation, sponsorship by the health care agency, attractive format, short length, ease of filling out and returning, and inducements for replying. The best response is from people interested in the topic.

Content analysis of charts and care plans is a common method of data collection. It is a method of observation and measurement that is systematic, objective, and quantitative. Frequency of occurrences usually is noted on a checkoff list. Descriptive statements can then be given about frequency of occurrences and changes in conditions. Unfortunately, it can take a long time to review records; classification systems may be too ambiguous for a phenomenon to fit a category; the chart chosen may not represent the phenomenon; and prejudices in the scoring method can bias the results.

Sampling

Sampling is a technique of selecting a sample from the whole population being studied. Evaluators want to be able to generalize their conclusions concerning the quality of care given the total population. Adequacy of sample size is important, especially with small samples, if the quality assurance committee members are to have confidence in their inferences. The more homogeneous the population, the smaller the sample size necessary to be representative. Budgetary and time restrictions greatly influence sample size.

The best sampling technique is *random sampling,* which allows each patient an equal chance to be included in the sample. A table of random numbers that can be located at the back of most statistics books is frequently used. To use this method, patient records are numbered. Evaluators close their eyes and point to a number on the table to start the selection. They then systematically progress by row or column until the appropriate number of records is selected. A roulette wheel can be used. The wheel is spun, and the charts of the patients whose numbers are chosen by the pointer are selected for review. The wheel is repeatedly spun until the desired sample size has been reached. A third possibility is to put pieces of paper with a chart number or patient name on each into a large container. The evaluator draws a piece of paper, rotates the papers, and draws another until the desired sample size is reached.

Systematic sampling consists of selecting every-*n*th patient. Selection can be according to admission, discharge, or an alphabetical listing. The evaluator makes a random start and then selects systematically. The size of the interval is determined by the percentage of the population desired in the sample size. For example, if one wants the sample to be 10% of the population, the evaluator chooses every tenth patient.

Stratified sampling divides the population into sections and then takes a random sample from each section to ensure that important variables are represented. For instance, patients may be classified according to body systems by the major diagnosis. If 30% of hospital admissions are classified as cardiovascular cases, 30% of the sample would be drawn from those cases.

Cluster sampling uses small samples from various sections of the population. A certain number of audits may be selected from each hospital unit. Instead of randomly selecting 100 patient charts, 10 charts may be randomly selected from each of 10 hospital units.

Multistage sampling randomly selects some percentage of the population and then randomly samples smaller subunits. For instance, in a large hospital system, the evaluator would randomly select which hospitals are to be audited. Next, the specialty area to audit within the selected hospitals is randomly selected. Finally, the specific units within those specialty areas and the specific patients on those units are randomly chosen.

Incidental or *convenience sampling* uses readily available subjects. The families of patients who happen to be in the coffee shop at a particular time or patients who happen to be in their rooms at a particular time may be interviewed.

The sample mean is not truly representative of the total population average. It is an attempt to approximate it. The difference between the mean or average of the sample and the total population is the sampling error.

Analysis of Data

Simple scoring is preferred and can be subjected to descriptive measures. Frequency distribution indicates how many times observations were assigned to specific categories. Measures of central tendency can be calculated from the frequencies. The *mean* is the average. It is calculated by adding all the scores and dividing that sum by the total number of scores. The *mode* is the most frequently occurring score, and the *median* is the score in the middle with half the number values above it and half below it (Burns and Grove, 1996; Campbell and Stanley, 1963; Polit-O'Hara, Hunger, and Polit, 1996).

HISTORY OF REGULATORY INFLUENCES AND CHANGING REGULATIONS

Health insurance can be traced to the seventeenth century in London where workers could pay to ensure that their family members would receive health care if needed. That worked well until the cholera epidemic in 1831, when there were insufficient funds to meet the needs of so many sick people.

Health care in the United States was simple before the depression of the 1930s. Most of the medical practices were simple remedies, as there were no medicines or advanced technologies. The fee for service was typically paid at the end of the visit and may have been a trade, like a chicken for the health care. Most people could afford the medical care. Hospitals were supported by charitable donations, but people who received charitable care often got

less quality of care than those who paid did. However, during the depression most people in the United States could not afford medical care, and many hospitals closed because of the drop in charitable donations. There was no insurance or local, state, or federal funding to defray costs. There was some disability insurance where the employer continued to pay a portion of a sick employee's salary, but there was no assistance for medical costs.

Technological advances and the development of antibiotics during the 1940s advanced the ability to improve health, but unfortunately the cost was prohibitive for most people in the United States. A prepaid payment system that would relieve the burden on the sick person during an illness and ensure that the physician and hospital expenses were paid was envisioned. The first known insurance in the United States was in Oklahoma in 1927 when a physician had people in the community buy shares from the physician to build the hospital and then qualify to receive any needed medical care. A prepaid program for teachers was started at Baylor University Hospital in Dallas in 1929. A prepaid program for municipal employees underwritten by a Kaiser insurance company was also started that year in Los Angeles. While physicians, hospitals, and legislators resisted prepaid health care programs, the American Hospital Association (AHA) developed national standards to govern those programs in 1933. Physicians, legislators, and hospitals collaborated to introduce the Blue Cross Plan in 1939.

There was a period of health care expansion from the 1940s through the 1960s, much of which was supported by the federal government. The Hill-Burton Act (The Hospital Survey and Construction Act of 1946) was the beginning of extensive federal subsidization for health care resources. That facilitated medical education and research and technological progress. Policies focused on an increase in access to quality health care. The Hill-Burton Act stimulated hospital building. Medicare and Medicaid were introduced in 1965 to support the right to quality health care for individuals who were elderly, poor, or age 65 or older and entitled to Social Security or a railroad retirement. The Social Security survey of 1963 found that about half of the retirees had no private health insurance, and it was common for a worker to lose employer-sponsored health insurance at retirement.

While insurance companies were afraid to insure the elderly, legislation was passed to extend Medicare coverage to permanently and totally disabled people in 1973. Part A is totally funded by federal funds and covers inpatient care. Part B is voluntary, partially funded, and covers outpatient services. The large enrollment, inflation, and increasing technology increased the costs to the federal government. Medicaid, which aids states in providing health care to the poor, is a companion to Medicare. While it provides federal funding to states, states are responsible for the administrative operation.

By the early 1970s the federal government understood that it could not afford unlimited coverage for unlimited numbers of enrollees in Medicare. Cost containment policies such as utilization review, rate control, and control of capital expenditures were addressed. In 1972 the Social Security Act was amended to create the Professional Standards Review Organization (PRSO). Physicians reviewed Medicare patients to control health care utilization and costs. The Economic Stabilization Program, which was a federal program to control rates with individual states responsible for rate control, was in effect from 1971 to 1974. The National Health Planning and Resources Development Act of 1974 authorized and established a national certificate-of-need (CON) program to control capital expansion in health care.

The federal government could not meet the health care costs by regulations alone, so it started combining market and regulatory strategies in the early 1980s. The Omnibus Budget Act of 1981 and the Tax Equity and Fiscal Responsibility Act (TEFRA) of 1982 combined the strategies. These laws permitted HMOs to offer competitive medical plans and encouraged competition. The TEFRA Act of 1982 set operating cost per case and required development of a prospective pricing system. The Peer Review Improvement Act of 1982 repealed the PSRO Program and started the Peer Review Organization (PRO). The Social Security Amendment of

1983 encouraged prospective pricing based on DRGs to control utilization and costs. The National Health Planning and Resource Development Act was repealed in 1986, consequently repealing the CON requirement. Civilian Health and Medical Programs of the Uniformed Services (CHAMPUS) was given authority to reimburse institutional providers based on DRGs in 1984. The Consolidated Omnibus Budget Reconciliation Act of 1985 went into effect in January 1987 and required all Medicare-participating hospitals to accept patients from CHAMPUS. The PRO reviews Medicare and CHAMPUS using the same generic screening tools. Legislation was facilitating competition between health care services (Koch and Fairly, 1993; Kreider and Haselton, 1997).

For nearly a century various groups have recommended proposals for health care reform. In 1915 a group recommended a focus on prevention and sharing of health care costs by employers, employees, and the government. In 1932 a commission encouraged doctors to form group practices to share responsibility for cost-effective, high-quality health care. In 1933 President Franklin Roosevelt initiated the Social Security Act, which he intended to include national health insurance. In 1946 President Harry Truman introduced a plan for national health reform, declaring that health is a right, not just a privilege. In 1972 President Richard Nixon advocated that employers take responsibility and contribute to their workers' health care. In 1993 President Bill Clinton advocated a bold health care reform.

President Clinton outlined six principles basic to the Health Security Act: (1) security—guaranteeing comprehensive benefits to everyone in the United States; (2) simplicity—cutting red tape and consequently simplifying the system; (3) savings—controlling the costs of health care; (4) quality—making health care better; (5) choice—preserving and increasing the options available; and (6) responsibility—making everyone responsible for health care.

Security is accomplished by providing every person in the United States with a comprehensive health benefits package that cannot be taken away.

Simplicity is achieved by reducing paperwork, which wastes time and costs billions of dollars. Savings can be achieved through group purchasing. Quality involves emphasizing keeping well and giving consumers information to judge quality themselves. Choice means the right to choose one's health care provider to protect the doctor-patient relationship. Responsibility means that every employee and every employer contribute to the cost of health care (The White House Domestic Policy Council, 1993).

The Clinton health care reform plan was complex and coherent, with interlocking parts that fit together logically. There was an emphasis on universal health care coverage and broad, comprehensive coverage that includes preventive care, prescriptive medications, mental health services, home health benefits, and long-term care. It was designed to slow the current rate of increase in health care costs until they are comparable to the rate of inflation while providing access to economical, high-quality health care. The Clinton plan did not pass legislation, but it did facilitate the momentum toward managed care, including HMOs, IPAs, and PPOs, which are characterized by prepayment, comprehensive coverage, and preventive care.

Quality standards are often set by professional bodies and promulgated through codes of ethics, standards of care, standards of performance, and practice guidelines, which can be monitored through accreditation, peer review, and certification processes. State boards of nursing help enforce standards under each state's nurse practice act. Multiple associations in nursing have developed standards using different criteria and formats that have lead to confusion. The American Organization of Nurse Executives, American Association of Colleges of Nursing, National League for Nursing, and the American Nurses Association have joined efforts to coordinate and standardize formats and criteria for certification and practice standards (Rocchiccioli and Tilbury, 1998). The American Nurses Association has a set of ANA Nursing Standards, including Standards of Clinical Nursing Practice and standards for such areas of nursing as addictions, nurse administrators, advanced practice, car-

diac rehabilitation, college health, community health, continuing education and staff development, correctional facilities, developmental disabilities or mental retardation, diabetes, forensics, genetics, gerontological nursing practice, home health, nursing informatics, oncology, otorhinolaryngology, parish nursing, pediatric clinical nursing, psychiatric-mental health, and respiratory nursing. They outline standards of care including the following: (1) assessment, (2) diagnosis, (3) identification of outcomes, (4) planning, (5) implementation, and (6) evaluations. Their standards of professional performance include the following: (1) quality of care, (2) performance appraisal, (3) education, (4) collegiality, (5) ethics, (6) collaboration, (7) research, and (8) resource utilization. ANA (1995, 1996a) has also published *Nursing Quality Indicators* and *Nursing Care Report Card for Acute Care* to help assess risk and improve quality of care.

The three voluntary accrediting agencies for community health nursing are the Community Health Accreditation Program (CHAP) of the National League for Nursing, The National HomeCaring Council, and JCAHO. CHAP is one of two organizations nationwide authorized to provide home care accreditation, and in 1998 it became the first accrediting organization in the nation to be deemed an authority for Medicare hospices (NLN, 1998). JCAHO accreditation is also voluntary for long-term care. Nursing homes are required to meet state and federal licensing standards. Federal and state surveys and regulatory activities have increased since the Omnibus Budget Recognition Act (OBRA) was passed in 1987 and implemented in 1990.

JOINT COMMISSION ON ACCREDITATION OF HEALTHCARE ORGANIZATIONS

The Joint Commission on Accreditation (JCOA) was established in 1948. It became the Joint Commission on Accreditation of Hospitals (JCAH) in 1951 and was renamed the Joint Commission on Accreditation of Healthcare Organizations (JCAHO) in 1987. This voluntary, independent accrediting organization published the first hospital accreditation standards in 1953. In 1965 the Health Care Financing Administration (HCFA) gave the Joint Commission deemed status and gave their standards the benchmark of quality and meeting most of Medicare standards. In 1970 the JCAH changed its standards from review of minimum requirements to optimum level of care, and in 1975 it required every hospital to have a plan for quality assurance using explicit, measurable criteria that could be used in retrospective audits of care documented in medical records. In 1979 the standards were written that stressed a coordinated, organization-wide program for medical and nursing quality assurance. The structure and process standards stressed quality assurance activities that focused on problems whose solutions would have a big effect on patient care outcomes. It established a quality assessment standard in 1980 that has since been revised. In 1985 standards replaced the broad, problem-based approach with narrower systematic monitoring and evaluation of important aspects of patient care. The standards focused on specific departments, with each conducting its own systematic monitoring and evaluation that were conducted by concurrent audits of both patient care processes and medical records so that problems could be resolved while the patient was still hospitalized. In 1988 the quality assurance standards for nursing were revised to be evaluated objectively against preestablished standards and criteria. The results needed to be analyzed to determine problem areas and a plan developed to correct practice deficiencies. Reevaluation of the effectiveness of the corrective action was expected. In 1991 JCAHO published a 10-step process for the assessment, measurement, and improvement of quality of care: (1) assign responsibility, (2) delineate scope of care, (3) identify important aspects of care, (4) identify indicators, (5) establish thresholds for evaluation, (6) collect and organize data, (7) evaluate care, (8) take action to improve care, (9) assess actions and document improvement, and (10) communicate information.

By 2000 there were enormous changes in response to a rapidly changing environment and health care arena. There was a focus on continuous monitoring of performance; use of active, collaborative multidisciplinary teams; more randomized data selection for review; reporting of aggregate data; use of computers to manage and analyze data; linkages between patient, organization, and structure functions; sentinel events; root causes; performance improvement and sustained performance leading to continuous quality improvement; surveying physician practices that are part of a system; and random, unannounced surveys.

The Joint Commission used to publish yearly accreditation manuals for hospitals, which identified general administrative policies and procedures and standards. In the late 1990s the Joint Commission published *CAMH: Comprehensive Accreditation Manual for Hospitals—The Official Handbook,* which is a looseleaf notebook containing accreditation policies, standards, scoring, aggregation rules, and decision rules. The manual has three sections containing 15 functional chapters (JCAHO, CAMH Update 4, November 1998 UM-5):

Section One: Patient-Focused Functions
    Patient rights and organization ethics
    Assessment of patients
    Care of patients
    Education
    Continuum of care
Section Two: Organization Functions
    Improving organization performance
    Leadership
    Management of the environment of care
    Management of human resources
    Management of information
    Surveillance, prevention, and control of infection
Section Three: Structures With Functions
    Governance
    Management
    Medical staff
    Nursing

The manual contained 488 standards in 1999. The manual has quarterly updates to continue to incorporate additional accreditation information. There are also monthly "Briefings on JCAHO."

Any hospital may apply for Joint Commission accreditation to assess the hospital's compliance with standards. Compliance is determined from verbal information, on-site observations, and documents. Scores can be as follows (JCAHO, CAMH Update 4, November 1998, UM-10):

Score 1   Substantial compliance indicates that the hospital consistently meets all major provisions of the standard and the intent.

Score 2   Significant compliance indicates that the hospital meets most provisions of the standard and the intent.

Score 3   Partial compliance indicates that the hospital meets some provisions of the standard and the intent.

Score 4   Minimal compliance indicates that the hospital meets few provisions of the standard and the intent.

Score 5   Noncompliance indicates that the hospital fails to meet the provisions of the standard and the intent.

NA   Not applicable indicates that the standard does not apply to the hospital.

The manual contains the following (JCAHO, CAMH Update 4, November 1998 UM-6 & -7):

- Standards state expectations that must be met for accreditation purposes.

- Intent statements explain the rationale, meaning, and significance of the standards and expectations that must be met for accreditation purposes.

- Examples of implementation outline strategies, activities, or processes that can be used to meet the intent of standards.

- Examples of evidence of performance provide insight into the sources a surveyor may seek as evidence that the hospital organization complies with standards.

- Scoring scale reflects the five levels of standards compliance.

- Scoring question focuses on the performance expectation of the standard.

- Scoring identifies the levels of compliance with standards and intents.

- Aggregation summary contains directions for determining the set scores from the individual scores to standards in a grid and for determining the grid element score from the set scores.

Improving performance involves designing the processes, monitoring performance through data collection, analysis of current performance, and improving and maintaining improved performance. Criteria to set priorities from the numerous opportunities for improvement include selecting high-risk, high-volume, or problem-prone processes to monitor and improve. Once improvement strategies have been implemented, the performance should be measured again (JCAHO, CAMH Update 3, August 1998, PI-1). Patient-focused functions indicate that each patient's rights should be respected and business should be conducted in an ethical manner (JCAHO, CAMH Refreshed Core, January 1998, RI-1). Assessment should be done to identify the kind of care needed to meet the patient's initial and changing needs (JCAHO, CAMH Refreshed Core, January 1998, PE-1). Hospital care is just part of an integrated system of care levels, health care practitioners, settings, and services along a continuum of care. Activities and processes should be coordinated within the continuum of care (JCAHO, CAMH Refreshed Core, January 1998, CC-1). Patient and family education should be done to promote health behavior, support recovery, and enable patients to make decisions about their own care (JCAHO, CAMH Refreshed Core, January 1998 PF-1).

Organization functions include ensuring that the organization designs processes and monitors, analyzes, and improves them to improve patient care (JCAHO, CAMH Update 3, August 1998). Leadership should plan, design, direct, integrate, coordinate, and improve services (CAMH Update 3, August 1998). Leadership should also manage and improve the environment of care for the patients, staff members, and others in the hospital (JCAHO, CAMH Update 1, February 1998). Leaders are responsible to hire competent staff and to create a culture that facilitates staff self-development and continued learning (JCAHO,

CAMH Update 3, August 1998). Management of information involves increasing collaboration and information sharing to enhance patient care while balancing security and ease of access and using aggregate data and comparative data to assess opportunities for improvement (JCAHO, CAMH Refreshed Core, January 1998). Surveillance, prevention, and control of infections both acquired in the hospital and brought to the hospital are important (JCAHO, CAMH Refreshed Core, January 1998).

Governance of the hospital involves developing the mission, vision, policies, and bylaws that govern the organization (JCAHO, CAMH Update 3, August 1998). Management includes the responsibilities of the chief executive officer and executive management and the relationship between the chief executive officer and the governing body (JCAHO, CAMH Refreshed Core, January 1998). Medical staff members are expected to actively participate and provide professional leadership (JCAHO, CAMH Refreshed Core, January 1998). The nurse executive participates in the hospital's leadership functions and helps provide a sufficient number of qualified nursing staff members to provide quality health care (JCAHO, CAMH Refreshed Core, January 1998).

In the mid-1980s the Agenda for Change created a performance-based accreditation system that is flexible and patient focused and facilitates improvement of patient health outcomes, but since then the measuring of health care quality has changed dramatically. Setting expectations, collecting data, and assessing how well those expectations are met are steps to measuring performance to obtain information for decision making and improvement. Standards are sets of expectations against which current and future performance can be compared. They focus on doing the right things. They identify the functions and processes that need to be used to reach good patient outcomes. On the other hand, indicators focus on the organization's past performance. They are quantitative measures used to collect and organize data about the functions and processes related to outcomes that provide early warning signs of undesirable patterns and trends,

thus identifying performance-improvement opportunities (JCAHO, CAMH Refreshed Core, January 1998, USI-1-2).

Employer groups, insurance companies, governmental agencies, and the public have expressed needs for comparative performance data and meaningful information about patient outcomes. Consequently, the Joint Commission has developed an indicator measurement system (IMSystem) that includes indicators about cardiovascular care, infection control, medication use, obstetrical care, oncology care, perioperative care, and trauma care. The system requires collection of only the elements that are required for the indicators and often uses data already collected by most health care organizations (JCAHO, CAMH Refreshed Core, January 1998 IMS).

The Joint Commission understands that hospitals must meet the requirements for multiple agencies and organizations that set standards and regulations for the health care industry and that that can absorb resources that could otherwise be used to provide and improve patient care. The Joint Commission has tried to identify duplications between standards of different organizations to simplify the compliance expectations. Consequently, hospitals can use the Occupational Safety and Health Administration (OSHA) incidence reports (OSHA 200 log) to demonstrate that the facility is measuring and tracking adverse events (JCAHO, CAMH Refreshed Core, January 1998, SCA-1).

The Joint Commission's triennial, on-site survey process will evolve to include performance measurement data to assess continuous quality improvement of outcomes. Health care customers want objective data that allow comparison between providers to guide the purchase of quality care for a fair price. The implementation of a more objective, data-driven accreditation process that includes outcomes data will be incremental over several years (JCAHO, CAMH Update 4, November 1998, PM-1).

Many strategies are being used to deal with unannounced, random surveys. They focus on keeping all employees involved in the process. Education about continuous quality improvement can be done starting with senior officers, managers, and supervisors and moving to all employees. Interdisciplinary teams can be formed for each chapter of the *Comprehensive Accreditation Manual for Hospitals,* with its quarterly updates to deal with the standards for that chapter. Each team can have a captain or chair. The team can meet monthly to quarterly to identify how those standards are met and to generate action plans and reports. They can brainstorm ways to improve quality. People can attend JCAHO surveys of sister hospitals. Posters highlighting key elements of certain standards can be posted in bathrooms or near cafeteria lines. People can do mock surveys or role-play, where they ask each other questions as if they were the surveyors. Random questions could be asked to people in the cafeteria line. People could be rewarded for right answers with a free drink or free dessert. People could visit all shifts each day with questions. Questions can be put into weekly newsletters. Quality improvement results can be posted at the nurse's station. Outside survey consultants, videotapes, audiotapes, computer programs, books, newsletters, games such as Jeopardy, and storyboard fairs about performance improvement projects have been used (Briefings on JCAHO, March 1997 and June 1999).

People can be informed of JCAHO accreditation results through direct personal contact, called staff meetings, e-mail, newsletters, cards, letters, signs, and posters. Organizations with which the agency does business can be called or sent letters (Briefings on JCAHO, March 1997).

ORYX is an attempt to track outcome measures by computer. At first different hospitals submitted different data. Consequently, data could not be compared. There is evolution toward core measures for all (Briefings on JCAHO, November 1998, p. 12; Kreider and Haselton, 1997).

A sentinel event is an unexpected outcome involving a death or serious physical or psychological injury that needs immediate investigation and response. Accredited organizations are expected to identify and respond to all sentinel events occurring in the organization by doing a thorough and credible root-cause analysis, implementing improvement to reduce risk, and monitoring the effectiveness of the improvements. Organizations that complete acceptable root-cause analyses for sentinel events will not be placed on accreditation watch (JCAHO, CAMH Update 3, August 1998, AC-5).

Self-reporting a sentinel event to the Joint Commission is not required. It is recommended that it be kept confidential and not reported to the media. State law protection of privileged and confidential information against the new voluntary self-reporting requirements should be checked before approving institutional sentinel event policies. JCAHO recommends appointing a JCAHO surveyor who will conduct an on-site sentinel event investigation as an ad hoc member to one of the hospital's peer review committees as a temporary appointment for the sole purpose of reviewing the root-cause analysis to preserve confidentiality. Other steps to safeguard the confidentiality of root-cause analysis reports include the following: (1) stamp "confidential and privileged" on every page of a sentinel event report, (2) to ensure peer review privilege, have all documents developed by qualified peer review committee members, (3) if the hospital's attorney can establish that the document is protected as "attorney work—product in anticipation of litigation" or "attorney/client privileged information," have each root-cause analysis reviewed by counsel, (4) keep the report generic by not identifying the patient or provider, (5) remove identifications in reports to JCAHO, and (6) consult the legal council if JCAHO requires a review of root-cause analysis to confirm that the information remains protected (Briefings on JCAHO, April 1998, p. 7). The Health Care Quality Improvement Act of 1986 provides basic protection for physicians who participate in peer review. JCAHO is trying to get further legislation to protect peer review information. In the meantime, many hospitals are hiring external third-party peer reviewers to conduct the peer review because hospitals can indemnify the outside reviewers to protect them from any legal liability (Briefings on JCAHO, September 1998, p. 7).

Sentinel events could include but are not limited to death or major permanent loss associated with a medication error; inpatient suicide; elopement; any procedure performed on the wrong patient, wrong side, or wrong body part; perinatal death; assault or homicide; patient falls; or hemolytic transfusion reaction involving blood group incompatibilities. Other high-risk areas include infant abduction, restraints/seclusion, and falls (JCAHO, BOJ's guide to 1999 standards and scoring, p. 13).

OUTCOME AND ASSESSMENT INFORMATION SET

The Outcome and Assessment Information Set (OASIS) is a group of data elements that (1) represent core items of a comprehensive assessment for adult home care patients and (2) form the basis for measuring patient outcomes for purposes of outcome-based quality improvement (OBQI). It is a major component of Medicare's partnership with home care. It is intended to foster and monitor improved home health care outcomes and to be an integral part of the revised conditions of Participation for Medicare-certified home health agencies (HHAs). It was developed over a 10-year period, with most data items derived from an HCFA-funded national research program that was co-funded by the Robert Wood Johnson Foundation to develop a system of outcome measurement for home health care. The items were then refined through iterations of clinical and empirical research, with additional items that were deemed essential for patient assessment added later by a work group of home health care experts. OASIS data can be used for the following: (1) to measure patient outcomes, (2) to do patient assessment and care planning for individual adult patients, (3) to prepare aggregate statistics, and (4) to facilitate performance improvement. HCFA has ruled that HHAs are to collect OASIS data and are to report that data to their state survey agency. OASIS data are to be electronically transmitted to the state system. State agencies are responsible for collecting and preparing OASIS data for retrieval by a central repository (HCFA Web site, accessed February 18, 1999).

RISK MANAGEMENT

Health care risk management is quite new. Losses were low before 1965, when the case of Darling v. Charleston Community Memorial Hospital set a precedent for holding hospitals directly liable for failure of administrators or staff to properly monitor and supervise health care delivery in the hospital. States also began to liberalize their workers' compensation laws into no-fault programs that facilitated an increase in claim settlements. Hospitals then started creating alternatives to commercial malpractice insurance including self-insurance. Medicare required self-insured hospitals to have risk management programs. The Joint Commission started requiring risk management programs in 1989. Several states require reporting of any event that resulted in harm to the safety or life of a patient or employee (Vestal, 1995).

Risk management involves the development and implementation of strategies to prevent patient injury, minimize financial loss, and preserve agency assets. Risk management focuses on liability control. It assesses areas in which claims can be prevented. By reducing the frequency and severity of injuries to patients, the likelihood of litigation can be decreased and litigation costs lessened. The risk management process includes risk identification, analysis, treatment, evaluation, and follow-up (Stull and Pinkerton, 1988).

The first step in risk management is identifying potential risks for accidents, injury, and financial loss. Energy should be put into preventive activities such as providing a safe physical environment, fostering customer satisfaction, and providing high-quality service. The present institution-wide monitoring system should be reviewed. The completeness of the monitoring system should be evaluated, including audits, committee minutes, incidence reports, patient questionnaires, and oral complaints. Whether additional systems need to be implemented to provide data for risk management control should be determined.

After data have been collected, they should be analyzed to determine the frequency and severity of problems in general categories. Then a plan to reduce the risks as much as possible should be developed and implemented. Safety procedures should be reviewed, and laws and codes related to patient care, consent, and safety should be monitored. Needs for personnel, patient, and family education should be identified and education implemented. The results of the risk management program should be evaluated and reported to appropriate groups. Risk management programs should include customer satisfaction, safety and security, continuous quality improvement, and liability control (Decker and Sullivan, 1992; Grohar-Murray and DiCroce, 1997; Marrelli, 1993; Martin and Tate, 1997; Paolella, 1995; Rocchicciolo and Tilbury, 1998; Yandrick, 1996; Yoder-Wise, 1999).

CUSTOMER SATISFACTION

The dissatisfied customer is the one most likely to pursue litigation. Therefore it is important to identify incidents that might lead to claims, educate patients and their families about the care, and handle patient complaints. To handle complaints, listen and let the patients express themselves before speaking. Do not become defensive. Avoid reacting emotionally. Negotiate. Ask for the patient's expectations and explain what you can or cannot do. Agree on actions to be taken and a time frame. Follow through. A caring attitude can be very effective. It is also important to teach personnel about customer relations and how to prevent and handle complaints.

SAFETY AND SECURITY

A safety and security program should provide safety for patients, their families and other visitors, and personnel. Risks from custodial negligence should be controlled. There should be plans for natural disasters, fire, electrical shock, and power loss. There should be an equipment maintenance program (Stull and Pinkerton, 1988).

National Safety Council

The safety movement began in ancient times with the Egyptians, Greeks, and Romans, and in the Middle Ages guidelines were established regarding working conditions. The safety movement became a major force in industry during the Industrial Revolution. In 1913 the National Council for Industrial Safety (later renamed the National Safety Council) was founded. It developed a forum to develop national standards. Other groups also formed and started keeping statistics on accident and injury rates in industry.

Occupational diseases and safety issues were identified, and methods to control hazardous and toxic materials and to protect the people who handle them were developed. On-the-job safety issues received serious attention. Since World War II, the safety movement has not only reduced injuries and deaths but has also shown administrators that money spent on safety measures returns a profit of up to several hundred percent.

The National Safety Council encourages cooperation among labor, management, and government to develop legislation and upgrade safety standards. The National Safety Council seeks to improve investigative methods and supports special research projects. Changes in the workforce, new technologies and their hazards, environmental hazards, blood-borne diseases, and drug and alcohol abuse are challenges for the future.

The mission of the National Safety Council is to promote health and protect life by providing assistance, knowledge, and expertise to safety professionals in all areas. Moral responsibility exists in a philosophy of accident prevention. The employer is responsible for ensuring a safe, healthful work environment, and employees are accountable for following safety guidelines and standards (National Safety Council, 1992).

Occupational Safety and Health Act

The purposes of the Occupational Safety and Health Act of 1970 and the Mine Safety and Health Act of 1977 are to ensure safe and healthful working conditions and to preserve the nation's human resources. They established nationwide guidelines and standards for the first time. The Secretary of Labor and the Occupational Review Committee are responsible for administration and enforcement of the acts. Research and education activities are the responsibility of the Secretary of Health and Human Services and are implemented by the National Institute for Occupational Safety and Health (NIOSH). The Assistant Secretary of Labor for Occupational Safety and Health acts as the chief of the Occupational Safety and Health Administration (OSHA). OSHA monitors the following: (1) development of standards about occupational health and safety, (2) development of health and safety regulations, (3) inspections and investigations to check the status of compliance, and (4) citations and proposals for penalties for noncompliance with the standards.

OSHA's primary responsibilities are as follows: (1) to promulgate, modify, and revoke health and safety standards; (2) to approve or reject state plans for programs; (3) to require employers to keep records of safety and health data; (4) to conduct investigations and inspections and to issue citations and propose penalties; (5) to petition the courts to restrain imminent danger situations; and (6) to provide educational programs, consulting, funding for state plans, and statistical records of illnesses, injuries, and accidents.

The Occupational Safety and Health Review Commission (OSHRC) is a three-member quasijudicial board that hears cases when OSHA actions are contested by employees and employers. The committee decisions can be reviewed by state and federal courts.

NIOSH is the federal agency responsible for research, education, and training. The representatives can inspect agencies and ensure compliance but are not authorized to enforce OSHA regulations. The main functions of NIOSH are as follows: (1) to develop educational programs, (2) to develop occupational health and safety standards, and (3) to conduct research. The responsibility to establish research methods and conduct statistics surveys is with the Bureau of Labor Statistics.

With few exceptions, OSHA applies to every employer in all 50 states and all U.S. possessions who has one or more employees and who engages in business affecting commerce. All local, state, and federal government employees and mine operators and their employees are exempt from coverage.

Under OSHA the employer is responsible for providing a safe, healthful work environment and for complying with the applicable standards. The employees must comply with applicable standards. The employer is liable for the state and federal sanctions for violating standards. Employees are subject to their employer's sanctions.

All standards promulgated by OSHA are published in the Federal Register. OSHA requires employers to keep records of all occupational illnesses and accidents and to report either to OSHA or to the state plan within 48 hours. OSHA can grant two types of variances from the standards: temporary and permanent. Employers must show just cause for either variance and inform the employees of the application.

Workplace inspections are usually conducted without prior notice. Investigations of imminent dangers are top priority, followed by catastrophic and fatal accidents, followed by employee complaints regarding hazards and reinspections. General inspection procedures include an opening conference, a walk-through documenting alleged violations, interviews with workers, and a closing session. Citations and penalties vary according to the seriousness of the violation. Violation citations are to be posted near where the violation occurred. If an employer wants to contest a case, the area office that initiated the action should be contacted. OSHA encourages states to assume responsibility for administering and enforcing occupational safety and health laws. Areas needing regulations include but are not limited to blood-borne pathogens, lifting guidelines, confined-space regulations, ergonomic guidelines, respiratory guidelines, and egress.

Administrators need to identify the tasks to be performed, identify the tools necessary, evaluate the environment in which the tasks will be performed, assess the organization in which this takes place, and make necessary changes to provide a safe work environment for the employee (Kavianian and Wentz, 1997; National Safety Council, 1992).

LIABILITY CONTROL

Policies and procedures for handling incidents and claims should be developed and implemented. Some incidents may relate to medication errors, falls, procedures (particularly invasive procedures), patient or family refusal of treatment, and patient or family dissatisfaction with care. Because of the negative connotation of the word incident, some agencies use the term *event, occurrence,* or *situation* instead. Filing an incident report is not admitting guilt. It is reporting something that is not a part of routine care.

It is preferable that incident report forms contain questions that can be answered yes or no or by multiple choice. Narrative should be limited. The observer should give a factual, nonjudgmental account of what was seen, heard, felt, or smelled. No impressions, interpretations, or opinions should be stated. All of the information needed should be in one place.

Documentation is critically important. The quality of the documentation often determines the outcome of lawsuits. Medical records are legal documents that can be introduced in court. Nurses and other personnel must be well versed in accurate and comprehensive documentation. Nurses should also know how to testify in court and how to serve as expert witnesses (Stull and Pinkerton, 1988).

Tort law is the branch of civil law that concerns legal wrongs committed by one person against the person or property of another. Torts may be intentional or unintentional.

Negligence is an unintentional tort that involves harm resulting from the failure of people conducting themselves in reasonable and prudent ways. Carelessness is not thinking before one acts or not paying attention. One can be careful and still be negligent for not acting as prudently as others would in the same circumstances.

Malpractice is negligent acts of people with specialized education. Malpractice reflects negligence, but not all negligence is malpractice. When people are held legally responsible for their negligent acts, they are legally liable and may be required to pay for damages. Medical malpractice refers to the negligent acts of any health care professional when conducting patient care responsibilities. Nursing malpractice refers specifically to nurses conducting their patient care responsibilities. Common causes of malpractice claims against nurses are medication errors from misreading the medication order or not clarifying an incomplete or ambiguous order and technique in giving injections.

Negligent conduct depends on the act itself and the surrounding circumstances, including the following: (1) the nature of the nursing function, (2) the nurse's qualifications to perform the function, (3) the urgency of the situation, and (4) the foreseeable harm if the care is not implemented. The emergency room nurse is not held to the same standards of care expected under more normal circumstances. Being a minor does not exempt a nurse from liability for acts of malpractice, and the nurse's state of mind and physical condition are not considered relevant.

The rule of personal liability means that people are responsible for their own tortious conduct even when someone else may share that liability under some other law. Supervisors will not usually be held liable for the negligent acts of those they supervise because all professional persons are held liable for their own negligent behavior. However, a supervisor may be found guilty of negligence for making an assignment beyond a worker's capabilities without giving adequate supervision in carrying out the delegated functions. If a supervisor believes that certain staffing will jeopardize patient safety and potentially precipitate litigation, the position should be documented and the hospital administrator informed.

The doctrine of respondeat superior applies to the U.S. government because the government has agreed to be sued for negligent acts of its employees under the Federal Tort Claims Act (FTCA). By virtue of special statutory enactments, nurses employed by the Veterans Administration and the U.S. Public Health Service have complete immunity from personal liability for acts of negligence in the implementation of their government responsibilities. However, the aggrieved patients may sue the government for injuries they have sustained. Occupational health nurses are potentially exposed to a greater risk of being sued for negligent conduct than other nurses because of the joint effect of the doctrine of respondeat superior and workers' compensation laws. Workers' compensation laws usually prevent an employee from suing an employer, so the aggrieved employee can sue only the nurse.

A nurse is legally required to implement medical procedures ordered by a licensed physician or a physician assistant acting on behalf of the physician employer unless the nurse has reason to believe harm would result from doing so. Failure to carry out the physician's order will subject the nurse to liability for subsequent harm to the patient if there is not reason to question the order. Consequently, nurses must know how to implement the procedure and the effect of the procedure on the patient. When nurses question physician's orders, they should tactfully question the physician. If the physician is insistent, the nurse should take the matter to the supervisor or responsible hospital official. Patient safety is of utmost concern. The nurse has a legal responsibility not to follow the order when there are reasonable grounds to believe that the action would harm the patient.

Consent is not legally required when immediate care is necessary to save the life and consent cannot be obtained either from the patient or an authorized legal representative. Constructive consent or consent implied by law is effective. Minors are not legally capable of giving valid consent to medical treatment, but minors who live apart from their parents and are married are considered emancipated and are capable of giving consent. The law presumes every adult is mentally competent until adjudicated otherwise. After people have been declared mentally incompetent in a judicial proceeding, they cannot give valid consents. When patients have been deemed clinically incompetent but not legally incompetent, nurses should seek the participation of the patient's next of kin in making decisions. When family members cannot agree, treatment should be postponed until a legal guardian is appointed with the authority to make the necessary medical decisions.

Informed consent is given by the patient who fully understands what is being consented to. Consent may be given orally or in writing. Both are legally effective, but it is advisable to get the consent in writing. The patient must be told the nature of the proposed treatment, alternative treatments possible, and the risks involved to be able to give an informed consent. Liability or negligence can result if the dangers of a procedure are minimized to obtain the patient's consent.

Most false-imprisonment cases in health care involve locking mentally ill patients in their rooms. An agency can be held liable for the conduct of a nurse-employee who unlawfully confines or detains a patient against the patient's will because of the doctrine of respondeat superior.

The plaintiff is the complaining party in a malpractice suit. The defendant is the answering party. All nursing malpractice suits consist of the following elements: (1) a claim that the nurse owed the plaintiff a special duty of care; (2) a claim that the nurse was expected to meet a specific standard of care; (3) a claim that the nurse's failure to meet that standard of care resulted in harm to the patient; and (4) a claim for money damages to compensate the plaintiff for the harm sustained (Bernzweig, 1990).

Battery is an intentional tort involving unpermitted and intentional contacts with one's person or extension of the body to clothing, object in the hand, car, and so forth. A hostile intent of the defendant is not necessary. It is the absence of the plaintiff's consent to the defendant's contact that is the issue. Direct contact with the plaintiff is not necessary, and the personal integrity exists even when the plaintiff is under anesthesia or asleep. The defendant is liable for all harm, including unforseeable consequences from the conduct.

Assault involves mental disturbance of personal integrity, including fright and humiliation. It does not include actual contact.

Grounds for civil actions regarding assault and battery include forcefully handling an unconscious patient, forcing a patient out of bed to walk, forcing a patient to submit to treatment even if a consent had been signed because resistance implies withdrawal of consent, lifting a protesting patient from bed to a stretcher or chair, threatening to strike or striking a child or adult unless in self-defense, and in some states performing alcohol, blood, urine, or other health tests for presumed drunken driving without consent. Some states have implied consent statutes in motor vehicle codes for the privilege of driving. Intentional torts such as assault and battery often are not covered in malpractice insurance.

Nurses have legal obligations to protect the patient's rights to privacy and confidentiality. Privacy is not public. It is secret. Confidential information is not to be divulged even in a court of law. Courts have limited access to patient records and to charter members of the health care team, including all nurses, attending physicians, technicians, orderlies, therapists, social service workers, patient advocates, ward clerks, and assigned house officers. Consultants, chaplains, and students are not charter members and should not participate in rounds, examinations, or conferences about patients unless the patient has given prior permission. Administrative personnel are permitted to review patient records without prior consent for staffing, statistical analysis, and quality of care review. It is recommended that a JCAHO surveyor who will conduct an on-site sentinel event investigation be appointed as an ad hoc member to one of the hospital's peer review committees, making that person a "charter member." Many health care organizations are hiring external third-party peer reviewers to conduct peer reviews because organizations can indemnify the outside consultants to protect them from any legal liability. The attending physician is the only one to retain the right to review the record after discharge without consent of the patient or surrogate. Adequate information needs to be transferred with a patient to guarantee continuity of care. Although the consent of the client is not necessary, it is a good practice. Transfer agreements between the discharging and receiving institutions specifying the exchange of information necessary for continuity of care are appropriate. Advances in technology, computerized medical databases, and telehealth systems have raised concerns about patient privacy and confidentiality of health care information (Dienemann, 1990; Gillies, 1994).

Defamation is verbal or written communication that injures someone's reputation. Oral defamation is slander, and written defamation is libel. Slander is less weighty than libel. It is appropriate for health care organizations to have policies and procedures for how customers can register complaints in an objective and confidential way. Health care organizations have been sued for unfavorable evaluations, termination notices, and information shared with prospective employers (Dienemann, 1990; Douglas, 1996).

There are legal considerations to managing a diverse workforce. People are protected from overt and subtle discrimination by Title VII of the Civil Rights Act of 1964. People have a responsibility to be fair and just. Diversity in language, word meanings, accents, and dialects lead to misunderstanding. People from unassertive cultures may be reluctant to ask questions. Cultural differences can lead to conflict and unfulfilled expectations. Managers can learn about cultural diversity and increase their own sensitivity, role model cultural sensitivity, and develop a comprehensive cultural diversity program for staff (Marquis and Huston, 1998).

TESTIFYING

Testifying under oath can be a terrifying experience, but understanding procedures and a few rules can make the experience less stressful. Appearance is important. One should dress neatly and conventionally. A business suit is usually appropriate. If one is testifying just before, after, or during a shift, a uniform is appropriate.

A pleasant demeanor is also important. One should project a polite, sincere, and cooperative image. One should know the facts before testifying. It is appropriate to review the record, particularly the part one is responsible for. The health care agency record should never be falsified. It may be helpful to make a sketch or diagram if placement of persons and objects is important.

The court recorder records everything said, so one should enunciate clearly. Questions must be answered orally because nodding the head and other nonverbal responses are difficult to record and subject to interpretation. One is likely to be asked for personal and professional information such as residence, age, marital status, educational background, grades received, and employment history. One should be sure the question is understood before answering it. Making an inaccurate response because the question was not understood can adversely affect the outcomes. Pausing before answering the question is appropriate to formulate an answer and to allow time for an attorney to raise objections. If the attorney objects to a question, one should refrain from responding until the issue is resolved. The lawyer will direct the witness if an answer is required. One should keep answers brief, tell the truth, and answer only the question asked. One should try to give favorable facts and avoid such questionable words as think, guess, and maybe. Sometimes matters of amount, distance, and time are crucial. One should not be forced into guessing. If unable to make a reliable judgment, "I don't know" is an appropriate response. When asked to identify an exhibit such as a medical record, one should scrutinize it carefully and indicate whether it is recognized or not. Whoever calls one as a witness has the first opportunity to ask questions. Afterward, the opposing party's attorney has the opportunity to ask questions (Kilmon, 1985).

EXPERT WITNESSES

Because malpractice litigation has increased and physicians are serving as expert witnesses for nursing less than they did before the 1970s, nurses are increasingly acting as expert witnesses. Some state nurses associations are developing resource banks of nurse expert witnesses. Nurses may need to submit a letter of intent describing their qualifications as a nurse expert, résumé, and letters of reference. Some state nurses associations provide continuing education regarding legal issues and being an expert witness to ensure a pool of adequately prepared expert witnesses.

Attorneys often want to meet experts before selecting them. They also need résumés and letters of reference. Attorneys often contact experts by telephone and provide brief case summaries. Then the nurse must decide which cases to accept. The case must match the expert's area of expertise. Experts should review only records that are within their specialty. The expert compares the facts of the case with standards of care and offers a professional opinion. The expert should understand clearly whether the attorney wants the expert to defend the nurse or dispute the nurse's credibility. The cases selected should not involve matters concerning places where the expert has worked or people with whom the expert has worked because the issue of bias could be raised. Fees negotiated should include time required to review the records, write a report, and provide testimony (Salmond, 1986).

CHAPTER SUMMARY

Chapter 15 covered the following:
History of Continuous Quality Improvement
Quality Management Heroes
Continuous Quality Improvement
    Tools and Processes for Continuous Quality Improvement
Program Evaluation
    Calendar of Events
    Committee Selection and Functions
    Conceptual Framework
    Review of the Literature
    Program Evaluation Model
    Instrument Development
    Sources of Internal and External Invalidity
    Research Designs
        Experimental designs
        Quasiexperimental designs
    Methods of Data Collection
    Sampling
    Analysis of Data
History of Regulatory Influences and Changing Regulations
Joint Commission on Accreditation of Healthcare Organizations
Outcome and Assessment Information Set
Risk Management
Customer Satisfaction
Safety and Security
    National Safety Council
    Occupational Safety and Health Act

Liability Control
Testifying
Expert Witnesses

REFERENCES

Aguayo R: *Dr. Deming: the American who taught the Japanese about quality,* New York, 1990, Carol Publishing.

Albrecht S: *Crisis management for corporate self-defense,* New York, 1996, American Management Association.

American Nurses Association: *Nursing care report card for acute care,* Washington, DC, 1995, The Association.

American Nurses Association: *Nursing quality indicators: definitions and implications,* Washington, DC, 1996a, The Association.

American Nurses Association: *Nursing quality indicators: guide for implementation,* Washington, DC, 1996b, The Association.

American Nurses Association: *Standards of clinical nursing practice,* ed 2, Washington, DC, 1998, The Association.

American Nurses Association: *1999 House of Delegates materials,* Washington, DC, 1999, The Association.

Band WA: *Touchstones: ten new ideas revolutionizing business,* New York, 1994, John Wiley & Sons.

Bernzweig EP: *The nurse's liability for malpractice: a programmed course,* St. Louis, 1990, Mosby.

Berwick DM: Sounding board: continuous quality improvement as the ideal in health care, *NEJM* 320(1):53-56, 1989.

Brassard M, Ritter D: *The memory jogger II,* Methuen, Mass, 1994, GOAL/PAC.

Burns N, Grove SK: *The practice of nursing research: conduct, critique, & utilization,* Philadelphia, 1996, WB Saunders.

Campbell DT, Stanley JC: *Experimental and quasi-experimental designs for research,* Chicago, 1963, Rand McNally.

Cofer JI, Greeley HP: *Continuous quality improvement for health information management,* Marblehead, Mass, 1998, Opus Communications.

Crosby PB: *Quality is free: the art of making quality certain,* New York, 1979, McGraw-Hill.

Crosby PB: *Quality without tears: the art of hassle-free management,* New York, 1984, Penguin Group.

Crosby PB: *Let's talk quality,* New York, 1989, McGraw-Hill.

Crosby PB: *Completeness: quality for the 21ˢᵗ century,* New York, 1992, Dutton.

Decker PJ, Sullivan EJ: *Nursing administration: a micro/macro approach for effective nurse executives,* Norwalk, Conn, 1992, Appleton & Lange.

Deming WE: *Quality, productivity, and competitive position,* Cambridge, Mass, 1982, Massachusetts Institute of Technology Press.

Dienemann J: *Nursing administration: strategic perspectives and application,* Norwalk, Conn, 1990, Appleton & Lange.

Donabedian A: Criteria and standards for quality assessment and monitoring, *Qual Rev Bull* 3:99-108, 1986.

Douglas LM: *The effective nurse leader and manager,* ed 5, St. Louis, 1996, Mosby.

Foley M and the Center for Labor Relations: *Key terms in collective bargaining,* Washington, DC, American Nurses Association.

Fuller J: *Managing performance improvement projects: preparing, planning, and implementing,* San Francisco, 1997, Pfeiffer.

Gift RG, Mosel D: *Benchmarking in health care: a collaborative approach,* Chicago, 1994, American Hospital Publishing.

Gillies DA: *Nursing management: a systems approach,* ed 3, Philadelphia, 1994, WB Saunders.

Grohar-Murray ME, DiCroce HR: *Leadership and management in nursing,* Stamford, Conn, 1997, Appleton & Lange.

Hagan J: *Management of quality: strategies to improve quality and the bottom line,* New York, 1994, Business One Irwin.

Hammer M: *Beyond reengineering: how the process-centered organization is changing our work and our lives,* New York, 1996, HarperBusiness.

Harbour JL: *The process reengineering workbook: practical steps to working faster and smarter through process improvement,* White Plains, NY, 1994, Quality Resources.

Health Care Financing Administration: *OASIS overview* (http://www.hcfa.gov/medicare/hsqb/oasis/hhoview.htm), accessed Feb. 18, 1999.

Hein EC: *Contemporary leadership behavior: selected readings,* ed 5, Philadelphia, 1998, Lippincott.

Huber D: *Leadership and nursing care management,* Philadelphia, 1996, WB Saunders.

Hunt VD: *Managing for quality: integrating quality and business strategy,* Homewood, Ill, 1993, Business One Irwin.

Jackson M, Twaddle G: *Business process implementation: building workflow systems,* Reading, Mass, 1997, Addison-Wesley.

Joint Commission on Accreditation of Healthcare Organizations: *Transitions from QA to CQI,* Oakbrook Terrace, Ill, 1991, JCAHO.

Joint Commission on Accreditation of Healthcare Organizations: *Briefings on JCAHO,* Oakbrook Terrace, Ill, June 1996-April 1999, JCAHO.

Joint Commission on Accreditation of Healthcare Organizations: *Briefings on JCAHO: BOJ's guide to 1999 standards and scoring,* Mablehead, Mass, 1999, Opus Communications.

Joint Commission on Accreditation of Healthcare Organizations: *CAMH: comprehensive accreditation manual for hospitals—the official handbook,* CAMH Updates, Oakbrook Terrace, Ill, Jan 1998-Feb 1999, JCAHO.

Jones JW: *High-speed management: time-based strategies for managers and organizations,* San Francisco, 1992, Jossey-Bass.

Juran JM: Product quality: a prescription for the West. Part I. training and improvement programs, *Man Rev* 70:8-14, 1981.

Juran JM: *Juran on planning for quality,* New York, 1988, Free Press.

Juran JM: *Juran on leadership for quality: an executive handbook,* New York, 1989, Free Press.

Juran JM: *Juran on quality by design: the new steps for planning quality into goods and services,* New York, 1992, Free Press.

Juran JM, Goyna FM Jr, Bingham RS Jr, editors: *Quality control handbook,* New York, 1979, McGraw-Hill.

Karlof B, Ostblom S: *Benchmarking: a signpost to excellence in quality productivity,* New York, 1993, John Wiley & Sons.

Kavianian JR, Wentz CA: *Occupational and environmental safety engineering and management,* New York, 1997, John Wiley & Sons.

Kilmon EL: Do you swear to tell the truth? *Nurs Econ* 3:98-102, March-April 1985.

King B, Schlicksupp H: *Idea edge: transforming creative thought into organizational excellence,* Methuen, Mass, 1998, GOAL/QPC.

Kirk R: *Managing outcomes, process, and cost in a managed care environment,* Gaithersburg, Md, 1997, Aspen.

Koch MW, Fairly TM: *Integrated quality management: the key to improving nursing care quality,* St. Louis, 1993, Mosby.

Kreider NA, Haselton BJ: *The systems challenge: getting the clinical information support you need to improve patient care,* Chicago, 1997, American Hospital Publishing.

Land G, Jarman B: *Breakpoint and beyond: mastering the future—today,* New York, 1992, HarperBusiness.

Lerbinger O: *The crisis manager: facing risk and responsibility,* Mahwah, NJ, 1997, Lawrence Erlbaum Associates.

Loveridge CE, Cummings SH: *Nursing management in the new paradigm,* Gaithersburg, Md, 1996, Aspen.

Marquis BL, Huston CJ: *Leadership roles and management functions in nursing: theory and application,* ed 2, Philadelphia, 1996, Lippincott.

Marquis BL, Huston CJ: *Management decision making for nurses: 124 case studies,* Philadelphia, 1998, Lippincott.

Marrelli TM: *The nurse manager's survival guide: practical answers to everyday problems,* St. Louis, 1993, Mosby.

Martin J: *The great transition: using the seven disciplines of enterprise engineering to align people, technology, and strategy,* New York, 1995, American Management Association.

Martin P, Tate K: *Project management memory jogger,* Methuen, Mass, 1997, GOAL/PAC.

McCloskey LA, Collett DN: *A primer guide to total quality management,* Salem, NH, 1993, GOAL/QPC.

Mears P: *Healthcare teams: building continuous quality improvements,* Delray Beach, Fla, 1994, St Lucie Press.

National League for Nursing: *National League for Nursing 1998 annual report,* New York, 1998, The League.

National Safety Council: *Accident prevention manual for business and industry,* Chicago, 1992, The Council.

Nicholas JM: *Competitive manufacturing management: continuous improvement, lean production, customer-focused quality,* Boston, 1998, Irwin McGraw Hill.

Oddo F, editor: *Coach's guide to the memory jogger II,* Methuen, Mass, 1995, GOAL/QPC.

Paolella MA: *Auditing health care benefits: how to manage costs and minimize risk,* New York, 1995, John Wiley & Sons.

Phillips JJ: *Handbook of training evaluation and measurement methods,* ed 3, Houston, 1997, Gulf.

Polit-O'Hara D, Hunger BP, Polit DF: *Essentials of nursing research: methods, appraisals, and utilization,* Philadelphia, 1996, Lippincott-Raven.

Ritter D, Brassard M: *The creativity tools memory jogger: a pocket guide for creative thinking,* Lawrence, Mass, 1998, GOAL/PAC.

Rocchiccioli JT, Tilbury MS: *Clinical leadership in nursing,* Philadelphia, 1998, WB Saunders.

Saba VK, McCormick KA: *Essentials of computers for nurses,* ed 2, New York, 1996, McGraw-Hill.

Salmond SW: Serving as an expert witness, *Nurs Econ* 4:236-239, Sept-Oct 1986.

Sandras WA: *Just-in-time: making it happen,* Essex Junction, Vt, 1989, Oliver Wright.

Smith R: *The 7 levels of change: create, innovate and motivate with the secrets of the world's largest corporations,* Arlington, Tex, 1997, Summit.

Stowell DM: *Sales, marketing, and continuous improvement: six best practices to achieve revenue growth and increase customer loyalty,* San Francisco, 1997, Jossey-Bass.

Stull MK, Pinkerton SE: *Current strategies for nurse administrators,* Rockville, Md, 1988, Aspen.

Swansburg RC: *Management and leadership for nurse managers,* ed 2, Boston, 1996, Jones & Bartlett.

Swansburg RC, Swansburg RJ: *Introductory management and leadership for nurses: an interactive text,* Boston, 1999, Jones & Bartlett.

Tappen RM: *Nursing leadership and management: concepts and practice,* ed 3, Philadelphia, 1995, FA Davis.

Thomas PR, Gallace LJ, Martin KR: *Quality alone is not enough,* New York, 1992, American Management Association.

Ulrich D: *Human resource champions: the next agenda for adding value and delivering results,* Boston, 1997, Harvard Business School Press.

Vestal KW: *Nursing management: concepts and issues,* ed 2, Philadelphia, 1995, Lippincott.

Walton M: *The Deming management method,* New York, 1986, Putnam.

Walton M: *Deming management at work,* New York, 1990, Putnam's Sons.

Wheatley M: *Understanding just in time,* Hauppauge, NY, 1997, Barron's.

White House Domestic Policy Council: *Health security: the president's report to the American people,* Washington, DC, 1993, The White House Domestic Policy Council.

Yandrick RM: *Behavioral risk management: how to avoid preventable losses from mental health problems in the workplace,* San Francisco, 1996, Jossey-Bass.

Yoder-Wise PS: *Leading and managing in nursing,* ed 2, St. Louis, 1999, Mosby.

BIBLIOGRAPHY

Arikian VL: Total quality management: applications to nursing service, *JONA* 21:46-50, June 1991.

Blue CL: Preventing back injury among nurses, *Orthop Nurs* 15:9-22, Nov-Dec 1996.

Bobnet NL, Ilcyn J, Milanovich PS et al.: Continuous quality improvement: improving quality in your home care organization, *JONA* 23:42-48, Feb 1993.

Breda KL: Professional nurses in unions: working together pays off, *J Prof Nurs* 13:99-109, March-April 1997.

Burns JP: Performance improvement with patient service partners, *JONA* 28:31-37, Jan 1998.

Chally PS, Loriz L: Ethics in the trenches: decision making in practice: a practical model for resolving the types of ethical dilemmas you face daily, *AJN* 98(6):17-20.

Collins JC, Porras JI: *Built to last: successful habits of visionary companies,* New York, 1997, HarperBusiness.

DiBenedetto DV: Occupational hazards of the health care industry: protecting health care workers, *AAOHN J* 43:131-137, March 1995.

Dienemann J: *Continuous quality improvement in nursing,* Washington, DC, 1992, American Nurses Association.

Dowd K: *Beyond value at risk: the new science of risk management,* New York, 1998, John Wiley & Sons.

Edwards JE et al.: *How to conduct organizational surveys,* Thousand Oaks, Calif, 1997, Sage Publications.

Elliott PP: Violence in health care: what nurse managers need to know, *Nurs Manage* 28:38-42, Dec 1997.

Ellis JR, Hartley CL: *Managing and coordinating nursing care,* ed 2, Philadelphia, 1995, Lippincott.

Elnitsky C, Nichols B, Palmer K: Are hospital incidents being reported? *JONA* 27:40-46, Nov 1997.

Hardy VS, Forrer J: A comprehensive quality management approach, *Nurs Manage* 27:35, 38, Jan 1996.

Harwood CC: *Kick down the door of complacency: seize the power of continuous improvement,* Boca Raton, Fla, 1998, St. Lucie Press.

Huda A, Wise LC: Evolution of compliance within a fall prevention program, *J Nurs Care Qual* 12:55-63, Feb 1998.

Ingersoll GL: Evaluation research, *Nurs Adm Q* 20:28-39, Summer 1996.

Johnson JH, Olesinsi N: Program evaluation: key to success, *JONA* 25:53-60, Jan 1995.

Karas BE, Conrad KM: Back injury prevention interventions in the workplace: an integrative review, *AAOHN J* 44:189-196, April 1996.

Kim KT, Graves PB, Safadi GS et al.: Implementation recommendations for making health care facilities latex safe, *AORN J* 67:615-616, 618, 621-624, March 1998.

Kobs A: A 'sourcebook' for leaders, *Nurs Manage* 29:23-25, Aug 1998.

Lawler EE III: *From the ground up: six principles for building the new logic corporation,* San Francisco, 1996, Jossey-Bass.

Lawler EE III, Mohrman SA, Ledford GE Jr: *Creating high performance organizations: practices and results of employee involvement and total quality management in fortune 1000 companies,* San Francisco, 1995, Jossey-Bass.

Lippman H: Legally speaking: expect to hear about unions, *RN* 54:67-72, Oct 1991.

Mandler TY, Gordon MS: When does a nurse become a "supervisor" under federal law? *Recruit Reten Restruct Rep* 10:5-7, March-April 1997.

Mapel L: Nursing unions: are they necessary? *Kansas Nurs* 71:1-2, April 1996.

Mark BA, Sayler J, Smith CS: A theoretical model for nursing systems outcomes research, *Nurs Adm Q* 20(4):12-27, 1996.

McCloskey JC, Mass M, Huber DG et al.: Nursing management innovations: a need for systematic evaluation, *Nurs Econ* 12:35-42, Jan-Feb 1994.

McKeon T: Performance measurement: integrating quality management and activity-based cost management, *JONA* 26:45-51, April 1996.

Meyer C: *Fast cycle time: how to align purpose, strategy, and structure for speed,* New York, 1993, Free Press.

O'Neil E, Coffman J, editors: *Strategies for the future of nursing: changing roles, responsibilities, and employment patterns of registered nurses,* San Francisco, 1998, Jossey-Bass.

Phillips JJ: *Return on investment in training and performance improvement programs,* Houston, 1997, Gulf.

Reiley P, Seibert CP, Miller NE et al.: Implementation of a collaborative quality assessment program, *JONA* 24:65-71, May 1994.

Rummler GA, Brache AP: *Improving performance: how to manage the white space on the organization chart,* San Francisco, 1995, Jossey-Bass.

Sapin BJ, Nguyen B: Are you protected under the NLRA? ANA fights to safeguard RNs' right to speak out, organize . . . *Nurs Trends Issues* 2:1-10, July 1997.

Schaffer RH: *The breakthrough strategy: using short-term successes to build the high performance organization,* New York, 1988, HarperBusiness.

Schultz AW: Evaluation of a clinical advancement system, *JONA* 23:13-19, Feb 1993.

Sherman JJ, Malkmus MA: Integrating quality assurance and total quality management/quality improvement, *JONA* 24:37-41, March 1994.

Smith HL, Discenza R, Piland NF: Reflections on total quality management and health care supervisors, *Health Care Superv* 12:32-45. 1993.

Smith PW, Rusnak PG: SHEA/APIC position paper. Infection prevention and control in the long-term-care facility, *Infect Control Hosp Epidemiol* 18:831-849, Dec 18, 1997.

Stahl DA: Managing risks in subacute care, *Nurs Manage* 28:26-27, Oct 1997.

Verhey MP, Ferretti CK: Quality management in a school-based nursing center: program development and implementation, *J Nurs Care Qual* 10(3):59-67, 1996.

Wakefield BJ et al.: Research utilization: nurses' perceptions of why medication administration errors occur, *MEDSURG Nurs* 7:39-44, Feb 1998.

Warren IB, Rozell BR: Supplemental staffing: nurse manager views of costs, benefits, and quality of care, *JONA* 25:51-57, June 1995.

Western P: QA/AI and nursing competence: a combined model, *Nurs Manage* 25:44-46, March 1994.

Yandrick RM: *Behavioral risk management: how to avoid preventable losses from mental health problems in the workplace,* San Francisco, 1996, Jossey-Bass.

Zabel AM, McGrew AB: Ergonomics: a key component in a CTD control program, *AAOHN J* 45:350-360, July 1997.

CASE STUDY

You are the evening charge nurse caring for 20 critically ill patients with the help of one LPN and two aides. There are many medications and treatments to give. You do not think it is possible for you and the LPN to do all of the medications and treatments and do not believe the aides are qualified to do most of the work that needs to be done. What are you going to do?

Critical Thinking Activities for this chapter begin on page 524.

APPENDIX

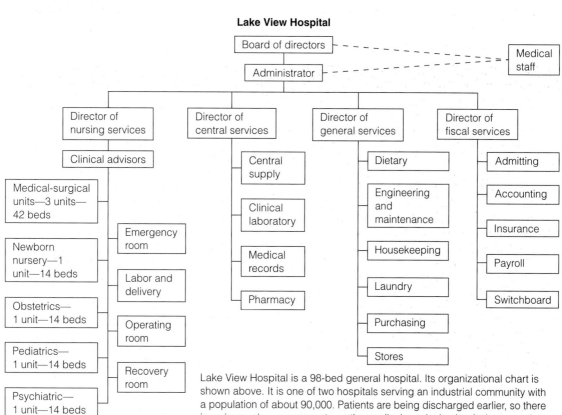

Lake View Hospital

Board of directors — — — — — — — — — — — Medical staff

Administrator — — — — — — — — — — —

Director of nursing services | Director of central services | Director of general services | Director of fiscal services

Clinical advisors

Medical-surgical units—3 units—42 beds

Newborn nursery—1 unit—14 beds

Obstetrics—1 unit—14 beds

Pediatrics—1 unit—14 beds

Psychiatric—1 unit—14 beds

Emergency room

Labor and delivery

Operating room

Recovery room

Central supply

Clinical laboratory

Medical records

Pharmacy

Dietary

Engineering and maintenance

Housekeeping

Laundry

Purchasing

Stores

Admitting

Accounting

Insurance

Payroll

Switchboard

Lake View Hospital is a 98-bed general hospital. Its organizational chart is shown above. It is one of two hospitals serving an industrial community with a population of about 90,000. Patients are being discharged earlier, so there is an increasing vacancy rate on the medical-surgical units. At the same time there is an increasing demand for geriatric services and ambulatory care. Demands for home health have also increased.

Organizational chart for Lake View Hospital

INDEX

Page numbers followed by *b* indicate boxes, those followed by *t* indicate tables, and those followed by *f* indicate figures.

CHAPTER 1: COMMUNICATIONS

1. Reflective Journal: Make observations in a clinical setting or reflect on past experiences. What communication system is in place? Describe it. Interview a staff nurse or manager about what barriers to communication are problems. Ask a staff nurse or manager what she thinks could be done to improve communications. What type of difficult people are involved? How are people dealing with them? How might they better deal with them? What do you think are the barriers to communication and what could be done to improve communications? Do transactional analysis on some interactions you have observed. What games have you observed during a certain time at a specific place?

2. Computer Activity: Look for related articles and information on the Web. Share your findings with colleagues.

3. Use Worksheet 1-1, "Distinguishing Between Facts and Inferences."

4. Draw five squares connected differently on each of two pages. One person stands with her back to the class and describes how the squares are connected. Classmates are to draw squares as described without feedback. A second person stands facing the class and describes how five squares are connected. Classmates are to draw the squares as described. Questions and answers are allowed. Compare the accuracy of both methods. Was there a difference? If so, which method produced the more accurate outcomes?

5. Using Worksheet 1-2, note the additions, deletions, and distortions as a story is told from one volunteer to another.

6. Using Worksheet 1-3, choose how you would handle a rumor about cutting wages. If possible, form a small group(s). Students explain the rationale for their choices one by one around the group and then try to come to consensus.

7. In class write scenarios for working with difficult people. What might be the causes of their behavior? How should you handle it as it is occurring? Assume roles with classmates and role-play how to handle difficult people, using Worksheet 1-4.

8. Keep a diary of some of your interactions with others. Do transactional analysis on them and analyze whether you were passive, aggressive, or assertive. If you were passive or aggressive, decide how you could have behaved assertively.

9. Write a script for the use of broken record and role-play it with a classmate. Write additional scripts as desired and role-play them.

10. Someone is criticizing the nursing staff and the institution in general. Write a script for using negative inquiry and role-play it with a classmate.

Worksheet 1-1

Distinguishing Between Facts and Inferences

A fact is information that can be verified. An inference is a statement that seems to be factual but needs to be verified by information that is not readily available. When inferences are mistaken for facts, communication shortcuts occur and the receiver assumes things that are not stated nor intended. This interferes with effective communications. In the story below, you will see how difficult it is to distinguish a fact from an inference and how easily people can jump to conclusions.

Anderson, the manager, called to an employee who was coming through the ward door 15 minutes after starting time. Anderson asked the employee to come into her office and said:

> I am glad to see that you were able to make it in today despite the transportation problems. I have been thinking about talking to you concerning your many latenesses and absences. As you know, we have specific rules here that say an employee must call in if she expects to be more than 10 minutes late. I have to begin to take some corrective steps when an employee is late more than three times in any 1 month. I know that getting the two children to school sometimes makes it difficult for you to come in on time, but still I must ask you to do something to avoid this situation in the future. The rules provide for a written warning and then suspension before dismissal. If you continue to be absent or late, I will have to follow these rules much as I would regret to do that. Please help me avoid such unpleasantness.

You may refer back to the story. Without discussion, decide whether you would classify each statement as a "fact" or an "inference." Indicate your decision by placing an x in the appropriate space. Try to finish within 3 minutes. Then group participants discuss why they chose "fact" or "inference."

	Fact	Inference
1. The employee to whom the story referred was late that day.		
2. The employee is a woman.		
3. There were transportation problems affecting the employee that day.		
4. The employee has two children.		
5. The employee takes the two children to school.		
6. The manager needs to give the employee a written warning.		

Worksheet 1-2

Rumor Observation Form

Five volunteers should leave the room. The leader calls in the first volunteer and reads the following statement after saying, "I just saw the accident but cannot wait to report it because I am due at work":

> The ambulance, heading west, was turning right at the intersection to go to the hospital when a red sports car convertible, heading east, attempted to turn left. When the drivers noticed that they were both turning into the same lane, they both honked their horns but continued to turn without slowing down. In fact, the sports car seemed to speed up just before the crash.

The first volunteer calls in the second and tells the story. Then the second volunteer calls in the third and tells the story, and so on until the fourth volunteer reports the accident to the fifth volunteer, the policeman. The audience notes the additions, deletions, and distortions with each reporting and then discusses the findings.

Volunteer	Additions	Deletions	Distortions
1.			
2.			
3.			
4.			
5.			

From *A handbook of structured experiences for human relations training*, Volume II, J. William Pfeiffer and John E. Jones, Editors, La Jolla: University Associates Publishers, Inc. 1974.

Worksheet 1-3

Managing Rumors

The institution where you are working is rightsizing. Productivity is being evaluated. A rumor that wages are going to be cut is circulating. Anxiety is increasing, and negative behavior is developing. As the manager, how will you handle this situation?

a. Play it cool and hope the rumor will be discovered to be false.
b. Let the rumor starters stop it.
c. Use influential people.
d. Hold a departmental meeting.
e. Use formal notice.
f. Start a counter-rumor.
g. Spread the word through the supervisors.

Working With Difficult People

Plan strategies for dealing with difficult people.

	Strategies
Hostile-aggressive	
Complaining	
Negative	
Unresponsive	
Overly nice	

CHAPTER 2: STRESS MANAGEMENT

1. Reflective Journal: Identify what time and stress management techniques you are using. Review others and decide if there are others you should try. Plan your strategies for experimenting with additional time and stress management techniques. Write your personal mission statement. Identify up to seven roles. Identify up to four goals for each role. Schedule your priorities into your calendar.

2. Computer Activity: Look for information about stress management, time management, and delegation on the Web. Share your findings with colleagues.

3. Create a scenario or consider a real situation and use Worksheet 2-1 to plan effective delegation.

4. Using Worksheets 2-2 and 2-3, list your major stressors and the symptoms that indicate that you are stressed. Reflect on your major stressors and consider ways to prevent stress, such as leaving the house a few minutes earlier to avoid heavy traffic or getting a credit card so you do not have to worry about having enough cash when you need to buy gas for the car.

5. Look at the list of values in Worksheet 2-4 and indicate whether each one is of high, medium, or low value to you.

6. Write three of your goals. Evaluate each one for its consistency with your values.

7. Pause for a moment and think about how you are feeling: calm, excited, happy, hopeful, or satisfied; or angry, anxious, confused, depressed, embarrassed, or frustrated.

8. Look at the jokes in the newspaper. Start a file of jokes and review it periodically. Watch a situation comedy on television. Go to a funny movie or read a funny book.

9. To practice time management, record what you do every 15 minutes for a typical week and assess how you spent your time. Identify time wasters.

10. Set a goal and plan strategies to accomplish it.

11. Assess your peak and low times and plan your schedule.

12. Prepare a daily "to do" list.

Worksheet 2-1

Effective Delegation Tool

1. Identify the task to be accomplished:

2. Identify the skill or educational level needed to complete the job:

3. Identify the person best able to complete the job in terms of capability and time available:

4. Write a clear description of what you want the employee to do:

5. Identify the outcome you expect and by when:

6. Describe the degree of responsibility and authority that the employee will have:

After presenting the necessary information to the employee, have her repeat what has been delegated.

Worksheet 2-2

Stressors

List your major stressors:

School/work: Personal:

1.   1.

2.   2.

3.   3.

4.   4.

5.   5.

Worksheet 2-3

Symptoms of Stress

List the symptoms that indicate you are stressed:

1.

2.

3.

4.

5.

Now list strategies you might employ to help you manage your stress. Describe why each strategy might work well for you.

1.

2.

3.

4.

5.

Worksheet 2-4

Values

Rate the values listed below as high, medium, or low value to you.

Value	High	Medium	Low
Affection			
Duty			
Expertise			
Health			
Independence			
Leadership			
Parenthood			
Pleasure			
Power			
Prestige			
Security			
Self-realization			
Service			
Wealth			

CHAPTER 3: DECISION-MAKING PROCESS AND TOOLS

1. Reflective Journal: Make observations in a clinical setting or reflect on past experiences. Answer the following questions: What creative thinking techniques have you observed being used? What decision-making tools have you observed being used? How are ethical issues addressed in an agency with which you are familiar? What departments are represented? Is there a nurse member on this committee? How does the committee function?

2. Computer Activity: Look for information about the various decision-making tools and related topics on the Web. Share your findings with colleagues.

3. Using Worksheet 3-1, problem solve the situation in the case study about personnel raises on p. 74.

4. Using Worksheet 3-2, determine what your decision in the case study about personnel raises on p. 74 might be given different ethical viewpoints.

5. Identify a problem or try to generate a list of uses for a pencil. Divide the class in half. Half the class uses brainstorming to solve the problem or generate a list of uses for a pencil. The other half uses brainwriting for the same assignment. Compare the results. Discuss your feelings about using the techniques.

6. Do some self-assessing and determine your own level of moral development—premoral, conventional, or autonomous.

7. Develop a Gantt chart to do an assignment, prepare for a test, do your housework, or perform a similar task. Write the steps that must be accomplished down the left side of the page. Put a time frame across the top of the page. Put a line through the grid when the step is in process and an X where it is completed.

8. Draw a PERT chart for the activities involved with a new addition to a health care facility. Consider completion of the building; ordering equipment and supplies; recruitment, selection, and orientation of staff; development of goals; development of budget; and admission of the first patients.

9. Use a decision tree to decide when and where to have a unit holiday party. Consider your alternatives, such as having the party in the afternoon or evening; having it at the health care agency, a private residence, or a public place; including only those employed at the agencies or including their families as well. Estimate the probable consequences. See Figure 3-2 on p. 65 and 3-3 on p. 66 as examples.

Worksheet 3-1

Problem-Solving Tool

Define the problem:

Explore alternatives and expected results from each alternative. Consider the time to implement, cost of implementation, and probability of acceptance of the implementation.

What is the most desirable alternative?

Ethical Decisions

Given a problem, what would your decision be using the following ethical philosophies?

Utilitarianism—greatest amount of good and happiness for the most people or least amount of harm

Egoism—best for oneself without regard for others

Formalism—golden rule

Rule ethics—obedience to laws, rules, professional codes, and authority

Fairness—benefit to the least advantaged

CHAPTER 4: MOTIVATION AND MORALE

1. Reflective Journal: Reflect on several motivation theories and identify which one explains what motivates you the best. Explain why. Do any not apply to you? If so, what? Ask a nurse manager what she does to motivate workers. Ask some colleagues what motivates them.

2. Computer Activity: Look for information about the various motivation theories on the Web. Share your findings with colleagues.

3. List five needs that you have now and place them in Maslow's classification.

4. Place those same needs in Alderfer's classification.

5. Make two columns on a sheet of paper. In one column list what was happening when you had job satisfaction. In the second column list what was happening when you had job dissatisfaction. Do these lists support Herzberg's theory or not?

6. Using Worksheet 4-1, identify the valence and expectancy of three things you want. How do they affect your motivation?

7. Think about something you need to do. Do you receive any reinforcement for doing it? How does the response you get affect your motivation?

8. Have you ever felt you were being treated inequitably? If so, how did you respond? Was your behavior consistent with equity theory?

9. Review the list of beliefs in McGregor's Theory X and Theory Y. How do you classify your philosophy?

Valence, Expectancy, and Motivation

List three things that you want, and then identify the valence, expectancy, and motivation of each.

Want	Valence	Expectancy	Motivation

CHAPTER 5: POWER, POLITICS, NEGOTIATIONS, AND LABOR RELATIONS

1. Reflective Journal: Make observations in a clinical setting or reflect on past experiences. What is your major source of power? What is the major source of power for someone else you know? Have you ever communicated with a legislator? If so, how? How might you get more involved in politics? Have you participated in a negotiation or observed negotiations? If so, were hard and/or soft tactics used? Were principled negotiations used? If so, how? Were dirty tricks used? If so, what ones? How did they work? Have you observed aspects of collective bargaining? What happened?

2. Computer Activity: Look up information about power, politics, negotiations, and/or labor relations on the Web. Share your findings with colleagues.

3. Using Worksheet 5-1, identify your sources of power and make a list of those sources.

4. Form a small group in class. Develop a scenario of a situation that requires negotiations. Choose sides and practice principled negotiations.

5. Using Worksheet 5-2, identify strategies for negotiating with parties in each quadrant.

6. Form small groups and discuss the manager's role in the four phases of unionization. Use Worksheet 5-3 to help you identify the characteristics of the four phases.

7. Outline the decertification process by using Worksheet 5-4.

8. Interview a union member about the pros and cons of unions. Use Worksheet 5-5 to help you identify the pros and cons of the collective bargaining process in general.

Worksheet 5-1

Sources of Power

List your sources of power.

1.

2.

3.

4.

5.

6.

7.

8.

Worksheet 5-2

Negotiating Strategies

Using the following grid, identify strategies for negotiating with parties with differing amounts of agreement and trust.

	High agreement	Low agreement
Trust	1.	1.
	2.	2.
	3.	3.
	4.	4.
	5.	5.
Distrust	1.	1.
	2.	2.
	3.	3.
	4.	4.
	5.	5.

Worksheet 5-3

Phases of Unionization

Describe four phases of unionization.

Phase 1:

Phase 2:

Phase 3:

Phase 4:

Worksheet 5-4

Decertification Process

Outline the steps in the decertification process.

Step 1:

Step 2:

Worksheet 5-5

Advantages and Disadvantages of Collective Bargaining

Identify advantages and disadvantages of collective bargaining:

Advantages	Disadvantages
1.	1.
2.	2.
3.	3.
4.	4.
5.	5.
6.	6.
7.	7.
8.	8.

CHAPTER 6: CONFLICT MANAGEMENT

1. Reflective Journal: Reflect on an organizational setting. What are the most common sources of conflict in that setting? How do people respond to the conflict? What kind of conflict do you have in your life? How do you handle it? What might you do differently to get even better results?

2. Computer Activity: Look up information related to conflict on the Web. Share your findings with colleagues.

3. Think of a situation in which you have had to deal with conflict. What were the sources of conflict? Would avoiding, accommodating, compromising, collaborating, or competing be the best way to deal with the conflict? What would be symptoms if you used the chosen mode too much?

4. Form a small group in class and use nominal group process to solve a problem, decide on class content, decide on possible class activities, set goals, and so forth.

5. Do role negotiations for a small group project.

6. Using Worksheet 6-1, make a decision chart for a small group project.

Worksheet 6-1

Decision Chart

Make a decision chart for a small group project, inserting the appropriate code in the blocks for each group member's tasks.

Names

Tasks

Codes:
   M Manages the process
   C Consulted
   D Makes decision
   I Informed of the decision

CHAPTER 7: THEORIES OF LEADERSHIP

1. Reflective Journal: Make observations in a clinical setting or reflect on past experiences. Answer the following questions: How would you describe your leadership style? What are some leadership styles you have observed? Did they seem appropriate to the situation and why? To what styles do you respond best? How could you become a more transformational leader?

2. Computer Activity: Look up information related to various leadership theories or management eras. Share your findings with colleagues.

3. Using Worksheet 7-1, write your philosophy of leadership and discuss it with a classmate.

4. Using Table 7-1 on p. 143, describe the atmosphere where you work or study.

5. Using Figure 7-1 on p. 144, consider your maturity level, where you fit on the four-quadrant model, and what type of leadership you want and need.

6. List five major desires. In which categories of Maslow's hierarchy of needs do they belong? Do your needs fluctuate from time to time?

7. Make a list of what was happening when you felt job satisfaction and another list of what was happening when you felt job dissatisfaction. Compare and contrast the lists. Do they support Herzberg's motivation hygiene theory?

8. Consider the characteristics of Theory X and Theory Y managers. Which would you rather work with? Which do you want to be? What can you do to become the type of manager you want to be?

Worksheet 7-1

Philosophy of Leadership

Write your philosophy of leadership, using the questions below to guide you:

• What characteristics or traits does an effective leader possess?

• What specific behaviors does an effective leader exhibit?

• What activities are appropriate to a leader?

CHAPTER 8: STRATEGIC AND OPERATIONAL PLANNING

1. Reflective Journal: Make observations in a clinical setting or reflect on past experiences. Answer the following questions: What is the agency vision? What values are supported? What is the department of nursing's philosophy? Is it consistent with the larger organizational mission or philosophy? How is this nursing philosophy implemented on a unit? Does the organization have a strategic plan?

2. Computer Activity: Look for related articles and information on the Web.

3. Using the Lake View Hospital case study on p. 193, complete the following tasks:

a. Consider current trends and do a situation audit using Worksheet 8-1. Hypothesize about the information not provided in the case study based on what is happening in your community.

b. Do a SWOT analysis using Worksheet 8-2.

c. Write the purpose of Lake View Hospital.

d. Write the philosophy for Lake View Hospital.

e. Develop the goals and objectives for one of the units.

f. Write a policy for Lake View Hospital.

g. Write a procedure for Lake View Hospital.

Worksheet 8-1

Situation Audit

Criteria	Past	Present	Future
Clients			
Competition			
Market share			
Environment			
Demographics			
Economics			
Laws			
Politics			
Technology			
Facilities			
Finances			
Human resources			

Worksheet 8-2

SWOT Analysis

Strengths

Weaknesses

Opportunities

Threats

CHAPTER 9: FINANCIAL MANAGEMENT, COST CONTAINMENT, AND MARKETING

1. Reflective Journal: Make observations in a clinical setting or reflect on past experiences. Answer the following questions: What are the sources of revenue for the agency? What is the unit charge for nursing services (for example, hours of care, room rates)? What is the cost to a patient for 24 hours of care or per visit or other appropriate charge unit? Does the cost vary with the amount and type of care (ICU for example)? Do Medicare, Medicaid, and private insurances reimburse the hospital at the same rate for the same care? What are the differences in reimbursement, and how is the deficit handled? Does the organization have a marketing plan? Who is responsible for the plan, if anyone?

2. Computer Activity: Search the Web for items about health care financing, budgeting, and marketing. Share your interesting findings with classmates or other colleagues.

3. Assess your personal financial situation using Worksheets 9-1, 9-2, and 9-3. Make a list of ways you could control costs for your personal budget.

4. Form small groups in class and brainstorm ways nurses can control hospital expenses.

5. One member of the class can get a list of costs of supplies and equipment from a local health care agency and share it with other class members.

6. Form a small group in class and perform a brief marketing audit of your nursing program by answering the following questions: What geographical area is served? Who are the potential students? What services are provided? Who are the competitors? How do the services compare? How do the prices compare? In what location is the service provided? How accessible is it to students? How far will students travel to obtain the service? Will faculty travel to provide the service? How is the nursing program promoted?

7. Identify the market segment for your nursing program—nursing students; educational level—associate degree, baccalaureate degree, graduate degree; functional area—practice, teaching, administering, researching, consulting; and practice area—general, medical, surgical, maternal, child, psychiatric, geriatric, community health, home care.

8. Form a small group in class and brainstorm ways you could increase the publicity for your nursing program and recruit more people into the profession.

9. Draw a grid depicting the Boston consulting firm's potential growth and profitability opportunities.

10. Using Worksheet 9-4, which depicts the life cycle in the first column and the Boston group's classification in the second column, identify the appropriate high or low profitability and growth opportunity for the life cycle and related Boston group's classification in the third column.

11. Form small groups. Using Worksheet 9-5, identify a situation in a health care agency with which you are familiar and list all the costs you can think of that are associated with it. Identify whether each cost is variable, semivariable, fixed, or semifixed.

12. Using Worksheet 9-5, identify your educational expenses and identify whether each cost is variable, semivariable, fixed, or semifixed.

Assessment of Assets and Liabilities

Assets	Amount
Checking accounts	$_____
Savings accounts	_____
Certificates of deposit	_____
Money-market funds	_____
Other savings	_____
Stocks	_____
Bonds	_____
Mutual funds	_____
Market value of home	_____
Other real estate	_____
Cash value of life insurance	_____
Surrender value of annuities	_____
Equity in retirement funds	_____
Equity in profit sharing plans	_____
IRAs	_____
Keoghs	_____
Collectibles	_____
Precious metals	_____
Antiques	_____
Automobiles	_____
Household furnishings	_____
Furs and jewelry	_____
Loans receivable	_____
Other assets	_____

Liabilities

Liabilities	
Current bills	$_____
Credit card balance	_____
Mortgage balance	_____
Home equity loan	_____
Auto loans	_____
Student loans	_____
Other debts	_____
Current net worth	
(assets minus liabilities)	$_____

Worksheet 9-2

Personal Cash Flow

Income		Monthly	Annually
Take-home pay		$_____	$_____
Bonuses		_____	_____
Self-employment income		_____	_____
New income from rental property		_____	_____
Interest		_____	_____
Dividends		_____	_____
Other		_____	_____
	Total	$_____	$_____

Expenditures			
Rent or mortgage		$_____	$_____
Property taxes		_____	_____
Income taxes		_____	_____
Credit card payments		_____	_____
Auto insurance		_____	_____
Homeowner's insurance		_____	_____
Food		_____	_____
Utilities		_____	_____
Furnishings		_____	_____
Transportation		_____	_____
Child care		_____	_____
Clothing and personal care		_____	_____
Medical bills		_____	_____
Dental bills		_____	_____
Educational expenses		_____	_____
Entertainment, recreation		_____	_____
Gifts		_____	_____
Contributions		_____	_____
Pocket money		_____	_____
Miscellaneous		_____	_____
	Total	$_____	$_____
Surplus or deficit (income minus expenditures)		$_____	$_____

Worksheet 9-3

Financial Goal Priorities

	Short term (1 year)	Medium term (1-5 years)	Long term (5-10 years)	Longest term (over 10 years)
Buy a car				
Buy a home				
Make home improvements				
Change jobs				
Start a business				
Have children				
Pay for children's education				
Ensure adequate disability income				
Provide for survivor in event of death				
Take dream vacation				
Buy vacation home				
Reduce debt				
Increase charitable giving				
Achieve adequate retirement income				
Take early retirement				
Other				
Other				

Worksheet 9-4

Cycle Profitability and Growth Opportunities

Life cycle	Boston group's classification	High or low profitability; high or low growth opportunity
Introduction	Question mark	
Growth	Rising stars	
Maturity	Cash cows	
Market decline	Dogs	

Worksheet 9-5

Costs

1. Briefly describe the situation in the space below:

2. In the chart below, list each separate cost that is associated with the situation described above and identify whether it is variable, semivariable, fixed, or semifixed.

Cost	Variable	Semivariable	Fixed	Semifixed

CHAPTER 10: ORGANIZATIONAL CONCEPTS AND STRUCTURES

1. Reflective Journal: Make observations in a clinical setting or reflect on past experiences. Answer the following questions: What is the organizational structure at the facility? How does the structure support the organizational purposes? Where is the top nursing position in the organization? Compare the nursing position with those of medicine and other powerful departments. Outline the similarities and differences in management responsibilities between first-level, middle-level, and top-level nursing managers in the agency.

2. Computer Activity: Check the Web for health care networks, matrices, decentralization, and other concepts of interest to you. Share some of your interesting findings with colleagues.

3. Draw a formal organization chart of the agency where you work. Note the span of management, flat or tall structure, decentralization or centralization, and line authority.

4. Observe the chain of authority and who influences whom where you work. Does the reality match the formal structure?

5. Consider how you would use line or staff authority to improve a procedure where you work.

6. Identify the organizational structure for at least one organization. Using Worksheet 10-1, identify the advantages and disadvantages of the structure.

7. Using Worksheet 10-2, decide whether principles of organization are implemented in a structure you identified.

8. Organizations are faced with a rapidly changing environment and greater competition than ever before. The more equalitarian relationships between managers and associates, the growing need for collaboration and shared decision making, and erosion of hierarchy and authority as the basis for influence increase the need for managers to enhance their personal power by acquiring technical knowledge and expertise. Identify what you will do to acquire technical knowledge and expertise.

Worksheet 10-1

Advantages and Disadvantages of Structure

List the advantages and disadvantages of the organizational structure.

Advantages	Disadvantages
1. _____	1. _____
2. _____	2. _____
3. _____	3. _____
4. _____	4. _____
5. _____	5. _____
6. _____	6. _____
7. _____	7. _____
8. _____	8. _____
9. _____	9. _____
10. _____	10. _____
11. _____	11. _____
12. _____	12. _____
13. _____	13. _____
14. _____	14. _____
15. _____	15. _____

Worksheet 10-2

Principles of Organization

List principles of organization and check if the structure designed meets or does not meet the principle.

List principles of organization	Met	Not met
1.	_____	_____
2.	_____	_____
3.	_____	_____
4.	_____	_____
5.	_____	_____
6.	_____	_____
7.	_____	_____
8.	_____	_____
9.	_____	_____
10.	_____	_____

CHAPTER 11: ORGANIZATIONAL CULTURE AND CHANGE

1. Reflective Journal: Make observations in a clinical setting or reflect on past experiences. Answer the following questions: Is the organization going through changes? What are some of them, if any? How are people responding?

2. Computer Activity: On the Web look for articles and other information related to organizational culture and change and share your findings with colleagues.

3. All organizations express cultural traits in rituals and symbols that serve to communicate and perpetuate the values, beliefs, and behaviors of the organization's members. Within organizations subcultures develop that reflect more specific traits of specific occupational groups. Registered nurses (RNs) form an occupational group because they engage in the same sort of work and get their professional identity from that work. They may do activities together outside the work area. Using Worksheets 11-1 and 11-2, identify some rituals and symbols of the organization in general and RNs more specifically in an organization with which you are familiar.

4. Identify a change you would like to make in your life. Using Worksheet 11-3, apply Lewin's force-field analysis. Identify the restraining forces and the driving forces. Plan strategies to weaken the restraining forces and strengthen the driving forces.

5. Identify a group to which you belong. List the norms. What are the do's and don'ts? List what you would like the norms to be. Identify culture gaps, using Worksheet 11-4.

Worksheet 11-1

Rituals

List rituals in general and registered nurse–specific rituals:

Rituals in general	RN-specific rituals
1.	1.
2.	2.
3.	3.
4.	4.
5.	5.
6.	6.
7.	7.
8.	8.
9.	9.
10.	10.

Worksheet 11-2

Symbols

List symbols of the organization in general and registered nurse–specific symbols:

Symbols in general	RN-specific symbols
1.	1.
2.	2.
3.	3.
4.	4.
5.	5.
6.	6.
7.	7.
8.	8.
9.	9.
10.	10.

Worksheet 11-3

Force-Field Analysis

Identify a change you want to make: _____

Identify the driving forces and the restraining forces:

Driving forces	Restraining forces
1.	1.
2.	2.
3.	3.
4.	4.
5.	5.

Plan strategies to strengthen the driving forces and weaken the restraining forces.

Strengthen driving forces	Weaken restraining forces
1.	1.
2.	2.
3.	3.
4.	4.
5.	5.

Worksheet 11-4

Culture Gaps

List the organizational norms, what you would like the norms to be, and identify culture gaps.

Organizational norms	Desired norms	Culture gaps
1.	1.	1.
2.	2.	2.
3.	3.	3.
4.	4.	4.
5.	5.	5.
6.	6.	6.
7.	7.	7.
8.	8.	8.
9.	9.	9.
10.	10.	10.

CHAPTER 12: SELECTION AND DEVELOPMENT OF PERSONNEL

1. Reflective Journal: Make observations in a clinical setting or reflect on past experiences. Discuss the hiring or staffing process in an organization. What criteria are used in making hiring decisions? Who makes the decisions? Identify strengths and weaknesses of the process. Describe the continuing education and certification requirements for nurses working in an organization. What is the manager doing to ensure that these objectives are met? Reflect on your career stage and developmental activities. Compare that with the usual career stages.

2. Computer Activity: Look for articles or other information related to selection and development of personnel. Share your findings with colleagues.

3. In preparation for hiring a staff nurse, use Worksheets 12-1 and 12-2 to identify essential and desirable qualities and to determine if the candidate has them or not.

4. In preparation for hiring a staff nurse for the unit, use Worksheet 12-3 to prepare a grid of topics to explore, including open-ended questions, self-appraisal questions, and direct questions to get at what you consider important topics.

5. Write an advertisement for the staff nurse position on your unit. Decide what modes you are going to use to recruit nurses for your unit.

6. Form dyads in class and interview each other for specific positions.

7. Update your résumé. Start or maintain a file of your accomplishments.

8. Using Worksheet 12-4, identify what new employees need to know.

9. Using Worksheet 12-5, list your interests and skills.

10. Draw your career map.

11. Design your business card.

12. Using Worksheet 12-6, "Group Roles Grid," identify the number of times members of a group play various roles during a class activity or group meeting.

13. Identify the stage of development of a group to which you belong.

Worksheet 12-1

Systematic Selection Chart

Qualities	Essential	Desirable
Background		
Education		
Training		
Achievements		
Aptitudes		
Work experience		
Relevant		
Stable		
Personality		
Interpersonal relationships		
Temperament		
Attitudes		
Values		
Mental		
Intelligence		
Motivation		
Interests		
Aspirations		
Energy level		
Physical		
Appearance		
Health		
Special		
Other points		

Worksheet 12-2

Qualification Assessment Form

Does the applicant have:

Essential quality	Yes	?	No	Comments
BS nursing education				
1 yr nursing experience				
Desirable quality				
Community health experience				
Health education experience				

Worksheet 12-3

Interview Grid

Prepare a grid of topics to explore, including open-ended, self-appraisal, and direct questions

Topics	Open-ended questions	Self-appraisal questions	Direct questions

Orientation

Identify what the new employee needs to know or be oriented to and who should orient the employee to each topic.

Orientation topic	Orienter

Worksheet 12-5

Interests and Skills

List your interests and skills as a basis for planning your future.

Interests	Skills
1.	1.
2.	2.
3.	3.
4.	4.
5.	5.
6.	6.
7.	7.
8.	8.
9.	9.
10.	10.

Worksheet 12-6

Group Roles Grid

Names

Roles

Initiator-contributor								
Information seeker								
Opinion seeker								
Information giver								
Opinion giver								
Elaborator								
Coordinator								
Orienter								
Critic								
Energizer								
Procedural technician								
Recorder								
Gatekeeper								
Encourager								
Harmonizer								
Compromiser								
Follower								
Group observer								
Standard setter								
Aggressor								
Dominator								
Recognition seeker								
Special interest pleader								
Blocker								
Self-confessor								
Help seeker								
Playboy								

CHAPTER 13: STAFFING AND SCHEDULING

1. Reflective Journal: Make observations in a clinical setting or reflect on past experiences. Identify the nursing model and staffing schedules used in the facility. What factors determine the assignment of personnel? How is the work of the unit or department organized? Identify the responsibilities of key persons in the unit. Describe the patient classification system used, if any. How does the patient classification system relate to staffing, budgeting, and quality assurance?

2. Computer Activity: Check the Web for information about assignment systems, home care, long-term care, health promotion clinics, nurse practitioners, and managed care, and share your findings with colleagues.

3. Identify the patient care delivery mode for at least one health care setting with which you are familiar. Use Worksheet 13-1 to help you identify the basic characteristics of the patient care delivery modes discussed in this chapter.

4. Form dyads to compare and contrast three patient care delivery modes.

5. Form small groups and discuss the relationship between managed care and case management.

6. Form a small group with two or three classmates and do the following activities:
   a. List at least six policy issues related to staffing schedules.
   b. Describe the pros and cons of centralized and decentralized scheduling, using Worksheet 13-2.
   c. Identify at least three different staffing patterns and discuss the pros and cons of each, using Worksheet 13-3.

Patient Care Delivery Modes

List characteristics of the following patient care delivery modes:

Case method
1.
2.
3.
4.
5.

Functional nursing
1.
2.
3.
4.
5.

Team nursing
1.
2.
3.
4.
5.

Modular nursing
1.
2.
3.
4.
5.

Primary nursing
1.
2.
3.
4.
5.

Case management
1.
2.
3.
4.
5.

Managed care
1.
2.
3.
4.
5.

Centralized and Decentralized Scheduling

Identify the pros and cons of centralized and decentralized scheduling

	Centralized	Decentralized
Pros	1. 2. 3. 4. 5.	1. 2. 3. 4. 5.
Cons	1. 2. 3. 4. 5.	1. 2. 3. 4. 5.

Worksheet 13-3

Staffing Patterns

Identify at least three staffing patterns and the pros and cons of each.

Staffing patterns	Pros	Cons
1. _____	a.	a.
	b.	b.
	c.	c.
	d.	d.
	e.	e.
2. _____	a.	a.
	b.	b.
	c.	c.
	d.	d.
	e.	e.
3. _____	a.	a.
	b.	b.
	c.	c.
	d.	d.
	e.	e.

CHAPTER 14: EVALUATION AND DISCIPLINE OF PERSONNEL

1. Reflective Journal: Make observations in a clinical setting or reflect on past experiences. Answer the following questions: When and how are personnel evaluated? Is there a process for disciplinary action in place? If so, what is it? Discuss how your agency handles chemically impaired employees. What are the policies and procedures regarding chemically impaired employees in the agency? What is the manager's role? What are the criteria for notification to the nursing administration and board of nursing? Who is responsible for notifying them?

2. Computer Activity: Check the Web for information about types of performance appraisal, discipline, and behavior modification. Share your findings with colleagues.

3. Evaluate an evaluation tool and share your assessment with a classmate. Use Worksheets 14-1 and 14-2 to help you in this process.

4. Practice an appraisal interview with a classmate. Evaluate classroom participation by the appraisal interview style of your choice. Discuss how it felt to appraise and be appraised in that manner.

5. Fill out Worksheet 14-3 to help you distinguish between the various methods of personnel evaluation. Then write a script for an authoritative and an equal–working-relationship appraisal interview. Arrange furniture accordingly and role-play the scripts with a classmate.

6. Using Worksheet 14-4, identify a behavior that you would like to change. Determine your baseline behavior. Graph the frequency. Plan reinforcement and extinction strategies.

7. Share your behavior modification plan with a classmate and solicit positive reinforcement from that classmate.

8. Offer your support of a classmate's behavior modification plan.

9. Use Worksheets 14-5, 14-6, and 14-7 to help you distinguish between different types of problem employees and types of employee counseling.

10. In class discuss experiences with substance abusers. What were the symptoms of the abuse? How was the situation handled? How might it have been handled?

11. Have at least one classmate contact the state nurses association for information about the peer review committee. Have a guest speaker from the state nurses association peer review committee or the state board of nursing. Discuss the differences between roles of the state nurses association and the state board of nursing regarding chemical dependency.

12. Role-play handling an angry employee.

Worksheet 14-1

Purposes of Personnel Evaluation

List at least five purposes of personnel evaluation.

1.

2.

3.

4.

5.

Worksheet 14-2

Errors in Performance Evaluation

List at least six common errors in performance evaluation.

1.

2.

3.

4.

5.

6.

Methods of Personnel Evaluation

Describe five methods of personnel evaluation.

1.

2.

3.

4.

5.

Worksheet 14-4

Behavior Modification

Behavior to change: _____

Baseline behavior:

Times	Sunday	Monday	Tuesday	Wednesday	Thursday	Friday	Saturday
12 AM							
1							
2							
3							
4							
5							
6							
7							
8							
9							
10							
11							
12 PM							
1							
2							
3							
4							
5							
6							
7							
8							
9							
10							
11							

List reinforcement strategies:

List extinction strategies:

Worksheet 14-5

Problem Employees

list at least three types of problem employees and briefly describe their behavior.

1.

2.

3.

Worksheet 14-6

Employee Counseling

Describe at least three types of employee counseling.

1.

2.

3.

Worksheet 14-7

Outplacement Counseling

Explain outplacement counseling, using the following questions as guidelines:

1. What is the purpose of outplacement counseling?

2. What are some potential sources of outplacement counseling?

   a.
   b.
   c.
   d.
   e.

3. What services might be useful to the terminating employee as a part of outplacement counseling?

CHAPTER 15: CONTINUOUS QUALITY IMPROVEMENT, RISK MANAGEMENT, AND PROGRAM EVALUATION

1. Reflective Journal: Make observations in a clinical setting or reflect on past experiences. Describe the continuous quality improvement program in a health care facility. What tools and processes are used for continuous quality improvement? What procedures are used to monitor for risk management? Who is responsible for the program? Have there been lawsuits against the agency? Is the agency unionized?

2. Computer Activity: Search the Internet for information about such topics as continuous quality improvement, risk management, American Nurses Association standards, JCAHO, and OASIS.

3. Evaluate the research design of a research report related to management.

4. Form small groups. Identify research designs and discuss the invalidity problems that are controlled and those that are not.

5. Fill out Worksheets 15-1 and 15-2 to help reinforce your knowledge of risk and risk management.

6. Inquire about the customer satisfaction program at a local health care facility.

7. Interview someone who serves on a committee for continuous quality improvement about the business conducted by that committee.

8. Watch a movie or television program involving a court case to become more familiar with the proceedings.

9. Review rules to remember when testifying by filling out Worksheet 15-3.

Worksheet 15-1

Risk Management Process

Briefly describe the five steps in the risk management process.

1.

2.

3.

4.

5.

Worksheet 15-2

Potential Risks

Identify at least three sources for identifying potential risks.

1.

2.

3.

Worksheet 15-3

Testifying

List rules to remember for testifying.

1.

2.

3.

4.

5.

6.